D1309947

MONITORING IN RESPIRATORY CARE

Monitoring in Respiratory Care

ROBERT M. KACMAREK, Ph.D., R.R.T.
Assistant Professor
Department of Anesthesia
Harvard Medical School
Director, Respiratory Care
Massachusetts General Hospital
Boston, Massachusetts

DEAN HESS, M.Ed., R.R.T.
Instructor, Department of Anesthesia
Harvard Medical School
Assistant Director, Respiratory Care
Massachusetts General Hospital
Boston, Massachusetts
Formerly, Assistant Director
Department of Research
York Hospital
York, Pennsylvania

JAMES K. STOLLER, M.D.
Medical Director
Head, Section of Respiratory Care
Department of Pulmonary and Critical Care Medicine
Cleveland Clinic Foundation
Cleveland, Ohio

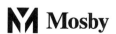 Mosby

St. Louis Baltimore Boston Chicago London Philadelphia Sydney Toronto

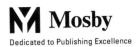

Mosby

Dedicated to Publishing Excellence

Sponsoring Editor: David K. Marshall
Assistant Editor: Julie Tryboski
Assistant Director, Manuscript Services: Frances M. Perveiler
Production Manager: Karen Halm

Copyright © 1993 Mosby–Year Book, Inc.
A Year Book Medical Publishers imprint of Mosby–Year Book, Inc.,

Mosby–Year Book, Inc.
11830 Westline Industrial Drive
St. Louis, MO 63416

All rights reserved. No part of this publication may be reproduced, stored in a retrieval system, or transmitted, in any form or by any means, electronic, mechanical, photocopying, recording, or otherwise, without prior written permission from the publisher. Printed in the United States of America.

Permission to photocopy or reproduce solely for internal or personal use is permitted for libraries or other users registered with the Copyright Clearance Center, provided that the base fee of $4.00 per chapter plus $.10 per page is paid directly to the Copyright Clearance Center, 21 Congress Street, Salem, MA 01970. This consent does not extend to other kinds of copying, such as copying for general distribution, for advertising or promotional purposes, for creating new collected works, or for resale.

1 2 3 4 5 6 7 8 9 0   97 96 95 94 93

Library of Congress Cataloging-in-Publication Data

Monitoring in respiratory care / [edited by] Robert M. Kacmarek, Dean
   Hess, James K. Stoller.
        p.   cm.
      Includes bibliographical references and index.
      ISBN 0-8151-4963-8
      1. Respiratory intensive care.   2. Patient monitoring.   3. Blood
   gases—Analysis.   I. Kacmarek, Robert M.   II. Hess, Dean.
   III. Stoller, James K.
      [DNLM: 1. Monitoring, Physiologic—methods.   2. Respiratory Tract
   Diseases—therapy.   WF 141 M744]
   RC735.R48M66   1992   92-49174
   616.2'075—dc20   CIP
   DNLM/DLC
   for Library of Congress

RC735
.R48
M66
1993

For Gram

R. K.

For Susan, Terri Anne and Lauren, who were there when I was not and encouraged me to be all that I am

D. H.

To Terry, for her unwavering support; Jake, for the joy; and my parents, Alfred and Nickie, for love and guidance

J. S.

JUN 1 1995

CONTRIBUTORS

Lisa J. Arguin, B.S.
Clinical Engineering Manager
Department of Respiratory Care
Massachusetts General Hospital
Boston, Massachusetts

Tim Blanchette, M.S., R.R.T.
Respiratory Therapist
Department of Pulmonary Medicine
Maine Medical Center
Portland, Maine

Richard D. Branson, R.R.T.
Clinical Instructor
Department of Surgery
University of Cincinnati Medical Center
Cincinnati, Ohio

Daniel P. Brutocao, M.D.
Pediatric Intensivist
Deaconess Medical Center
Sacred Heart Medical Center
Spokane, Washington

Nausherwan K. Burki, M.D., Ph.D., F.R.C.P.
Professor of Medicine
University of Kentucky
Chief, Division of Pulmonary and Critical
  Care Medicine
Department of Medicine
University of Kentucky Medical Center
Lexington, Kentucky

Robert S. Campbell, R.R.T.
Critical Care Coordinator
Department of Respiratory Care
University of Cincinnati Medical Center
Cincinnati, Ohio

Robert L. Chatburn, R.R.T.
Instructor, Department of Pediatrics
Case Western Reserve University
Director of Respiratory Care
Rainbow Babies and Childrens Hospital
Cleveland, Ohio

Alfred F. Connors, Jr., M.D.
Associate Professor of Medicine
Case Western Reserve University
Director, Medical Intensive Care Unit
Division of Pulmonary Critical Care
  Medicine
Metro Health Medical Center
Cleveland, Ohio

Jeffrey B. Cooper, Ph.D.
Associate Professor
Harvard Medical School
Director, Anesthesia Technology
Department of Anesthesia
Massachusetts General Hospital
Boston, Massachusetts

John Cunningham, Ph.D.
Associate Professor and Head
  Department of Nutrition
University of Massachusetts
Amherst, Massachusetts
Associate in Surgery
Surgical Services
Massachusetts General Hospital
Boston, Massachusetts

Michael J. Decker, C.R.T.T.
Technical Director
Laboratory for Technology Assessment
Case Western Reserve University
Cleveland, Ohio

Thomas D. East, Ph.D.
Associate Professor of Anesthesiology,
   Bioengineering and Medical Informatics
Department of Anesthesiology
University of Utah School of Medicine
Salt Lake City, Utah

C. Gregory Elliott, M.D.
Associate Professor of Medicine
University of Utah School of Medicine
Medical Director
Respiratory Care
LDS Hospital
Salt Lake City, Utah

Reed M. Gardner, Ph.D.
Professor, Department of Medical
   Informatics
University of Utah
Co-Director, Medical Informatics
LDS Hospital
Salt Lake City, Utah

Mary E. Gilmartin, B.S.N., R.R.T.
Pulmonary Clinical Nurse Specialist
National Jewish Center for Immunology
   and Respiratory Medicine
Denver, Colorado

Takahisa Goto, M.D.
Clinical Fellow in Anaesthesia
Harvard Medical School
Clinical Fellow in Anaesthesia
Massachusetts General Hospital
Boston, Massachusetts

**Loren Greenway, B.S., B.A., R.R.T.,
   R.C.P.**
Administrative Director Respiratory/
   Hyperbaric Services
LDS Hospital
Cottonwood Hospital
Alta View Hospital
Salt Lake City, Utah

Eileen P. Hall, B.S., B.M.E.
Clinical Engineering Manager
Department of Biomedical Engineering
Massachusetts General Hospital
Boston, Massachusetts

Kathy W. Harris, M.P.H., R.R.T.
Administrative Director of Pulmonary
   Medicine
Maine Medical Center
Portland, Maine

Dean Hess, M.Ed., R.R.T.
Instructor, Department of Anesthesia
Harvard Medical School
Assistant Director, Respiratory Care
Massachusetts General Hospital
Boston, Massachusetts
Formerly, Assistant Director
Department of Research
York Hospital
York, Pennsylvania

Robert M. Kacmarek, Ph.D., R.R.T.
Assistant Professor
Department of Anesthesia
Harvard Medical School
Director Respiratory Care
Massachusetts General Hospital
Boston, Massachusetts

William R. Kimball, M.D., Ph.D.
Assistant Professor of Anesthesiology
Harvard Medical School
Assistant Anesthetist
Massachusetts General Hospital
Boston, Massachusetts

Patricia B. Koff, M.E., R.R.T.
Developmental Coordinator
Division of Pulmonary Sciences and
   Critical Care Medicine
University of Colorado Health Sciences
   Center
Denver, Colorado

M. Jeffrey Mador, M.D.
Assistant Professor of Medicine
State University of New York at Buffalo
Staff Physician
Buffalo Veterans Administration Medical
   Center
Buffalo, New York

Kevin McCarthy, R.C.P.T.
Technical Director
Pulmonary Function
Cleveland Clinic Foundation
Cleveland, Ohio

David P. Meeker, M.D.
Staff Physician
Department of Pulmonary and Critical
　Care Medicine
Cleveland Clinic Foundation
Cleveland, Ohio

P. Pearl O'Rourke, M.D.
Associate Professor
University of Washington
Director, PICU
Children's Hospital
Seattle, Washington

Susan Redline, M.D., M.P.H.
Associate Professor of Medicine
Division of Pulmonary and Critical Care
　Medicine
Case Western Reserve University
University Hospitals of Cleveland
Cleveland, Ohio

Ray Ritz, R.R.T.
Assistant Director
Respiratory Care
Massachusetts General Hospital
Boston, Massachusetts

John W. Salyer, R.R.T.
Director of Respiratory Care
Primary Children's Medical Center
Salt Lake City, Utah

Kingman P. Strohl, M.D.
Professor of Medicine
Case Western Reserve University
Division Chief
Pulmonary Division/Critical Care
　Medicine
University Hospitals of Cleveland
Cleveland, Ohio

James K. Stoller, M.D.
Medical Director
Head, Section of Respiratory Care
Pulmonary and Critical Care Medicine
Cleveland Clinic Foundation
Cleveland, Ohio

Richard Teplick, M.D.
Associate Professor of Anesthesia
Harvard Medical School
Director, Division of Critical Care
Department of Anesthesia
Massachusetts General Hospital
Boston, Massachusetts

Martin J. Tobin, M.D.
Professor of Medicine
Loyola University Stritch School of
　Medicine
Maywood, Illinois
Program Director
Division of Pulmonary and Critical Care
　Medicine
Edward Hines Jr. Veterans
　Administration Hospital
Hines, Illinois

Carlos A. Vaz Fragoso, M.D.
Director, Pulmonary Lab
Danbury Hospital
Danbury, Connecticut

John M. Walsh, M.D., M.S.
Assistant Professor of Medicine and
　Physiology
Loyola University Stritch School of
　Medicine
Maywood, Illinois

Herbert P. Wiedemann, M.D.
Chairman, Department of Pulmonary and
　Critical Care Medicine
Cleveland Clinic Foundation
Cleveland, Ohio

Gary Wiederhold, A.A.S.
Technical Training Instructor
Technical Support Representative
Puritan Bennett
Olathe, Kansas

FOREWORD

Both technically and conceptually, respiratory care is more compex than ever before. With our new modes and ventilator capabilities, wider use of vasoactive drugs, and more aggressive adjustments of body fluid compartments and chemical composition, we routinely manipulate vital functions more directly and more rapidly than was possible a short generation ago. We also carry out these manipulations in more settings and under more diverse conditions—in prehospital emergency care, in the intensive care unit, during intrahospital transport, in magnetic resonance imagers, in aircraft, and in patients' own homes

This expansion of respiratory care has created a great need not only for knowledgeable, well trained clinicians, but also for devices and techniques for *monitoring*—both of our patients and of what we do to them. Monitoring today consists of the continuous or repetitive assessment of a patient, that patient's physiologic status, and the function of life-support and other apparatus, for the purposes of guiding management decisions and assessing their effects. Fortunately, hand in hand with the expansion of technical capability in management has also come greatly increased monitoring capability. We can now monitor respiratory gases breath-by-breath, over many breaths, or within the course of a single breath; we can track changes in arterial, peripheral capillary, and mixed venous oxygenation as they occur; we quantitate global and regional perfusion; we measure energy expenditure and monitor the patient's work of breathing.

Yet these enhanced monitoring capabilities are both boon and bane. Artifact and outlier confuse both monitor and clinician. An intubated but stable patient coughs and rolls over in bed, triggering loud alarms in three or four separate monitoring devices and aggravating the stress of the ICU environment for both patient and caregiver. Monitoring is sophisticated and often life-saving, but it is far from ideal.

And monitoring information per se is not patient assessment. Data do not manage patients. Monitoring information is useful only to the extent that it enables a skilled clinician to utilize it in appropriate patient care. This requires considerably more than reading numbers from a computer screen, LED display, or strip recorder. It requires a thorough understanding of what is being monitored and why, of how the monitor works, and of what its output *means* in the management of this patient.

Fortunately for clinicians, this heretofore daunting task has just been made a lot easier. This book exactly addresses the problems I have just described, and it does so with comprehensiveness and authority never before offered. Its authors are experts not only in the technical aspects of monitoring but also in teaching its implications and practical implementation. They cover in detail the principles of measurement and monitoring, the chemical, physical, and physiological underpinnings of monitoring as applied at the bedside, as well as the practical "how-to," aspects required for clinical application.

This book will be indispensable to physicians, respiratory care practitioners, nurses, and all students whatever their level and focus within respiratory care. The editors are to be congratulated for recognizing a need, conceiving such an ideal response to this need, and assembling a cast of contributors who have so thoroughly and appropriately responded.

David J. Pierson, M.D.
Medical Director, Respiratory Care
Harborview Medical Center
Professor of Medicine
University of Washington
Seattle, Washington

PREFACE

Our ability to provide respiratory care to patients at all levels of illness has dramatically increased over the last decade. Along with this growth in therapeutics has been a corresponding growth in our ability to monitor the effects of specific interventions. The purpose of this text is to discuss the various respiratory care monitoring techniques currently available and to provide a comprehensive reference book on all aspects of monitoring in respiratory care, exhaustively covering each aspect in state-of-the-art chapters. Extensive referencing is included with each chapter to assist the reader in locating original work in each area.

We believe this text will be extremely useful to all clinicians who provide respiratory care in both critical and noncritical care areas, whether their specific career developed along the lines of medicine, respiratory therapy, or nursing. We also believe this book is especially useful for all students of respiratory care. The reader will find specific details on individual approaches to monitoring, as well as consolidated approaches to monitoring in specific settings.

The text has been developed in four sections: (1) Overview and Engineering Principles; (2) Invasive Monitoring Techniques; (3) Noninvasive Monitoring Techniques; and (4) Integration of Monitoring Into Various Clinical Settings. Section 1 is designed to provide an overview of general engineering and physical principles common to all respiratory care monitors. Section 2 details the specific physiologic and technologic features of invasive monitoring used in respiratory care (indices of oxygenation, hemodynamic monitoring, and work of breathing), while Section 3 details commonly used noninvasive monitors of respiratory function (oximetry, transcutaneous gas monitoring, capnography, indirect calorimetry, respiratory inductance plethysmography, airway waveforms, lung volumes, and cardiovascular function). Section 4 is designed to integrate the material from the first three sections into their clinical application in varying settings. Discussions of monitoring of respiratory function from the neonatal ICU, to home care, to monitoring at altitude are presented.

Regardless of their level of expertise, readers will find information directly useful in their clinical practice across a wide range of clinical settings.

Robert M. Kacmarek, Ph.D., R.R.T.
Dean Hess, M.Ed., R.R.T.
James K. Stoller, M.D.

CONTENTS

Chapter 1

Perspectives on Monitoring in Respiratory Care

Dean Hess, M.Ed., R.R.T.

Robert M. Kacmarek, Ph.D., R.R.T.

James K. Stoller, M.D.

INTRODUCTION

Monitoring in respiratory care is ubiquitous and ranges from simple and noninvasive monitors such as the spirometer on a ventilator to complex and invasive monitors such as the pulmonary artery catheter. Since the introduction of the Swan-Ganz catheter[1] in 1969, use of both invasive and noninvasive monitoring has increased exponentially.

Noninvasive monitoring in respiratory care became very popular in the 1980s. Before the early 1970s, arterial blood gases and pH were infrequently measured, but we now measure oxygen tension (Po_2), carbon dioxide tension (Pco_2), and oxygen saturation noninvasively and continuously. Much of this technologic advance is the result of microprocessors. The microprocessor has increased the speed and sophistication of data acquisition and manipulation and has allowed the miniaturization of monitoring equipment.

DEFINITION OF TERMS

Monitoring is the activity of continuously, or nearly continuously, evaluating the physiologic function of a patient in real time in order to guide management decisions (e.g., when to make therapeutic interventions) and to assess the impact of treatment.[2]

Monitoring differs from *measurement* because monitoring is a continuous, or at least nearly continuous activity, while measurements take place intermittently. Thus, continuous electrocardiography (ECG) in the intensive care unit (ICU) satisfies the definition for monitoring, but arterial blood gas analysis is intermittent and therefore is a measurement. Sometimes the distinction between monitoring and intermittent measurement is less distinct. For example, the pulmonary artery catheter can be used to continuously *monitor* pulmonary artery pressure and intermittently *measure* pulmonary artery occlusion pressure and cardiac output.

Another criterion for monitoring is that it be done in real time. Thus Holter monitoring, though continuous, would not meet this criterion for monitoring because it does not provide real-time information. A *clinical analyzer* uses body fluid or tissue that has been removed from the patient to perform a measurement.[3] A clinical analyzer typically serves many patients, whereas a monitor is dedicated to a single patient.

Monitoring may be invasive or noninvasive. Invasive monitors penetrate the body of the patient (e.g., pulmonary artery pressure monitoring, systemic arterial pressure monitoring, intracranial pressure monitoring, and esophageal pressure monitoring). Noninvasive monitors do not penetrate the body; they typically rest on the skin of the patient or sample inspired and expired gases. Though nonpenetrating, noninvasive monitoring should not be assumed to be harmless. For example, heated transcutaneous Po_2 and Pco_2 electrodes can produce skin burns,[4] and the pulse oximeter probe can produce pressure necrosis.[5]

Monitoring in respiratory care goes beyond monitoring of respiratory functions. Because of critical interactions between the lungs and other organs, monitoring in respiratory care subsumes related monitoring (e.g., cardiac, neurologic, and renal function).

WHY THE CURRENT INTEREST IN NONINVASIVE MONITORING?

There is considerable interest in monitoring in all aspects of respiratory care—adult acute care, neonatal/pediatric care, and home care. This interest arises from four basic goals: (1) to detect potentially adverse events early, (2) to intervene to avoid adverse sequelae, (3) to avoid invasive procedures, and (4) to obtain continuous real-time data.

Despite this interest, whether monitoring can prevent adverse events by "early detection" remains an appealing but unproven outcome. Certainly, avoiding invasive testing is desirable whenever possible. Risks of infection from indwelling devices, transmission of disease (e.g., hepatitis and HIV infection) to both patient and health care provider, excessive blood loss from gratuitous sampling, thrombus formation, and distal embolization are completely avoided by noninvasive monitoring,[6] even though noninvasive monitoring occasionally causes some harm.

In theory, continuous monitoring should detect events that might go unnoticed with intermittent measurement. However, new information about moment-to-moment variability in clinical parameters raises the obvious question: What degree of variation really matters?[7, 8] As with many ICU treatment modalities, the technical ability to monitor currently outstrips clinical understanding of when to monitor.

Despite these aforementioned uncertainties about the benefits of monitoring, clear-cut advantages of monitoring include rapid acquisition of data (i.e., in real time), lessened suspicion that monitoring itself alters the events being monitored (e.g., withdrawal of an arterial blood gas can be associated with acute hyperventilation), and, for noninvasive techniques, lower risks of invasive complications. Manufacturers have avidly promised these advantages of monitoring and have waged successful marketing campaigns that have caused monitoring equipment to proliferate. Lest the monitoring "tail wag the dog," manufacturers are reminded that monitoring should remain clinically sensible and that the impetus for better monitoring should be a clinical need rather than a technologic opportunity.

HOW MUCH MONITORING IS NEEDED?

This is an important question for clinicians, administrators, and health care policymakers. Many clinicians want to be able to monitor every possible parameter—adopting a "more is better" attitude. Administrators and health care policymakers, on the other hand, become justifiably concerned with the costs associated with this approach to monitoring.

With some monitors, clinicians may not understand what the displayed numbers mean and may not use the information appropriately.[9, 10] A clinician's optimal use of the information obtained by monitoring often lags behind the introduction of the monitor into clinical practice. Many clinicians take the displayed results at face value, with little understanding of how the data were collected, how the data were processed inside the *black box*, and what restrictions limit the usefulness of the results. This can be problematic in patient care, examples of which include:

- Transcutaneous P_{O_2} (Ptc_{O_2}) and P_{CO_2} (Ptc_{CO_2}) values may not be valid indicators of arterial P_{O_2} (Pa_{O_2}) and P_{CO_2} (Pa_{CO_2}) in patients with low cardiac output.[11]
- Use of pulse oximetry to evaluate patients for home oxygen may exclude some patients from reimbursement who would qualify based on blood gas results.[12, 13]
- Pulse oximetry may not detect arterial desaturation in patients with high carboxyhemoglobin levels.[14]
- End-tidal P_{CO_2} (Pet_{CO_2}) may be a poor indicator of Pa_{CO_2} in patients with pulmonary disease characterized by increased dead space.[15]
- Pulmonary artery occlusion pressure may be a poor reflection of left atrial pressure and left ventricular end-diastolic volume (preload) with high levels of positive end-expiratory pressure (PEEP).[16]

Clinicians need to be certain that they clearly understand the application and limitations of the monitors they use, because the unappreciated limitations of the monitor can cause inappropriate clinical decisions.

One goal of monitoring is to assure that the benefits of monitoring outstrip any associated risks, especially when monitoring devices encourage frequent sampling. For example, the number of arterial blood gases obtained in critically ill patients may correlate more with the presence of an arterial catheter than the clinical condition of the patient.[17] The Swan-Ganz catheter has been used for more than 20 years, and there remains considerable controversy regarding the appropriate application of this monitoring device.[18-20] The clinical significance of changes in newer measurements with a Swan-Ganz catheter (e.g., mixed venous oxygen saturation, right ventricular ejection fraction) are even more unclear. Although professional organizations such as the American Association for Respiratory Care[21] and the Society for Critical Care Medicine[22] have provided guidelines for the use of some monitors, clear professional guidelines for using most monitoring systems are lacking. In the absence of standard guidelines or their awareness, decisions to use a particular monitor are usually based on the clinician's personal experience or bias or on institutional tradition.

Another concern in using monitors is to ensure that the monitoring activities do not distract the clinician's attention from the patient being monitored. Frequently, we do so much monitoring that one clinician is needed to care for the monitors and another to care for the patient. Sometimes we seem to spend more time monitoring monitors than caring for patients. There is nothing worse than watching a patient deteriorate while the staff tries to ensure that the monitoring equipment is working properly. Finally, the lure of data from monitors can divert attention away from the patient being monitored. For example, in a study by Mok et al.,[23] transcutaneous Po_2 and pulse oximetry were performed on a group of clinically normal infants, all of whom were free of cardiopulmonary disease. Based on the monitoring results alone, some of these *normal* babies would have been given supplemental oxygen.

Data overload can occur with excessive monitoring. When presented with excessive data, some clinicians tend to ignore all of it rather than choose that which is most useful at the time. Others focus only on specific data, potentially choosing the wrong data. In either case, the monitoring does not benefit the patient. East et al.[24] reported that the number of individual categories of information available for decision-making in the ICU can exceed 200 per patient, which outstrips the clinicians' capacity to integrate and analyze the data. The role of computerized decision-making to assist with this task is being explored,[25] but it is too early to know how successful this might be in the future.

Another problem with excessive monitoring is the increased probability of false-positive alarms. In other words, the more monitors that are used, the more likely it becomes that a false-positive alarm will occur. For example, if the incidence of false-positive alarms with a noninvasive monitor is 5%, then the probability of a correct (true-positive) alarm is 0.95. If two monitors with a false-positive rate of 5% are used, then the probability of both monitors giving a correct response is 0.90 (0.95 × 0.95). If 20 monitors are used, the probability of all monitors giving a correct response is $(0.95)^{20}$ or 0.36 and, more importantly, the probability that at least one monitor is giving a false-positive alarm is 64%! Although these calculations may be somewhat exaggerated (e.g., the false-positive rate may be less than 5%, and the monitor results may not be completely independent of each other), the point remains that the likelihood of encountering a false-positive alarm increases as the number of monitors used increases. This becomes confusing to those caring for the patient, who are faced with the decision to either treat the patient or ignore the monitor. This has been demonstrated with the clinician's use of pulmonary function test results, where it has been shown that the percentage of subjects with at least one abnormal test increases as the number of tests performed increases.[26]

Most clinicians would agree that a monitor is performing well if it has a sensitivity for detecting adverse events of 100% (i.e., a false-negative rate of 0%) and a specificity of 95%

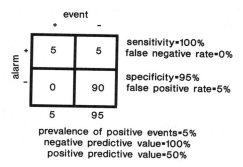

FIG 1–1.
The relationship between positive and negative adverse events and positive and negative monitor alarm conditions. Because the frequency of positive adverse events is low, the positive predictive value is relatively low (i.e., rate of false positive alarms is relatively high).

(i.e., a false-positive rate of 5%). If the prevalence of adverse events is only 5%, the positive predictive value of the monitor will be 50% (Fig 1–1). In other words, half of the monitor alarms will be false alarms! Unfortunately, this encourages clinicians caring for the patient to ignore the alarms.

The issue of excessive alarms related to clinical monitoring has been addressed in several published papers. In an evaluation of auditory alarms during anesthesia, Kestin, Miller, and Lockhart[27] found that 75% of all alarms were spurious, and only 3% indicated risk to the patient. In that study, 99% of the alarms originated from the pulse oximeter, ECG, and blood pressure monitors. In a study evaluating the utility of pulse oximetry in a surgical ICU, Bentt et al.[28] found that a pulse oximeter alarm could be present up to 47% of the time, or 28 min/hr. They concluded that appropriate use of pulse oximetry may be compromised in the ICU because of these frequent false alarms.

Another concern in using monitors is that the monitoring device can fail. In a study evaluating intraoperative pulse oximetry failure, it was found that the failure rate of this monitoring system was low (about 10%) in the relatively controlled environment of the operating room.[29] Anecdotally, the failure rates of monitoring systems in the ICU are much higher. However, this has not been studied systematically or reported in the biomedical literature. Some monitoring systems, such as capnographs and transcutaneous monitors, seem to be especially prone to failure in the ICU environment.

Although respiratory monitoring is often very useful in patient care, it should not be performed simply because it is technically possible. Because there are virtually no data to show that the addition of monitoring (of any variable) alters outcome in any way, the decision to monitor, like any other clinical decision, should be based on therapeutic objectives and careful weighing of expected benefits versus possible risks of monitoring. Overall, we need to be careful with respiratory monitoring (e.g., pulse oximetry) to avoid the temptation of overmonitoring. Just because a pulse oximeter (or any other respiratory monitor) is useful in the care of *some* patients does not justify its routine use for *all* patients.

THE USE OF MONITORS FOR SPOT CHECKS

Recently, the tendency has arisen to substitute noninvasive monitor spot checks for intermittent invasive measurements. The principal example of this is use of pulse oximetry as a substitute for blood gas measurements. This practice, although not condemned, must be carefully evaluated. Pulse oximeters, and most other noninvasive monitors, only evaluate a single parameter. In the case of the pulse oximeter, only arterial oxygen saturation is evaluated. Unlike arterial blood gases, pulse oximetry provides no information about ventilation or acid-base status. Noninvasive monitors (e.g., pulse oximeters) frequently lack the same accuracy and precision of the measurements that they replace. For the sake of being easy to use, monitors typically do *not* adhere to the same rigorous calibration and quality control procedures that are applied to laboratory measurements like blood gases. Differences also exist in the accuracy and precision of monitors made by different manufacturers[30] and between individual units from the same manufacturer—situations that can cause different results at different times on the same patient without any accompanying change in the patient's clinical state.

THE FINANCIAL IMPACT OF MONITORING

In this era of cost containment, the costs associated with respiratory monitoring must be considered. In the past 10 years, several published papers have addressed the issue of costs associated with noninvasive monitoring, the thrust of which has been that noninvasive monitoring of oxygenation by transcutaneous oxygen monitoring or pulse oximetry results in fewer arterial blood gas measurements and, thus, lower cost. However, the financial impact of many other types of respiratory monitoring has not yet been addressed.

In 1985, Peevy and Hall[31] reported that introducing transcutaneous oxygen monitoring into their neonatal intensive care unit reduced the costs of care by more than $100,000 over a 4-year period. This reduction was attributed primarily to fewer arterial blood gas analyses (2.13 arterial blood gas analyses/patient-day before transcutaneous monitoring versus 1.28 arterial blood gas analyses/patient-day after introduction of transcutaneous monitoring). Beachy and Whitfield[32] also reported a reduction in arterial blood gas analyses as a result of transcutaneous oxygen monitoring, but they did not analyze the possible cost savings associated with this.

King and Simon[33] evaluated the use of pulse oximetry for tapering supplemental oxygen in hospitalized patients. Use of pulse oximetry to taper oxygen resulted in significantly fewer arterial blood gas analyses compared to a control group in which oxygen was tapered by conventional means (51 blood gas analyses in 13 control patients versus 16 blood gas analyses in 16 oximetry patients). King and Simon[33] speculated that this would result in a cost savings of about $18,000/year in their 20-bed pulmonary ward and $146,000/year in the entire hospital. Kellerman et al.[34] reported the impact of pulse oximetry on arterial blood gas analysis in their emergency department. In this study, pulse oximetry resulted in a 43% reduction in the number of arterial blood gas analyses, with an estimated decrease in laboratory charges of $95,000/year.

Bone and Balk[35] described an 8-bed noninvasive respiratory care unit at Rush-Presbyterian-St Luke's Medical Center in Chicago as "a cost effective solution for the future." Although their paper describes cost-reducing features such as reduced nurse-patient ratios, no specific cost savings were provided. Krieger et al.[36] have also described a noninvasive monitoring unit for long-term ventilator patients, in which the principal respiratory monitoring technique is respiratory inductive plethysmography (RIP). Placing long-term ventilator patients in that unit, rather than keeping them in the ICU, resulted in an estimated cost reduction of $203.25/patient-day or $106,000/year. However, it is important to note that this cost savings was the result of transferring patients out of the ICU rather than the result of employing RIP *per se*. To the extent that RIP is not needed to ensure safe transfer of the patient to the long-term unit, the cost savings may be even greater.

Despite the apparent appeal of cost savings with noninvasive monitoring, several cautions seem warranted. First, as pointed out by Finkler,[37] the use of patient charge data rather than actual costs can lead to misleading conclusions about health care costs. Second, to our knowledge, no studies have shown that respiratory monitoring actually shortens hospital length of stay or improves patient outcomes. Finally, unless monitoring has a clear-cut value for patient care, the benefit of substituting noninvasive techniques for invasive monitoring is doubtful. To claim a cost savings when one form of unnecessary (albeit noninvasive) monitoring is substituted for another equally unnecessary measurement is faulty logic.

THE FUTURE OF MONITORING

Most clinicians would agree that monitoring is an integral part of respiratory care. Although monitoring has generally advanced the care of patients with respiratory problems, much of the support for monitoring is anecdotal, with little scientific evidence that monitoring has enhanced patient outcome.

The respiratory care community would benefit from a clarification of the role of monitoring (i.e., how much and what type of monitoring is appropriate). Because of the increasing financial pressures on the health care delivery system, we must determine when monitoring is necessary and cost-effective, and when it is not. Though controlled trials are the recommended strategy for evaluating this issue, entrenched appeal for noninvasive monitoring in respiratory care may frustrate appropriate trials. In the absence of such trials, professional guidelines for the use of respiratory monitors are needed.

The future will bring more technologic advances in respiratory monitoring. Manufacturers will certainly continue to introduce new monitors, some of which will probably provide useful data, while others will not. Practitioners should preserve a critical and rigorous approach to newly introduced devices. Care must be exercised not to accept solutions (i.e., new monitors) for which there is no problem (i.e., no clinical application) or that society cannot afford. We must balance technical capability, clinical usefulness, and cost (Fig 1–2).

In the context of a critical attitude, what promising advances in monitoring are likely to affect practice over the next decade? Systems using point-of-care (POC) devices,[38, 39] which provide measurements and monitoring at the bedside rather than remote laboratories, show

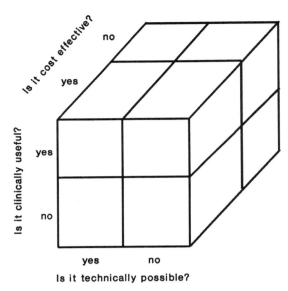

FIG 1–2.
When evaluating the potential use of a monitoring system, one should consider technical capability, clinical usefulness, and cost. One should select monitors that are technically feasible, clinically useful, and cost-effective.

promise in this regard. Two forms of POC testing are already in common use—bedside hand-held blood glucose monitoring devices (originally designed for at-home use by diabetics) and pulse oximetry. With POC technology, blood gases, electrolytes, glucose, and hematocrit can be determined on whole blood samples of less than 0.5 mL in fewer than 90 seconds.[38] The major attractiveness of these devices is that they provide rapid results, allowing treatment and monitoring of response in a nearly real-time manner. The principal disadvantage of these devices is that accuracy and precision are often compromised in favor of cost and rapid results.

As with other modalities, POC measurements have an appropriate role if their limitations are appreciated. As with traditional laboratory devices, methods of calibration, quality control, quality assurance, documentation, and proficiency testing should be applied to POC testing devices. New POC testing devices have recently become available for measuring activated partial thromboplastin time (aPTT), for bedside immunoassay of cardiac enzymes (rapid CK-MB), and for theophylline. Before widespread use, critical assessment of POC devices should be performed and guidelines for appropriate use should be prepared.

Another technology likely to have a future impact on respiratory monitoring is *in vivo* monitoring of arterial blood gases and pH.[3, 40–42] These devices have evolved from systems that are used for monitoring blood gases and pH in extracorporeal membrane oxygenation systems during open heart surgery. Although these systems can use electrochemical electrode systems (miniaturized electrodes similar to those found in blood gas analyzers), they typically use optode microsensing. An optode is a sensor that operates via optical detection of altered light.

For *in vivo* monitoring of blood gases and pH, fluorescent optodes are being developed. This optode is an optic fiber with a fluorescent dye at one end. Components of the fluorescent chemical are activated when exposed to an appropriate light intensity. A fluorescent dye will either augment or quench fluorescence as the concentration of a specific analyte (e.g., O_2, CO_2) changes around the dye. Several designs of *in vivo* optode blood gas monitoring systems are under development. The first design consists of an indwelling system passed through an arterial catheter. The second design requires withdrawal of blood from an arterial catheter into the measurement chamber and flushing of the blood back into the patient after measurement.

Many questions will need to be answered before the use of *in vivo* blood gas monitoring systems can be endorsed. Are these devices sufficiently accurate and precise? Is the drift in measurements over time acceptable? What calibration and quality control methods are needed? Because these devices require the presence of an arterial line, will this result in unnecessary arterial catheterization and associated complications? Are these expensive patient-dedicated devices cost-effective? Currently, it seems that *in vivo* blood gas monitoring devices are likely to be of benefit to only a very small number of critically ill patients.

Undoubtedly, new monitoring devices besides POC devices and indwelling continuous blood gas monitors will become available. As with these and all monitoring modalities, clinicians will be challenged to clarify the adequacy of new modalities as substitutes for traditional techniques, their safety and detailed cost, and the circumstances under which clinical use will be optimized.

SUMMARY

Monitoring in respiratory care is physiologically, technologically, and economically complex. Appropriate use of this technology requires a thorough understanding of these complexities. The purpose of this book is to provide the reader with the knowledge base needed to use wisely the information provided by the vast array of monitors used in respiratory care.

REFERENCES

1. Swan HJC, Ganz W, Forrester J, et al: Catheterization of the heart in man with use of a flow-directed balloon-tipped catheter. *N Engl J Med* 1970; 283:447–451.
2. Hess D: Noninvasive monitoring in respiratory care—present, past, and future: An overview. *Respir Care* 1990; 35:482–498.
3. Shapiro BA: In-vivo monitoring of arterial blood gases and pH. *Respir Care* 1992; 37:165–169.
4. New W: Pulse oximetry versus measurement of transcutaneous oxygen. *J Clin Monit* 1985; 1:126–129.
5. Berge KH, Lanier WL, Scanlon PD: Ischemic digital skin necrosis: A complication of the reusable Nellcor pulse oximeter probe. *Anesth Analg* 1988; 67:712–713.
6. Lemen RJ, Quan SF: Intravascular line placement in critical care patients, in Fallat RJ, Luce JM (eds): *Cardiopulmonary Critical Care Management.* New York, Churchill Livingstone Inc, 1988, pp 113–143.
7. Thorson SH, Marini JJ, Pierson DJ, et al: Variability of arterial blood gas values in stable patients in the ICU. *Chest* 1983; 84:14–18.

8. Hess D, Agarwal NN: Variability of blood gases, pulse oximeter saturation, and end-tidal carbon dioxide pressure in stable, mechanically ventilated trauma patients. *J Clin Monit* 1992; 8:111–115.

9. Connors AF, Dawson NV, McGaffree DR, et al: Assessing hemodynamic status in critically ill patients: Do physicians use clinical information optimally? *J Crit Care* 1987; 2:174–180.

10. Bowton DL, Scuderi PE, Harris L, et al: Pulse oximetry monitoring outside the intensive care unit: progress or problem? *Ann Intern Med* 1991; 115:450–454.

11. Tremper KK, Barker SJ: Transcutaneous oxygen measurement: Experimental studies and adult applications. *Int Anesthesiol Clin* 1987; 25:67–96.

12. Carlin BW, Clausen JL, Ties AL: The use of cutaneous oximetry in the prescription of long-term oxygen therapy. *Chest* 1988; 94:239–241.

13. Golish JA, McCarthy K: Limitation of pulse oximetry in detecting hypoxemia (abstract). *Chest* 1988; 94:50S.

14. Barker SJ, Tremper KK: The effect of carbon monoxide inhalation on pulse oximetry and transcutaneous PO_2 *Anesthesiology* 1987; 66:677–679.

15. Yamanka MK, Sue DY: Comparison of arterial-to-end-tidal PCO2 difference and deadspace/tidal volume ratio in respiratory failure. *Chest* 1987; 92:832–835.

16. Berryhill RE, Benumof JL: PEEP-induced discrepancy between pulmonary arterial wedge pressure and left atrial pressure: The effects of controlled vs. spontaneous ventilation and compliant vs. noncompliant lungs in the dog. *Anesthesiology* 1979; 51:303–308.

17. Muakkassa FF, Rutledge R, Fakhry SM, et al: ABGs and arterial lines: The relationship to unnecessarily drawn arterial blood gas samples. *J Trauma* 1990; 30:1087–1095.

18. Robin ED: Death by pulmonary artery flow-directed catheter: Time for a moratorium? (editorial). *Chest* 1987; 92:727–731.

19. Robin ED: The cult of the Swan-Ganz catheter. Overuse and abuse of pulmonary flow catheters. *Ann Intern Med* 1985; 103:445–449.

20. Robin ED: Defenders of the pulmonary artery catheter. *Chest* 1988; 93:1059–1066.

21. Hess D: The AARC clinical practice guidelines. *Respir Care* 1991; 36:1398–1401.

22. Task Force on Guidelines, Society of Critical Care Medicine. Guidelines for standards of care for patients with acute respiratory failure on mechanical ventilatory support. *Crit Care Med* 1991; 19:275–278.

23. Mok JYQ, Hak H, McLaughlin FJ, et al: Effect of age and state of wakefulness on transcutaneous oxygen values in preterm infants: A longitudinal study. *J Pediatrics* 1988; 113:706–709.

24. East TD, Morris AH, Wallace CJ, et al: A strategy for development of computerized critical care decision support systems. *Intern J Clin Monit Comput*, in press.

25. East TD: Computers in the ICU: Panacea or plague? *Respir Care* 1992; 37:170–180.

26. Vedal S, Crapo RO: False positive rates of multiple pulmonary function tests in healthy subjects. *Bull Eur Physiopathol Respir* 1983; 19:263–266.

27. Kestin IG, Miller BR, Lockhart CH: Auditory alarms during anesthesia monitoring. *Anesthesiology* 1988; 69:106–109.

28. Bentt LR, Santora TA, Leverle BJ, et al: Accuracy and utility of pulse oximetry in the surgical intensive care unit. *Curr Surg* 1990; 47:267–268.

29. Fruend PR, Overand PT, Cooper J, et al: A prospective study of pulse oximetry failure. *J Clin Monit* 1991; 7:253–258.

30. Hannhart B, Michalski H, Delorme N, et al: Reliability of six pulse oximeters in chronic obstructive pulmonary disease. *Chest* 1991; 99:842–846.

31. Peevy KJ, Hall MW: Transcutaneous oxygen monitoring: Economic impact on neonatal care. *Pediatrics* 1985; 75:1065–1067.

32. Beachy P, Whitfield JM: The effect of transcutaneous PO_2 monitoring on the frequency of arterial blood gas analysis in the newborn with respiratory distress. *Crit Care Med* 1981; 9:584–586.
33. King K, Simon RH: Pulse oximetry for tapering supplemental oxygen in hospitalized patients: Evaluation of a protocol. *Chest* 1987; 92:713–716.
34. Kellerman AL, Cofer CA, Joseph S, et al: Impact of portable pulse oximetry on arterial blood gas test ordering in an urban emergency department. *Ann Emerg Med* 1991; 20:130–134.
35. Bone RC, Balk RA: Noninvasive respiratory care unit: A cost effective solution for the future. *Chest* 1988; 93:390–394.
36. Kreiger BP, Ershowsky P, Spivak D, et al: Initial experience with a central respiratory monitoring unit as a cost-saving alternative to the intensive care unit for medicare patients who require long-term ventilator support. *Chest* 1988; 93:395–397.
37. Finkler SA: The distinction between cost and charges. *Ann Intern Med* 1982; 96:102–109.
38. Chernow B: The bedside laboratory. A critical step forward in ICU care. *Chest* 1990; 97:183S–184S.
39. Misiano DR, Meyerhoff ME, Collison ME: Current and future directions in the technology relating to bedside testing of critically ill patients. *Chest* 1990; 97:204S–214S.
40. Miller WW, Gehrich JL, Hansmann DR, et al: Continuous in vivo monitoring of blood gases. *Lab Med* 1988; 10:629–635.
41. Shapiro BA, Cane RD: Blood gas monitoring: Yesterday, today, and tomorrow. *Crit Care Med* 1989; 17:573–581.
42. Shapiro BA, Cane RD, Chomka CM, et al: Preliminary evaluation of an intra-arterial blood gas system in dogs and humans. *Crit Care Med* 1989; 17:455–460.

Chapter 2

Fluid Mechanics

William R. Kimball, M.D., Ph.D.

INTRODUCTION

As life progressed from unicellular to multicellular organisms, methods of transporting nutrients to and removing waste products from the cells became necessary. This led to the evolution of circulatory systems. As these large multicellular organisms adapted to life out of water, ventilatory systems evolved.

The cardiovascular and respiratory systems obey the laws of fluid mechanics. This chapter will discuss basic properties of fluids, the laws that govern these fluids, and special modifications of these laws that occur in man and other vertebrates. Knowledge of the laws of fluid mechanics is necessary both to understand how the circulatory and respiratory systems work and to understand the principles of the measurement techniques used to monitor these two systems. While fluid mechanics comprises a separate discipline in physics and entire textbooks are dedicated to this topic, this chapter will discuss only the basic concepts.

BASIC PROPERTIES OF FLUIDS

A fluid is a substance that assumes the shape of the container holding it, and it will readily change its shape if the shape of the container changes. Fluids have two intrinsic properties: density and viscosity.

Density

The density of a fluid represents the mass of fluid contained within a defined volume. Gases are less dense than liquids, while water is less dense than mercury. Ideal fluids cannot be compressed; their density is constant. Real fluids, especially gases, change their density if the forces placed on them are sufficiently large. Only severe physiological conditions cause compression, leading to changes in density. This discussion will consider conditions where fluids are incompressible. Density, represented by the Greek letter ρ, is expressed as grams per cubic centimeter, kilograms per liter, or slugs (pounds mass) per cubic foot.

Viscosity

Viscosity represents the property of a fluid to resist flow. While an ideal fluid possesses no viscosity, all real fluids are viscous. During flow, all parts of the fluid may not move at identical flow rates, so adjacent elements of fluid may be required to slip past each other. The force impeding slippage between adjacent fluid elements moving at different velocities is proportional to viscosity. Gases have lower viscosities than liquids, while water has a lower viscosity than motor oil. The Greek letter μ represents viscosity.

One common unit for measuring viscosity is the poise, which has the units

$$1 \text{ poise} = 1 \text{ dyne} \cdot \text{sec/cm}^2$$

Relative viscosity compares the viscosity of a liquid to the viscosity of water. Different units measuring viscosity, and the multipliers used to convert between them, are given in Table 2–1.

Viscosity can be determined by moving a plate of area A at a constant velocity u along a fluid whose height is h (Fig 2–1). If the force F necessary to move this plate is constant, and the fluid rests on an infinitely large stationary surface of material similar to the plate, the viscosity will be given by the relation

$$\mu = F \cdot h/(A \cdot u) = (F/A)/(u/h) \tag{2-1}$$

Another definition of viscosity considers the ratio of shear stress, the force causing two adjacent layers of fluid to move past each other (force/area), to the rate of strain, the variation in velocity of moving fluid elements caused by a force (u/h).

If two identically shaped plates are moved at the same velocity through two fluids of equal height, then the more viscous fluid will require a greater force to maintain the velocity of the plate. For two identically shaped plates moved by equal forces, the more viscous fluid will sustain a lower velocity gradient (change in velocity with height, u/h) than the less viscous fluid.

TABLE 2–1.
Viscosity Conversions

	Poise	lb/ft · sec	lb/in. · sec	kg/m · hr
Poise gm/cm · sec	1	6.72×10^{-2}	5.6×10^{-3}	3.6×10^2
lb/ft · sec	14.88	1	8.33×10^{-2}	5.36×10^3
lb/in. · sec	178.6	12	1	6.43×10^4
kb/m · hr	2.78×10^{-3}	1.87×10^{-4}	1.56×10^{-5}	1

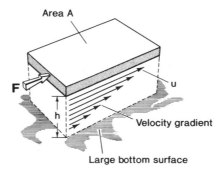

FIG 2–1.
Viscosity of a fluid. Motion of a plate of area *A* through an otherwise stationary fluid requires that a force *F* be applied to the plate. This force is proportional to the velocity of the plate, *u,* and to the depth of the fluid, *h*. The fluid in contact with the plate must move at the same velocity as the plate, while the fluid more distant from the plate will move at a slower velocity. The velocity of the fluid in contact with the bottom surface of the container must be zero. When the plate, moving at a constant velocity, produces a linear change in the velocity of the fluid per unit depth of a homogeneous fluid, the fluid is a Newtonian fluid.

A Newtonian fluid is a homogeneous fluid, such as air, water, or alcohol, whose viscosity is constant and whose change in velocity is a linear function of the height of the fluid (u/h = a constant). One biological fluid, blood, is non-Newtonian. Its properties will be considered later in this chapter.

BASIC PARAMETERS OF FLUID MECHANICS: PRESSURE, FLOW, RESISTANCE

A fluid can pass through a passage of any shape. The ability of a fluid to move or flow through a passage relates directly to the forces generating the flow and to the forces impeding the flow. For a fluid moving within a long tube at a constant flow rate Q, the force, which is both distributed over the cross-sectional area of the tube and is parallel to the direction of the fluid flow, is the driving pressure. Both the resistance of the tube and the properties of the fluid produce forces that impede the fluid flow. The pressure difference between two points within the tube, for example, for points A and B in Figure 2–2, equals the product of the flow through the tube, Q, and the resistance of the tube, R:

$$P_A - P_B = \Delta P = Q \cdot R \qquad (2–2)$$

Pressure

Pressure is the driving force. It is the force acting perpendicular to a unit area of surface. One property of a pressure acting on an enclosed, nonmoving fluid is that the pressure applied to

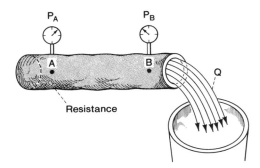

FIG 2–2.
Fluid flowing past two points, A and B, in a channel or pipe produces a pressure drop that is related to the bulk flow of the fluid, *Q*, and to the resistance of the channel or pipe. Resistance is depicted by the nonuniformity of the channel walls.

the fluid is transmitted equally to every particle of the fluid and to the walls of the container. This phenomenon is known as the *law of Pascal*.

Atmospheric pressure is commonly employed as a reference and as a calibration pressure. One approach to measuring atmospheric pressure employs a barometer, a vertical tube filled with a fluid, usually mercury, which is occluded at one end while the open end rests in a basin of the same fluid (Fig 2–3). Atmospheric pressure is the distance in millimeters between the top of the mercury in the tube and the top of the mercury in the basin (e.g., 760 mm Hg). Therefore, pressure is given by the relationship:

$$P = \rho \cdot g \cdot h \qquad (2\text{--}3)$$

where ρ is the density of the fluid, g is the gravitational acceleration constant, and h is the height of the fluid. Other units of pressure measurement include centimeters of water, dynes per square centimeter, Newtons per square meter (Pascals), pounds per square inch, or atmospheres. Table 2–2 lists different units of pressure measurement and factors used to convert between these measurements.

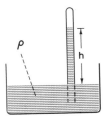

FIG 2–3.
A barometer measures atmospheric pressure. The height of the fluid, *h*, is affected by its density ρ and by atmospheric pressure, which at sea level varies only slightly with weather conditions.

TABLE 2–2.
Pressure Conversions

	Pascal	bar	lb/in.^{2}	lb/ft^2	atm	mm Hg	cm H$_2$O
Pascal	1	10^{-5}	1.45×10^{-4}	0.0209	9.87×10^{-6}	7.5×10^{-3}	0.0102
bar	10^5	1	14.5	2088.5	0.987	750.6	1020
lb/in.^{2}	6895	0.069	1	144	0.068	51.7	70.3
lb/ft^2	47.88	4.79×10^{-4}	6.94×10^{-3}	1	4.72×10^{-4}	0.359	0.488
atm	1.01×10^5	1.013	14.7	2116	1	760	1.034×10^3
mm Hg	133.3	1.33×10^{-3}	1.93×10^{-2}	2.785	1.32×10^{-3}	1	1.36
cm H$_2$O	98.07	9.80×10^{-4}	1.42×10^{-2}	2.047	9.67×10^{-4}	0.735	1

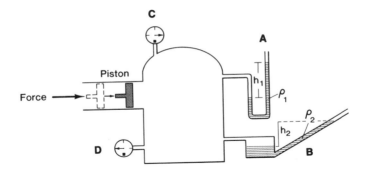

FIG 2–4.
Types of manometers. When a piston connected to a large chamber is advanced, producing an increase in chamber pressure, the four pressure measuring devices (A–D) connected to the chamber must each measure the same pressure change. **A,** U-tube manometers determine pressure as the difference in height between the two limbs of the U-tube. When one limb of the manometer is open to atmospheric pressure, the manometer measures changes in pressure that differ from atmospheric pressure. The more dense the fluid in the manometer, ρ_1, the smaller the height difference for a given pressure change, h_1. If the two limbs of the U-tube are of equal diameter, then the pressure difference can be determined by measuring either the change in height of one limb relative to the level where no pressure difference was applied to the manometer, or the height difference between the two limbs of the manometer. **B,** Slanted tubes can magnify small pressure differences compared to the height of a fluid in the reservoir. A very small tube or a very wide reservoir mouth assures the reference level will remain constant. **C,** Gauges measure a pressure change by converting the pressure to the displacement of a diaphragm. A gear mechanism converts the displacement of the diaphragm into motion of a needle on a scale. The measurement of "absolute pressure" adds the change in pressure within the chamber to atmospheric pressure. **D,** This gauge measures only the pressure change within the chamber relative to atmospheric pressure, similar to the manometers. This pressure is "gauge pressure."

Pressure is also measured as the difference in the height of a fluid in a U-tube manometer as in Figure 2–4, A, or as the height above a reference level as in Figure 2–4, B, or by reading the scale of a gauge as in Figure 2–4, C or D. According to the law of Pascal, the application of a force to a piston of area A transmits the pressure equally to all parts of the fluid within the chamber, to the manometers connected to the chamber wall, and to the gauges attached to the other wall of the chamber. The difference in height of the fluid in the manometer (Fig 2–4, A), represents the pressure within the chamber, P_{chamber}, compared to atmospheric pressure, P_{atm}. Thus,

$$P_{\text{chamber}} - P_{\text{atm}} = \text{force/area} = \rho \cdot g \cdot h \qquad (2–4)$$

where h refers to the height difference between the two limbs of the liquid column in the U-shaped tube. Since one end of the U-tube manometer is open to the atmosphere, this pressure difference employs atmospheric pressure as a reference. Other manometers measure pressure as the difference in height above the reservoir level of the fluid. Height is measured parallel to the direction of the gravitational field. For the slanted manometers of Figure 2–4, B, the height is the vertical height, not the length of the fluid column. When fluid density cannot be reduced, a slanted tube can provide improved resolution of small pressure changes.

Gauges employ a deformable diaphragm to convert pressure into the motion of a needle. The motion of the needle depends on the deformability of the diaphragm and amplification ratio of the gears that convert the diaphragm deformation into needle movement. If either the diaphragm or the gear ratio changes, the measurement will be inaccurate unless the measuring scale is also changed. Gauges can use atmospheric pressure as a reference (Fig 2–4, D), similar to the manometers in Figures 2–4, A and B, or they can measure *absolute pressure*, which is pressure referenced to zero (Fig 2–4, C). Absolute pressure becomes the pressure in the chamber added to atmospheric pressure. The term *gauge pressure* implies that atmospheric pressure is the reference pressure. Biological systems commonly employ measurements of gauge pressure. Pressure measurements can be presumed to represent gauge pressure, where the reference pressure is atmospheric pressure, unless stated otherwise.

Flow

Flow is the volumetric measurement of fluid movement. Conversion factors used to convert between different measures of volume are listed in Table 2–3. The volume passing a location and the time during which the fluid movement is measured will define the flow. Some units of measurement are cubic centimeters per second, liters per minute, or gallons per hour. Table 2–4 lists the different units of flow measurement and the factors used to convert between them.

Although flow considers the volumetric measurement of fluid movement, another method addresses the velocity of a fluid element of small but finite volume. While a fluid may move at a volumetric flow rate Q through a tube of cross-sectional area A, the average velocity of each fluid element u is represented by

$$u = Q/A \qquad (2\text{–}5)$$

In a steadily moving fluid, individual fluid elements may move at veolicities either faster or slower than the average velocity. In addition, the direction of motion of an individual fluid element may be quite different from the general direction of the fluid motion.

TABLE 2–3.
Volume Conversions

	liter	gallon	in.³	ft³	cm³	m³
liter	1	0.264	61.02	0.0353	10^3	10^{-3}
gallon	3.785	1	231.1	0.134	3.78×10^3	3.78×10^{-3}
in.³	0.0164	4.33×10^{-3}	1	5.79×10^{-4}	16.39	1.64×10^{-5}
ft³	28.32	7.481	1.73×10^3	1	2.83×10^4	2.83×10^{-2}
cm³	10^{-3}	2.65×10^{-4}	0.061	3.53×10^{-5}	1	10^{-6}
m³	10^3	264.6	6.10×10^4	35.3	10^6	1

TABLE 2–4.
Flow Conversions

	liter/sec	gal/hr	ft³/min	cm³/sec	m³/sec
liter/sec	1	951.1	2.119	10^3	10^{-3}
gallon/hr	1.05×10^{-3}	1	449.5	10.51	1.05×10^{-5}
ft³/min	0.472	2.22×10^{-3}	1	473	4.73×10^{-4}
cm³/sec	10^{-3}	9.52×10^{-2}	2.11×10^{-3}	1	10^{-6}
m³/sec	10^3	9.52×10^4	2.11×10^3	10^6	1

Flow Patterns and Streamlines

While the bulk movement of a fluid is referred to as *flow*, the pattern each individual fluid element follows determines the *flow pattern*. A flow pattern can be studied by continuously adding a marker substance to the flowing fluid. For example, jets of smoke can be added to a gas, while a dye can be injected into a liquid. A streamline denotes the path the marker follows. A streamline is parallel to the direction of flow, and usually will be parallel to the vessel wall. Fluid cannot cross a streamline. The paths of the marker show how the elements of the fluid are flowing relative to other elements of the fluid. "Laminar flow" occurs when the trail of the marker remains sharply defined and immobile at any specific point in a steadily moving fluid, as in Figure 2–5, A. However, if the streamlines at a given point move randomly in a sinuous manner, perpendicular to the direction of the bulk flow, or if the marker mixes with the fluid and cannot be identified within the flowing fluid, then no streamline remains defined and the flow pattern has developed the characteristics of "turbulent flow," as in Figure 2–5, B. For laminar flow the fluid elements move in layers. Each layer may move at a velocity that differs

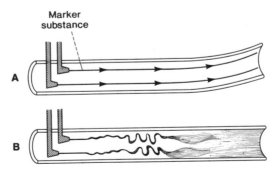

FIG 2–5.
Flow patterns. **A,** During laminar flow a marker substance added to a flowing fluid remains stationary and follows gradual changes in the direction of the flow. **B,** During turbulent flow the paths of the marker substance become unsteady. These paths may move perpendicular to the walls defining the flow direction, or the marker may become dispersed within the flowing fluid, eventually becoming unrecognizable or totally mixed within the fluid.

from its adjacent layer. If laminar flow occurs in a tube, then each very thin concentric fluid layer must slide past the adjacent layers.

Resistance

The pattern of flow, either laminar or turbulent, markedly affects the measurement of resistance produced by a flowing fluid. Resistance is defined as pressure divided by flow. It denotes many factors that act together to retard the movement of a fluid. The pattern of flow is one factor influencing the value of resistance. Resistance, as defined above and in Figure 2–2, is represented by

$$R = (P_B - P_A)/Q. \qquad (2\text{--}6)$$

It is expressed in units such as centimeters of water per cubic centimeter per second, or millimeters of mercury per liter per second.

Resistance Configurations

Resistance elements can be arranged sequentially in the direction of flow, called *series*, or they can be arranged next to each other with all elements having the same input pressure and the same output pressure, called *parallel*.

When elements are arranged in series (Fig 2–6, A), the resistances are additive. Since the flow is constant from point A to point D, the pressure difference between points A and B is given by

$$P_A - P_B = Q \cdot R_A \qquad (2\text{--}7)$$

where R_A is the resistance of the first element. Similarly R_B and R_C are the differences in pressure between point B and point C, and between point C and point D, respectively. However, the total pressure drop defines the total resistance, R_T, thus

$$P_A - P_D = Q \cdot R_T = Q \cdot (R_A + R_B + R_C) \qquad (2\text{--}8)$$

where

$$R_T = R_A + R_B + R_C \qquad (2\text{--}9)$$

is the sum of the resistance of each unit.

For elements arranged in parallel (Fig 2–6, B), the input pressure P_i and the output pressure P_o are the same for all elements, but the flow for each element, Q_1, Q_2, and Q_3, will be proportional to their respective resistances R_1, R_2, and R_3. Therefore,

$$P_i - P_o = Q_1 \cdot R_1 = Q_2 \cdot R_2 = Q_3 \cdot R_3 \qquad (2\text{--}10)$$

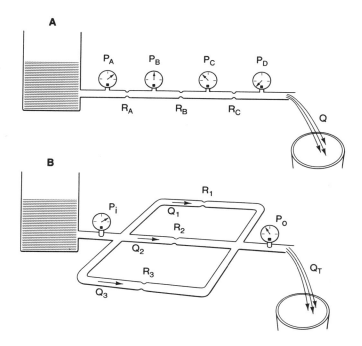

FIG 2–6.
Series and parallel resistances. **A,** Resistances connected in series have a common flow Q, but the pressures near the resistances P_A, P_B, P_C, and P_D, decrease progessively and in proportion to the resistances R_A, R_B, and R_C. The total resistance is the sum of the individual resistances. **B,** When resistances are connected to the same input and output pressures, P_i and P_o, the total flow, Q_T, is split between each pathway. The flow through each pathway, Q_1, Q_2, or Q_3, is proportional to the resistance of the individual pathway, R_1, R_2, or R_3. The sum of the resistances of parallel pathways is less than the resistance of any pathway.

but since the total flow, Q_T, is the sum of the flows, total flow becomes

$$\begin{aligned} Q_T &= Q_1 + Q_2 + Q_3 \\ &= (P_i - P_o)/R_1 + (P_i - P_o)/R_2 + (P_i - P_o)R_3 \\ &= (P_i - P_o)/R_{\text{sum}} \end{aligned} \qquad (2\text{--}11)$$

where R_{sum} is expressed as

$$1/R_{\text{sum}} = 1/R_1 + 1/R_2 + 1/R_3. \qquad (2\text{--}12)$$

For resistances arranged in parallel, the total resistance will be less than the resistance of the pathway with the least resistance. If three equal resistances were placed in parallel, then the resistance of the three would be one-third the value of either of the resistances.

An example of a series system is the gastrointestinal circulation system where arterial blood flows through the intestinal capillary bed before reaching the capillary bed of the liver and then joining flow in the inferior vena cava. An example of a parallel system is the systemic circulation, where the capillary beds of multiple organ systems (heart, kidneys, brain, etc.) are placed between the left and right hearts. For the respiratory system any device placed over the mouth or nose provides a series resistance. Parallel resistors are uncommon in the respiratory system, although the resistances of the mouth and the nasal passages are arranged in series.

EFFECT OF FLOW PATTERN ON RESISTANCE

Established Laminar Flow in Pipes

While flow patterns are either laminar or turbulent, *Poiseuille* flow is a special form of laminar flow that develops when a fluid flow is constant and slow, and the fluid has traveled a long distance inside a smooth tube of constant diameter. These conditions permit sufficient time for the flow pattern to develop. The resistance between two points along a pipe during Poiseuille flow, as in Figure 2–2 between points A and B, is described by *Poiseuille's* law:

$$R = \frac{8L}{\pi r^4}\mu \qquad (2-13)$$

where r is the radius of the pipe, L is the distance between the two points for the resistance measurement, and μ is the viscosity of the fluid. Clearly, the radius of the pipe is very important in determining the resistance to fluid flow. Poiseuille's law describes a fluid velocity profile that is parabolic, as in Figure 2–7. This parabolic velocity profile is a special form of laminar flow.

Nonlaminar Flow

Any change in velocity of a fluid requires an acceleration or deceleration. This can occur only when a force acts on the fluid element. Two forces that act on a fluid are its resistive and its

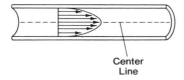

Center
Line

FIG 2–7.
Velocity profile of Poiseuille flow. During established laminar flow the velocity of individual fluid elements increases as the elements move near the center of the channel. Friction prevents movement of the fluid in contact with the wall of the channel, and viscosity determines the increase in velocity of fluid elements more distant from the wall. Maximum velocity occurs in the center of the channel.

inertial properties. The resistive force on a fluid relates to its viscosity μ, while the inertial force acting on a fluid relates to its density ρ.

When a fluid flows past a sudden increase in area, as in Figure 2–8, A, or a sudden decrease in area, as in Figure 2–8, B, the flow profile will be disrupted. If the flow profile before the change in tube size were laminar, then when the fluid reaches the downstream tube the flow pattern will become disrupted. While the fluid in the center of the tube might continue flowing as if there were no area change, the fluid flowing near the wall of the tube before the widening would have to flow laterally toward the more distant wall as in Figure 2–8, A, or toward the center of the tube as in Figure 2–8, B. These changes in the flow lines create a lateral acceleration. This lateral acceleration could disrupt the flow patterns, creating turbulent flow. If the tube downstream of the diameter change were of constant size and if Poiseuille flow had existed before a sudden widening, Poiseuille flow would be likely to redevelop downstream of the disruption in Figure 2–8, A. For the downstream tube of Figure 2–8, B, the flow pattern could either remain turbulent, or could eventually return to laminar flow. Whether laminar or turbulent flow persists after the area change is determined by the value of the Reynolds number.

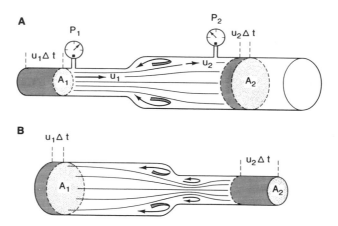

FIG 2–8.
Streamlines at a sudden change of pathway area. **A,** Sudden increases in cross-sectional area disrupt flow patterns. Since velocity must remain zero at the walls and the velocity of the center of the stream cannot change instantaneously, although average velocity will decrease as soon as the channel widens, areas of turbulence will develop as the flow moves to encompass the entire width of the channel. These laterally directed forces will disrupt flow patterns. During any area change, when density remains constant, mass transfer must be identical. Mass transfer is the product of mean fluid velocity, its density, the cross-sectional area of the passage, and the amount of time allowed for the mass transfer. Pressure changes are described by Bernoulli's law, as described in the text. **B,** Sudden decreases in cross-sectional area also alter flow patterns by deflecting peripheral flow to the center of the tube and by accelerating the elements. A steady flow before the constriction may produce unsteadiness, which will not resolve after the restriction.

Reynolds Number for Determining Flow Patterns

Sometimes fluid flowing in a long straight tube can spontaneously become turbulent. Four factors are important to determine the tendency of fluid flow to become turbulent: viscosity (μ), density (ρ), mean fluid velocity (u), and the diameter of the vessel (d). The Reynolds number *Re* determines the relationship of these four factors, where

$$Re = \frac{\rho \cdot u \cdot d}{\mu} \tag{2–14}$$

For homogenous fluids when *Re* <2000 flow will become laminar, while for *Re* >3000 flow will usually become turbulent. Highly viscous fluids will tend to dampen flow instabilities, while large velocities, densities, or wide diameter tubes will tend to promote propagation of these instabilities. In the example of Figure 2–8, B, where the tube narrows suddenly, Poiseuille flow could only redevelop if the Reynolds number distal to the narrowing were less than the critical number, Re <2000, and if the tube were sufficiently long to allow the flow pattern to redevelop.

While the Reynolds number considers flow within a tube distant from either branching or changes in cross-sectional area, both factors can produce turbulent flow near this type of geometric change, as in Figure 2–8, even for Re somewhat less than 2000. Thus, while the Reynolds number can be used as a guide to predict turbulence, geometric factors downstream of the point under consideration can produce turbulence, although the turbulence may not be self-sustaining.

Turbulent flow is common in pathological conditions. Heart murmurs caused by a stenotic aortic or mitral valve are the audible manifestations of turbulent flow. Similarly, the wheezing heard during a forced expiration in an asthmatic patient or a patient with chronic obstructive pulmonary disease may represent turbulent airflow.

Kinematic Viscosity

The Reynolds number employs both viscosity and density when assessing the tendency of a flow to become turbulent. Two other variables, flow velocity and the diameter of the passage, are also required. To simplify calculation of the Reynolds number when different fluids are used in the same setting, kinematic viscosity ν (Table 2–5), which is the ratio of fluid viscosity

TABLE 2–5.
Kinematic Viscosity Conversions

	stoke	ft²/hr	in.²/sec	m²/hr
stoke	1	3.875	0.155	0.36
ft²/hr	0.258	1	0.04	0.0929
in.²/sec	6.452	25	1	2.323
m²/hr	2.778	10.76	0.4306	1

to density ($\nu = \mu/\rho$), replaces the two separate values of viscosity and density. The Reynolds number becomes

$$Re = (u \cdot d)/\nu$$

Values for viscosity and density of some common substances are included in Table 2–6.

Measurement of Flow

During laminar flow according to the law of Poiseuille, resistance is constant and the pressure drop along a tube is linearly related to the mean fluid velocity u. Yet, during turbulent flow, resistance depends more on the velocity of flow, and the pressure drop along a tube is proportional to the square of the mean velocity, $u = Q/A$. Thus, the pressure drops for these two types of flow are:

$$\Delta P \propto u \qquad \text{Laminar flow}$$

$$\Delta P \propto u^2 \qquad \text{Turbulent flow}$$

When measuring the pressure drop along a tube with a region of turbulence, as in Figure 2–8, the pressure drop can be determined by an equation first described by Rohrer,

$$\Delta P = k_1 \cdot u + k_2 \cdot u^2 \qquad (2\text{--}15)$$

where both k_1 and k_2 are constants.

One device commonly used to measure flow is the venturi meter, Figure 2–9, A. It is a tube with a gradual narrowing and then a gradual widening. These gradual changes in size

TABLE 2–6.
Viscosity and Density of Common Substances

Compound		Viscosity (poise)	Density (gm/ml) or (gm/cm^3)
ethanol	at 0° C	1.773×10^{-2}	0.80625
	at 37° C	0.952×10^{-2}	0.775
H_2O	at 0° C	1.787×10^{-2}	0.99984
	at 37° C	0.692×10^{-2}	0.99333
mercury	at 0° C	1.685	13.596
	at 37° C	1.484	13.505
castor oil	at 0° C	53	0.969
	at 37° C	3.4	
air	at 0° C	1.708×10^{-4}	1.2929×10^{-3}
	at 37° C	1.881×10^{-4}	1.1423×10^{-3}
bone			1.7021
sugar			1.59

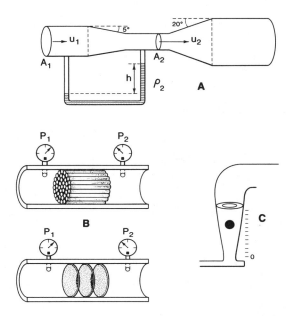

FIG 2–9.
Flow measurement devices. **A,** Venturi meters employ a gradual decrease in channel area to maintain laminar flow while creating a velocity change and thus a pressure change. The difference in flow between the wide and the narrow area determines a pressure drop that is proportional to the initial flow. **B,** Pneumotachographs are resistors placed within flowing fluid. These resistors are commonly multiple parallel capillary tubes or fine mesh screens. The pressure drop across the stream is proportional to the flow, provided the flow pattern remains laminar. A pneumotachograph is commonly employed to measure respiratory airflow, but the screens or capillary tubes must be kept free of secretions and water vapor condensation. **C,** Rotameters measure flow as it passes through a tapered tube. The flow of the fluid lifts a bobbin, which measures flow along a scale calibrated for the specific fluid.

avoid creating turbulence when the tube narrows or widens. A 5-degree angle with the axis of the tube meets this criterion for widening, while a 20-degree angle with the axis will be an appropriate rate of flow convergence. The narrowing also must keep the Reynolds number from exceeding its critical value at the neck of the tube. Under these conditions, the velocity of the fluid at the inlet of the venturi meter can be determined from the height difference of the fluid in the U-tube manometer. This relationship is developed in the discussion of Bernoulli's law in Equations (2–18) through (2–21).

A second device for measuring flow is the pneumotachograph (Fig 2–9, B). It is routinely used to measure respiratory airflow. Pneumotachographs either consist of a group of fine-mesh screens, placed perpendicular to the direction of flow and completely spanning the flow channel, known as a screen pneumotachograph, or they consist of a group of thin-walled capillary tubes placed parallel to the direction of flow and also completely spanning the flow channel, known as a Fleisch pneumotachograph. Either the screens or the capillary tubes provide a resistance that creates a pressure drop as the fluid passes through the resistance. The difference in pressure before and after the resistance will be directly proportional to flow if the flow is laminar.

Flow can also be measured using a rotameter (Fig 2–9, C). This is a vertical tube of gradually increasing cross-sectional area with a weighted element resting within the center of the tube. As flow increases through the vertical tube, the weight is lifted by the gas movement around the weight.

Each rotameter is specific for its range of flow and for the gas it measures. If either the flow tube or the weight is changed, or if a different gas passes through the rotameter, the flow measurement will be inaccurate. For low flow rates the measurement error will be primarily dependent on the difference in viscosities between the gas flowing through the rotameter and the viscosity for which the rotameter was designed. For high flow rates, differences in density between the gas in use and the intended gas is the primary factor determining the measurement error.

LAWS OF FLUID MECHANICS

Archimedes' Principle

An object placed into a fluid usually either floats or sinks. An object that floats has buoyancy. Markers that float in the ocean or in lakes and are used to locate hazards or channels are called buoys and employ the principle of buoyancy. When the buoy rests in water the force the buoy exerts on the water must be balanced by the force the water exerts on buoy. Archimedes noted that the force an object immersed in a fluid exerts on the fluid is equal to the amount of fluid displaced.

Conservation of Mass

Neither blood nor respired air moves at constant velocity, nor do they flow through long straight tubes. Both the respiratory and circulatory systems have many bifurcations and changes in cross-sectional area. When the cross-sectional area of a tube changes, the mass of fluid entering a tube must equal the mass of fluid leaving the tube in the same amount of time, Δt. That is, by conservation of mass

$$\rho_1 \cdot u_1 \cdot A_1 \cdot \Delta t = \rho_2 \cdot u_2 \cdot A_2 \cdot \Delta t \qquad (2\text{–}16)$$

where u_1 and u_2 are the mean velocities of flow before and after the change in cross-sectional area from A_1 to A_2, and ρ_1 and ρ_2 are the densities of the fluid. Since incompressible fluids maintain constant density, as the cross-sectional area of a tube changes, as in Figure 2–8, the average velocity of the fluid must change in proportion to the change in cross-sectional area.

For a fixed time period during incompressible flow, the principle of conservation of mass becomes

$$u_1 \cdot A_1 = u_2 \cdot A_2 \qquad (2\text{--}17)$$

or the change in velocity of fluid motion is inversely proportional to the change in the area through which it passes.

Bernoulli's Law

Many biological systems produce fluid movement upward or downward in the gravitational field of the earth. The changes in height of the fluid also affect the pressures driving these fluids. An analysis of these factors, initially developed by Daniel Bernoulli, can be derived using the principle of conservation of energy. If pressure acts on a small volume V, then PV is work that must be added to potential energy to obtain total energy within a system. Bernoulli's law suggests that

$$P + \rho \cdot g \cdot h + \tfrac{1}{2} \cdot \rho \cdot u^2 = \text{constant}, \qquad (2\text{--}18)$$

since volume is constant during incompressible flow. In this relationship P denotes absolute pressure, ρ denotes density, g is gravitational accleration, h is the height of the fluid column, and u is the velocity of the fluid element under consideration. Bernoulli's law would determine the difference in pressure between the two ends of a tapered tube with openings at different heights to be

$$P_1 - P_2 = \tfrac{1}{2} \cdot \rho \cdot (u_2^2 - u_1^2) + \rho \cdot g \cdot (h_2 - h_1) \qquad (2\text{--}19)$$

where u_1 and u_2 are the mean velocities of the fluid at the entrance and exit of the tube, respectively, and h_1 and h_2 are the heights of the entrance and exit of the tube. This solution neglects the pressure loss due to the resistance of fluid movement in the tube.

For the venturi meter of Figure 2–9, A, Bernoulli's law can be applied to one point before the convergence and to another point after the convergence:

$$P_1 + \tfrac{1}{2} \cdot \rho \cdot u_1^2 = P_2 + \tfrac{1}{2} \cdot \rho \cdot u_2^2 \qquad (2\text{--}20)$$

The central axis of this venturi meter is horizontal, so $h_1 = h_2$. If the difference in pressure between points 1 and 2 were measured by a U-tube manometer with a fluid of density ρ_2 and the areas of both the wide and narrow portions of the venturi tube were A_1 and A_2, respectively, then the velocity of the fluid entering the meter, u_1, would be determined as

$$u_1 = A_2 \cdot \left[\frac{2 \cdot (\rho_2 - \rho_1) \cdot g \cdot h}{\rho_1 \cdot (A_1^2 - A_2^2)} \right]^{1/2} \qquad (2\text{--}21)$$

where $P_1 - P_2 = (\rho_2 - \rho_1) \cdot g \cdot h$, ρ_1 is the density of the flowing fluid and ρ_2 is the density of the fluid in the manometer.

Stokes' Law

When a sphere moves through a stagnant fluid of zero viscosity, the streamlines around the sphere form a symmetrical pattern and the force on the upstream face of the sphere equals the force on the downstream face of the sphere. For a real fluid where viscosity is finite, a greater force will be exerted on the face of the sphere that faces the direction of flow. This force difference is *viscous drag*, and will act to move the sphere in the direction of the fluid flow. Drag for a sphere can be calculated using Stokes' law. This relationship determines the force on the sphere in an incompressible fluid with finite viscosity as

$$F = 6 \cdot \pi \cdot \mu \cdot r \cdot v \qquad (2-22)$$

where μ is the viscosity of the fluid, r is the radius of the sphere, and v is the velocity of the sphere relative to the velocity of the fluid before the fluid is disturbed by the sphere.

Stokes' law and Archimedes' principle apply to red blood cells (RBCs) in blood, since blood is a suspension of particles in a fluid, plasma. The *sedimentation rate*, the rate of settling of red blood cells in plasma, is the terminal velocity of RBCs in plasma. It is determined by setting the sum of the buoyant force of the RBC plus the drag of the RBC equal to the weight of the RBC. Sedimentation rate is frequently used to assess the presence of human diseases, although it is not diagnostic of any specific disease.

Laplace's Law

Since flow in small blood vessels will be laminar and obey Poiseuille's law, minimal changes in vessel radius can markedly affect the pressure drop along the vessel. Both the amount of elastic tissue in the vessel wall and the activity of the smooth muscle in the vessel wall influence vessel diameter. These two factors comprise the circumferential tension T in the vessel wall. According to the law of Laplace wall tension T for a cylinder can be computed from the relationship:

$$T = \text{P} \cdot r$$

where P is the transmural pressure, the pressure difference between the inside and the outside the vessel, and r is the radius of the inner surface of the vessel. The larger the radius, the larger the wall tension. Wall tension is the force exerted radially, around the circumference of the vessel. If pressure within a vessel were to increase, then wall tension would increase. If the increase in wall tension exceeded both the contractile force produced by the smooth muscle tissue and the recoil force produced by the elastic tissue, the vessel might expand until the point at which the wall would tear along the longitudinal axis of the vessel.

For a sphere, Laplace's law becomes

$$T = P \cdot 2r$$

and the wall tension is twice that of the tension of a cylinder.

PHYSIOLOGIC ISSUES IN FLUID MECHANICS

Rheological Properties of Blood

While the sedimentation rate is one property unique to RBCs in blood, the measurement of viscosity expresses another, more important effect of red blood cells on blood. As discussed previously viscosity is proportional to the force required to slide one fluid element past another fluid element at a different velocity. The viscosity of a Newtonian fluid during laminar flow may be determined using Poiseuille's equation by measuring the pressure drop along a tube of known length and radius. While viscosity of a Newtonian fluid will remain unchanged throughout a wide range of tube lengths and radii, it will be affected by altering temperature.

For a non-Newtonian fluid such as blood, viscosity will vary with tube diameter, flow rate, and the hematocrit. Since blood is a fluid composed of a nearly homogeneous plasma component and a particulate component (primarily red blood cells, but including white blood cells and platelets), the ratio of the viscosity of blood to the viscosity of plasma increases progressively as the hematocrit increases. The viscosity of blood may exceed twice the viscosity of plasma when the hematocrit (the ratio of red blood cell volume to total blood volume) reaches polycythemic levels, hematocrits exceeding 65%. Yet, depending on the velocity of flow and the diameter of the vessels, the ratio between the viscosity of blood and of plasma is widely variable.

One further property of blood is that the ratio of viscosity of blood to the viscosity of water decreases in vessels with a diameter of less than 0.3 mm. This diameter is within the range of microscopic blood vessels; arterioles have diameters smaller than 0.3 mm. Additionally, the viscosity of blood in perfused tissue is much greater than the viscosity of blood in a conventional capillary viscometer of 0.3 mm or less. Fahraeus and Lindqvist described these effects in 1931. They ascribed these results to a separation of blood flow in small vessels; RBCs would flow along the axis (or in the center) of the vessel whereas plasma would flow near the wall of the vessel. Since flow at the vessel wall must be zero, the greatest velocity gradient must occur in the plasma, which has the lowest viscosity. The red blood cells clump in the center of the stream where shear forces are minimal. Migration of red blood cells to the center of the vessel is enhanced for highly deformable cells that aggrregate strongly. Low pH, low oxygen tension and high carbon dioxide tension reduce RBC deformability. Rigid cells, such as sickle cells, migrate poorly to the center of vessels, possibly leading to vessel obstruction. In small vessels with deformable red cells, the plasma lubricates the flow of the cells through the vessel, and the red cells actually traverse the vessel faster than the plasma. When blood flow is very slow, as in veins, then aggregation may continue until large clusters of red blood cells, called *rouleau*, are created. Very slow rates of shear, such as those that occur in veins, result in large increases in viscosity since the red blood cells are distributed uniformly between the vessel walls. Thus, the major determinant of resistance in veins is viscosity, not vessel geometry.

Flow Limitation

In some physiologic systems when driving pressure increases, flow will increase until a certain flow is achieved; above this pressure further increases in pressure will not increase flow. This phenomenon is called *flow limitation*. It occurs in the respiratory, cardiovascular, and urinary systems.

A simple example of a flow-limiting system is shown in Figure 2–10, A. The piston generates a pressure within a chamber. Fluid exits the chamber through an orifice that supports a tube with elastic walls. This tube can be compressed by a pressure that is greater on its outer surface than on its inner surface. As pressure increases within the chamber, the flow generates both a pressure drop along the inner surface of the tube and a pressure difference across the wall of the tube. This pressure difference across the tube wall causes the tube to collapse and flow velocity to increase. As flow velocity increases the pressure drop increases, which further compresses the tube lumen and leads to a further increase in flow velocity. Eventually, the increase in driving pressure, with decreases in tube cross-sectional area, directly matches the increase in pressure drop along the collapsible tube, so that volumetric flow will not increase further. In this setting flow cannot exceed some maximal value regardless of whether driving pressure within the chamber is increased or whether pressure (suction) at the outlet is decreased (increased).

For the respiratory or urinary systems, a distensible reservoir (lungs or bladder) is connected to the Starling resistor. Since the volume inside the reservoir will affect both the pressure inside the reservoir and the pressure inside the collapsible tube, as well as the net force applied across the collapsible tube wall, the maximal flow will depend on the volume of the reservoir. This is schematically shown in Figure 2–10, B. A piston (muscle) applies pressure equally to the outer and inner surfaces of the elastic reservoir and to the distensible wall of the tube. If the reservoir is distended, the box is not pressurized, and flow at the chamber opening is occluded, then both the reservoir and tube are larger than their unpressurized sizes due to the recoil pressure within the reservoir. When the obstruction to emptying is released and the box is pressurized, both the reservoir and the tube will be compressed. The reservoir will be compressed by the box pressure, while the tube will be compressed by the box pressure and by the venturi effect of the flow through the distensible tube. (For simplicity, this discussion assumes the reservoir volume remains constant, independent of flow through the tube.) Flow will increase and the compresssing pressure within the box acting on the distensible tube will eventually exceed the effect of the distending pressure from the reservoir on the compressible tube. Further increases of box pressure produce a condition similar to that in Figure 2–10, A,

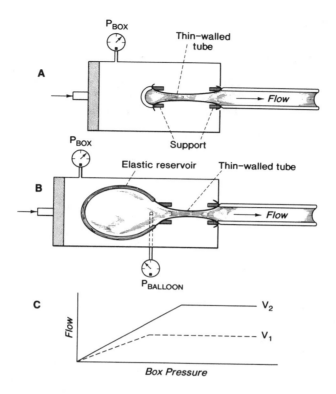

FIG 2–10.
Starling's resistor. **A,** A thin-walled, distensible tube supported at each end but subjected to the pressure creating the flow, P_{box}, will experience a decrease in the aperture of the tube as flow increases. Reductions of tube aperture further increase flow velocity if the driving pressure remains constant. **B,** Starling resistor mechanisms occur physiologically in the lungs and urinary system. An elastic reservoir is connected to the chamber end of the distensible tube, and the whole system is compressed by muscular effort, either the chest wall muscles for the lung, or the abdominal muscles for the bladder. The elastic reservoir causes maximal flow to be dependent on the volume (recoil pressure) of the reservoir. **C,** The flow through a Starling resistor rises as box pressure increases until a maximum flow is achieved. At this point any increase in box pressure is dissipated by an increase in the disruption of the flow, so that no increase in flow rate occurs. Maximal flow will be greater for a larger reservoir volume, V_2, than for a smaller reservoir volume, V_1.

where box pressure and flow are the primary determinants of the compressive forces on the distensible tube.

When the flow from this system is compared for two different reservoir volumes, V_1 and V_2, as in Figure 2–10, C, then the reservoir with the larger volume, V_2, will have a larger flow for any given value of pressure inside the box. But for either reservoir volume, flow will reach a maximum as box pressure increases. Thus, while flow limitation may occur in a collapsible tube, the maximal flow will depend on the volume within the reservoir that is sustaining the flow.

NOMENCLATURE

Symbols

A	Cross-sectional area
g	Gravitational acceleration constant
h	Height
F	Force
L	Length
P	Pressure
Q	Flow, volumetric
R	Resistance
Re	Reynolds number
r	Radius
T	Tension (force per unit length)
V	Volume
v	Velocity

Greek

Δ	Difference
μ	Viscosity
ν	Kinematic viscosity
π	Ratio of circumference to diameter
ρ	Density

BIBLIOGRAPHY

Berne RM, Levy MN: *Cardiovascular Physiology*. St. Louis, CV Mosby Co, 1967.

Fahraens R, Lindquist T: The viscosity of blood in narrow capillary tubes. *Am. J. Physiol.* 96:562– 568, 1931.

Halliday D, Resnick R: *Fundamentals of Physics*, ed 2. New York, Wiley, 1981.

Honig, CR: *Modern Cardiovascular Physiology*. Boston, Little, Brown & Co, 1981.

Pedley TJ, Drazen JM: Aerodynamic theory, in Macklem, PT, Mead J (eds); *Handbook of Physiology*, Sec 3, The Respiratory System, Vol III, Mechanics of Breathing, Part 1, American Physiological Society, Bethesda, MD, Baltimore, Waverly Press, 1986, pp 41–54.

Pedley TJ, Schroeter RC, Sudlow MF: Gas mixing in the airways, in West JB (ed); *Lung Biology in Health and Disease*, Vol 3, Bioengineering Aspects of the Lung. New York, Marcel Dekker, 1977, pp 163–265.

Schmid-Schonbein H: Microrheology of erythrocytes, blood viscosity and the distribution of blood flow in the microcirculation, in Guyton AC, Cowley AW (eds): *International Review of Physiology*– Vol 9, Cardiovascular Physiology. Baltimore, University Park Press, 1976.

Sears FW, Zemansky MW, Young HD: *College Physics*, ed 6. Reading, MA, Addison Wesley, 1985.

Smith JJ, Kampine JP: *Circulatory Physiology: The Essentials*. Baltimore, Williams and Wilkins, 1980.

Streeter VL: *Fluid Mechanics*, ed 4. New York, McGraw Hill, 1966.

Strandness, Jr, DE, Sumner DS: *Hemodynamics for Surgeons*. New York, Grune and Stratton, 1975.

Chapter 3

Sensors and Transducers

Reed M. Gardner, Ph.D.

INTRODUCTION

Terminology

According to Webster, a sensor is "any of various devices designed to detect, measure, or record physical phenomena, as radiation, heat, blood pressure, etc., and to respond, as by transmitting information, initiating changes, or operating controls." A transducer is "any of various devices that transmit energy from one system to another."[1] The number and type of transducers used by the medical profession is large and diversified. Physicians, nurses, respiratory therapists, and other clinicians caring for critically ill patients are confronted with some of the most sophisticated medical instrumentation in all of medical care. It seems that each year new methods and technologies are found for measuring parameters previously thought to be impossible or improbable.

The task of covering all the sensors and transducers that clinicians might encounter is daunting. A recent medical device encyclopedia further illustrated the size of the task[2]—it is comprised of four volumes and has more than 250 articles and nearly 2500 pages of text! From those articles, 33 are directly applicable to respiratory care, and include topics such as oxygen sensors, nitrogen analyzers, and colorimetry. More detailed background material and basic theory can also be found in the scientific literature and in texts on bioinstrumentation.[3–5]

For centuries, without medical instruments, physicians and other health care professionals relied on only their five senses (sight, hearing, smell, taste, and touch). Today's medical instruments use sensors and transducers and signal processing equipment to convert information about patients into a form that humans can perceive and understand. One of our primary concerns when making a measurement is to know its accuracy. The *accuracy* of a measured quantity is the true value minus the measured value divided by the true value (usually expressed as a percentage). True values are seldom known exactly, but a reference value traceable to the National Institute of Standards and Technology is usually used. The *precision* of a measurement expresses the number of distinguishable alternatives from which a given result is selected. A weight of 75.2 kg is more precise than a weight of 75 kg. High precision does not imply high accuracy. *Resolution* is the smallest incremental quantity that can be measured with certainty. *Reproducibility* is the ability of an instrument to provide the same output for an equal input.

Medical instrumentation will have both *static* (pertaining to bodies or forces at rest or in equilibrium—opposite of dynamic) and *dynamic* (pertaining to dynamics; active—opposite of static) requirements. Static requirements usually refer to the performance of an instrument involving very low frequency events such as measurement of body weight. Dynamic requirements refer to dynamically changing measures that vary at high frequency, such as the arterial blood pressure or airflow from a rapidly breathing patient.

Instrumentation systems may have one or many of the components shown in Figure 3–1. The primary flow of information is from left to right. The physical quantity, property, or condition that the system measures is called the *signal*. Most medically important signals can be grouped into the following categories of biopotentials: electrocardiogram (ECG), pressure (blood pressure), flow (expiratory airflow), displacement (chest wall movement), impedance (chest wall bioimpedance), temperature (core body temperature), and chemical concentrations (K^+ or Po_2).

Transducers/Sensors

A transducer or sensor converts one form of energy to another. The final signal is usually electrical since the technology for amplifying and displaying electrical signals is well developed. The transducer should respond to only the form of energy present in the signal, to the exclusion

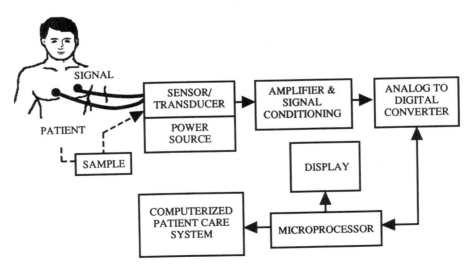

FIG 3–1.
Block diagram of a generalized instrumentation system. The transducer converts energy or information from the signal to another form of energy—usually electrical. The signal is then processed and displayed so that humans and computers can perceive the information.

of all others. In the real clinical situation this is seldom exactly possible, but can usually be accomplished well enough to provide useful information. The ideal transducer should interface with the patient in such a way that minimizes the energy extracted, while being minimally invasive. Many transducers have a primary sensing element such as a diaphragm, which converts pressure to displacement that is then sensed with variable resistive elements called strain gauges. Transducers can be something as conceptually simple as ECG electrodes. However, other transducers may require an energy source—for example, a dc voltage for a pressure gauge or pulses of electrical energy to activate the light sources in a pulse oximeter.

Amplifier and Signal Conditioning and Analog-to-Digital Conversion

Seldom can the output from a transducer be directly attached to the display device. Usually signals from transducers are small (in the milli- or microvolt range) and must be amplified and often filtered to remove unwanted signals. Most medical devices use only simple amplifiers and filters and then convert the desired signal to a digital form using an *analog-to-digital converter* (ADC). ADCs convert "analog" signals, such as an ECG, to digital form, usually with 10-bit (1 part in 1024) resolution at rates of from 100 to 300 times per second.

Ohm's law is a basic law of physics that relates voltage and current to resistance (analogous to the relationship between gas pressure, flow, and resistance). Figure 3–2 is a diagram of a simplified electrical/ mechanical circuit. The two types of current are dc (direct current) or

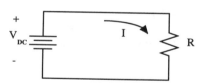

FIG 3–2.
Simplified diagram of an electrical/mechanical circuit showing the relationship of voltage and current to resistance (electrical) and pressure and flow to resistance (gas flow). Also the idea of conductance (the inverse of resistance) is presented.

$$\text{Voltage} = V = IR$$

where I = current and R = resistance.

$$\text{Pressure} = P = FR$$

where F = flow and R = resistance.

$$R = V/I \text{ (electrical)} \quad R = P/F \text{ (gas flow)}$$

Conductance $= 1/R = I/V$ (electrical) or $= F/P$ (for gas flow).

battery circuits and ac (alternating current). In the United States, household current is 60 Hz (hertz, cycles per second). Figure 3–3 shows two simplified circuits with dc and ac excitation. Just as there is a resistance to dc flow, there is an electrical impedance related to capacitors and inductors. (Electrical impedance is defined as the apparent resistance in a circuit to the flow of alternating current, analogous to the actual resistance to a direct current.) Equations for the electrical impedances of the simplified ac circuits are shown in Figure 3–3.

Microprocessors

With microprocessors being inexpensive and reliable, the technology of signal processing, transmission, and display is accomplished with these devices. These microprocessors can take signals such as arterial blood pressure and in real time derive and display heart rate and systolic, diastolic, and mean blood pressures. These systems also compensate for undesirable transducer characteristics (e.g., nonlinearities) or they may average repetitive signals to reduce noise. Similar examples exist for respiratory care with ventilatory rate, mean airway pressure (MAP), and peak and plateau pressures.

Display and External Transmission

The results of the measurement process are displayed to the user in a form that is easily perceived. The usual forms of display are graphical plots, but display can also be in the form of digital results. For example, from a ventilator one might see the respiratory rate and tidal volume displayed. In recent years it has become even more important to transmit and store data in a computerized "charting" system so they can be shared with a diverse medical data user group. Typically, the clinical or blood gas laboratory is required to transmit data to the

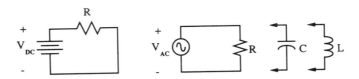

FIG 3–3.
Two simple dc and ac circuits. Note that AC circuits or circuits that have time-varying signals can have two additional electrical elements, capacitors (C) and inductors (L). These elements have "impedance factors" as shown.

$$X_c = \frac{1}{2\pi fc}$$

where *f* is the frequency in hertz.

$$X_L = 2\pi f L$$

intensive care unit (ICU). Just as the clinical staff in the ICU needs to know the laboratory results, they also need to know respiratory care charting results. In fact, the blood gas laboratory must know the F_{IO_2} and other ventilator parameters to make a reasonable interpretation of the blood gas results. With computerized expert systems becoming common, a high-priority task will be the sharing of respiratory care data.[6-13]

HOW COMMONLY USED TRANSDUCERS WORK

Pressure Transducers

Strain gauges are devices that allow measurement of a change in the dimensions, displacement, or deformation of an object. Electrical strain gauges are used extensively in pulmonary and cardiovascular monitoring to measure pressures, flows, and temperatures. Several types of electrical strain gauge pressure transducers are available: resistance, inductance, capacitance, and semiconductor transducers. Each of these pressure transducers has a diaphragm sensing element that deforms when pressure is applied. Depending on the type, the movement of the diaphragm is sensed by a change in resistance, inductance, or capacitance. The electrical resistance gauge is the most widely used. Recently, several pressure transducers have been made using electronic integrated circuit technology. These transducers are accurate, very reliable, inexpensive (< $20), and disposable.[14-16] Figure 3–4 shows a diaphragm pressure transducer with resistive sensing elements attached. Figure 3–4, B shows, with the motion of the diaphragm greatly exaggerated, how an applied pressure causes the resistor wires to be stretched (increasing resistance) or relaxed (decreasing resistance). Volume displacements of pressure transducers used for measuring blood pressure are typically of the order of 0.1 mm³ per 100 mm Hg applied. Thus the approximate displacement of the 4×4 mm pressure transducer diaphragm would be only 0.00625 mm with 100 mm Hg applied or 0.0000626 mm for each mm Hg applied!! This is indeed a very small displacement.

Figure 3–4, C, shows schematically how resistors are "etched" onto the surface of semiconductor materials using integrated circuit technology. The semiconductor "chip" becomes the diaphragm. Typically these semiconductor devices are very small (less than 4×4 mm).

Transducers for measuring blood pressure have recently been standardized by the American National Standards Institute (ANSI).[14] They have sensitivities of 5 μV per volt of excitation per mmHg pressure applied. Thus if 5 V of dc is applied, an output of 25 μV per mm Hg pressure applied is generated—a rather small signal. For measurements of airway pressures and pressures across Fleisch pneumotachometers, signal levels even smaller are produced, and errors caused by instabilities of pressure transducers and amplifiers become problematic.

Figure 3–5 shows a pressure transducer that measures the movement of the change in inductance by use of a moving magnetic armature attached to the diaphragm. This type of transducer is called a *linear variable inductance transducer* (LVDT), and it requires ac excitation. The resistive pressure transducer can be excited with either dc or ac voltage excitation.

Figure 3–6 shows a capacitance-type pressure transducer. Here the diaphragm moves the two plates of the capacitor closer together, causing the capacitance to increase. Capacitive transducers must also be energized with ac excitation.

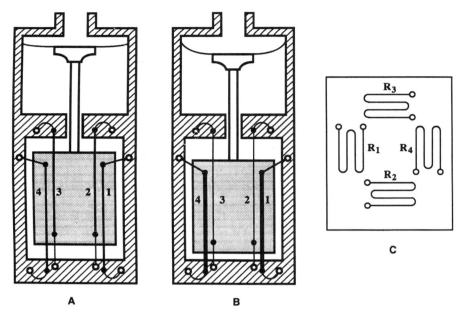

FIG 3–4.
Resistive strain gauge pressure transducer. Elements 1, 2, 3, and 4 are resistive wires. **A,** no pressure is applied. **B,** Pressure is applied to the transducer—the movement of the diaphragm is greatly exaggerated to illustrate the operating principle. **C,** Layout of resistors on a semiconductor "chip" for a modern disposable pressure transducer.

The principles used by electrical resistance strain gauges were discovered in 1856 by Lord Kelvin. He noted that the resistance of a metal wire increased with increasing strain and that different materials had different sensitivities to strain. Strain gauges usually use a Wheatstone bridge configuration (Fig 3–7), which is made up of four resistors that change resistance when a pressure is applied. Typically, two of the resistors increase their resistance and two decrease their resistance as shown in Figure 3–4, B. By configuring the transducer in this way, its ouput voltage is increased by four compared with a transducer where only one of the resistors changes with the pressure applied. The four active resistors in a typical pressure transducer are designed to have nearly the same resistance and are physically near each other. As a result, an unwanted change in "zero" or sensitivity is minimized because if the temperature increases slightly, each of the resistors increases its resistance proportionally, thus maintaining its "zero" point.

Temperature Transducers

Measurement of body temperature has been an important part of health care for centuries. Today it remains one of the simple, yet reliable, parameters measured in combination with other indicators to assess the state of health. For the respiratory and critical care clinician, the

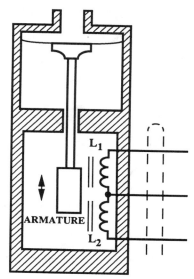

FIG 3–5.
LVDT (inductive) pressure transducer.

measurement of respiratory gas temperatures and body core temperatures to compensate for the temperature dependency of Po_2, Pco_2, and pH probes is essential.[17]

Each special application for monitoring temperature may have a unique need. For example, the classic mercury-in-glass thermometer may perform adequately for an occasional noninva-

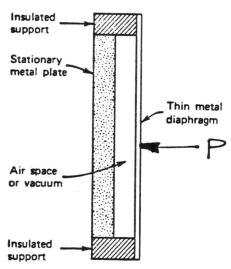

FIG 3–6.
Capacitance-type pressure transducer.

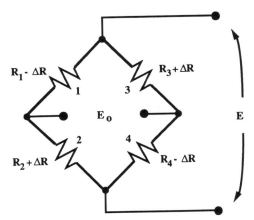

FIG 3–7.
Resistive pressure transducer configured as a Wheatstone bridge. Note from Figure 3–4 that elements 1 and 4 decrease in resistance (shorten) as pressure is applied, while elements 2 and 3 increase in resistance (elongate). The term *Eo* is the output voltage from the transducer and *E* is the excitation voltage.

sive measurement of body temperature, but these are not appropriate where size, speed of response, and breakage are considerations. Thermocouples or thermistor sensors are convenient electronic substitutes that offer small size and fast response at relatively low cost.

Thermistors

A thermistor is small in size and has a high resolution and rapid response for blood temperature measurement at a point along an indwelling catheter (e.g., thermodilution cardiac output monitoring with a Swan-Ganz catheter). A thermistor sensor is fabricated by forming a powdered semiconductor material (usually a metal oxide) into a small bead around two lead wires, or by sintering the semiconductor into a pellet shape, then coating its opposite faces with conducting electrodes.[17] The resistance of the resulting thermistor has a large variation with temperature. Unfortunately, the resistance-temperature curve is nonlinear (Fig 3–8). However, the unique and stable characteristics of thermistors are easily determined. Thermistors can be manufactured to very small sizes (of the order of 0.2 mm in diameter), to have fast response times (<0.1 seconds), and to have a temperature range of 100°C. They can be pretrimmed to be interchangeable within ±0.1°C of each other. Thermistors have a much higher sensitivity than thermocouples and thus have better resolution. Their primary disadvantage is their nonlinearity.

Thermocouples

When two dissimilar metals such as copper and constantan are placed in contact with each other, a small voltage can be measured across the metallic contact junction.[17] This voltage varies with temperature and can be used to measure body temperatures. For the biological temperature range, the combination of copper and constantan (an alloy of 55% copper and

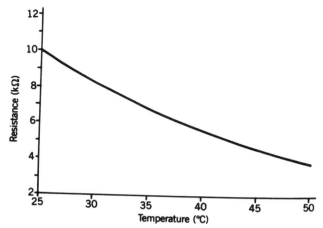

FIG 3–8.

Resistance versus temperature for a thermistor pellet that has a nominal resistance of 10 kΩ at 25°C. (*From Christensen DA: Thermometry, in Webster J (ed): Encyclopedia of Medical Devices and Instrumentation. New York, Wiley-Interscience, 1988, Vol 4, pp. 2759–2765. Used by permission.*)

45% nickel) is appropriate. These are T-type thermocouples and have a sensitivity of about 43 μV/°C. They have good linearity over the temperature range of 25 to 50°C, they are inexpensive, and they have good stability.

Spectrophotometry/Colorimetry

Colorimetry is based on the observation that molecules absorb light. The wavelengths and efficiency of absorption depend on both the structure of the molecule and its environment, making absorption of light a useful tool for characterizing both small molecules and macromolecules such as hemoglobin. Colorimetric methods use these light-absorbing spectral properties to measure the presence and concentration of substances.[18] Figure 3–9 is a block diagram of a spectrophotometer/colorimeter. Figure 3–10 shows the almost linear absorption of infrared radiation at 4.26 μm when shined through a 4-mm-thick sample of CO_2.

The probability of light absorption at a single wavelength is described by the Beer-Lambert law. The passage of light through any given thickness of any substance results in absorption of a constant fraction of the incident light. In differential equation form this is stated as:

$$dI/I = - KC\ dL$$

where dI/I is the fraction of light absorbed by a layer of thickness dL, K is a constant that depends on the properties of the substance, and C is the concentration of the absorbing substance. Integrating the above equation yields:

$$\ln(I_o/I) = KCL$$

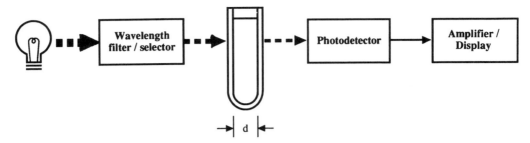

FIG 3–9.
Block diagram of a spectrophotometer/colorimeter.

where ln is the natural logarithm, L is the path length, I_o is the initial intensity, and I is the final intensity of light after passing through the sample. The quantity (I/I_o) is known as the transmittance (T). Optical density (OD) (also called absorbance) is related to T by the equation:

$$OD = -\log T = \text{Absorbance}$$

A plot of OD as a function of concentration is ideally a straight line.

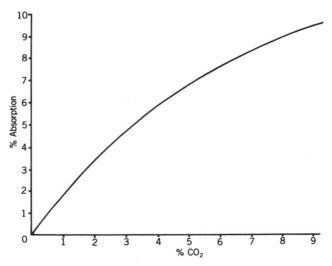

FIG 3–10.
Absorbance versus concentration for infrared radiation shined through a cuvette of CO_2. (*Ref. [19]*)

Blood Gas Analyzers

pH Electrode

The measurement of pH is accomplished by using a special glass electrode that generates an electrical potential when solutions of differing pH are placed on the two sides of its membrane. pH is measured in virtually every blood gas analyzer using these glass electrodes (Fig 3–11). The glass used in the electrode is a member of the class of ion-specific electrodes that react only with a specific ion. The pH glass sensor, introduced in the early 1900s, was the first example of an ion-selective electrode. The Nernst equation that follows applies to this thin ion-specific glass. Therefore, the voltage across the membrane (E) changes by 61.5 mV/pH unit at body temperature (37°C). Since the range of physiological pH is only about 0.6 pH units, the change in voltage for the entire pH range is only 36.9 mV. The pH meter must be capable of accurately measuring changes of about 0.1 mV. In typical blood gas analyzers, the pH of very small samples (20 μL) can be measured.

The Nernst equation for the hydrogen ion (H^+) is:

$$EH^+ = (RT/F) \cdot \ln [(H^+_o)/(H^+i)]$$

where R is the gas constant, F is Faraday's constant, and T is the absolute temperature (kelvin).

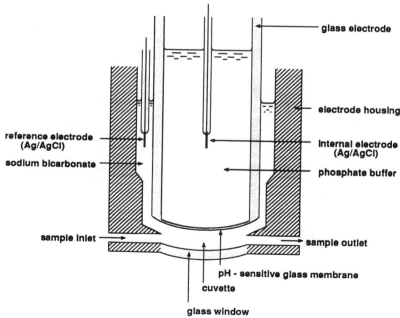

FIG 3–11.
pH electrode.

At body temperature (37°C) the quantity (RT/F) is 61.5 mV. Therefore, at body temperature the above equation becomes:

$$EH^+ = 0.0615 \cdot \log_{10} [H^+]$$

where $\log_{10} [H^+]$ is defined as a pH unit.

P_{CO_2} Electrode

The CO_2 electrode was first described by Stow and his colleagues [19] in 1957, and was later improved by Severinghaus and Bradley.[20, 21] The basic idea of the electrode is to allow an unknown CO_2 sample to equilibrate with an aqueous solution, and then measure the pH. Figure 3–12 shows that a P_{CO_2} electrode consists of a glass pH electrode covered with a Teflon or Silastic membrane. A thin layer of water containing salt and bicarbonate ion is held between the glass and the Teflon by a spacer (nylon stocking or filter paper are also used as spacers).

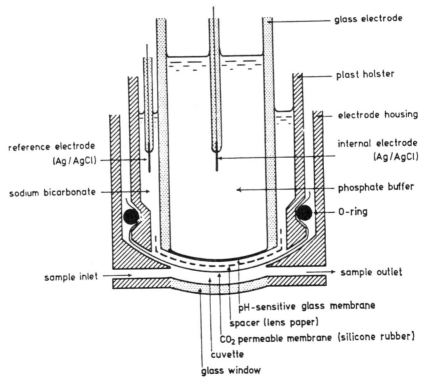

glass electrode

plast holster

electrode housing

internal electrode (Ag/AgCl)

reference electrode (Ag/AgCl)

phosphate buffer

sodium bicarbonate

O-ring

sample inlet

sample outlet

pH-sensitive glass membrane

spacer (lens paper)

CO_2 permeable membrane (silicone rubber)

cuvette

glass window

FIG 3–12.
Severinghaus P_{CO_2} electrode. With earlier electrodes the spacer element, shown here as lens paper, was actually a nylon "gauze" made from a nylon hose worn by women.

The CO_2 gas molecules from the sample diffuse through the Teflon membrane and react with water to form hydrogen ions and bicarbonate:

$$CO_2 + H_2O \rightarrow H_2CO_3 \rightarrow H^+ + HCO_3^-$$

Using a reference electrode in contact with the water film permits the measurement of the resulting pH. With low-bicarbonate concentrations, the measured pH is then determined by the Henderson-Hasselbalch equation:

$$pH = pK + \log([HCO_3^-]/[CO_2])$$

or in simplified form:

$$pH = C - \log[P_{CO_2}]$$

The electrode senses a pH change of 1 pH unit for a tenfold change in P_{CO_2}. The P_{CO_2} can be measured over the range of 10 to 90 mm Hg—the range of clinical interest.

PO2 Electrode

Oxygen was first measured in 1774 by the French chemist Antoine-Laurent Lavoisier. More than 100 years later, Danneel, working in Walther Nernst's laboratory, showed that dissolved oxygen reacted with electrodes in solution when a voltage was applied between the electrodes. However, it was not until 1925 that Jaroslav Heyrovski made the application of oxygen polarography practical, for which he earned the 1959 Nobel prize.[22, 23] Figure 3–13 shows the basic Leland Clark electrode introduced in 1956 on which the designs of most contemporary P_{O_2} electrodes are based. Clark had the idea of covering the sensor with a membrane to increase the stability of P_{O_2} readings and to minimize the effects of fluid flow past the electrode. The Clark electrode consists of a tiny (25-μm) platinum wire sealed in glass with the tip exposed by polishing. The tip is covered with an oxygen-permeable membrane, usually polypropylene. The Clark polarographic sensor, with about $- 0.7$ V applied, gives a current output that is almost exactly linearly related to P_{O_2}. The amount of oxygen extracted from the sample is very small, so stirring of the sample is not required.[24] The polarographic electrode must be calibrated to establish linearity, drift, response time, zero current level, and flow sensitivities. Most often this is done by using 100% oxygen, room air, and a known gas mixture.[23] The oxygen electrode can be used with oxygen in a gaseous or liquid phase and does not require equilibration with a blood sample. The output current of the P_{O_2} electrode is linear within $\pm 1\%$ from 0 to 100% oxygen. At sea level this is a range from 0 to 760 mm Hg.

Severinghaus and Astrup, two of the pioneers of blood gas analysis, have written a historical review of blood gas instrumentation development; the reader is referred to this excellent series.[25-31]

CO Oximetry

The basis of oximetry of multiple hemoglobin measures is dependent on the optical absorption spectra of hemoglobin (Hb), carboxy (carbon monoxide) hemoglobin (COHb), and methemo-

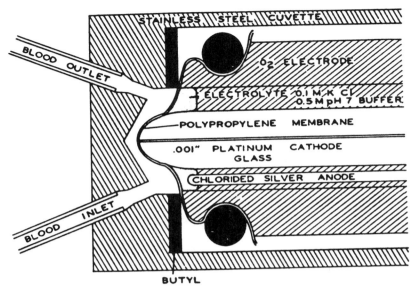

FIG 3–13.
Clark PO$_2$ electrode. (*From Severinghaus JW: Blood gas concentrations in* Handbook of Physiology. *Bethesda, MD, American Physiological Society, 1965, Sec 3, Vol 2, Chap 61, pp 1475–1487. Used by permission.*)

globin (MetHb). By measuring the optical absorption at multiple wavelengths, all of the above-mentioned parameters can be measured.

Continuous Oximetry

The basis for continuous So$_2$ measurement relies on the difference in optical absorption spectra of Hb and Hbo$_2$ (Fig 3–14). As a result, various optical methods for measuring oxygen saturation have been developed using two or more wavelengths in the near-infrared region: LAMBA1, where the largest difference in light absorption between Hb and Hbo$_2$ exists (about 660 nm), and LAMBDA2 at the wavelength where the two hemoglobins have the same absorbance (805 nm). The 805-nm wavelength, where the two hemoglobins have the same absorbance, is called the *isosbestic wavelength* (Fig 3–14). This principle is used to measure hemoglobin concentrations, oxygen saturation, and the saturation of carboxyhemoglobin and methemoglobin in laboratory blood gas analyzers. Modifications and engineering extrapolation of these principles are applied to the pulse oximeter.

Fiber-Optic Reflection Oximeters

The first report[29, 32] of the measurement of oxygen saturation by reflected light from blood was described in 1949. It was not until fiber-optic catheters and inexpensive light sources and

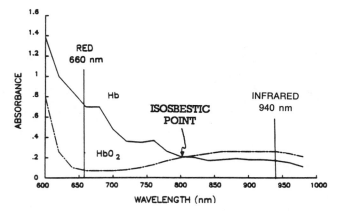

FIG 3–14.
Optical absorption spectra of Hb, Hbo₂, and Hbco in the visible and near-infrared wavelength regions. (*From Gardner RM: Pulse oximetry: Is it monitoring's "silver bullet"? J Cardiovasc Nurs 1987; 1:79–83. Used by permission.*)

detectors became available that this mode of measuring oxygen saturation became widely used.[33] Mixed venous oxygen saturation measurements are now made for selected patients with disposable fiberoptic Swan-Ganz catheters using this technology.[34]

Pulse Oximeters

A recent and major advancement in oximetry has been accomplished with the pulse oximeter.[31, 35–46] Contemporary pulse oximeters use two light-emitting diodes (LEDs) to shine light through a variety of body locations (fingers, ears, or nose) where a small photodiode detects the transmitted signal (See Chapter 10—Pulse Oximetry). These inexpensive disposable probes and their associated processing and display capability have revolutionized oxygen saturation monitoring.[31, 36]

Figure 3–15 shows a block diagram of a pulse oximeter. The specific red and infrared wavelengths of light are generated by LEDs. These LEDs are ubiquitous, being used first in digital watches and now often used for displays on intravenous pumps. The receiving photodiode detects the light from the pulsations of the red and infrared light sources after they have been transmitted and absorbed by the tissue. A typical signal generated by one of the pulsating light sources is shown in Figure 3–16. It has been observed that when the pulsatile components of the light are less than 0.5% of the steady (dc) component, the system's accuracy falls.

Oxygen saturation can now be measured noninvasively between 50 to 100% with an accuracy of about 2.5% (ISD). Pulse oximeters do not, however, measure other types of hemoglobin such as carboxyhemoglobin or methemoglobin. Pulse oximetry has revitalized oximetry, which is a reversal of a trend started when the oxygen electrode became available and Po_2 measurements became feasible. Severinghaus and Astrup have stated "Pulse oximetry is arguably the most significant technologic advance ever made in monitoring the well-being and safety of patients during anesthesia, recovery, and critical care."[31]

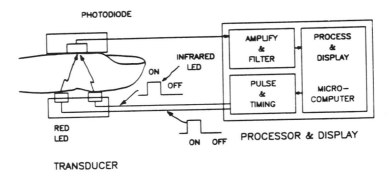

FIG 3–15.
Schematic block diagram of a pulse oximeter showing the transducer with its red and infrared LEDs and the photodiode detector. Each LED is pulsed several times each second, and the pulses are received by the photodiode. The signals from the photodiode are processed by the microcomputer and shown on a display. (*From Gardner RM: Pulse oximetry: Is it monitoring's "silver bullet"? J Cardiovasc Nurs 1987; 1:79–83. Used by permission.*)

Continuous Respiratory Gas Measurement

Two types of gas sampling techniques are used to analyze respiratory gases from a patient's airway circuit: mainstream (in line) and sidestream (diverting) (See Chapter 12—Capnography). Mainstream sampling uses a transducer housed in an airway connector placed "in line"

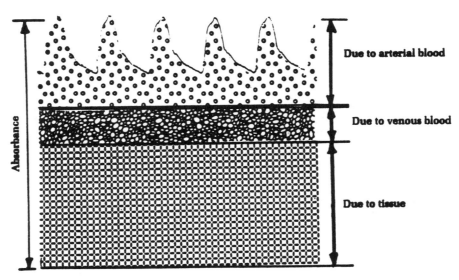

FIG 3–16.
Pulsatile light output from the photodiode generated from one of the LED input signals. The typical plethysmographic signal is superimposed on the nonspecific absorption signals. The pulsatile signal is processed to give nearly beat-by-beat oxygen saturation. (*From Gardner RM: Pulse oximetry: Is it monitoring's "silver bullet?" J Cardiovasc Nurs 1987; 1:79–83. Used by permission.*)

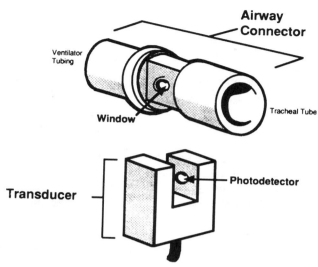

FIG 3–17.
Schematic of in-line continuous mainstream infrared CO_2 gas analysis method. (*From Szaflarski NL, Cohen NH: Use of capnography in critically ill adults. Heart Lung 1991; 20:363–374. Used by permission.*)

with the patient's breathing circuit. Figure 3–17 is an illustration of an in-line infrared CO_2 measurement system. Sidestream or diverting sampling systems actively withdraw gas from the patient's airway via a sampling tube to the analyzer. Figure 3–18 shows a schematic of a sidestream sampling method. For the sidestream method, a small internal diameter tube must be used to allow for rapid gas withdrawal,[47] and gas analysis takes place in an external sensor. Because the gas sample must be transported to the external sensor, unavoidable transit times

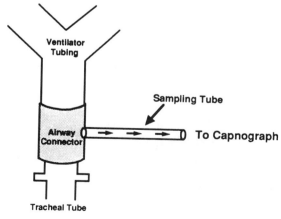

FIG 3–18.
Schematic of sidestream continuous gas sampling method. (*From Szaflarski NL, Cohen NH: Use of capnography in critically ill adults. Heart & Lung 1991; 20:363–374. Used by permission.*)

of as long as a few seconds may occur. Also, gas sampling requires that water vapor and airway secretions not interfere with the flow of gases to the external transducer.

CO_2 *Gas Analyzers*

CO_2 can be measured in its gaseous form and in blood and tissues. The measurement technology is usually different for each measurement. In its gaseous form, CO_2 is usually measured in a respiratory circuit using infrared absorption, while measurements of Pco_2 in blood are usually made with an electrode system. Since the two use rather different methodologies and sensors, each will be discussed.

Just as Pco_2 electrodes can be used in blood gas machines, they can also be used to measure respiratory gases. Because the response time of the CO_2 electrodes is slow and because the electrodes are somewhat temperamental, they are seldom used for continuous gas analysis.

Various gases and liquids absorb power (energy) in specific regions of the electromagnetic spectrum, as has already been discussed for spectroscopy and colorimetry. Figure 3–19 shows that CO_2 has an infrared absorption peak at 4.26 μm, which is almost clear of other potentially interfering gases such as nitrogen, oxygen, nitrous oxide, halothane, and water.[21] The relationship between %CO_2 and optical density (absorption) is almost linear. The technical tasks that must be solved to make CO_2 gas sensors successful are (1) choosing the appropriate pathlength to give the best compromise of sensitivity and linearity, (2) choosing an appropriate infrared light emitter—a task greatly simplified because of the need to develop infrared emitters for transoceanic fiber-optic communications, and (3) choosing an appropriate detector to sense the infrared signal—again a technology that is now within reason because of the semiconductor sensor revolution and the need for better worldwide optical fiber communications.[21]

As a result of emitter and transducer developments, the ability to measure CO_2 in line in ventilators is becoming common practice. Previous sensors required the use of a rotating "chopper wheel" that had multiple filters and reference gases on its circumference. Because it is now possible to measure CO_2 at 4.26 μm and water at 1.45 μm, the measurement of respiratory gases is now possible under normal clinical situations.

O_2 *Gas Analyzers*

Continuous O_2 analyzers have long been used in breathing circuits to ascertain that patients were receiving the desired level of oxygen therapy. The polarographic oxygen sensor (Po_2 electrode) is the most common gas-composition sensor used in respiratory care. The polarographic Po_2 electrode, such as that used for continuous ventilator gas analysis, is much the same as the sensor used in blood gas analyzers. The response time of these sensors is usually in the range of 30 to 360 seconds, depending on the membrane uses.

Some oxygen sensors such as the yttria-stabilized zirconia electrode, illustrated in Figure 3–20, incorporate a solid electrolyte.[48, 49] The zirconia crystals demonstrate oxygen-ion conduction at temperatures above 600°C. The crystal has a thin layer of porous platinum on each side that forms the electrodes. When the sample gas has a different concentration than the reference gas, a voltage difference (V) is generated across the crystal. The equation for the potential is:

$$V = \frac{RT}{4\text{F}} \cdot \ln\left[\frac{P_{(sample)}\,O_2}{P_{(reference)}\,O_2}\right]$$

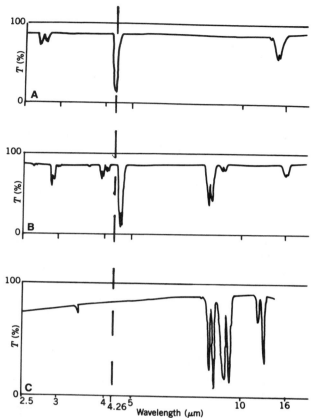

FIG 3–19.
Transmission spectrums in the infrared region for **A**, CO_2, **B**, nitrous oxide, and **C**, halothane. Note that CO_2 has a good absorption peak at 4.26 μm that is independent of the other two anesthetic gases. (*From Coombes RG, Halsall D: Carbon dioxide analyzers, in Webster J (ed): Encyclopedia of Medical Devices and Instrumentation. New York, Wiley-Interscience, 1988, Vol 1, pp. 556–569. Used by permission.*)

where F is the Faraday constant and T is the operating temperature of the cell (kelvin).

Fuel or galvanic cells are another large class of commonly used oxygen sensors.[49] These devices require no external power and are essentially batteries whose output current is a function of the Po_2. A diagram of the fuel cell sensor is shown in Figure 3–21. The fuel cell usually has a gold cathode and a lead anode immersed in potassium hydroxide (KOH) electrolyte. The reactions are:

$$O_2 + 2H_2O + 4e^- \rightarrow 2H_2O_2 + 4e^- \rightarrow 4OH^- \text{ (cathode)}$$
$$2Pb + 6OH^- \rightarrow 2PbO_2H^- + 2H_2O + 4e^- \quad \text{(anode)}$$

The oxidation of lead to lead hydroxide at the anode provides the four electrons necessary for

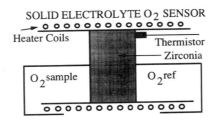

FIG 3–20.
Zirconium cell solid-state oxygen sensor. (*From East TD: What makes noninvasive monitoring tick? A review of basic engineering principles.* Resp Care 1990; 35:500–519. Used by permission.)

the reduction of oxygen at the cathode. Because the lead and hydroxide are consumed in the process, fuel cells have a finite life of about three months when exposed to 100% oxygen and about 15 months when exposed to room air.

The paramagnetic method makes use of a principle of oxygen described by Linus Pauling (it is sometimes called the *Pauling principle*). Oxygen exhibits an unusual attraction to an applied magnetic field—a phenomenon known as *paramagnetic susceptibility*. Figure 3–22 illustrates the basic function of a paramagnetic analyzers.[48, 49] A reference gas is passed through two symmetrical pathways joined in the middle by a differential pressure transducer. A strong pulsating electromagnetic field (EMF) is placed on one pathway just before the gas outlet, and the sample gas is injected at the junction of the two pathways near the outlet. If the sample gas has a higher paramagnetic affinity than the reference gas, it will be attracted to the magnetic field and produce a restricted flow in that pathway. This restriction produces a pressure gradient between the pathway that is proportional to the difference in Po_2 between the reference and the sample gas. The paramagnetic sensor is fast, having a response time of less than 200 ms. As a result, the sensor is ideally suited for fast, breath-to-breath applications.

Multiple Gas Analyzers

We often need to measure multiple gases from patients. For example, in anesthesiology it is important to measure oxygen, carbon dioxide, nitrogen, and the anesthetic gases.[50] Other

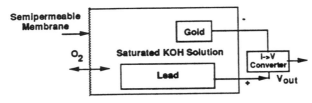

FIG 3–21.
Fuel cell oxygen sensor. (*From East TD: What makes noninvasive monitoring tick? A review of basic engineering principles.* Resp Care 1990; 35:500–519. Used by permission.)

DIFFERENTIAL PRESSURE
PARAMAGNETIC OXYGEN SENSOR

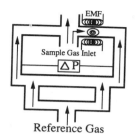

FIG 3–22.

Paramagnetic oxygen sensor. (*From East TD: What makes noninvasive monitoring tick? A review of basic engineering principles. Resp Care 1990; 35:500–519. Used by permission.*)

applications in pulmonary function laboratories and ICUs have also been described. Most of the multiple gas analyzers currently available use a sidestream sampling method.

A mass spectrometer is a device that separates a stream of charged particles (ions) into a spectrum according to their mass-to-charge ratios and determines the relative abundance of each type of ion present.[51] Medical mass spectrometers have been used extensively in pulmonary medicine. Figure 3–23 shows the elements of such a mass spectrometer. These devices are "leaky" vacuum tubes that usually take a sample of gas from ventilator or anesthesia circuits. The sample inlet has a capillary tube that is often made of Teflon. Gas is drawn through this tube by a vacuum pump. A small amount of gas in the inlet chamber "leaks" into the ionization chamber, where a stream of electrons bombards the sample and causes the molecules to lose electrons and become positive ions. These positive ions are then focused and accelerated with electrical fields into the strong magnetic field of the dispersion chamber. The dispersion chamber is also fitted with collectors. The molecules measured are collected by appropriately placed collectors. A current proportional to the number of molecules collected is the fraction of the gas mixture the molecule represents.

Mass spectrometers are used in pulmonary function laboratories, anesthesia, some ICUs, and for continuous blood gas analysis. They have the distinct advantage that they can synchronously measure multiple respiratory gases and trace gases to enable measurements of complex pulmonary function in the clinical pulmonary function laboratory and during anesthesia.[52–57] Mass spectrometers have gained wide use in anesthesia monitoring. They help the anesthesiologist determine if the anesthesia delivery system is functioning correctly, the level of anesthesia, the patient uptake of anesthetic gas, and some indication of the physiological status of the patient. Multiplexed mass spectrometers (Fig 3–24) are used for anesthetic gases in surgery and in some ICUs.

Gas chromatography is a method of separating gas mixtures into their various components by forcing them through a long, narrow column packed with either solid or liquid material.[48] *Chromatography* was the term originally given to this method because substances were identified by the color of the reaction with the material lining the column. However, more sophisticated and diverse methods of separation are now used, and most do not rely on color to identify the substance.

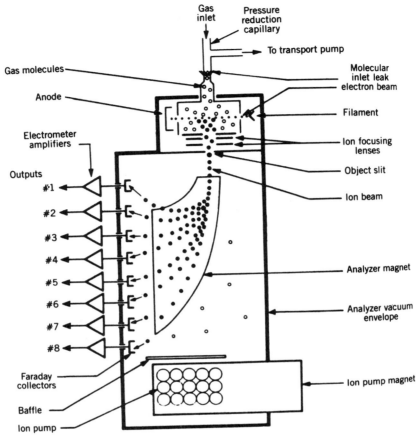

FIG 3–23.
Magnetic sector-type mass spectrometer showing its ion pump and vacuum chamber. (*From Sodal IE, Clark JS, Swanson GD: Mass spectrometers in medical monitoring, in Webster J (ed):* Encyclopedia of Medical Devices and Instrumentation. *New York, Wiley-Interscience, 1988, Vol 3, pp. 1848–1859. Used by permission.*)

A gas chromatograph consists of a sample port leading to a chamber where the sample is heated.[48] Heating removes the problem of water vapor in the sample. The sample is then added to a known concentration of a reference gas, usually helium for respiratory measurements. The sampled gas is forced by a pump through a long, narrow column. The material in the column separates the gases based on their molecular weight and viscosities. Each gas arrives at the detector at a distinct time (Figure 3–25). A peak is seen for each gas as it reaches the detector. The area under the peaks is proportional to the gas concentration. An advantage of the gas chromatograph is that only small samples are needed. However, the analysis takes from 15 minutes to 2 hours. Thus the method is not applicable for breath-by-breath analysis.

Raman spectroscopy is a versatile method of molecular analysis first postulated by Adolf

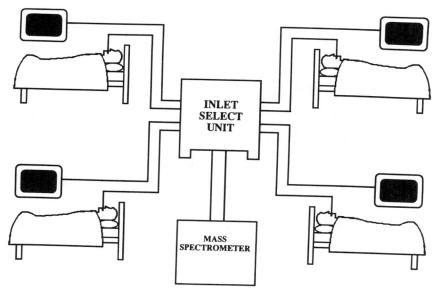

FIG 3–24.
A multiplexed mass spectrometer patient monitoring system that services four patients.

Smekal in 1923, and first observed by Sir Chandrasekhara Venkata Raman in 1928.[48, 58–60] When light collides with gas molecules, the photon loses energy to the gas molecule and subsequently has less energy and, consequently, a longer wavelength (lower frequency). The magnitude of this wavelength shift corresponds to the vibrational and rotational energies of

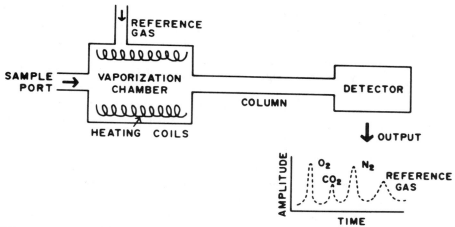

FIG 3–25.
Gas chromatograph multiple gas analyzer. (*From East TD: What makes noninvasive monitoring tick? A review of basic engineering principles.* Resp Care *1990; 35:500–519. Used by permission.*)

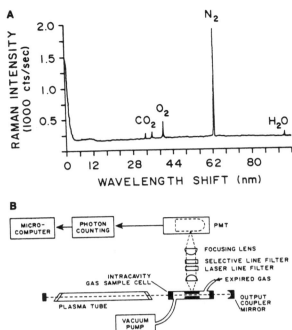

FIG 3–26.
A, Raman scatter spectrum for a typical sample of expired respiratory gas. **B,** System for Raman spectrographic analysis of expired respiratory gases. (*From East TD: What makes noninvasive monitoring tick? A review of basic engineering principles.* Resp Care 1990; 35:500–519. Used by permission.)

the molecules and is different for each gas. A Raman spectrum for a typical expired sample of respiratory gas is shown[48, 58] in Figure 3–26. The amplitudes of the peaks are proportional to the concentration of the gas present. Gas concentrations are measured by isolating the specific characteristic Raman wavelengths for each of the gases by using multiple optical wavelength filters. The magnitude of the Raman signal is small, but by using high-intensity light sources such as lasers, the signal levels are good and thus low concentrations of gases such as anesthetic agents can be measured.[59] The Raman scattering takes place almost instantaneously (about 10 picoseconds) so that breath-to-breath measurements are possible—they are limited only by the dynamics of the sidestream sampling mechanism.

Using a sidestream sampling technique, a multigas monitor based on acoustic principles was recently introduced.[48] The device measures all gases and vapor concentrations except oxygen by a special infrared absorption technique called *photoacoustic spectroscopy.* A precision microphone detects the energy the gases absorb; it "listens" as they expand and contract. Oxygen concentration is determined by magnetoacoustic techniques. The manufacturer (Brüel & Kajaer) claims that the sensing system requires less frequent calibration and that it is more accurate than more conventional infrared techniques.

Gas Flow/Volume

Gas Flow

Various gas flowmeters are available: rotameters, ultrasonic and thermal flowmeters, and pneumotachographs. Rotameter-type flowmeters place a small turbine in the flow path. For steady flows with uniform gas composition, this type of flowmeter can be calibrated to be very accurate. Unfortunately, with the rapidly varying flows and variable gas compositions found in respiratory measurements, this type of flowmeter is often too inaccurate to be useful. Ultrasonic flowmeters have also been used for gas flow, but they also suffer from limitations similar to the rotameter. Thermal flowmeters employ a sensing elements such as metal wires, metal films, and thermistors whose resistance changes with temperature. Flowmeters that use a single, temperature-compensated, heated wire (the so-called "hot-wire" anemometer) with linearizing circuits provide good unidirectional flow indications. Respiratory gas flowing in either direction "cools" the wire, which in turn requires more energy to heat it and maintain a constant temperature. The unidirectional flow measuring capability is a major limitation of the hot-wire anemometer.[3, 61]

One of the most popular and accurate respiratory flowmeters is the 1925 Fleisch pneumotachograph, named after its inventor.[62] This device depends on the measurement of a pressure drop across a flow resistor. The flow resistor is usually either a screen or a series of capillary tubes in parallel. Figure 3–27 shows a Fleisch pneumotachometer with a screen and parallel tubes in series. This fixed resistor in the flow path causes a pressure drop that is (nearly) linearly

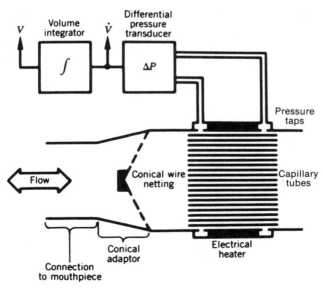

FIG 3–27.
Fleisch pneumotachometer. A linear resistance-flow element.

related to flow. The equation for Poiseuille's law describes the pressure-flow characteristic of the Fleisch pneumotachograph:

$$P_1 - P_2 = \frac{8uLF}{\pi r^4}$$

where $P_1 - P_2$ is the pressure drop across the flow head, u is the gas viscosity, L is the length of the device, r is the radius of the device, and F is the flow. A differential pressure transducer senses the pressure drop. The nearly linear pressure-flow characteristic is limited to the laminar flow region, where the Reynolds numbers is less than 2000 (Fig 3–28). Although the pressure-flow relationship (resistance) appears linear in Figure 3–28, the conductance characteristic of the Fleisch flowmeter is nonlinear, as seen in Figure 3–29. Figure 3–30 shows that the addition of the screen upstream (Fig 3–27) causes important changes in the conductance characteristics of the Fleisch flowmeter.

As noted in Poiseuille's equation, the output of the Fleisch pneumotachograph is directly proportional to the viscosity of the flowing gas. These viscosity variations are gas composition and temperature dependent. For example, the resistance of the Fleisch can increase by 12.5% when the gas composition changes from room air (20.9% O_2) to 100% O_2. Figure 3–31 shows the conductance-flow characteristics for a Fleisch pneumotachometer with varying O_2–N_2 gas mixtures (from room air to 100% O_2). Figure 3–32 shows that the relative resistance with

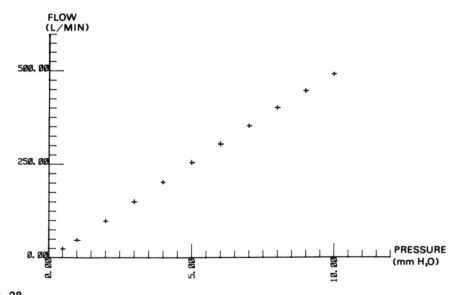

FIG 3–28.
Flow-pressure curve of a typical Fleisch No. 3 pneumotachometer provided by the manufacturer. (*From Yeh MP et al: Computerized determination of pneumotachometer characteristics using a calibrated syringe. J Appl Physiol: Respir Envir Exercise Physiol 1982; 53:280–285. Used by permission.*)

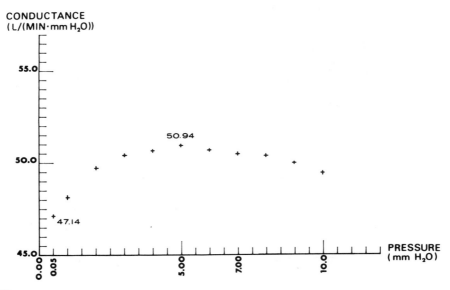

FIG 3–29.
Conductance-pressure curve for the same pneumotachometer as Figure 3–28. (*From Yeh MP et al: Computerized determination of pneumotachometer characteristics using a calibrated syringe. J Appl Physiol: Respir Envir Exercise Physiol 1982; 53:280–285. Used by permission.*)

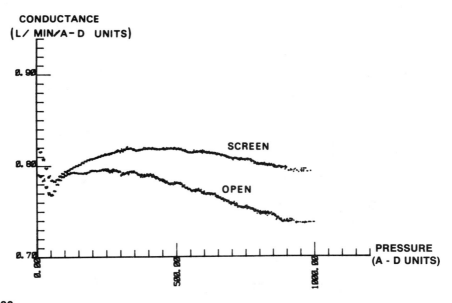

FIG 3–30.
Conductance characteristics of the same pneumotachometer with a wide-open upstream geometry (open curve) and with the manufacturer's upstream metal screen (screen curve). See Figure 3–27 for position of screen. (*From Yeh MP et al: Computerized determination of pneumotachometer characteristics using a calibrated syringe. J Appl Physiol: Respir Envir Exercise Physiol 1982; 53:280–285. Used by permission.*)

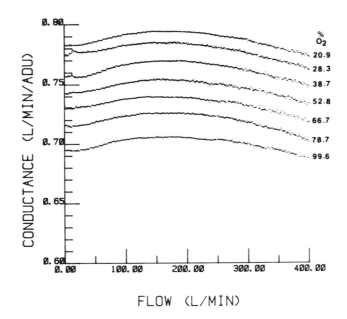

FIG 3–31.
Relative conductances with room air and O_2–N_2 gas mixtures. Note that the flow-conductance curves have the same shape. (*From Yeh MP et al: Effects of O_2, N_2 and CO_2 composition on nonlinearity of Fleisch pneumotachograph characteristics. J Appl Physiol: Respir Envir Exercise Physiol 1984; 56:1423–1425. Used by permission.*)

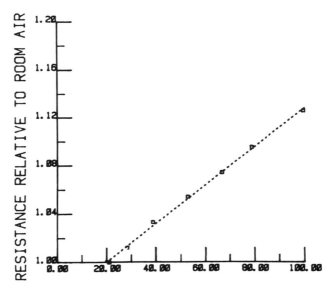

FIG 3–32.
Relative resistance of O2–N2 gas mixtures compare to room air. (*From Yeh MP et al: Effects of O_2, N_2 and CO_2 composition on nonlinearity of Fleisch pneumotachograph characteristics. J Appl Physiol: Respir Envir Exercise Physiol 1984; 56:1423–1425. Used by permission.*)

varying O_2 concentrations is linear. Yeh et al.[63, 64] have developed methods for accurately linearizing and calibrating Fleisch pneumotachographs to within about 1%.

Figure 3–33 shows a schematic diagram of a variable orifice flow-measuring device. The device has a nonlinear flow-pressure characteristic. However, the characteristic is highly reproducible. Because of its nonlinear flow-pressure characteristics, computerized "linearization" methods are used.[48]

The Wright respirometer is an example of a rotating-vane, or turbine, flow-measuring device. The flow of gas through the device turns the turbine at a rate dependent on the flow.[48] The movement of the turbine can be either mechanically or electronically coupled to a display device. If a mechanical mechanism is used, the turbine is linked to a mechanical display meter. If the rotations are sensed electronically, typically electronic pulses are generated by means of the turbine interrupting a beam of light. Each pulse is counted and is proportional to the flow. The inertia of the turbine makes it slow to respond and somewhat inaccurate for measuring breath-to-breath flow rates.

Thermal-element flowmeters use sensors such as thermistors and metal wires (hot-wire flowmeter) to sense flow.[48] The hot-wire anemometer uses a small heated element in the pathway of the gas flow. The current needed to maintain the element at constant temperature is measured and is proportional to the gas flow that cools the element. One limitation of most thermal-element flowmeters is that they are unidirectional. If measuring the direction of the flow is important, then directional valves and multiple flowmeters are used.

The two types of ultrasonic flowmeters are the transit-time and vortex-shedding types.[48] Figure 3–34 shows a diagram of the transit-time ultrasonic flowmeter. The time it takes the ultrasonic pulse to travel upstream and downstream changes, and it is based on gas flow, gas temperature, the speed of sound (c), the length of the pathway (L), and the angle of the sensors in relation to the stream as shown in these equations:

$$T_u = t_{upstream} = \frac{L}{c - v^*\cos(\beta)}$$

$$T_d = t_{downstream} = \frac{L}{c + v^*\cos(\beta)}$$

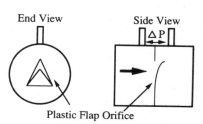

FIG 3–33.
Variable orifice flow transducer. (*From East TD: What makes noninvasive monitoring tick? A review of basic engineering principles. Resp Care 1990; 35:500–519. Used by permission.*)

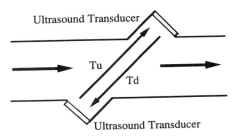

FIG 3–34.
Transit-time ultrasonic flowmeter. (*From East TD: What makes noninvasive monitoring tick? A review of basic engineering principles.* Resp Care *1990; 35:500–519. Used by permission.*)

The vortex-shedding flowmeter (Fig 3–35) places obstructions in the airway so that whirlpools of gas (vortices) are produced.[48] The principle of vortex shedding has been known since 1878. The frequency at which vortices are shed is related to the flow of the gas past the obstruction. An ultrasonic transmitter is placed perpendicular to the flow. The ultrasonic signal is modulated by the frequency of the vortices, and flow is thus detected. The measurement is independent of gas density, viscosity, temperature, pressure, and conductivity. The design of the obstruction and the surrounding structures are primary factors that affect the calibration and linearity of this type of flowmeter. Vortex-shedding flowmeters are unidirectional.

Peak Flowmeters

Wright and McKerrow first reported the use of a simplified peak flowmeter in 1959—the Wright peak flowmeter.[65] Since that time this peak flowmeter has become the standard against which all other peak flowmeters have been tested and compared. In 1978 Wright described a simplified "mini-Wright" peak flowmeter.[66] This development and the competitive environment of modern medical instrumentation have lead to the proliferation of inexpensive peak

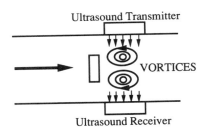

FIG 3–35.
Vortex-shedding ultrasonic flow transducer. (*From East TD: What makes noninvasive monitoring tick: A review of basic engineering principles.* Resp Care *1990; 35:500–519. Used by permission.*)

flowmeters. As a consequence, there have been a large number of reports in the literature comparing each new peak flowmeter with the original "Wright peak flowmeter," or espousing the advantage of the latest peak flowmeter.[67] There is some confusion about which is adequate or even best. As a result, the National Asthma Education Panel recently made recommendations on diagnosing asthma[68] and established technical standards and testing methods for peak flowmeters.[69]

Eight different models of peak flowmeters were recently tested using many different peak flow detecting technologies. The results of this testing showed—to the credit of the instrument manufacturers—that the quality, accuracy, and reproducibility of currently available peak flowmeters is surprisingly good.[67]

Gas Volume/Spirometers

Although the output of flowmeters can be integrated over time to obtain volume, several simpler and more accurate volume-measuring devices known as *spirometers* have been developed.[70–73] Basically, spirometers are calibrated containers that collect respiratory gases as they are exhaled. The simplest of these was used in the mid-1800s and was simply an inverted cylindrical "bell" that used a water bath as a seal. The vertical displacement of the bell and its known cross-sectional area were used to measure volume. More recently, recorders were added to spirometers with a time base so that the more dynamic characteristics of volume and flow could be easily determined. The American Thoracic Society (ATS) has taken the leadership to standardize spirometers used in pulmonary function laboratories.[72]

Spirometers are devised using a variety of technologies; a water seal, as described above; a rolling seal, in which a cylinder moves horizontally with a very thin (usually plastic) seal; a wedge bellows; and a variety of flow sensors. Recently, the characteristics of a wide variety of spirometers have been measured.[73] Most, but not all, commercially available spirometers meet the ATS requirements.

Plethysmography

Plethysmographs measure volume. When it is impossible or inconvenient to measure the volume of body parts such as the gas in the lungs or blood in the lower leg, plethysmographs are used. For measurement of thoracic gas volume, a body plethysmograph is frequently used.[70, 71] For a volume of gas at constant temperature, the product of pressure (P) and volume (V) is a constant (Boyle's law). The patient is seated in a body plethysmograph, with the nose occluded, breathing quietly, through a tube to the outside. When the subject is breathing at functional residual capacity (FRC) the airway is closed, trapping the gas in the lung at near FRC. The subject then gently pants against a closed shutter at about two times per second. The pressure at the mouth is measured as is the volume change in the body box, which is measured via either a plethysmograph or a spirometer. The pressure and volume signals measured with the appropriate transducers are then applied to allow measurement of lung volume. Plethysmography for the legs and other body parts applies the same transducers and principles.

Biosensors and Electrochemical Sensors

Biosensors are sophisticated descendants of the canary in the coal mine.[74, 75] Modern biosensors have evolved as a result of two disparate disciplines: information technology with its microcomputers and optical fibers, and molecular biology. With such sensors, faster measurements can now be made at the bedside at potentially less expense than with current clinical laboratory measurements. Leland C. Clark, Jr., inventor of the oxygen electrode, is credited with developing the first biosensor.[74] Clark extended his "oxygen electrode" to measure blood glucose by coating his electrode with a gel containing a biocatalyst. Currently, roughly 100 different enzymes are used in biosensors, and the future points to an ever-increasing number. In the future, miniature disposable implantable biosensors, and eventually noninvasive biosensors, may become available to detect many of the body's chemical and gas measurements.

VENTILATORS: AN INTEGRATED INSTRUMENTATION COMPLEX

The modern ventilator is a place where many of the transducers discussed in this chapter come together. Today's ventilator is a complex unit of sensors, electronics, microcomputers, and software engineering.[76] These ventilators can be modified easily by a simple software change to provide almost any new mode of ventilation and to collect information from a variety of sensors. This information can be displayed, stored, and manipulated in a variety of ways—limited only by the imagination of software engineers. Ventilators of the future will likely have plug-in modules to perform pulse oximetry, breath-by-breath infrared CO_2 analysis, mixed venous oximetry, and perhaps even noninvasive blood pressure monitoring. Communications capabilities to provide convenient and practical electronic interfaces with other monitoring devices will become common.

Computer-aided protocols may eventually find their way into ventilators.[76] The need for better and more consistent respiratory monitoring has been pointed out by many investigators.[76-81] Before these computer protocols can be applied, however, dramatic improvements must occur in the automatic acquisition processing and recording of data.[76] Dealing with only the "raw" signals coming from the transducers, with the "artifacts/noise" and the complexity of signals, is likely to stymie progress with standardized computerized protocols. The transducers we currently have available to us in respiratory monitoring are sufficiently robust, accurate, and stable at present to allow computer-driven protocols to be developed. However, understanding the complexity of signal versus noise will be a difficult task—one that will require the efforts of the larger pulmonary community to solve. Such an activity will require careful review of the problems and the development of standard methodologies so that a medical consensus can be achieved. The future for respiratory care monitoring is bright and the challenges achievable. We must now develop a strategy and "team" to improve the quality of monitoring, not just the quantity of signals we measure.

REFERENCES

1. *Webster's New World Dictionary* (1980).
2. Webster JG (ed): *Encyclopedia of Medical Devices and Instrumentation*. New York, John Wiley & Sons, 1988.
3. Webster JG (ed); *Medical Instrumentation: Applications and Design*. Boston, Houghton-Mifflin Co, 1978.
4. Cobbold RSC: *Transducers for Biomedical Measurements: Principles and Applications*. New York, John Wiley & Sons, 1974.
5. Carr JJ, Brown JM: *Introduction to Biomedical Equipment Technology*. New York, John Wiley & Sons, 1981.
6. Andrews RD et al: Computer charting: An evaluation of a respiratory care computer system. *Respir Care* 1985; 30:695–707.
7. Gardner RM: Patient-monitoring systems, in: Shortliffe EH, Perreault LE (eds): *Medical Informatic: Computer Applications in Health Care*. Reading, MA, Addison-Wesley Publishing Co, 1990, pp. 366–399.
8. Hawley WL, Tariq H, Gardner RM: Clinical implementation of an automated medical information bus in an intensive care unit. *SCAMC* 1988; 12:621–624.
9. Shabot MM: Standardized acquisition of bedside data: The IEEE P1073 medical information bus. *Intl J Clin Monit Comput* 1989; 6:197–204.
10. Gardner RM et al: Medical Information Bus: The key to future integrated monitoring (editorial). *Intl J Clin Monit Comput* 1989; 6:205–209.
11. Scott F: Computers play important role in critical care. *ADVANCE Resp Therapists* 1989; 2:1–3, 24.
12. Gardner RM, Hawley WH, East TD, Oniki T, Young HFW: Real time data acquisition: Recommendations for the Medical Information Bus (MIB) *Intl J Clin Monit & Comput*, 1991; 8:251–258.
13. Gardner RM: Computerization and quality control of monitoring techniques, in: *Contemporary Management in Critical Care #4: Respiratory Monitoring*. Martin J. Tubin, Editor. Churchill Livingston, 1991, pp. 197–211.
14. Gardner RM, Kutik M: American National Standard for interchageability and performance of resistive bridge type blood pressure transducers. ANSI 1986.
15. Gordon VL, et al: Zero stability of disposable and reusable pressure transducers. *Med Instr* 1987; 17:81–91.
16. ECRI. Disposable pressure transducers (evaluation). *Health Devices* 1988; 17:75–94.
17. Christensen DA. Thermometry, in Webster J (ed): *Encyclopedia of Medical Devices and Instrumentation*. New York, Wiley-Interscience, 1988, Vol 4, pp. 2759–2765.
18. Mandel R, Shen W: Colorimetry, in Webster J (ed); *Encyclopedia of Medical Devices and Instrumentation*. New York, Wiley-Interscience, Vol 2, pp. 771–779.
19. Stow RW, Baer RF, Randall B: Rapid measurement of the tension of carbon dioxide in blood. *Arch Phys Med Rehabil* 1957; 38:646–650.
20. Severinghaus JW, Bradley AG: Electrodes for blood PO_2 and PCO_2 determination. *J Appl Physiol* 1958; 13:515–520.
21. Coombes RG, Halsall D: Carbon dioxide analyzers, in Webster J (ed): *Encyclopedia of Medical Devices and Instrumentation*. New York, Wiley-Interscience, Vol 1, pp. 556–569.
22. Mylrea KC: Oxygen sensors, in Encyclopedia of Medical Devices and Instrumentation. Volume 3:2169–2174; J. Webster (ed). Wiley-Interscience, New York 1988.
23. Mendelson Y: Blood gas measurement, transcutaneous. In Encyclopedia of Medical Devices and Instrumentation. Volume 1:448–460; J. Webster (ed). Wiley-Interscience, New York 1988.
24. Severinghaus JW: Blood gas concentrations, in *Handbook of Phyiology*. Bethesda, MD, American Physiological Society, 1965, Sec 3, Vol 2, Chap 61, pp. 1475–1487.

25. Severinghaus JW, Astrup PB: History of blood gas analysis. IV. Leland Clark's oxygen electrode. *J Clin Monit* 1986; 2:125–139.
26. Severinghaus JW, Astrup PB: History of blood gas analysis. I. The development of electrochemistry. *J Clin Monit* 1985; 1:180–192.
27. Severinghaus JW, Astrup PB: History of blood gas analysis. II. pH and acid-base balance measurements. *J Clin Monit* 1985; 1:259–277.
28. Severinghaus JW, Astrup PB: History of blood gas analysis. III. Carbon dioxide tension. *J Clin Monit* 1986; 1:60–73.
29. Severinghaus JW, Astrup PB: History of blood gas analysis. VI. oximetry. *J Clin Monit* 1986; 2:270–288.
30. Severinghaus JW, Astrup PB: History of blood gas analysis. V. Oxygen measurement. *J Clin Monit* 1986; 2:174–189.
31. Severinghaus JW, Honda Y: History of blood gas analysis VII. Pulse oximetry. *J Clin Monit* 1987; 3:135–138.
32. Wood EH, Geraci JE: Photoelectric determination of arterial oxygen saturation in man. *J Lab Clin Med* 1949; 34:387–401.
33. Johnson CC et al: A solid state fiberoptics oximeter. *J Assn Adv Med Instrum* 1971; 5:L77–83.
34. Divertie MB, McMichan JC: Continuous monitoring of mixed venous oxygen saturation. *Chest* 1984; 85:423–428.
35. Merrick EB, Hayes TJ: Continuous, non-invasive measurements of arterial blood oxygen levels. *Hewlett-Packard J* 1976; 28:2–9.
36. Gardner RM: Pulse oximetry: Is it monitoring's "silver bullet"? *J Cardiovasc Nurs* 1987; 1:79–83.
37. Wukitsch MW, Petterson MT, Tobler DR, et al: Pulse oximetry: Analysis of theory, technology, and practice. *J Clin Monit* 1988; 4:290–301.
38. Blackwell GR: The technology of pulse oximetry. *Biomed Instr Technol* 1989; 23:188–193.
39. Kelleher JF: Pulse oximetry. *J Clin Monit* 1989; 5:37–62.
40. Yelderman M, New W, Jr: Evaluation of pulse oximetry. *Anesth* 1983; 59:349–352.
41. Mendelson Y, Kent JD, Shahnarian A, et al: Simultaneous comparison of three noninvasive oximeters in healthy volunteers. *Med Instr* 1987; 21:183–188.
42. Cecil WT, Thorpe KJ, Fibuch EE, et al: A clinical evaluation of the accuracy of the Nellcor N-100 and Ohmeda 3700 pulse oximeters. *J Clin Monit* 1988; 4:31–36.
43. Hanning CD: "He looks a little blue down this end": Monitoring oxygenation during anaesthesia. *Br J Anaesth* 1985; 57:359–360.
44. Morris RW et al: The prevalence of hypoxemia detected by pulse oximetry during recovery from anesthesia. *J Clin Monit* 1988; 4:16–20.
45. Rothfusz ER, Kitz DS, Andrews RW, et al: O2 Sat, HR and MAP among patients receiving local anesthesia: How low/high do they go? *Anesth Analg* 1988; 67:S189.
46. Mendelson Y, Kent JC: Variations in optical absorption spectra of adult and fetal hemoglobins and its effect on pulse oximetry. *IEEE Trans Biomed Eng* 1989; 36:844–848.
47. Szaflarski NL, Cohen NH: Use of capnography in critically ill adults. *Heart Lung* 1991; 20:373–374.
48. East TD: What makes noninvasive monitoring tick? A review of basic engineering principles. *Resp Care* 1990; 35:500–519.
49. Kocache R. Oxygen analyzers, in Webster J (ed): *Encyclopedia of Medical Devices and Instrumentation*. New York, Wiley-Interscience, 1988, Vol 4, pp 2155–2160.
50. Gravenstein JS: Monitoring in anesthesia, in Webster J (ed): *Encyclopedia of Medical Devices and Instrumentation*. New York, Wiley-Interscience, 1988, Vol 3, pp. 1932–1950.
51. Sodal IE, Clark JS, Swanson GD: Mass spectrometers in medical monitoring, in Webster J (ed):

Encyclopedia of Medical Devices and Instrumentation. New York, Wiley-Interscience, 1988, Vol 3, pp 1848–1859.

52. Matalon S, Erickson J, Mosharrafa M, et al: A method for the in vitro measurement of tensions of blood gases with a mass spectrometer. *Med Instr* 1975; 9:133–135.

53. SARAcap CO2, O2 and N2O Respiratory Monitor Biomedical Systems—Mary Polizzi, Specification materials, PPG Biomedical Systems Inc., St. Louis, MO. 1987, pp. 1–10.

54. Gardner RM, Clemmer TP: Selection and standardization of respiratory monitoring equipment. *Respir Care* 1985; 30:560–569.

55. Sodal IE, Swanson GD, Micco AJ, et al: A computerized mass spectrometer and flowmeter system for respiratory gas measurements. *Ann Biomed Eng* 1983; 11:83–99.

56. Brantigan JW, Dunn KL, Albo D: A clinical catheter for continuous blood gas measurement by mass spectrometer. *J Appl Physiol* 1976; 40:443–446.

57. Severinghaus JW, Ozanne G: Multi-operating room monitoring with one mass spectrometer. *Acta Anaesthesiol Scand Suppl* 1978; 70:168–187.

58. East TD, East KA: Nitrogen analyzers, in Webster JG (ed): *Encyclopedia of Medical Devices.* New York, Wiley-Interscience, 1988, Vol 4, pp. 2052–2058.

59. VanWagenen RA, et al: Dedicated patient monitoring of anesthetic and respiratory gases by Raman scattering. *J Clin Monit* 1986; 2:215–222.

60. Long DA: *Raman Spectroscopy.* New York, McGraw-Hill, 1977.

61. Buess C, Boutellier U, Koller EA: Pneumotachometers, in Webster J (ed): *Encyclopedia of Medical Devices and Instrumentation.* New York, Wiley-Interscience, 1988, Vol 4, pp. 2319–2324.

62. Fleisch A. Der pneumotachograph: Ein apparat zur beischwindigkeigregistrierung der atemluft. *Pfluegers Arch* 1925; 209:713–722.

63. Yeh MP et al: Computerized determination of pneumotachometer characteristics using a calibrated syringe. *J Appl Physiol: Respir Envir Exercise Physiol* 1982; 53:280–285.

64. Yeh MP, Adams TD, Gardner RM, et al: Effects of O_2, N_2 and CO_2 composition on nonlinearity of Fleisch pneumotachograph characteristics. *J Appl Physiol: Respir Envir Exercise Physiol* 1984; 56:1423–1425.

65. Wright BM, McKerrow CB: Maximum forced expiratory flow rate as a measure of ventilating capacity. *Br Med J* 1959; 2:1041–1047.

66. Wright BM: A miniature Wright peak flowmeter. *Br Med J* 1978; 2:1627–1628.

67. Gardner RM, Crapo RO, Jackson BR, et al: Evaluation of accuracy and reproducibility of peak flow meters at 1400 meters. *Chest*, 1992; 101:948–952.

68. National Asthma Education Program (NAEP) Expert Panel: Diagnosis and management of asthma. Bethesda, MD, National Heart, Lung and Blood Institute, February 4, 1991.

69. National Asthma Education Program, Statement on technical standards for peak flow meters. Bethesda, MD, National Heart, Lung and Blood Institute, February 4, 1991.

70. Petrini MF. Pulmonary function testing, in Webster J (ed): *Encyclopedia of Medical Devices and Instrumentation.* New York, Wiley-Interscience, Vol 4, pp. 2379–2395.

71. Morris AH, Kanner RE, Crapo RO, et al: *Clinical Pulmonary Function* Testing. A Manual of Uniform Laboratory Procedures, ed 2, Intermountain Thoracic Society, Salt Lake City, Utah, July 1984.

72. Gardner RM, Hankinson JL, Clausen JL, et al: ATS statement on standardization of spirometry—1987 update. *Resp Care* 1987; 32:1039–1060.

73. Nelson SB, Gardner RM, Crapo RO, et al: Performance evaluation of contemporary spirometers. *Chest* 1990; 97:288–297.

74. Schultz JS: Biosensors. *Sci Am* 1991; 265:64–69.

75. Fogt EJ: Electrochemical sensors, In Webster J (ed); *Encyclopedia of Medical Devices and Instrumentation*. New York, Wiley-Interscience, 1988, Vol 2, pp. 1062–1072.
76. East TD: The ventilator of the 1990s. *Resp Care* 1990; 35:232–240.
77. Kafer ER et al: Ventilators for anesthesiology, in Webster J (ed): *Encyclopedia of Medical Devices and Instrumentation*. New York, Wiley-Interscience, 1988, Vol 4, pp. 2847–2858.
78. Quan SF: Ventilatory monitoring, in Webster J (ed): *Encyclopedia of Medical Devices and Instrumentation*. New York, Wiley-Interscience, 1988, Vol 4, pp. 2864–2877.
79. Milic-Emili J: Is weaning an art or a science? *Am Rev Respir Dis* 1986; 134:1107–1108.
80. Moser KM: Truths in historical perspective. *Heart Lung* 1987; 16:345–346.
81. Bone RC: Recent advances in pulmonary and critical care medicine. *Intern Med Spec* 1987; 8:90–103.

Chapter 4

Signal Processing and Data Display

Lisa J. Arguin, B.S.B.M.E.

Eileen P. Hall, B.S.B.M.E.

INTRODUCTION

Technology has changed dramatically over the past 40 years, with many technical advances and improvements. Such changes have revolutionized the way that physiologic signals are detected, processed, and displayed. In 1951, the first vacuum tube digital computers were introduced. Transistors, which became available by 1960, are a fraction of the size of vacuum tubes with equal capability, and quickly made the vacuum tube obsolete. By the early 1970s, the integrated circuit (IC), or chip, was produced. This changed the way in which electronic devices have been designed. An individual integrated circuit can house multiple components, many of which are transistors.[1] Figure 4–1 illustrates the progression of these striking physical changes in technology.

The purpose of this chapter is to describe what happens to a signal from the time of its detection to the time of its display. Equipped with this information, the clinician will be better able to assess the quality of data presented by bedside technology.

TERMINOLOGY

Data, devices, formats, signals, outputs, and recordings are often labeled as being either analog or digital. In the purest sense, *analog* describes anything that is continuous, whereas *digital* indicates discrete and discontinuous. A very simple illustration is that of a light bulb. If the light bulb is controlled by a dimmer switch so that continuous changes in brightness are evident, this would be considered an example of an analog device. On the other hand, a two-position light switch that is either in the on or off position would be considered digital. Although the light bulb itself is not a digital device, to the eye there are but two discrete states, on or off, which is unlike the continuous dimmer.

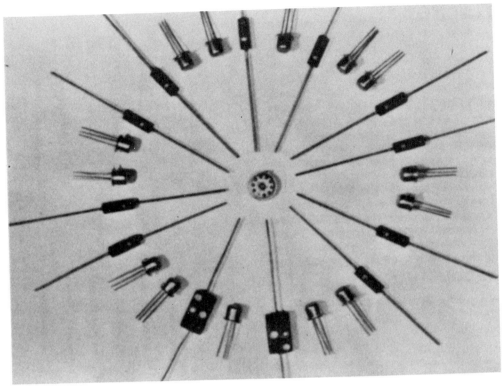

FIG 4–1.
In the middle is an integrated circuit and surrounding it are the discrete components required to build a circuit to perform the same task. (*From Boylestad R, Nashelsky L: Electricity, Electronics, and Electromagnetics: Principles and Applications. Englewood Cliffs, NJ, Prentice-Hall Inc, 1977. Used by permission.*)

Digital systems function in a binary manner and utilize devices that exist in only one of two states. These systems are either on or off, open or closed, high or low, yes or no, and, in the case of digital data, 1 or 0. Digital integrated circuits consist of basic building blocks known as logic gates, specifically OR, AND, NOT, and Flip-Flops. These circuits examine input data in the form of 1's and 0's and provide an output, either a 1 or a 0, depending on the gate used and the input configuration. Figure 4–2 identifies the symbols that are used for each of these circuits and the truth table for each. These logic circuits comprise the heart of most digital processing systems.[2]

All electronic devices utilize both hardware and software. Hardware consists of the physical components that comprise the device. That is, the computational equipment necessary for the information processing. Software is the set of programs, instructions, or routines that specify, augment, and support the programming and computer operations. In the design of present-day electronic devices, the cost and time associated with software development, validation, and implementation typically exceed that of hardware development.[1]

Truth Tables for AND, OR, and NOT Functions

A	B	$A \cdot B$	$A + B$	$\bar{A}$	$\bar{B}$
0	0	0	0	1	1
0	1	0	1	1	0
1	0	0	1	0	1
1	1	1	1	0	0

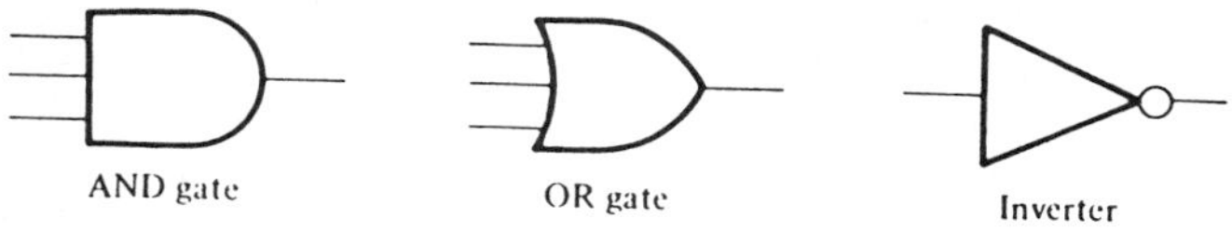

AND gate   OR gate   Inverter

FIG 4–2.
Depicted are the symbols used for AND, OR, and NOT (inverter) logic gates, as well as their truth tables. (*From Boylestad R, Nashelsky L: Electricity, Electronics, and Electromagnetics: Principles and Applications. Prentice-Hall Inc, 1977. Used by permission.*)

At the heart of every digital computer, such as the physiologic monitor, is a microprocessor. Microprocessors are classified as being x bits, where x can be 4, 8, 12, 16, 32, and, most recently, 64. The number of bits provides an indication of how quickly data can be processed. This is quite important when selecting the microprocessor for a system. The microprocessor consists of a control unit and an arithmetic-logic unit. The control unit coordinates data transfer and establishes the operating sequences. The arithmetic-logic unit conducts the arithmetic and logic processes. The logic circuits previously mentioned are used in this portion of the system.[1]

In addition to the control and logic units, a memory unit stores information. This information can be accessed for different functions and by different mechanisms. Read-only memory (ROM) stores information such as physiologic parameter processing programs. Information is programmed into this device ("burned-in") at the time of manufacture and cannot be altered. Although it can be "burned-in" only once, there is no limit as to the number of times that it can be accessed or read. A programmable ROM (PROM) is a memory device that can be programmed at any time by anyone, rather than only at the time of manufacture. Like ROM, it can be written to once only, after which its information can only be read and not reprogrammed. After it is programmed, a PROM functions like a ROM. An erasable PROM (EPROM) can have its data changed or erased using ultraviolet light, allowing new information to be programmed. Random-access memory (RAM) differs from ROM and PROM because there is no limit as to the number of times that it can be changed (read from and written to). This type of memory is called "random" because information can be accessed and stored at random, at any time, and in no particular sequence. Information such as an open file in a word processor, or real-time parameter values in a bedside monitor, are stored in RAM. The microprocessor and the memory units together are the central processing unit (CPU) of the computer.[1–4]

Because physiologic signals are typically very small (micro and millivolts), amplification is always necessary. When amplifying the input signal, it is crucial that signal distortion be at a minimum. Nonlinear distortion occurs when new frequencies are present in the output that were not part of the original input signal. Frequency distortion occurs when different frequencies are amplified differently (i.e., some more than others). Phase-shift distortion occurs when there is nonuniform phase shifting of signals at different frequencies.

Differential amplifiers are commonly used to amplify physiologic signals (e.g., ECG, EEG, and EMG). The concept behind this device is to amplify the difference between the two signal inputs while minimizing those signals that are common to both. Signals common to both are typically artifact and/or interference that is present in the system. Another type of amplifier is a *clamping amplifier*. The purpose of this device is to take the input signal and restrict the output signal amplitude to a defined range (e.g., ±3 V, 0 to 2 V). Clamping amplifiers are often found in circuits when the signal is converted from analog to digital.[2, 3]

Signals are often converted from analog to digital by devices called analog-to-digital converters (ADC). A signal must be in a digital form if it is to be used by a microprocessor, thus necessitating this conversion. One type of ADC converts the analog signal into a series of pulses that are proportional to the signal voltage. If the signal amplitude (voltage) varies with time, the converter must have an adequate sampling rate. If the sample rate is too slow, voltage changes will be missed and the signal will be misrepresented. Once processed, it is necessary to convert the digital signal back to an analog form so that it can be displayed or printed on an analog device. This is accomplished using a digital-to-analog converter (DAC). The numeric value of the digital signal that is presented in code is proportional to the magnitude, voltage, or current of the analog signal.[2]

In addition to being amplified and converted, signals are often filtered to eliminate unwanted signals. These unwanted signals may be other physiologic signals, electrical noise, or signals that were intentionally introduced into the system. Filters are generally categorized as low pass, high pass, or bandpass. *Low-pass filters* yield zero output for signals of higher frequencies than the specified cutoff frequency, and thus only allow low-frequency signals to pass. Conversely, *high-pass* filters eliminate unwanted signals whose frequencies fall below the filter's cutoff frequency. *Band-pass* filters are designed to allow only a certain range, or band, of signal frequencies to pass through with specific low and high cutoff frequencies. Band reject filters do the opposite of bandpass filters by rejecting signals within a certain range of frequencies. Figure 4–3 is a graphical representation of high-, low-, and bandpass filters. Each of these types of filters is found in medical devices, and each is vital if the desired signal is to be accurately represented.[2, 3]

Various other components found in device design also should be mentioned. Biophysical signals are often transmitted via modulation. The physiologic signal is termed the *modulating wave* and it is carried by another signal called the *carrier wave*. The carrier wave, which is usually a sinewave, will vary either its frequency, amplitude, or phase. Depending on the type of modulation, it will vary proportionally to the corresponding variations of the modulating wave's frequency, amplitude, or phase. A demodulator is the device used to recover the original modulating signal from the carrier. The AM radio is an everyday example of amplitude modulation where a high-frequency carrier is used for the transmission of audio signals. Figure 4–4 illustrates the concept of amplitude modulation. An integrator is a device whose gain changes with frequency because its output voltage is proportional to the integral of the input voltage.[2, 5]

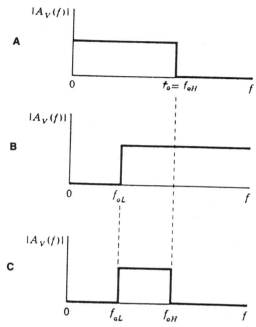

FIG 4–3.
Ideal filter characteristics for **A**, low-pass, **B**, high-pass, and **C**, bandpass filters. (*From Millman J, Halkias C: Integrated Electronics: Analog and Digital Circuits and Systems. New York, McGraw-Hill, 1972. Used by permission.*)

SIGNAL PROCESSING

The signal processing of three physiologic measurements will be discussed in this section. The first is impedance pneumography, which is the noninvasive technique most often used to measure respiration rate and to detect apnea. It was chosen for discussion because it is generally considered an unreliable measurement, yet it is extensively used. The second and third measurements both relate to hemodynamics. Hemodynamics is an extremely important parameter and is routinely monitored both noninvasively and invasively. The same information (systolic, diastolic, and mean values) is obtained for each. However, the actual data, respective levels of accuracy, and measurement methods are quite different. The signal processing for both methods is outlined and their differences, advantages, and disadvantages are compared.

Impedance Pneumography

Impedance pneumography is not a new measurement. It has been utilized by monitoring manufacturers for more than 20 years. This might lead one to believe that it is a tried and true

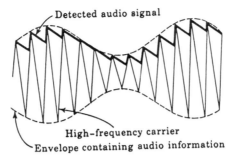

Detected audio signal

High-frequency carrier

Envelope containing audio information

FIG 4–4.
An amplitude-modulated wave and the detected audio signal. The carrier waveform is normally a sinusoid of much higher frequency than the triangular carrier wave depicted here. (*From Millman J, Halkias C: Integrated Electronics: Analog and Digital Circuits and Systems. New York, McGraw-Hill, 1972. Used by permission.*)

technique, and that it always yields accurate and reliable information. Unfortunately, this is not the case. Although impedance pneumography is incorporated into the most technically sophisticated monitors, the information that it presents should always be validated by the clinician.

Impedance pneumography is based on the assumption that air is nonconductive. This means that it has a high impedance and is resistive to current flow. Blood and other fluids found in the chest are conductive and offer a lower impedance compared to that of air. During inspiration, the relative amount of nonconductive air is greater than the amount of conductive blood and fluid, which results in significant transthoracic impedance. The opposite situation exists during exhalation. If a controlled electrical current is applied to the chest, there will be a change in measured voltage that is dependent on the change in the transthoracic impedance as determined by the patient's breathing pattern. Figure 4–5 is a simple block diagram of an impedance pneumography system.[6]

Most manufacturers of impedance pneumography use very similar methods. The following is a description of the signal processing common to these monitors. Specifics have been extracted from the Hewlett-Packard manual for the 78833 series neonatal monitor, the Hewlett-Packard manual for the M1002 ECG/Respiration module, and the Spacelabs manual for the 90418 ECG/Respiration module.

The measuring of respiration by impedance pneumography begins with a low-amplitude, high-frequency, approximate sinusoid signal on the order of tens or hundreds of kilohertz. The signal, which is often referred to as a carrier, must be at a high frequency so that it is out of the ECG bandwidth and so that tissue stimulation is avoided. The carrier signal is applied to one of the patient's ECG electrodes located on one side of the chest (usually right arm or right leg) and is received by another located on the other side (typically the left arm or the left leg). This facilitates the measuring of the signal across the patient's chest. The total impedance of the "system" consists of the patient's inherent body impedance, which is typically in the range of 1 to 4 kΩ, and the impedance change that is caused by respiration, which ranges between 0.25 to 1.0 Ω.[6, 7]

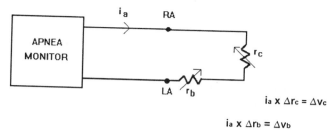

$$i_a \times \Delta r_c = \Delta v_c$$

$$i_a \times \Delta r_b = \Delta v_b$$

FIG 4–5.

Simplified respiration/apnea monitor-patient circuit. i_a = carrier frequency current generated by monitor; r_b = base impedance body; and r_c = impedance change primarily due to respiratory activity; however, other signals (e.g., cardiac activity and motion artifact) may also cause variation. (*From ECRI, Infant home apnea monitors. Health Dev 1987; 16:79–109. Used by permission.*)

   The carrier signal originates in the monitor as a square-wave that is converted to a sinewave by use of dividers and low-pass filters. It is applied to the patient via the ECG cable, wires, and electrodes. The two measuring electrodes are attached to a bridge network, and as the transthoracic impedance changes, so does the resultant voltage across the bridge. At this point the respiration signal is very small and must be amplified before further processing. A differential amplifier performs this function by amplifying the difference in voltage between the two measuring electrodes. Before the analog signal can be converted to digital it must be changed from an alternating signal to a unidirectional, or dc, signal. The carrier frequency must also be eliminated. Demodulators, integrators, and low-pass filters are used to accomplish these tasks. At this point in the process, the signal has been modified from the patient's respiration signal coupled with the original carrier signal, to a dc respiration signal only. It then goes to a clamping amplifier, which will limit the signal voltage necessary for the analog-to-digital conversion. Once converted, the signal is essentially a train of pulses whose widths are proportional to the voltage of the breaths in the original respiration signal. The components mentioned thus far are all classified as hardware. The software becomes involved with the signal when the conversion to digital is complete.

   A microprocessor, termed the *respiration microprocessor*, samples the digital signal and calculates the respiration rate and determines alarm conditions such as rate violations, apnea, and equipment faults. Like many parameters, such as ECG and oxygen saturation via pulse oximetry, the respiration rate is not calculated for every breath. It is a value that is calculated based on the number of breaths detected within a moving time window, which is usually a few seconds in duration. Many monitors define a breath as a signal that goes above and returns below a sensing threshold level. This level can be set automatically by the device or manually by the user. For rate violations, the microprocessor compares the calculated rate to the rate alarm settings as determined by the user (or the default settings) that are stored in the device's memory. Apnea is determined by calculating the duration between breaths compared to the delay time, again as set by the user or as compared to the device default settings. Equipment fault determinations, such as lead fail, are made by comparing the observed impedance level, which is predominantly the patient's base impedance, to the maximum tolerable levels as programmed in the software. Specific threshold levels for this vary, but most fall within the range of 1.5 to 3 KΩ. The microprocessor also evaluates trends, performs self-tests to ensure its own reliability, and prepares the signal for display.

The respiration microprocessor uses both ROM and shared memory. The ROM actually holds, or stores, the respiration program. For example, the impedance threshold that triggers a lead fail alarm is found here. The shared memory houses information such as the alarm limit settings programmed by the user. Information from both of these components is queried so that the respiration microprocessor can perform its functions.

After the respiration microprocessor, the signal is routed to another microprocessor that supervises the displayed information (numerics and waveforms) for all monitored parameters. The respiration wave information is housed in RAM and is then converted from a digital to an analog signal by a DAC. This is done because the signal must be in an analog form to be presented on an analog device such as a cathode-ray tube (CRT), which is the type of display typically used with critical care monitors. The numerical information is also stored in RAM and is converted from parallel to serial information. Both the analog waveform and the serial numerics are routed to a video driver, which is a device that controls the display. It is the responsibility of the display microprocessor to display information in the appropriate location and format, including status messages, graphs, parameter numerics, and waveforms. The respiration wave is displayed on a scale of centimeters per ohm and the digital rate is in breaths or respirations per minute. This is the end result as seen by the user after the raw signal has been obtained and processed. Specified accuracies for this measurement vary for each manufacturer, but are in the range of ± 2 to 5%. A block diagram of an impedance pneumography device is shown is Figure 4–6.

For many patients, this method of respiration monitoring is reliable. These are patients who have regular and easily distinguishable breathing patterns, exhibit a minimum of physical activity, and do not experience apneic episodes that are attributed to upper airway obstruction. Over the years, studies[8, 9] have been conducted that indicate that this is not a reliable method of detecting apnea caused by upper airway obstruction. It is also not an effective way of

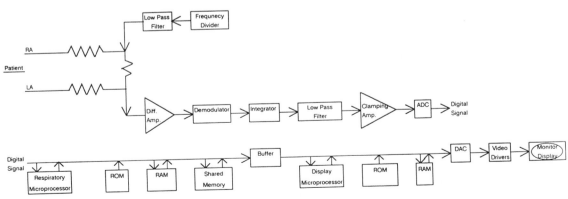

FIG 4–6.
Block diagram of respiration/apnea monitor that uses the impedance pneumography measurement method. (*Adapted from Hewlett-Packard technical manual for the 78833 series neonatal monitor.*)

monitoring patients that have very low level signals, such as in premature infants who require sensitivity settings to the point where cardiac activity is interpreted as breathing. In addition, vibrations from nearby equipment, patient movement, chest wall fluctuations due to cardiac impulses, and personnel movement may all cause conditions where the patient will be apneic, but the device will not so indicate.[6, 8–10]

Although there is little that can be done to improve these devices' ability to detect upper airway obstruction via impedance pneumography, there are measures that can be taken to avoid missed episodes due to motion and cardiac artifact. The first is to place the electrodes as far from the heart as possible in order to reduce the detection of impedance changes due to cardiac activity. Unfortunately, this may be somewhat difficult since the patient's ECG is also obtained with the same electrodes. Also, many patients have very restricted chest surface area, thus prohibiting ideal electrode placement. Another measure, which is most critical, is to set an appropriate sensitivity threshold. The magnitude of the impedance respiration signal is in the range of 0.3 to 1.0 Ω, and the frequency components of the waveform are typically less than 5 Hz. Therefore, the device should be designed such that the minimum sensitivity setting is greater than the maximum excursion due to cardiac activity. Also, the device should filter any signals with frequency components greater than 6 to 10 Hz. These features are incorporated into the design of most monitors. Another crucial safeguard that most monitors use is a coincidence alarm. This alarm is triggered if the respiration rate equals the heart rate and is controlled by one of the device's microprocessors that is constantly comparing these two measured rates.[6, 10]

Although there are limitations to this method, it also has some notable advantages. First, impedance pneumography is a very cost-effective measurement because it utilizes the ECG monitoring components. Essentially, the clinician is obtaining two measurements, ECG and respiration, for the cost of one. Second, it is a noninvasive measurement and there is no additional patient inconvenience. This is a significant factor when dealing with neonates. Third, its application is simple for the clinician. Typically, a good signal only requires optimal integrity of the electrodes, lead wires, cable, and proper lead placement.[6]

There are other methods of monitoring respiration such as respiratory inductive plethysmography (see Chapter 15), nose and throat thermistors, proximal airway pressure sensors (see Chapter 16), pulse oximetry (see Chapter 10), and end-tidal CO_2 monitoring (see Chapter 12). There are those who feel that these methods are more accurate and reliable than impedance pneumography. However, it is generally accepted that no other method is as simple, noninvasive, and cost-effective as impedance pneumography for the measurement of respiration and apnea.[8–10]

Blood Pressure Monitoring

Blood pressure measurement is useful to examine when discussing signal processing because a signal generated by a single physiologic phenomenon is detected in numerous ways with varying degrees of effort and accuracy. For example, the contraction of the ventricles results in a blood pressure pulse that can be detected through the use of a cuff and the clinician's hearing ability. On the other end of the spectrum is a much more sophisticated system that requires the use of a catheter inserted into a vessel, a tubing system, a blood pressure transducer, and a monitor. Generally, the methods used to measure blood pressure can be classified as either indirect and noninvasive or direct and invasive. Each method is appropriate in certain cases, depending on the clinical condition of the patient, and each has its advantages and limitations. The following is a technical discussion of the various methods of noninvasive and indirect measurement and invasive hemodynamic monitoring. The differences between the two types of measurements will be discussed relative to a comparison of results when using different methods on the same patient.

Noninvasive Blood Pressure Monitoring

Although arterial blood pressure can be monitored noninvasively, it has limitations. There are three noninvasive methods used to obtain basic blood pressure information: auscultation, palpation, and oscillometry.

Auscultation

As the name implies, auscultation depends on an individual's or device's ability to detect sound. It is the most widely used method. As can be seen in Figure 4–7, it is a simple technique that requires a pressure cuff attached to a sphygmomanometer, stethoscope, and listening device that is typically in the form of an observer's ear. The cuff is placed on the patient's arm and inflated to a level greater than the expected systolic pressure, so that the vessel is sufficiently occluded. The stethoscope is placed over the brachial artery and the cuff is gradually deflated at a rate of approximately 3 mm Hg/heart beat. The first pulsations detected via the stethoscope represent the systolic pressure. As the blood vessel continues to reopen to its normal state, the pulsations gradually decrease and diastolic pressure is represented by the cuff pressure at which no pulsations are detected. These "sounds" are commonly referred to as Korotkoff sounds, and it is generally accepted that they closely approximate arterial systolic and diastolic values. Mean arterial pressure (MAP) is not directly measured and must be calculated based on the measured systolic and diastolic values. A simple calculation (the standard triangular estimate) for MAP is typically employed:

$$MAP = DP + 1/3(SP - DP)$$

where DP is diastolic pressure and SP is systolic pressure. This technique will yield varying results, depending on the observer's ability to hear and coordinate sound detection with a simultaneous observation of the manometer.[11, 12]

Palpation

Palpation is similar to auscultation in that it uses a pressure cuff and a sphygmomanometer. In addition, results can vary depending on the observer's sensitivity, in this case tactile versus audio. A cuff is placed on an arm or leg and inflated to occlude the arterial vessel sufficiently. One or two fingers are placed on a pulse point distal to the cuff. The pulsation first detected

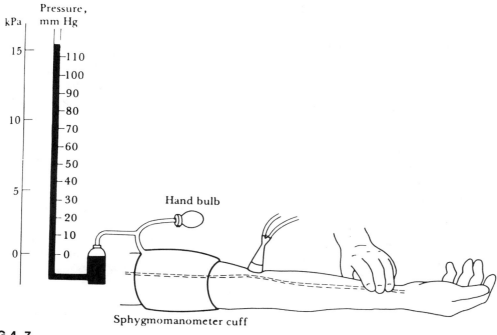

FIG 4–7.
Auscultation blood pressure measurement system. The handbulb inflates the sphygmomanometer cuff to a pressure greater than the patient's systolic blood pressure. Korotkoff sounds are detected using a stethoscope placed over a distal artery. (*From Rushmer RF: Cardiovascular Physiology. Philadelphia, WB Saunders, 1961. Used by permission.*)

represents the systolic pressure. A pulse transducer device such as a Doppler is often substituted for the clinician's fingers. This partially eliminates variability among users.

Oscillometry

Oscillometry is an automated method and, although it is the most complex, it is the most consistent and reproducible. An oscillometric device has a cuff and tubing, air pump, bleed valve, calibrated pressure transducer, signal processing components, and display device. The cuff serves the same purpose as in the previous techniques, and is applied by the clinician. This is the extent of interclinician variability. The cuff is automatically inflated to a predetermined level that is greater than most systolic pressures. If this predetermined level is not adequate to occlude the vessel completely, the device will reinflate the cuff to a greater pressure. Some noninvasive blood pressure (NIBP) monitors will automatically adjust the inflation pressure level after the systolic pressure has been determined. This is advantageous, however, only if the device is used continuously on one patient. The bleed valve then releases air from the cuff in step increments. These step increments are typically in the range of 3 to 6 mm Hg per step. The pressure transducer that is incorporated into the device monitors both the actual pressure in the cuff and the pulsations caused by the blood flow. Pulsations due to initial blood flow begin, increase in amplitude, and then rapidly decrease. The point at which the oscillations have reached maximum amplitude at the lowest pressure recorded by the transducer is considered to be the patient's MAP. Figure 4–8 illustrates both the cuff deflation pressure and the pressure oscillations due to blood flow. There are various methods used for determining systolic and diastolic pressures. Some use the point at which the oscillation amplitudes rapidly decrease as an index of diastolic pressure. Others determine the systolic pressure by the point at which the oscillation amplitudes suddenly increase. Others simply calculate one, and sometimes both, of these values. The method used to make these measurements is contained in the device's ROM. The monitor's microprocessor obtains the information and performs the necessary comparisons and calculations, and the results are then displayed for the clinician. Artifact rejection is a serious problem with this technique, because noise can often resemble pressure pulsations. Many manufacturers require that the device "see" two pulsations of relatively equal amplitude within one step in order to record the pressure. Figure 4–9 is a simplified block diagram of an oscillometric device.[11–13]

Oscillometric NIBP devices are used in hospitals, clinics, and even drugstores. They offer consistency, reproducibility, and time savings for the clinician. However, this measurement does have its limitations, which are discussed later in this chapter.

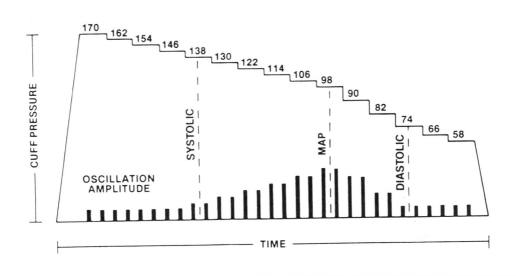

FIG 4–8.
The transducer in the Critikon Model 8100 Dinamap monitors both the cuff deflation pressure (*top waveform*) and the oscillations created by arterial blood flow (*lower portion of graph*). MAP is the point of maximum oscillation amplitude. (*From the Critikon Dinamap Model 8100 operator's manual. Used by permission.*)

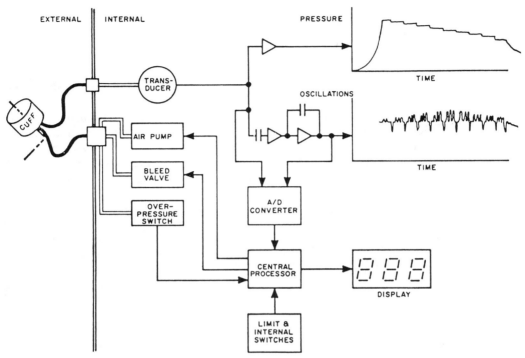

FIG 4-9.
Block diagram of the major components in an oscillometric NIBP device. The top right graph is the cuff pressure as controlled by the air pump and bleed valve. The lower right graph illustrates the pressure oscillations from blood flow as the arterial vessel reopens. (*From Ramsey M: Noninvasive automatic determinations of mean arterial pressure.* Med Biol Eng Comp 1979; 17:11–18. *Used by permission.*)

Invasive Blood Pressure Monitoring

The direct measurement of blood pressure is an example of a complex measurement that has been simplified by technological advances. It is interesting to study in terms of signal processing because of the complex nature of the waveform, the multiple components required for the measurement, and the critical factors involved in the accurate reproduction of the waveforms.

The basic features of an invasive blood pressure measurement system consist of the measured system or entity that provides the input signal, an input transducer, a signal conditioner, and an output transducer (usually in the form of a display where the clinician can obtain useful information for decision-making). The specific measured system for direct hemodynamic monitoring is the blood pressure of the patient at a specific physiological site (e.g., radial artery, right atrium, or pulmonary artery). The input signal is the pressure pulse that is a complex waveform resulting from the contraction of the ventricles and the traversal of the wave through the vasculature. The physiological signal is transmitted to the input transducer via a fluid-filled catheter that resides in the vessel at the measurement site and is connected to the transducer via fluid-filled tubing and stopcocks. From the transducer, the signal travels via a cable to the bedside monitor where it is conditioned and the blood pressure waveform and values are displayed. The morphology and magnitude of the waveform varies with the measurement site because of the effect of changes in vascular impedance as the pulse travels peripherally. Peripheral pressure waveforms have higher peaks and therefore higher systolic pressures than pressures measured centrally, as seen in Figure 4–10.

The pulsatile pressure is delivered to the transducer via an airtight, fluid-filled system. In general terms, a transducer converts a mechanical force into an electrical signal. In the specific case of blood pressure measurement, the transducer converts the patient's blood pressure to an electrical signal that is amplified, filtered, and displayed in meaningful terms for the clinician. A complete blood pressure measurement system from the patient to the monitor is illustrated in Figure 4–11.

The mechanical force of the patient's blood pressure causes a slight displacement of the mechanical component, a stiff diaphragm, in the transducer, which results in a proportional change in the electrical signal. The diaphragm is connected to a strain gauge, which realizes a change in resistance corresponding to a change in length due to the displacement. Note that current technology has allowed the measurement components to be contained in a small semiconductor chip. A more detailed description of the function of a transducer can be found in Chapter 3.

Requirements for Blood Pressure Catheter-Transducer Systems

The catheter-transducer systems used in blood pressure monitoring must be able to reproduce faithfully the complex physiological waveforms in order to ensure accurate measurement. These systems should be evaluated in terms of their frequency response. Catheter-transducer

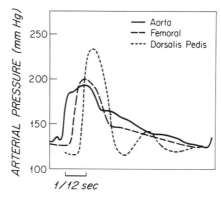

FIG 4–10.
Differences in pressure pulses at various physiological sites, both central and peripheral. The diagram illustrates the increase in the systolic peak as the waveform travels from the heart to the periphery.

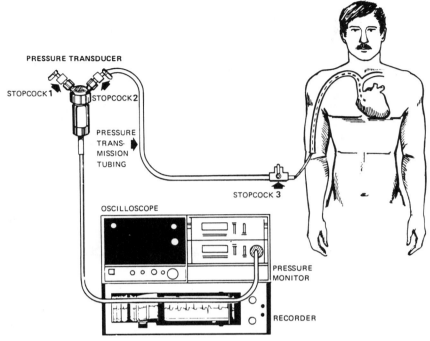

PRESSURE TRANSDUCER

STOPCOCK 1 | STOPCOCK 2

PRESSURE
TRANS-
MISSION
TUBING

STOPCOCK 3

OSCILLOSCOPE

PRESSURE
MONITOR

RECORDER

FIG 4–11.
Components of a blood pressure measurement system. The patient's pressure pulse provides the input signal, which is transmitted to the transducer via an indwelling fluid-filled catheter, a tubing system, and stopcocks. The transducer converts the mechanical force of the pressure pulse into an electrical signal, which is amplified, filtered, and displayed on the bedside monitor. (*From Schroeder, JS and Daily, EK. Techniques in Bedside Hemodynamic Monitoring, The C.V. Mosby Company, 1976. Used by permission.*)

systems fall into a category of systems known as underdamped, second-order dynamic systems. (The meaning of "underdamped" will be discussed in detail. The system is considered "second-order" because a second-order differential equation is needed to describe its dynamic response.) A similar type of system is one in which a mass is attached to a spring and the mass is pulled down and then released, resulting in oscillation of the system. This type of system is illustrated in Figure 4–12.

Underdamped second-order systems are characterized by three mechanical parameters: elasticity (the stiffness of the spring in the mass-spring system, or the stiffness of the transducer diaphragm in the catheter-transducer system), mass (the fluid in the tubing system), and friction (the movement of the fluid in the catheter and tubing system with each pressure pulse.)[14] These characteristics determine two parameters used in analyzing underdamped, second-order systems: the natural frequency and the damping coefficient. For the mass-spring system, the natural frequency is the number of oscillations of the mass per unit time. For a catheter-transducer system, the natural frequency refers to how rapidly the system oscillates.

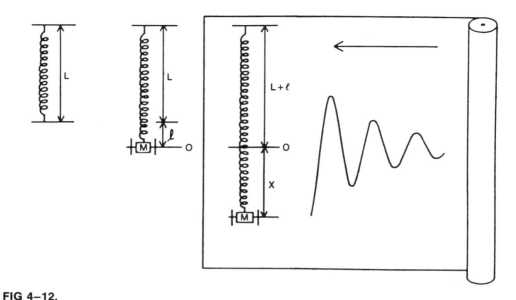

FIG 4–12.
A mass-spring system is shown at its equilibrium state. It is then displaced by a distance x and released. The resulting motion is recorded in time. The oscillations are characteristic of damped harmonic motion. The mass-spring system is an example of an underdamped second-order system. (*From Kleinman B: Understanding natural frequency and damping and how they relate to the measurement of blood pressure. J Clin Monit 1989; 5:137–147. Used by permission.*)

Because both of these systems exist in situations where friction is present, the frequency is known as the damped natural frequency. (In the absence of friction it would be called the undamped natural frequency.) Frictional forces affect how quickly the system returns to its resting position, which is indicated by the damping coefficient.

The degree of damping in the mass-spring system determines the motion of the mass, while for a catheter-transducer system it determines how well the system will accurately reproduce the waveform. The damping coefficient is the indication of the degree of damping. If there is no damping in a system, a mass will oscillate indefinitely. A small amount of damping (a damping coefficient equal to approximately 0.2) will result in some oscillation, with the mass eventually returning to rest. This type of system is considered underdamped. A sufficient amount of damping to just prevent oscillations (a damping coefficient equal to 1) would result in the mass returning to rest in a nonoscillatory fashion, similar to an exponential decay. This type of system is considered critically damped. An even greater amount of damping (damping coefficient >1) would result in the mass returning to rest in a similar manner, but in a longer time period than for a critically damped system. This system is considered to be overdamped. Finally, if the mass slightly overshoots the equilibrium position and then returns to rest (damping coefficient in the range of 0.4 to 0.6) the system is considered to be optimally damped. The various degrees of damping are illustrated[15] in Figure 4–13.

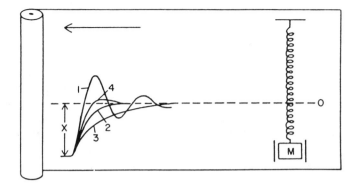

FIG 4–13.
The various degrees of damping of the mass-spring system are illustrated. The first curve (*1*) demonstrates underdamping, the second (*2*) shows critical damping, the third (*3*) illustrates overdamping, and the fourth (*4*) curve is an example of optimal damping. (*From Kleinman B: Understanding natural frequency and damping and how they relate to the measurement of blood pressure.* J Clin Monit *1989; 5:137–147. Used by permission.*)

If an external oscillatory force is applied to the system at a frequency close to the undamped natural frequency, the amplitude of the oscillations will greatly increase. The frequency of the force at which the amplitudes of the oscillations is maximum is the *resonant frequency*. Resonant frequency is illustrated in Figure 4–14. It occurs at the undamped natural frequency of the system.[15]

Due to the nature of the signal in blood pressure monitoring, it is crucial to ensure that it can be reproduced by the measurement system. The pressure pulse is a wave and therefore can be described in terms of frequency and amplitude. To analyze these physiological waves, the pulsatile signals are broken down into sinusoidal components. Thus, a pressure pulse can

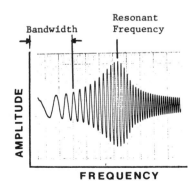

FIG 4–14.
A frequency sweep of an underdamped system shows the resonant frequency as the frequency at which maximum amplitude oscillation occurs.

be described as a sum of sinusoidal signals consisting of a fundamental frequency plus a number of harmonic frequencies, or multiples, of the fundamental frequency. The frequency of the periodic complex wave determines the frequency of the fundamental component.[7] The amplitude of the higher frequency components becomes progressively smaller as the harmonics increase. A measurement system must be able to reproduce adequately the fastest changing components of the wave in order to ensure its fidelity. Fidelity refers to the degree to which the output of a system accurately reproduces the essential characteristics of the input.

The frequency response of a blood pressure measurement system required for reproduction of the arterial pulse wave must extend from the fundamental frequency to the highest harmonic considered necessary for reproduction of the sharpest portions of the wave. The patient's heart rate in the case of blood pressure waveforms can be considered the primary determinant of the fundamental frequency. For example, if the patient has a heart rate of 60 beats per minute (bpm), then the fundamental frequency for reproducing the pressure wave would be one Hertz (i.e., 60 bpm/60 seconds per minute = 1 cycle/second, or 1 Hz). It is generally accepted that, for pulsatile physiologic waveforms, the fundamental frequency plus the first six harmonics will adequately reproduce the input signal. Figure 4–15 illustrates the harmonic components of a blood pressure waveform.

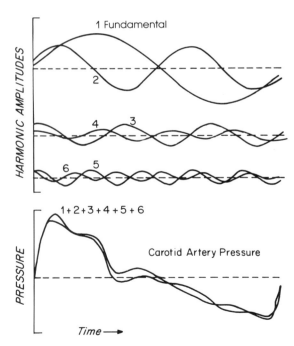

FIG 4–15.
Harmonic components of a physiological waveform. The illustrations at the top demonstrate the fundamental frequency and harmonics two through six. The bottom drawing illustrates the pressure waveform as a summation of these six harmonics.

If any of the frequencies contained in the pressure pulse approach the undamped natural frequency of the catheter-transducer system, the amplitudes of those frequencies will be augmented, resulting in false increases in the systolic peaks and, thus, incorrect measurements. Therefore, the requirement for accurate reproduction of the blood pressure waveform would be for the monitoring system to have a very high undamped natural frequency. The appropriate combination of natural frequency and damping varies depending on the patient's heart rate and the shape of the waveform. Higher heart rates and sharp fast-rising systolic peaks require higher undamped natural frequencies. The appropriate range of damping is dependent on the frequency of the system. Figure 4–16 shows the range of adequate dynamic response for a particular pressure waveform and heart rate. The higher the natural frequency, the greater the range of acceptable damping coefficients.[14]

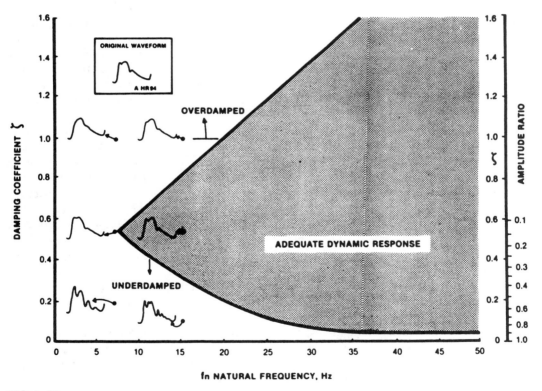

FIG 4–16.
The range of adequate natural frequencies and damping coefficients for a particular waveform and heart rate are shown in the shaded area. The effects of overdamped (loss of detail) and underdamped (overshoot and ringing) systems on the waveform are shown on the upper and lower left portions of the diagram respectively. (*From Gardner R. Direct blood presssure measurement—dynamic response requirements. Anesthesiology 1981; 54:321. Used by permission.*)

The dynamic requirements discussed above are influenced by certain situations and components of the catheter-transducer system. Dynamic response is affected by the increased compliance due to stopcocks and flush devices, which have a tendency to trap air bubbles. Extra lengths of tubing add mass to the system, which results in reduced dynamic response. Small air bubbles trapped in the tubing system add compliance to the system and may cause ringing, or overshoot, which results in false high systolic values. Conversely, large amounts of air or clotting can cause a loss of signal, resulting in a damped waveform, and falsely low systolic readings. Therefore, to maximize dynamic response, clinicians should ensure that the catheter-transducer systems used minimize the entrapment of air, utilize minimum tubing lengths, and employ the fewest number of components such as stopcocks as possible.

The Monitor

Some of the following technical specifics have been adapted from the HP 78350 series service manual. From the transducer, the electrical signal is sent to a monitor via a cable attached to a preamplifier. The excitation voltage is supplied to the transducer from the monitor via the transducer cable. The input signal from the transducer is transferred to an input amplifier with a proportional gain. Most monitors have the ability to detect whether the transducer has a sensitivity of 40 microvolts per volt per millimeter of mercury (μV/V/mm Hg) or 5 μV/V/mm Hg and will amplify the signal accordingly. Today, most transducers have a sensitivity of 5 μV/V/mm Hg. After amplification the signal is filtered before demodulation. A synchronous demodulator is used to rectify the signal using an operational amplifier that alternates between an inverting gain and a noninverting gain, using the excitation voltage for switching.[16]

An electronic filter is then used to remove the excitation frequency and leave the dc pressure signal. The cutoff frequency of low-pass filters used to restrict the bandwidth varies among the manufacturers of physiological monitors. Some monitors include filters that restrict the bandwidth to 12 Hz and lower in an effort to avoid amplitude distortion that occurs when pressure components have frequencies in the same frequency range as the resonant frequency of catheter-transducer systems. These filters attenuate frequencies above this range. As a result, useful and significant data contained in higher frequencies are lost, resulting in falsely low systolic pressure readings.[17]

The signal then travels by another amplifier to the system output and also to the analog-to-digital conversion stage. This stage uses a DAC and a comparator in a method based on successive approximations. The microprocessor supplies a number, and the DAC converts it to an analog signal, which is compared against the input voltage. The output of the comparator returns to the microprocessor for further processing. Monitors contain separate circuits for detection of a disconnection of the transducer from the monitor. Also, a DAC and amplifier are used to provide calibration, test, and zero compensation functions.[16]

The analog-to-digital converted pressure information is processed by the microprocessor in the digital circuits and the results are passed to a display board. The digital circuits also provide accurate storage and recall of the gain constant used by the internal software for the pressure signal display and output.[16]

Derivation of the Numeric Values from the Waveform

The pressure waveform is displayed on the monitor screen. It is often difficult, however, to determine the value of the pressure from the waveform if it is not displayed on a calibrated scale with adequate resolution. The monitor displays the digital values of the systolic, diastolic, and mean pressures as determined by a pressure algorithm that is implemented in software. The algorithm has some limited abilities in determining the sources of beat-to-beat variations in the pressure waveform, such as respiratory artifact in arterial pressures.

The algorithms for most monitors consist of two main processes. The first process is the detection of a heartbeat. The input to the algorithm is the pressure waveform and the output is the systolic, diastolic, and mean pressures for each beat. If the new pressures for each beat are continuously displayed, the values will constantly be changing at a fast rate and the clinician would not know which values to record. For this reason, the monitor evaluates the values and determines an appropriate average value for the display.

A simple rule can be used to determine this averaged value. When the mean pressure of the new beat is close to the mean pressure of the last beat, the new beat and the last beat are averaged using a weighting factor. A high weight is placed on the new beat in this case. When the new beat mean pressure differs from the mean value of the previous beat, a low weight is given to the new beat in the updated display value. Using this algorithm, stable beats are strongly preferred over unstable beats.[18]

When patients are mechanically ventilated, changes in the ventilation pattern produce changes in the pulmonary artery pressure without any apparent change in the patient's hemodynamic status. This problem can be reduced if beats are selected during the portion of the ventilatory cycle when the alveolar pressure is stable. The variation is generally minimized at the end of expiration. Changes in systemic arterial waveforms due to respiration, however, are clinically relevant. In this case, simple averaging of all the beats may be a better method than favoring end-expiratory beats.[19]

One algorithm that may be used in filtering beats for display is a variation of standard exponential averaging. It is described by the following equation:

$$\text{new filtered value} = \text{old filtered value} + (\text{new data point} - \text{old filtered value})/K$$

where K is the weighting factor for new data points.[19] The new data point is the pressure value of a new beat, the old filtered value is that which is displayed on the monitor, and K is the time constant of the filter. The greater the value of K, the lower the weight given to a new data point, and the more slowly the displayed value responds to changes in data. A greater time constant results in more stable displayed average values, but also slows the display response to substantial changes in pressure. Thus, there are two tasks for algorithms used in monitoring pulmonary artery pressures. First, it must identify beats that occur at or near the end of expiration; second, it must weight all beats so that the filtered, displayed value corresponds to the average of the end-expiratory beats.[19]

THE DISPLAY

The information must be displayed in a clear and meaningful way to be clinically useful. In the case of direct blood pressure monitoring, it is desirable to have both waveform information and digital values. The waveform information must be displayed on a calibrated scale to obtain accurate measurements. The information is also available to be printed for more careful examination and for a permanent record.

The traditional form of displays for direct hemodynamic monitoring has been an oscilloscope that uses a CRT. The CRT has been used for many years, and it provides a clear picture with minimal artifact. The CRT, however, is somewhat limiting because it is bulky, fragile, and requires a substantial amount of power. There are newer solid-state technologies that allow displays to have flat screens that are far less expensive.

One alternative to the CRT that uses less power and is less expensive is the liquid-crystal display (LCD). It gets its name from an organic material that has the optical properties of crystals and the fluidity of liquids. These displays do not generate light, but rather reflect it. The liquid-crystal molecules align themselves in the direction of an applied electric field. The alignment changes the liquid-crystal index of refraction and results in the color change that forms the display. The advantages of LCD displays are decreased weight and bulk, lower power consumption, and less expense. Its limitations include poor resolution and a narrow viewing angle.

Another type of technology that offers light weight and low power requirements is electroluminescent (EL) displays. These displays produce light by exposing a solid material to an intense electric field. The color of the light emitted is determined by the energy gap of the solid material. These displays have a better viewing angle than LCDs, but the resolution is not as good as that of a CRT.[20]

Differences Between Invasive and Noninvasive Monitoring of Arterial Blood Pressure

In the clinical environment, more than one method may often be used to measure blood pressure. For example, a patient may have an indwelling radial artery catheter placed to monitor blood pressure continuously, but a nurse may "check" the values obtained by using the auscultation method described above. Similarly, a nurse may attempt to "verify" the invasive pressure readings by using a combined technique that requires the occlusion of the brachial artery of the same arm as the indwelling radial catheter using a cuff. Detection of the systolic endpoint is established by using the waveform of the invasive line as displayed on the monitor as the distal sensor. The cuff pressure at the time of the first reappearance of the waveform is taken as the systolic pressure. Confusion results when clinicians expect values for pressures obtained from very different methods to agree.

Noninvasive indirect methods of blood pressure detection are completely different from invasive direct methods in terms of what is actually measured. Indirect methods measure flow or changes in volume of the cuff, while direct methods actually measure pressure. Each type of measurement is associated with a variety of sources of errors. Errors in measurement using invasive methods include failure to reference properly the transducer to atmospheric pressure and the appropriate physiological level, increased compliance and hence decreased frequency response due to excess air entrapment or extra lengths of tubing, and inappropriate filtering.

Most of the errors associated with noninvasive indirect methods are due to the observer or the technique. Sources of error for noninvasive methods include cuff size and placement, stethoscope application, deflation rate, detection sensitivity, detection endpoints, and respiratory variation. For noninvasive methods, the accuracy of the measurement is dependent on the appropriate cuff width for the subject's arm. A cuff that is too wide will yield false low measurements, while one that is too narrow will produce false high measurements. Additionally, the placement of the cuff on the arm is crucial because of hydraulic effects if the cuff is either too high or too low relative to the left ventricle. If the cuff is placed too high on the arm, the reading will be falsely low. If it is placed too low, the result will be falsely high measurements.

Additional errors are inherent in the auscultatory technique. If the stethoscope is applied with too much pressure, the artery will be distorted and sounds will be produced that will be heard below the subject's diastolic pressure, resulting in false low diastolic readings.[21] An appropriate rate of cuff deflation is crucial to ensure accuracy of noninvasive readings. The faster the deflation rate and the slower the heart beat, the greater the error. To ensure accuracy, the rate should be based on the heart rate, the most appropriate being 3 mmHg/beat. Figure 4–17 illustrates the importance of cuff deflation rate in detecting systolic pressure. Further error can be introduced by the observer's ability to hear. Accuracy will be affected by the differences in hearing among various observers. The specification of endpoints for diastole using auscultation are not well defined and have a tendency to change. For this reason, there may be discrepancies between diastolic measurements between observers. Finally, just as respiratory variations have an effect on invasive methods of measurement, they can also impact noninvasive readings that are taken at specific intervals, rather than continuously. For this reason it is important to time the measurements with the respiratory cycle to ensure the consistency.

Oscillometry has the potential for error in that the observer is not present during the measurement, so that artifact due to clinical or environmental factors is not eliminated and inaccurate measurements may result. Consistency is improved, however, because the rate of cuff deflation, detection sensitivity, and endpoint detection are all controlled by the device.

When making comparisons between measurements using different methods, several points should be considered. It should be realized that systolic detection in the form of Korotkoff sounds in the case of auscultation, or oscillations in the case of oscillometry, occurs after the artery has already begun to reopen due to cuff deflation. That is, at some point after systolic pressure. Thus, systolic measurements using noninvasive methods will always be somewhat lower than direct measurements due to differences in signal processing. Additionally, differences will result between the two types of measurements due to differences in the measurement sites. For noninvasive methods, the site is the brachial artery, while for invasive measurements the site is the radial artery. Studies have shown that systolic pressures measured invasively will be slightly higher than those measured noninvasively due to the difference in the physiological site of measurement. For all of the reasons outlined above, discrepancies generally exist between measurements performed using invasive and noninvasive techniques on the same

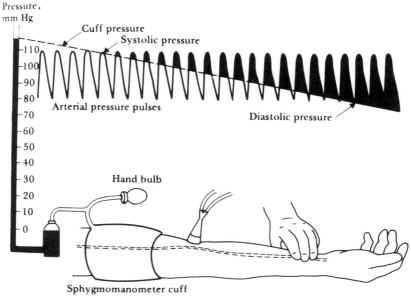

FIG 4–17.
Importance of cuff deflation rate in determining systolic pressure using indirect methods. Systolic pressure is slightly underestimated using these techniques. The faster the deflation rate, the greater the error. The appropriate deflation rate is dependent on the subject's heart rate (3 mm Hg per heartbeat). (*From Rushmer RF: Cardiovascular Physiology. Philadelphia, WB Saunders, 1961. Used by permission.*)

patient in close time proximity. Studies have shown that auscultation tends to underestimate systolic pressure as compared to direct methods by as much as 16 or 17 mm Hg, and overestimate diastolic pressure pressure by as much as 6 or 7 mm Hg when using the point of sound muffling as the endpoint.[22] Similarly, the oscillometric method tends to underestimate direct systolic pressure by approximately 9 mm Hg and overestimate direct diastolic pressure by approximately 9 mm Hg, while mean blood pressures correlate well.[23]

Most studies that investigate and quantify the differences between the two types of measurement used subjects who were critically ill. These were unstable patients who were either hypotensive or hypertensive. For these patients, the noninvasive techniques are less accurate. The differences between the signals and the manner in which they are processed to obtain the measurements used clinically should be taken into consideration when the clinician confronts conflicting data.

CONCLUSION

Monitoring technology has experienced dramatic changes over the last few decades. In fact, the monitors used in the 1970s bear little, and in some cases no, resemblance to those used today. Advances in technology have not only enabled more physiologic parameters to be measured, but the information is more accurate and consistent. Manufacturers who are involved with medical instrumentation have a responsibility to design devices that are user-friendly, cost-effective, reliable, and, above all, accurate. However, responsibility also rests with those who apply the technology. Understanding the limitations of a device is crucial to understanding its potential inaccuracies. Information should never be accepted blindly with no thought given to the question "Does this make sense?" Technology is merely a tool and should be regarded as such. Technical advances, coupled with sound clinical assessment and judgment, will continue to alter, and hopefully improve, patient care as it has done in the past.

REFERENCES

1. Fleming D, Feinberg B: *Handbook of Engineering in Medicine and Biology.* Cleveland, CRC Press, 1976.
2. Millman J, Halkias C: *Integrated Electronics: Analog and Digital Circuits and Systems.* New York, McGraw-Hill, 1972.
3. Webster J: *Medical Instrumentation: Application and Design.* Boston, Houghton Mifflin Co, 1978.
4. Graf R, Whalen G: *The Reston Encyclopedia of Biomedical Engineering Terms.* Reston, VA, Reston Publishing Co, 1977.
5. Oppenheim A, Willsky A: *Signals and Systems.* Englewood Cliffs, NJ, Prentice-Hall Inc., 1983.
6. ECRI, Infant home apnea monitors. *Health Dev* 1987; 16:79–109.
7. Geddes LA, Baker LE: *Principles of Applied Biomedical Instrumentation.* New York, John Wiley and Sons, 1989.
8. Warburton D, Stark A, Taeusch HW: Apnea monitor failure in infants with upper airway obstruction. *Pediatrics* 1977; 60:742–744.
9. Brouillette RT, Morrow AS, Weese-Mayer DE, et al: Comparison of respiratory inductive plethysmography and thoracic impedance for apnea monitoring. *J Pediat* 1987; 111:377–383.
10. Staewen W: Apnea monitoring basics. *Biomed Instrum Technol* 1991; 25:322–323.
11. Geddes LA: The indirect measurement of blood pressure. *Austral Phys Eng Sci Med* 1980; 3–2:66–82.
12. Gravenstein JS, Newbower RS, Ream AK, et al: *Essential Noninvasive Monitoring in Anesthesia.* New York, Grune and Stratton, 1980.
13. Ramsey M. Noninvasive automatic determination of mean arterial pressure. *Med Biol Eng Comp* 1979; 17:11–18.
14. Gardner, R: Direct blood pressure measurement—dynamic response requirements. *Anesthesiol* 1981; 54:227–236.
15. Kleinman, B: Understanding natural frequency and damping and how they relate to the measurement of blood pressure. *J Clin Monit* 1989; 5:137–147.
16. H-P 78354 monitor service manual, Hewlett-Packard, 1987.
17. Bruner JM: *The Handbook of Blood Pressure Monitoring.* Littleton, MA, PSG Publishing Co, Inc, 1978.
18. H-P 78553 module service manual, Hewlett-Packard, 1985.
19. Ellis DM: Interpretation of beat-to-beat blood pressure values in the presence of ventilatory changes. *J Clin Monit* 1985; 1:65–70.
20. Teschler L: New technology for flat displays. *Machine Des* July 23, 1991; pp 52–59.
21. Geddes LA: *Handbook of Blood Pressure Measurement.* Clifton, NJ, Humana Press, 1991.
22. Finnie KJC, Watts DG, Armstrong W: Biases in the measurement of arterial pressure. *Crit Care Med* 1984; 12:965–968.
23. Venus B, Mathru M, Smith R, Pham, CG: Direct versus indirect blood pressure measurements in critically ill patients. *Heart Lung* 1985; 14:228–231.

Chapter 5

Fundamentals of Metrology: Evaluation of Instrument Error and Method Agreement

Robert L. Chatburn, R.R.T.

"When you can measure what you are studying,
and express it in numbers, you have advanced
to the stage of science. When you cannot measure . . .
your knowledge is of a meager and unsatisfactory kind."

Lord Kelvin[1, 2]

INTRODUCTION

Modern monitors are like pushbutton phones; you can make a mistake ten times as fast as the old technology. Certainly they provide safe, quick, and convenient data for patient assessment. The utility of the assessment, however, is only as good as the accuracy of the biological signal. Clinicians must be familiar with the basic concepts of measurement theory in order to operate patient monitors and to evaluate new technology. The two fundamental concepts that should be understood are measurement error (relevant to the operation of patient monitors) and agreement between devices (relevant to the evaluation of new technology).

Issues related to error and agreement stem from the larger study of metrology (measurement science), which is concerned with the *truth* and *consistency* of observations. Truth relates to how closely the observations adhere to a "gold standard." In measurement theory (the theoretical branch of metrology), truth is called *validity*; in instrument science (the empirical branch) it is called *accuracy*. Accuracy, however, is not a static characteristic of measurements. Repeated measurements of a fixed quantity will exhibit variability in the degree to which the measured value reflects the true value. Although the individual values of repeated measurements change as a result of complex, random, and probably unknowable factors, as a group they often seem to follow a Gaussian or normal distribution. This observation leads to the concept of *consistency*, which relates to how closely the observations agree with one another when repeated. In measurement theory, consistency is defined in terms of *reliability*; in instrument science it is called *precision*.

As with other disciplines, the terminology of measurement science has developed rather haphazardly. This leads in some cases to ambiguity and outright contradiction. Although numerous standards exist for the various specialized areas of metrology, these are often not used because people who measure do not work within any particular field and because they are often not required to use standards. For example, many journals that report on measurement techniques do not specify the use of a particular nomenclature beyond the use of SI units.

In 1969, the Organisation Internationale de Metrologie Legale (OIML) issued a document entitled Vocabulary of Legal Metrology, Fundamental Terms. This document, in the French language, was translated by the British Standards Institution in 1971 as PD 6461. The following terms that predominate in common usage are taken from this translation[3]:

> *Discrimination (also called resolution):* the quality which characterizes the ability of the measuring instrument to react to small changes of the quantity measured
>
> *Accuracy:* the quality which characterizes the ability of a measuring instrument to give indications approximating to the true value of the quantity measured
>
> *Repeatability (also called precision):* the quality which characterizes the ability of a measuring instrument to give the same value of the quantity measured, not taking into consideration the systematic errors associated with the variations of the indications. Repeatability refers to short-term measurements with the same apparatus (i.e., the closeness of agreement among repeated measurements of the same variable under the same conditions).
>
> *Reproducibility:* repeatability determined by a long-term set of measurements or by different persons with different apparatus (i.e., the ability of the measurement system to maintain its output/input precision over a relatively long time).

Other commonly used terms that do not have official definitions will be discussed later.

The purpose of the following discussion is to explore the theoretical and practical aspects of metrology as they relate to method or device evaluation studies. Practical approaches to data analysis with examples will be presented for studies comparing measured values to known or true values and for studies comparing the results of two similar measurement systems.

MEASUREMENT THEORY

It has been said that measurement theory is the conceptual foundation of all scientific decisions.[4] Measurement provides the fundamental basis for research and development. The development of mechanical design involves three elements[5]: the inspirational, the rational, and the experimental. The inspirational is based on intuition and experience. Inspiration, guided by common sense, provides the creative impetus for development. The rational is based on laws of physics and mathematics. It provides the tools required to express the creative impulse. The experimental is based on measurement of the variables pertaining to the operation of the device or system under development. Experimental observation provides the feedback from reality. It is grist for the mill of developmental evolution.

Measurement is also a fundamental element of any control process. The concept of control requires the measured discrepancy between the actual and desired performances. Control systems must know magnitude and direction to react intelligently.

The two fundamental methods of measurement are *direct comparison* with a standard, and *indirect comparison* through the use of a calibrated system.[5] Measurements of length and weight are examples of the technique of directly comparing an object with an accepted standard (e.g., a ruler or standard mass). Ideally, the standard should be traceable (through three or four generations of copies) to the prototype kept by the National Institute of Standards and Technology (formerly called the National Bureau of Standards).

Indirect comparisons are made with some form of transducer connected to a chain of signal conditioning and display or recording devices. These components may be referred to as the measuring system. The system senses information about the measured object, then converts and displays the information in the form of an analogous displacement on a scale or chart or in digital format. The output is adjusted or *calibrated* by comparison to a known standard to provide truthful information about the physical quantity, property, or condition that the system measures (called the *measurand*).[6]

A calibration is said to be *traceable* if it can be traced back along a recorded line of increasingly more certain calibrations to the primary standard used in the SI system (usually through a network of laboratories that can perform the service). An instrument has no traceable validity if it cannot be proved at any time (especially after a failure) that its readings are in the official traceable line. Malfunction of an uncalibrated and nontraceable instrument means that previously collected data cannot be accepted because there is no way to reestablish the calibration to give the same readings after repair. Thus, ensuring traceability for an instrument is analogous to taking out insurance before a disaster occurs.[3]

The word *error* has two different meanings.[7] The primary use is to denote the difference between a measured value and the "true" one. The true value of a measurand is never actually determined, but rather is assumed either on the basis of comparison with a standard or by estimation from a series of measurements. Alternatively, error refers to the uncertainty in a measurement. An example is the expression 25 ± 3 mL, where ± 3 expresses the uncertainty in terms of some measurement of repeatability (e.g., the standard deviation of repeated measurements).

Every measurement is assumed to have errors associated with it, if for no other reason than that the true value of any quantity is unknowable. Even standards are simply the best estimate of a true value made from many carefully controlled measurements. In terms of measurement theory, errors fall into two categories: systematic errors and random errors.

Random errors occur in an unpredictable manner due to uncontrollable factors and cause measurements to both over- and underestimate the true value. The true value itself may vary slightly in a random fashion. As the number of repeated measurements of the same quantity increases, random errors tend to sum to zero. Hence the mean value of repeated measurements will converge on the true value. The central limit theorem of statistics says that both the sum and the mean of a set of random values will have an approximately normal distribution if the sample size is sufficiently large.[8] This provides the basis for establishing the probability of a given measurement value and hence the confidence in the reliability of our observations.

Systematic errors occur in a predictable (although not always controllable) manner and cause measurements to consistently either under- or overestimate the true value. Systematic errors are not affected by the number of repeated measurements made but can be reduced by proper calibration. Calibration, however, does not improve random error.

The effects of measurement errors may be expressed as:

$$\text{Measured value} = \text{True value} + (\text{Systematic error} + \text{Random error})$$

The observed measurement is seen as the sum of the true value and the errors.[9] The goal is to identify and minimize measurement errors.

Inasmuch as all measurements contain random and systematic errors regardless of how hard we try to eliminate them, they may be called "legitimate" errors. Specific sources of random and systematic errors, and techniques to minimize them, are discussed in the following section on instrumentation science.

One class of avoidable errors exists that may be considered "illegitimate,"[7] and should never be allowed to creep into measurements. These include blunders, or outright mistakes in reading instruments or in controlling the conditions of the experiment, and errors in performing calculations. So-called *chaotic errors* resulting from environmental disturbances (e.g., vibration or contaminating substances) that are of sufficient magnitude to obscure measurement data are also to be avoided.[5, 7]

INSTRUMENTATION SCIENCE

Instrumentation science involves the practical application of measurement theory to actual measurement systems. The instrumentation performance characteristics relating to error assessment are *accuracy* and *precision*.

Accuracy

Accuracy is a term whose definition is somewhat ambiguous, depending on how it is used. In general, accuracy refers to the maximum difference between a measured value and the true value,[5] and is often expressed as a percentage of the true value:

$$\text{Accuracy (\%)} = \frac{\text{Measured value} - \text{True value}}{\text{True value}} \times 100$$

Some authors[5, 10–13] define accuracy as a reflection of systematic error, or the difference between the mean value of a large number of repeated measurements and the true value (which is the definition of the statistical term *bias*). That is, an instrument that has high accuracy has low systematic error.[5, 7] However, there seems to be no logical reason to limit the definition of accuracy to systematic error. In fact, it appears to contradict the general definition of accuracy as the difference between the measured and true value (about which there is no disagreement) because the difference may always have some component of both systematic and random error. Also, as a practical matter, when a measurement is taken, all one really wants to say is that it probably is not incorrect by more than some specific amount. One recognizes the inherent uncertainty (i.e., random error) of a measurement and expects that to be included in the accuracy specification.

A more consistent definition of accuracy—and the one most commonly implemented by manufacturers—is that of maximum or total error (i.e., the sum of systematic and random errors) regardless of type, source, or direction (positive and negative random errors are assumed to be of the same magnitude).[1, 6, 14] Manufacturers use a variety of methods to arrive at accuracy specifications for their instruments. Yet they generally include random and systematic error in the specification as a worst case statistical estimate for a given reading (e.g., mean ± 2 standard deviations). However, some manufacturers specify the worst case accuracy as a nonstatistical value corresponding to the maximum error value found during the creation of a calibration curve (i.e., the largest horizontal distance from any data point to the curve[14]). Accuracy specifications may be related to a time frame (i.e., different specifications apply to 24-hour, 90-day, and 12-month time intervals after calibration) to account for drift.

Accuracy is commonly expressed as a percentage of the full-scale reading (Fig 5–1, A). For example, a reading of 80 on a scale of 0–100 may have a stated accuracy of ± 2% of full scale (i.e., ± 2% of 100), meaning that the true value may be as low as 78 and as high as 82. For instruments with digital readouts there may be a specification of ± a given number of digits. Both of these formats indicate a constant error. Alternatively, instrument accuracy may be specified in terms of a percentage of the actual reading (Fig 5–1, B), which indicates proportional error. (Constant and proportional errors are defined and explained below.) If accuracy (in %) is unqualified, full scale is assumed.[6] Accuracy may also be expressed in the form "±% full scale or ±% of reading, whichever is larger" (Fig 5–1, C). The significance of these different ways of specifying accuracy is detailed below.

Unfortunately, the common usage of the term accuracy is counterintuitive. An instrument that is considered highly accurate will have a low value for its accuracy rating and vice versa. The term inaccuracy more "accurately" describes the instrument's rating, although marketing managers mysteriously avoid this nomenclature.

Precision

A set of repeated measurements of the same quantity will generally exhibit some small differences among the observed values. Precision is defined as the degree of agreement among repeated results and is a quantification of random error.[1, 5, 7, 10] Dealing with the uncertainties of random error necessitates the use of statistical procedures. The most common way of assessing agreement, and hence specifying precision, is to calculate a statistic based on the

A

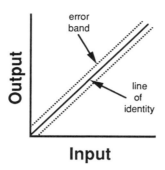

B

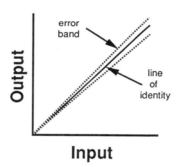

C

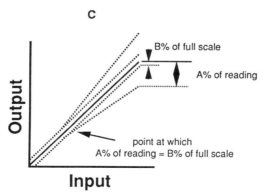

FIG 5–1.
Various conventions used to express the instrument inaccuracy specification. **A,** As ±% of full scale; **B,** a ±% of reading; **C,** as ±% of full scale or ±% of reading, whichever is greater.

difference between individual values and the mean value of the sample. The mean value of a sample of data is defined as:

$$\overline{X} = \frac{X_1 + X_2 + \cdots + X_n}{n} = \frac{1}{n} \sum_{i=1}^{n} X_i \qquad (5-1)$$

where n is the sample size. As the number of repeated measurements, n, increases toward infinity, the mean value of the measurements approaches the mean value of the theoretical population of all possible repeated measurements, μ, which is assumed to be the true value (assuming that systematic error is zero).[15] It follows that for any finite sample of data, not only do the individual values differ but the mean value differs from the true value. The variability in the raw data due to random error causes variability in the difference between the mean and true values. In any case, the sample mean is used as the best estimate of the true value, with large sample sizes being preferable.

The difference between an individual measurement and the mean (i.e., the deviation) is the random error of that particular measurement. Random error is assumed to follow a Gaussian or normal distribution and is usually quantitated in terms of the square root of the average squared deviation (i.e., the standard deviation S) for the group of repeated measurements:

$$S = \sqrt{\frac{1}{n-1} \sum_{i=1}^{n} (X_i - \overline{X})^2} \qquad (5-2)$$

When calculated according to Equation (5–2), the standard deviation of the sample is a point (i.e., single value as opposed to a range of values) estimate of the standard deviation of the theoretical population of repeated measurements, σ. (A point estimate is the best guess for the true value of a population parameter based on a single sample.)

Under the assumption of normality, it is possible to assign a probability to random error statements. We can either think in terms of the size of the random error itself or in terms of the scatter of the actual measurements around the mean value caused by random error. For example, we can say that 95% of the random errors will be smaller than 1.96 or approximately two standard deviations. Stated differently, 95% of individual measurements are expected to lie within the range of values from two standard deviations below the mean value to two standard deviations above the mean value. Such a range is referred to as the *error tolerance* or a *tolerance interval*.[12, 16] Because the tolerance interval includes the mean, or estimated true value, we can say that the tolerance interval is the range of values that contains the true value with a specific confidence level. A "two sigma" error (i.e., tolerance interval based on two standard deviations) is the one most commonly specified by manufacturers, although tolerance intervals using other multiples of the standard deviation are sometimes reported. Table 5–1 lists some random error estimates based on a normal distribution.

For a given set of measurements, as the tolerance interval widens the more confident we can be that it contains the true value. On the other hand, when comparing two or more sets of measurements or error specifications, the one with the smallest tolerance interval represents the greatest precision, assuming that the tolerance intervals are all defined the same way (e.g., as two sigma intervals). Remember that the tolerance interval will reflect either the variability

TABLE 5–1.
Error Estimates Based on a Normal Distribution

Name	Symbol	Confidence Level	Chance that a Single Value will be Greater
Probable error*	E_p	50%	1 in 2
Standard deviation†	σ	32%	1 in 3
Two sigma error	2σ	5%	1 in 20
	2.58σ	1%	1 in 100
Three sigma error‡	3σ	0.27%	1 in 370

* Also known as mean deviation (equal to 0.6745σ).
† σ represents the standard deviation of a population. (S represents the standard deviation of a sample taken from a population and is used as the best estimate of σ).
‡ Also called the practical maximum error of a single measurement.

of the method or of the quantity being measured or both *depending on the design of the experiment*.

Analogous to the tolerance interval is the concept of a *confidence interval*. As stated above, sample statistics such as the mean and standard deviation are point estimates of population parameters. Different samples will yield different values for these estimates. For example, the sample mean is assumed to have a normal distribution with a mean value equal to the population mean and a standard deviation ($S_{\overline{X}}$, also called the standard error of the mean) given by:

$$S_{\overline{X}} = \frac{S}{\sqrt{n}} \tag{5–3}$$

Thus, if we construct a range of values an appropriate number of standard errors above and below the sample mean, it will represent a confidence interval that contains the true value of the population mean 95% of the time:

$$\text{CI for } \mu = \overline{X} \pm t_{\alpha/2}\left(\frac{S}{\sqrt{n}}\right) \tag{5–4}$$

where t is the two-tailed t statistic for the desired confidence level and $n - 1$ degrees of freedom.

Confidence intervals can be constructed for the standard deviation as well as other statistics. Note that the difference between a tolerance interval and a confidence interval is that the former is a range of individual measurement values, whereas the latter is a range of calculated parameter values. As such, a tolerance interval is larger than a confidence interval.[12]

Precision should not be confused with resolution, defined as the smallest incremental quantity that can be measured.[6] Resolution is an inherent but often overlooked limitation of the ubiquitous digital display. A digit of such a display changes only when the sensor of the measurement device detects a change of some minimum amount. Any change less than this threshold amount is ignored. For example, digital pressure monitors for use with ventilators are often designed to read out in increments of 1.0 cm H_2O. When used to make repeated measurements of, say, the positive end-expiration measure (PEEP) level, they may give very precise (i.e., unvarying) readings but will not reflect pressure changes less than 1.0 cm H_2O due to vibrations caused by condensation in the ventilator delivery tubing. Of course, such small changes may be of no interest most of the time, but if they were, such a measuring device would be inappropriate.

Like accuracy, the common usage of the term *precision* is counterintuitive because a measurement considered to be highly precise has a small deviation from the true value and vice versa. To avoid further confusion regarding nomenclature, the term *inaccuracy* will be used to mean the total error of a measurement, *bias* to mean systematic error, and *imprecision* to mean random error. Therefore, a highly inaccurate measurement is one that is highly biased and/or highly imprecise (a scheme also used by Doebelin[14] and by Bourke et al.[17]). In terms of instrumentation science:

$$\begin{aligned} \text{Measured value} &= \text{True value} \pm \text{Bias} \pm \text{Imprecision} \\ &= \text{True value} \pm \text{Total error} \\ &= \text{True value} \pm \text{Inaccuracy} \end{aligned}$$

Thus we interpret an inaccuracy specification as meaning that any measurement of a known value will be within the given range with a given probability. The converse statement, that the true value will be within the same range from the measured value, is not always correct (see the section on Interpreting Error Specifications later in this chapter). Using this convention, if inaccuracy is positive, the measured value is said to overestimate the true value and vice versa. The effects of bias and imprecision on measurements are illustrated in Figure 5–2.

Imprecision

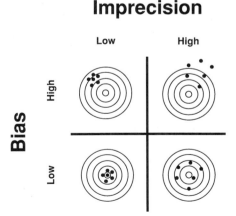

FIG 5–2.
An illustration of the effects of bias and imprecision (i.e., systematic and random error) using the analogy of target practice at a rifle range.

Severinghaus et al.[18, 19] have created an index of total error they call *ambiguity*. It is defined as the absolute sum of bias and precision (i.e., mean and standard deviation of error), preserving the sign when bias is significant at $P < 0.05$.

SOURCES OF ERROR: BIAS AND IMPRECISION

Having identified the two main categories of inaccuracy, bias and imprecision, the specific sources of these errors will be examined. First, however, it is important to review the concept of linearity and the related concept of calibration.

Linearity

Most instruments are designed to have a *linear* output. This means that a plot of the data representing the output of the device (i.e., the measured values) versus the input (i.e., the known or standard values) can be fit with a straight line. Furthermore, the ratio of output to input (referred to as *static sensitivity*[14]) remains constant over the operating range. The importance of linearity is that once a measurement system is calibrated with at least one known input, unknown input values will be faithfully represented by the output over the linear range.

The linearity (or rather nonlinearity) specification for a system can be assessed by first fitting the best straight line to the instrument's response curve over the range of acceptable input values. Then linearity is characterized as the maximum allowable deviation from this line expressed as a percentage of full scale, or as a percentage of the reading similar to the way that inaccuracy is specified (except that the linearity specification is relative to the best straight line thorugh the data, while accuracy is relative to the line of identity).[10, 14] For a device with negligible bias, the specification of nonlinearity is equivalent to the nonstatistical specification of overall accuracy (mentioned above) because the straight line that best fits the data is the line of identity. Thus, some commercial instruments give only a linearity specification and not an accuracy specification. On the other hand, an accuracy specification but not a linearity specification may be given if linear behavior of the device is implied by a fixed sensitivity specification.[14]

A more sophisticated procedure is to calculate the *harmonic distortion*. A nonlinear system will produce frequency components (harmonics) in the output that are not present in a sinusoidal input signal (which oscillates at the fundamental frequency). Harmonic distortion is calculated from the output signal as:

$$\text{Harmonic distortion} = \left(\frac{\text{Sum of the squares of amplitudes of all harmonics}}{\text{Square of amplitude of the fundamental frequency}} \right)^{\frac{1}{2}}$$

The higher the value for the harmonic distortion, the more nonlinear the system is judged to be.[9, 20, 21]

Calibration

When a measurement system is made, the manufacturer will often supply with it a calibration curve, which is simply a plot of the instrument's output for a series of known inputs. For devices like rotameters and flowmeters, these curves are necessary to convert the output of the device during use into accurate measurements because their performance (i.e., their output reading to input characteristics) cannot be changed. For other types of devices, such as electronic pressure transducers and gas concentration analyzers, it is possible to change the output to match known values. Thus, before the device is used it must be calibrated.

For a linear measurement system, calibration can be a simple two-step procedure. First the readout is set to zero while no input signal is applied to the instrument. (A modification of this is to select a known input signal having a low value on the readout scale such as the use of 21% oxygen during the calibration of an oxygen analyzer.) Next, the sensitivity (gain or slope) is set by applying an input signal of known value (such as 100% oxygen for an oxygen analyzer), preferably at the upper end of the output range, and adjusting the readout to this value (Fig 5–3. If the instrument has good linearity, the readouts for all input values between these two calibration points will be accurate. The measured values during an experiment will be very near the true values and the response curve will closely follow the line of identity.

If very accurate measurements are required over a limited range of the measurement scale, the device should be calibrated to a known value close to the value(s) of the quantity to be measured. It may then be possible to construct a new response curve and error rating for that portion of the scale which is expected to be used.

This leads to another question. What "gold standards" are appropriate for the calibration of monitoring equipment? Many monitoring devices measure pressure, volume, and flow. The primary calibration procedure for static pressure transducers is a liquid manometer; for volume transducers, a calibrated syringe, and for flow transducers, volumetric displacement (e.g., using a spirometer) by a constant flow over a known period of time, assuming that the spirometer and timing device are accurately calibrated. An alternative flow calibrating proce-

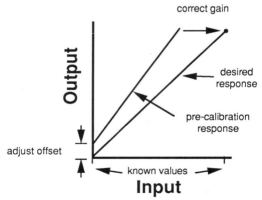

FIG 5–3.
The two-point calibration procedure. First the offset is adjusted then the gain is corrected.

dure is to connect the flow measurement system to a calibrated laboratory-grade rotameter.[5, 10] Such devices should be calibrated at known values spanning the entire range of expected measurements. In addition, dynamic as well as steady-state calibrations should be made when appropriate. A typical example of this is the American Thoracic Society recommendation for using standardized waveforms as inputs to pulmonary function evaluation equipment.[22]

Gas analysis devices are calibrated with reference gas mixtures, for which component concentrations are certified by the vendor. Partial pressure measurements are checked using values calculated from known gas concentrations and accurate pressure measurements. Analyzers should be checked for linearity and accuracy using at least three concentrations of gas over the entire range of the instrument.[10]

It is interesting to note that some widely used devices are not routinely calibrated. Their day-to-day performance is accepted solely on the blind faith that the manufacturer would not sell an inaccurate product or that the device operates the same as it did when new. Electronic thermometers and sphygmomanometers are two examples. Perhaps the most glaring example is the ubiquitous pulse oximeter. This device is used daily to make life support decisions, yet the user is not able to calibrate the output. Early models of the Hewlett Packard ear oximeter did include a filter that served as a standard, but current devices are not similarly equipped. One could argue that the accuracy of these devices is not critical. However, this depends on how they are used and the types of decisions they support. Aside from this, it seems imprudent to assume either the competence and good will of a manufacturer or the consistent performance of a device over extended periods of use. Investigation of these issues might prove interesting.

Sources of Bias

Constant Error.—If the zero point is not set correctly but the gain is correct, the instrument will be biased and will consistently read low or high over the entire scale. This form of bias is referred to as *constant* or *offset error* (Fig 5–4, A).[9, 11, 12, 23] *Drift error* is a form of time-dependent offset error in which the bias is minimal at the beginning, but increases over time as the instrument is used. Analog integrators are particularly susceptible to drift and need to be constantly re-zeroed.

Proportional Error.—On the other hand, if the zero point is set correctly but the gain is wrong, the bias will be dependent on the input level. The higher the true input value, the more error (either higher or lower than true value) there is in the measured value. This is known as *proportional error* (Fig 5–4, B).[9, 11, 12, 23] Constant and proportional errors can occur together or independently.

Range Error.—Even with proper calibration, other errors may arise. Range error occurs when the true value of the input signal is outside the operating range of the instrument (Fig 5–4, C). Signals that are either below or above the calibrated scale values may be clipped (i.e., the true value changes but the readout does not). A more insidious form of range error occurs when the instrument continues to give a readout for over-range values but with proportional

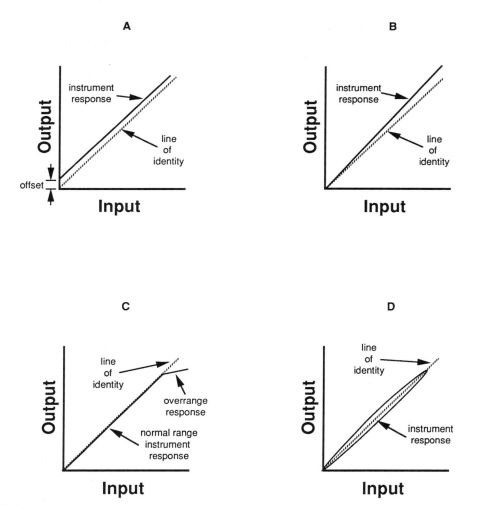

FIG 5–4.
Common sources of error in measurement systems. **A,** Constant systematic error; **B,** proportional systematic error; **C,** over-range error introduced when measurements are made beyond the highest calibrated level; **D,** hysteresis.

or hysteresis errors. In the worst case, the instrument may be damaged and fail when exposed to over-range conditions.

Hysteresis. — If an instrument gives a different reading for a given signal value depending on whether that value is approached from a larger or smaller reading (i.e., the input is decreasing or increasing), the device is said to show hysteresis (Fig 5–4, D).[9, 10] Hysteresis errors may be positive, negative, or a mixture of both. It is possible to mistake this form of error as being random error without a careful examination of the order in which observations are made.

Response Time. — Response time is a measure of how long it takes a device to respond to a step change (i.e., an instantaneous change from one constant level to another) in the measurand.[6] There are two accepted methods for stating response time. The first is simply to give the time constant, which is the time required for the device to read 63% of the step change (Fig 5–5, C).[24] For example, if an oxygen analyzer giving a stable reading in room air is

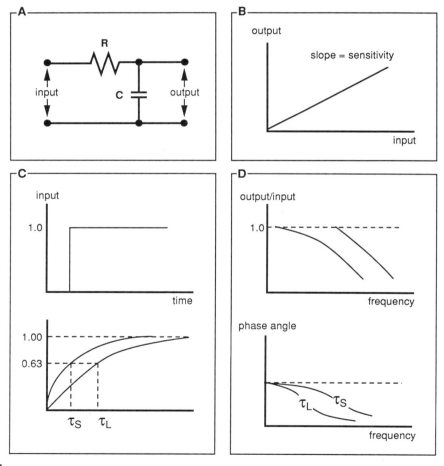

FIG 5–5.
A, A low-pass RC filter, an example of a first-order instrument (see *Respir Care* 1982; 27:276–281 for a practical application). **B,** Static sensitivity for constant inputs. **C,** Step response for long time constants (τ_L) and short time constants (τ_S). **D,** Sinusiodal frequency response for long and short time constants.

immediately exposed to 100% oxygen, the time constant is the time required for the meter to read 50% [i.e., $0.63 \times (100 - 21)$]. The advantage of specifying the time constant is that the time required to measure any given percentage of the step change can be calculated from the equation:

$$\text{Measured value } (\%) = 100A(1 - e^{-t/\tau})$$

where A is the magnitude of the step change, τ is time measured from the beginning of the step change, e is the base of the natural logarithm (≈ 2.72), and t is the time constant.

The other way of stating response time is to give the time necessary to reach 90% of the step change (sometimes modified as the time to go from 10 to 90%). For example, a 90% response time of about 100 ms is required for breath-by-breath analysis of respiratory gases.[10] Slow response times can cause errors during calibration if the user does not allow enough time for the instrument to stabilize at the known values. For practical purposes, it takes about five time constants to reach a steady-state value.

Frequency Response.—Frequency response is a measure of an instrument's ability to measure an oscillating signal accurately.[6, 10, 25] This performance characteristic is expressed in the form of two relations: (1) the measured signal amplitude (expressed as the ratio of output to input) as a function of signal frequency and (2) the phase shift (between the displayed signal and the actual signal) as a function of frequency. A device that is calibrated for a given frequency range may exhibit errors in the magnitude and timing of the measured signal if used at higher frequencies.[9] Measurement systems will generally either underestimate (attenuation) or overestimate (amplify due to resonance) the true signal amplitude as the frequency increases (Fig 5–5, D). Frequency response problems are especially evident for pressure and flow measurements and with instruments using analog meter readouts.[26–31]

Loading Error.—This type of error is of particular importance. A basic axiom of measurement theory is that "the measurement process inevitably alters the characteristics of both the source of the measured quantity and the measuring system itself, from which it must follow that there will always be some difference between the measured indication and the corresponding to-be-measured quantity."[5] For example, placing a pneumotachometer in a flow stream changes the flow rate because of the added resistance. Also, when electronic devices are coupled together, unrecognized electronic loading can occur and be quite serious.[10]

Environmental Conditions.—If a measurement system is used under significantly different conditions (e.g., pressure or temperature) than those under which it was calibrated and if no correction is made, systematic errors may result.[7] Typical examples are the effects of barometric pressure and humidity on polarographic oxygen electrodes and the effects of gas composition on pneumotachometers.

Operator Errors.—Between-observer variations in measurement technique and within-observer habits (such as always holding one's head to one side while reading a needle and scale having parallax) can result in bias.[7, 17] Human observers also exhibit what is known as "digit preference."[17, 32] Anytime an observer must read a scale, a guess must be made as to the last digit of the measurement. Most people tend to prefer some digits over others. For example, a blood pressure of 117/89 mm Hg is rarely recorded. Observers tend to prefer terminal digits of 5 and 10. Thus, readings such as 120/85 mm Hg are far more commonly recorded.[17]

A related issue is the way observers round numbers. For example, many people will round a number with a terminal digit of 5 to the next highest number. However, this will lead to a bias toward rounding up rather than rounding down if the data are contaminated by terminal digit bias. To avoid this, rounding of numbers with a terminal digit of 5 should be detemined by the digit to the left of the 5. If this digit is even, the number should be rounded down; if it is odd, the number should be rounded up.[33] Thus, 3.45 is rounded to 3.4 whereas 6.15 is rounded to 6.2. The choice of the appropriate number of significant digits to use when rounding results may also vary among observers, although guidelines are available.[33, 34] As a rule of thumb, for experiments involving 10 or fewer measurements, the precision (i.e., standard deviation) should be expressed with no more than two significant figures, and the standard error with one.[34] Errors of judgment, when important, can be minimized by implementing detailed research protocols.

Sources of Imprecision

Noise.—Numerous sources of random error introduce imprecision into measurements. All measurements are subject to some degree of noise, or minor, rapidly changing disturbances caused by a variety of environmental factors. Electronic and mechanical components of measurement systems are affected by temperature, pressure, and humidity changes as well as mechanical disturbances such as vibration. We are also continuously bathed in a sea of stray electromagnetic radiation (e.g., radio and television signals). Electronic devices are particularly susceptible to the ubiquitous "60 cycle noise" arising from electrical power lines. These disturbances may be difficult to trace and are not affected by calibration procedures. They are, however, usually considered to occur randomly so that their effects cancel out if enough repeated measurements are made. Noise can be particularly disturbing with weak signals that are highly amplified. The noise is amplified along with the signal such that a limit is eventually placed on the sensitivity of the measurement.

Nonlinearity.—Nonlinearity of the measurement system response is considered to cause imprecision because it will introduce an unpredictable error that varies over the operating range depending on the level of the input signal (in contrast to a proportional error, which is predictable). Many instruments in common usage in respiratory care are not ideally linear but are adequate for their intended applications. Errors due to nonlinearity can be minimized by calibrating at two points within the range in which most measurements will be made (Fig 5–6).

Operator errors can also be random. For example, within-observer variations may be caused by reading a dial at different angles, failing to judge the exact reading consistently, or slight variations in preparing transducers (e.g., transcutaneous electrodes) or samples.[17]

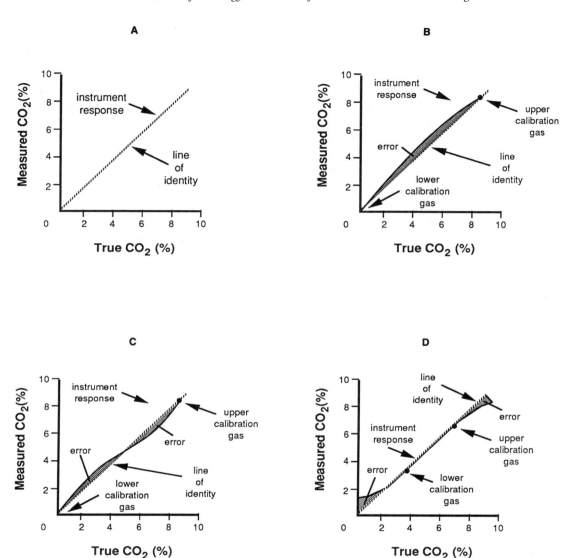

FIG 5–6.
Errors due to instrument nonlinearity. **A,** An instrument ideal response showing perfect linearity an proper calibration; **B,** logarithmic response characteristic of an unlinearized infrared CO_2 gas analyzer. Zero and gain are properly adjusted using a two-point calibration procedure but significant errors are introduced for measurements between the calibration points; **C,** partially linearized instrument. Calibration is the same as in **B; D,** partially linearized instrument with the same response characteristics as shown in **C** but calibrated with low and high gases in the range of expected measurements. (*From Norton,* Respir Care *1979; 24:131–137. Used by permission.*)

Even if the above sources of error are minimized, errors may be caused simply by the lack of a precise definition of the quantity to be measured.[7] A classic example of this in pulmonary physiology is the measurement of transpulmonary pressure. The definition of transpulmonary pressure requires that the pressure surrounding the lungs be measured. However, it is questionable whether this measurement can really be made even with a catheter in the pleural space. Measurements of esophageal pressure (assumed to reflect pleural pressure changes) only compound the potential errors.[35]

PROPAGATION OF ERRORS IN CALCULATIONS

Often, a physical quantity of interest is not measured directly, but is a function of one or more different measurements made from an experiment. For example, resistance and compliance of the respiratory system are not measured directly, but are calculated from measurements of pressure, volume, and flow. In such cases, the bias and imprecision of the calculated parameter depends on the bias and imprecision of the measurements.

Given two or more variables (e.g., X and Y) and their means and standard deviations (e.g., $\overline{X}$, S_X and $\overline{Y}$, S_Y) we are interested in estimating the mean and standard deviation of a calculated parameter Z (i.e., $\overline{Z}$ and S_Z). For this, the following equations have been suggested[7, 34]:

Scale factor: Let $Z = aX$, then:

$$\overline{Z} = a\overline{X} \qquad S_Z = aS_X$$

Sum or difference: Let $Z = X \pm Y$, then:

$$\overline{Z} = \overline{X} \pm \overline{Y} \qquad S_Z = \sqrt{S_x^2 + S_Y^2}$$

General linear combination: Let $Z = a + bX + cY + \ldots$, then:

$$\overline{Z} = a + b\overline{X} + c\overline{Y} + \ldots \qquad S_Z = \sqrt{(bS_X)^2 + (cS_Y)^2} + \ldots \qquad (5-5)$$

Logarithmic function: Let $Z = \log x$, then:

$$\overline{Z} = a \log \overline{X} \qquad S_Z = \frac{aS_X}{\overline{X}} \qquad (5-6)$$

General product: Let $Z = \alpha X^a Y^b$, then:

$$\overline{Z} = \alpha \overline{X}^a \overline{Y}^b \qquad S_Z = \overline{Z}\sqrt{\left(\frac{aS_X}{\overline{X}}\right)^2 + \left(\frac{bS_Y}{\overline{Y}}\right)^2 + \ldots} \qquad (5-7)$$

Note that the standard error of Z can be calculated by substituting the standard error in place of the standard deviation in the above equations for the general linear combination and the general product.[34]

INSTRUMENT PERFORMANCE EVALUATION STUDIES

Any evaluation of a measurement system must address one fundamental question: Is the inaccuracy of the system acceptable for the intended use? More specifically, we usually want to know how close a single measurement value will be to the true value and how much confidence can be placed in it. Before any judgment can be made, we must (1) have decided beforehand what level of inaccuracy is acceptable and (2) evaluate the inaccuracy of the system in question. These two components are both elusive and confusing. What follows is an attempt to summarize the major issues and provide a practical approach to performance evaluation experiments.

Some standard allowable total error for a given type of measurements is required before a particular device can be judged acceptable. Such standards may be generated in several ways:

1. On the basis of the intended application. For example, a simple oxygen analyzer used in an adult ICU may have an allowable error of ±2% of full scale because such a small discrepancy will have little clinical effect. However, measurement of oxygen concentration for the purpose of calculating gas exchange parameters requires much better accuracy. Norton[36] has shown that an error of 1% in the measurement of oxygen concentration leads to an error of 24% in the calculation of oxygen consumption and 32% in the calculation of respiratory exchange quotient. He therefore recommends an allowable error of 0.1% for oxygen analyzers used for these purposes. On the other hand, he demonstrates that an error of 5 mm Hg ($\approx$1%) in the measurement of barometric pressure leads to a negligible error ($\approx$0.02%) in the conversion of volume from ATPS to BTPS.
2. On the basis of the inaccuracy of similar, commonly used measurement systems (e.g., the acceptance of pulse oximetry on the basis of results comparable to *in vitro* oximeters)
3. By professional consensus (e.g., standards set by the American Thoracic Society and the International Standards Organization)
4. By arbitrary statistical methods (e.g., if the standard deviation of the measurement method is one-fourth or less of the normal population standard deviation, then analytic imprecision may be judged to be negligible[12]).

Note that even if the allowable error can be agreed on, it is important to know the value or range of values of measured quantities that represent cutoff points for medical decisions. For example, an imprecision in Ptco$_2$ readings of ±15 mm Hg might be reasonable for Po$_2$s above 100 mm Hg but would not be adequate for lower values in the range that might indicate hypoxemia.

There is a conspicuous lack of standards for measurement systems used in respiratory care. Clinicians generally accept with open arms whatever technology is developed. The philosophy seems to be that it is better to measure something with whatever accuracy the state-of-the-art will allow than to not be able to measure it at all. Yet this overlooks the possibility of doing harm by basing clinical decisions on inaccurate measurements. Sometimes incorrect information is worse than no information at all. One theoretical example is the possibility of increasing the incidence of retrolental fibroplasia in premature infants as a result of using pulse oximeters to wean FIO_2.

We need not and, perhaps, should not look outside of our own profession for standards regarding medical instrumentation. As one authority has already stated "One principle remains clear: If professional organizations do not take an active role and do not provide the assurance of quality and professional responsibility, then regulatory and governmental agencies will become actively involved in the process and will set the rules by which we practice our profession. Therefore, it is incumbent upon pulmonary professionals to take the lead and to prepare standards of practice for our profession."[37]

Assuming that some standard is available for a particular type of measurement, the next problem is to quantitate the level of inaccuracy that the system exhibits. Two general categories of studies are to be considered. One is the comparison of measured values to values that are assumed to be known with negligible error. Examples include the comparison of measured PO_2 to various known levels obtained from tonometered solutions, the comparison of electronic pressure transducer readings with readings from a water manometer, or the comparison of a pneumotachometer with flow rates indicated by a laboratory rotameter. In each case, the measurement system in question is first calibrated to manufacturer's directions and then its performance is compared to a source of known values or values measured with systems so accurate that their readings are assumed to give true values. Because the true values are assumed to be known in such studies, the objective is to estimate the total error or inaccuracy of a given measurement system.

The other type of study involves the comparison of one measurement system to another when both are measuring an unknown value. Usually, the purpose of such a study is to compare a new (perhaps quicker and less expensive) measurement system to an existing system whose performance has previously been judged acceptable. Some examples include the comparison of $PtcO_2$, $PtcCO_2$, and oxygen saturation measurements with measurements of blood samples. The true values of these variables in blood samples taken from patients are never known. They can only be estimated using accepted measurement systems that have been properly calibrated and maintained with strict quality control procedures. Therefore, the objective is to discern the *agreement* between the two systems.

GENERAL EXPERIMENTAL APPROACH

A complete examination of experimental design is beyond the scope of this discussion. In general, however, pairs of data (i.e., measured versus known values or values from two methods for a given level of input) should be gathered over a wide range of input levels (one data pair per input level). These data will provide information about bias and some information about imprecision. Additional data pairs may be gathered from repeated measurements at selected input levels (i.e., critical levels corresponding to cutoff points for making decisions) to provide better estimates of imprecision. The sample size for a given experiment will be limited by many practical factors. However, the larger the sample, the more closely the estimates of bias and imprecision will reflect the characteristics of the theoretical population, that is, of all observations made with a given measurement system.

Experiments should be planned with a consideration of the possible sources of bias and imprecision (discussed above). For example, to estimate the inaccuracy expected in the normal daily operation of a measurement system, data should be collected over the entire range of measurements that will be used clinically and over a period of days to account for errors due to the magnitude of measurements and to variations in environmental and operator factors, and even calibration errors. On the other hand, if the inaccuracy of the system alone is desired, repeated measurements of the same quantity should be made within a short time frame with all other confounding factors held as constant as possible.

EVALUATION OF INACCURACY[11, 12, 38]

Perhaps the most commonly recommended approach to the assessment of total error involves linear regression analysis. However, this approach is only appropriate if the data are judged to be linear.

Assessing Linearity

The first step in any analysis of comparison data is to make a scatter plot of the data. The data set should contain at least six known input levels that range from the lower to the upper limits of measurement and should include values near medical decision levels.[11] The measured value (dependent variable) is plotted on the Y-axis versus the known value (independent variable) on the X-axis with the line of identity drawn at 45 degrees. Assuming that the measurement system in question has been properly calibrated, the data should lie close to the line of identity. Linearity is assessed as a tendency for the data to follow a curved rather than a straight line. There is an alternative method of plotting the data that sometimes shows nonlinearities more clearly.[39] In this case, the difference between data pairs is plotted on the Y-axis versus the known value on the X-axis with a horizontal line drawn through zero difference. If the magnitude of the differences is not constant over the range studied, either a proportional error or a change in the imprecision has occurred. In either case, the standard error of the estimate (see below) may be misleading because it will increase as values of X increase. If porportional error is present, the coefficient of variation (i.e., the standard deviation of repeated measurement values divided by their mean value) will be constant over the range of measured values. However, in this case, it has been shown that if the coefficient of variation is less than 20%, the least-squares regression line is still correct.[40]

The plot of the data should be inspected for *outliers*, or values that depart from the expected distribution. Outliers at the upper and lower limit of the range will have a strong effect on the estimates of systematic error. Outliers near the center of the range will have a strong effect on the estimate of random error. Any of the sources of error mentioned previously can cause unusually large deviations from the desired linear relation. Outliers are identified as any measurement that is more than k standard deviations from the mean, where k is based on the sample size and the significance level (Table 5–2).[38] Any occurrence of an outlier should be examined for evidence of a real source of nonlinearity rather than a spurious error. The occurrence of more than 3 unexplained outliers per 100 observations suggest that there may be a serious problem with the measurement system.[12]

In some cases, a subjective judgment of the degree to which the data follow a straight line is sufficient.[11] However, a formal decision can be made based on statistical (e.g., chi square) analysis.[5, 12] If the data are found to be nonlinear, they may sometimes be put into a linear form using a mathematical (e.g., logarithmic) transformation.[12, 41]

Estimating Bias

Bias, or systematic error, can be estimated using linear regression analysis. The general idea of this procedure is to fit a linear equation of the form $Y = a + bX$ to the set of comparison data using the technique of least squares. (In this application of regression analysis, it is important to remember that X and Y values are two different estimates of the same quantity, and if there were no measurement error, they would be equivalent.) The least-squares method minimizes the sum of the squared deviations about the regression line (i.e., vertical distances from actual data points to the line).

Once the regression equation is derived, the predicted value of Y as a function of X, symbolized by $\hat{Y}$, can be calculated as

$$\hat{Y} = a + bX_0$$

where X_0 is the known (assumed "true") value for which a predicted value of Y is desired, and $\hat{Y}$ represents the estimated mean value of an indeterminate number of repeated measurements of X_0.

The derived parameters a (the estimate for the Y intercept) and b (the slope of the line) give estimates of constant and porportional systematic errors.[40] Thus, the difference between a predicted value and the associated true value represents the bias (i.e., mean total systematic error) of the measurement:

$$\text{Bias} = (\hat{Y} - X_0) \qquad (5\text{–}8)$$

Bias calculated in this way is a point estimate whose value will change with each new sample. (A point estimate is the best guess for the true value of a population parameter based on a single sample.) Alternatively, a confidence interval for bias may be expressed as the point estimate of bias plus or minus a multiple of the standard deviation of the mean:

$$\text{CI for bias} = (\hat{Y} - X_0) \pm t_{\alpha/2}\left(\frac{S}{\sqrt{n}}\right) \qquad (5\text{–}9)$$

TABLE 5–2.
Factors for Determining (a) Outliers in Raw Data;
(b) Tolerance Intervals; (c) Confidence Intervals
for the Standard Deviation of the Mean Value
(i.e., Standard Error of the Mean) of a Series of
n Measurements with a Known Standard
Deviation

(a)

n	Confidence Level 95% k	99% k
9	4.42	7.10
10	4.31	6.99
12	4.16	6.38
15	4.03	5.88
20	3.90	5.41
25	3.84	5.14
30	3.80	5.00
40	3.75	4.82
50	3.73	4.70

(b)

n	Confidence Level 95% k_1	99% k_1
2	19.22	96.17
4	3.25	5.69
6	2.25	3.24
8	1.90	2.52
10	1.72	2.18
12	1.61	1.97
14	1.51	1.84
16	1.48	1.75
18	1.44	1.67
20	1.40	1.62
25	1.34	1.52
30	1.30	1.45
35	1.27	1.40
40	1.25	1.37
45	1.23	1.34
50	1.21	1.31
100	1.14	1.20
1000	1.04	1.06
∞	1.00	1.00

(continued)

TABLE 5–2.
(Continued)

(c)	Confidence Level	
	95%	99%
n	$\dfrac{t_{\alpha/2}}{\sqrt{n}}$	$\dfrac{t_{\alpha/2}}{\sqrt{n}}$
6	1.05	1.65
8	0.84	1.24
10	0.72	1.03
12	0.64	0.90
15	0.56	0.70
20	0.47	0.64
25	0.41	0.56
30	0.37	0.50
40	0.32	0.43
50	0.28	0.38

where t is the two-tailed t statistic at the desired confidence level and $n - 1$ degrees of freedom, and S is an estimate of bias in the form of a standard deviation of the Y values. This estimate may be be obtained from linear regression data or from repeated measurements of a known quantity as explained below. The factor

$$\frac{t_{\alpha/2}}{\sqrt{n}}$$

may be found in Table 5–2.

Estimating Imprecision

Estimates Using Linear Regression Data.—If a linear equation is a good model of the data, then the regression line connects the mean values of hypothetical distributions of Y for each level of X (Fig 5–7). The distributions of the observed Y values are all assumed to be Gaussian, or normal, and to all have the same variance (standard deviation squared). The differences between the observed values of Y and those predicted by the regression equation are called *residuals*. Because the value predicted by the regression equation is the estimated mean value of repeated measurements and hence the best estimate of the true value X, the residuals represent the random errors of measurement. The standard deviation of the residuals (or standard error of the estimate, $S_{Y\cdot X}$) is an estimate of the standard deviation of repeated

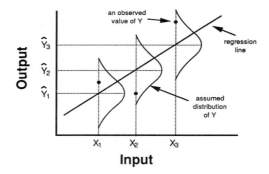

FIG 5–7.
A linear regression line connects the mean values of the hypothetical distributions of *Y* for each value of *X*. The variances, and hence the standard deviations of the distributions are assumed to be equal. Thus, calculation of the standard error of the estimate is equivalent to grouping together all the measured values into one distribution and calculating the standard deviation.

measurements of Y at any specific value of X[17, 40, 42, 43]:

$$S_{Y \cdot X} = \sqrt{\frac{\Sigma (Y - \hat{Y})^2}{n - 2}} \qquad (5-10)$$

Thus, $S_{Y \cdot X}$ is an estimate of the imprecision of measured values.

Estimates Using Repeated Measures. — Depending on the experimental conditions under which the data for linear regression were obtained and on the number of observations recorded, the use of the standard error of the estimate may not reflect the true imprecision associated with the measurement system. When only one observation is obtained for each input level, there is no information about the repeatability of the measurement (i.e., the variation in repeated measurements of the same quantity), just the implicit assumption that repeatability is the same over the entire range of measurement. To the extent that this assumption is incorrect, the use of the standard error of the estimate will be a poor estimate of random error for any particular measurement level.

Ideally, imprecision should be estimated from a separate experiment in which repeated measurements of a known value are made under conditions that potentially include all sources of random error (detailed earlier). The known value should represent, where applicable, a medical decision level. That is, a value below which one decision is made and above which some other decision is made. For example, a transcutaneous oxygen saturation of 88% is considered the level below which a patient requires supplemental oxygen and hence is eligible for Medicare reimbursement.[44]

The sample size for repeated measurements of a known value of X (total number of repeated measurements) should be no less than 20, with larger samples being preferable.[11] The data can be assessed for normality using either graphical (plotting the data on normal probability graph paper) or statistical (chi square or Kolmogorov-Smirnov) tests.[5, 12, 14] The standard deviation of the repeated measurements [from Equation 5–2] is calculated and used to estimate imprecision.

While the above procedure provides a good estimate of imprecision for one particular value of the measurand, we are more often interested in the general performance of the measurement system over its entire range. To carry the procedure to its logical extreme would require large samples of repeated measures at every value that the system could measure. For example, evaluation of a new digital oxygen analyzer (with readouts to the nearest whole percent) would require 20 or more repeated measurements of 80 known oxygen concentrations from 21 to 100% in increments of 1% (totaling at least 1600 measurements). These data would allow the construction of a look-up table that showed the standard deviation of repeated measurements at every level of the measurand.* Assuming that the variances of the repeated measurements at different concentrations of oxygen were not very different and were not related to the level of oxygen concentration, then such a table could be accurately summarized by taking the square root of the average variance. This estimate of imprecision could then be interpreted as the expected standard deviation from repeated measurements of any value of the measurand.

Of course, there is seldom either enough time or money to perform the above-described evaluation of a device, particularly in a hospital setting. Yet the concept can be made practical by simply reducing the number of repeated measurements at each level. The smallest number of measurements that will allow an estimation of the standard deviation is two. By taking duplicate measurements at each level of the measurand it will be more practical to increase the number of levels. This approach seems more feasible while maintaining some usefulness. It can be shown that the variance [standard deviation from Equation (5–2) squared] of a set of duplicate measurements is equal to one-half of the squared difference between the two measurements.[32] Thus, an estimate of the standard deviation of repeated measurements based on an average variance of a set of duplicate measurements, S_{dup} is given by:

$$S_{dup} = \sqrt{\frac{\sum_{i=1}^{n} d^2}{2n}} \tag{5–11}$$

where d is the difference between duplicates and n is the number of data pairs.[32]

A plot of the differences between the two repeated measurements should be examined and they should average to zero. If the mean difference is significantly different from zero, we can conclude that the first measurement is somehow affecting the second and the data cannot be used to assess precision.[45] Either a one-sample t test (testing the equivalence of the mean difference and zero) or a two-sample paired t test (testing the equivalence of the mean value from one set of measurements with the mean value of its duplicate) could be used for this.

Note that if the imprecision estimated from repeated measures turns out to be significantly smaller than that indicated by the standard error of the estimate, and the experiments are designed to include the same sources of random error, the linear model is not correct.[41] This may be checked statistically using an F test.[11, 41, 46]

---

* At least one manufacturer, Radiometer, has approached this level of description in their specification tables for blood gas analyzer electrodes (see ABL4 User's Handbook).

The choice of using replicate measurements spanning the entire range of input values is affected by many considerations. How many experimental runs are possible given limited resources? How many runs are justified by the importance of the problem? How many input levels should be chosen and how many repeat runs should be performed at each level? These study design issues (along with the effects of including repeat data in linear regression analyses) can be dealt with in quantitative terms and are explained quite well in the text by Draper and Smith[41] (pp. 51–55).

The estimates of imprecision described above are point estimates. A confidence interval for imprecision can be expressed as[47]:

$$\text{CI for } S = \left[\sqrt{\frac{(n-1)S^2}{\chi^2_{\alpha/2,n-1}}}, \sqrt{\frac{(n-1)S^2}{\chi^2_{1-\alpha/2,n-1}}} \right] \tag{5-12}$$

where S is some estimate of the sample standard deviation; $\chi^2_{\alpha/2,n-1}$ and $\chi^2_{1-\alpha/2,n-1}$ are chi-squared values with $n-1$ degrees of freedom. Weisbrot[12] provides a table that simplifies the use of Equation (5–12). It is derived from the $(n-1)$ and χ^2 terms in Equation (5–12) and the tables of χ^2 values created by Lindley et al.[48]

Estimating Tolerance Intervals

In assessing imprecision, we are frequently less interested in estimating parameters and more concerned about where *individual measurements* might fall. That is, we are interested in determining the range of values that should include the true value with a specified degree of confidence. If the true mean and standard deviation of an infinite number of repeated measurementes were known, then a two-sigma tolerance interval could be expressed as:

$$\text{TI} = \mu \pm 1.96\sigma$$

This interval includes exactly 95% of the observed measurements and thus we can say with 95% confidence that the true value lies within this range of values. In this special case, the confidence level coincides with the proportion of measurements encompassed by the tolerance interval. However, μ and σ are unknowable. Therefore, we must substitute the appropriate point estimates $\overline{X}$ and S. Because of the random error involved with estimating the population mean and standard deviation, the proportion of the population of measured values covered by the tolerance interval is not exact. As a result, the confidence level must be calculated based on the uncertainty of the point estimates of the population parameters. The tolerance interval is expressed as[38, 47]:

$$\text{TI} = \overline{X} \pm \alpha k_1 S \tag{5-13}$$

where k_1 is determined so that one can assert with the desired confidence that the true value lies within the specified tolerance limits.[47] The proportion of measurements that we wish to include in the tolerance interval is determined by the factor α in Equation (5–13). For most purposes a two-sigma tolerance interval is sufficient, meaning that 95% of the measurements should lie within the specified tolerance interval and thus $\alpha = 1.96 \approx 2$. When keeping imprecision to a minimum is desirable, an error tolerance of 99% is usually chosen, in which case $\alpha = 2.57$. If a three-sigma error tolerance is desired, only 0.27% of all measurements will lie outside of the tolerance interval and $\alpha = 3$. Values of k_1 as a function of confidence levels and sample sizes are given in Table 5–2 (modified from Wilpole and Myers[47]).

Because of the use of point estimates for the population mean and standard deviation, the tolerance interval given by Equation (5–13) is associated with a double probability. There is one probability *that a given measurement will lie within the specified interval* for a given set of measurements (determined by the factor α in the equation) and there is another probability (the confidence level) *that we will be correct* in assuming that a given measurement falls within the tolerance interval (determined by the factor k_1 in the equation). From the standpoint of making a medical decision, based on a single measurement, we would like to know the probability of making the correct decision. Assuming that the correct decision would be made if the measurement is accurate, then the probability of being right is the probability that the measurement inaccuracy is within the specified range. This probability is the product of the proportion of measurements included within the tolerance interval and the confidence interval. For example, if the two-sigma tolerance interval of a measuring device were known with 95% confidence, then the probability of making an accurate measurement would be $0.95 \times 0.95 = 0.90$.

The tolerance interval given by Equation (5–13) assumes that measurement errors are normally distributed. However, it is possible to define a tolerance interval that is independent of the shape of the underlying distribution: *For any distribution of measurements, the tolerance interval is given by the smallest and largest observations in a sample of size n, where n is determined so that one can assert with the desired level of confidence that at least the desired proportion of measurements is included between the sample extremes.*[47] Table 5–3 gives the required sample sizes for the desired confidence level and the desired proportion of measurements to be included in the tolerance interval.[47] For example, we must have a sample size of 130 measurements in order to be 99% confident that at least 95% of the measurements will lie between the smallest and largest observations in the sample.

TABLE 5–3.
Sample Size for Nonparametric Tolerance Limits

Proportion of Measurements Included in Tolerance Interval	Confidence Level	
	95%	99%
99.5%	947	1,325
99%	473	662
95%	93	130
90%	46	64
85%	30	42
50%	8	11

It is important to remember that the tolerance interval takes into consideration only the effects of random error, therefore it is a statement of measurement imprecision. If the effect of systematic error or bias is included, the total measurement error or inaccuracy may be estimated. On the other hand, if bias is negligible or can be corrected through calibration, the tolerance interval may be used as the inaccuracy specification for the measurement system.

Estimating Inaccuracy

With estimates of bias and imprecision, the total error or inaccuracy in the measurement of the known value X_0 can be estimated as follows:

$$\text{Inaccuracy} = \text{Bias} \pm \text{Imprecision} \qquad (5-14)$$
$$\text{Inaccuracy} = (\hat{Y} - X_0) \pm (\alpha k_1 S)$$

where $\hat{Y}$ is the estimated mean value of repeated measurements of a known quantity X_0, preferably at a medical decision level. (Of course, $\hat{Y}$ may be replaced by $\overline{X}$ if the data are from repeated measurements of only one level of the known quantity and thus linear regression analysis is not used.) Also, S may be any of the estimates of the standard deviation of repeated measurements described above, α is the factor determining the desired width of the tolerance interval, and k_1 is the factor accounting for the uncertainty of the estimates for mean and standard deviation (from Table 5–2). The confidence we have in this estimate of inaccuracy is that associated with our choice of k_1.

If the measurement system is properly calibrated, we would expect that the imprecision is larger than the bias, thus giving rise to both positive and negative values for inaccuracy (i.e., the $\pm$ gives rise to the best case and worst case inaccuracy). The absolute values of the positive and negative estimates of inaccuracy are examined and the larger is compared with the previously determined standard for allowable error. If the calculated inaccuracy is less than the allowable inaccuracy, implying that this level of error would not change the medical decision, the measurement system is deemed acceptable.[23]

If the allowable error is stated in terms of the component bias and imprecision, statistical methods can be used to test the acceptability of the calculated inaccuracy. The hypothesis that the bias is zero (i.e., the mean difference between the measured and true values is zero) can be evaluated with a t test. The hypothesis that the observed standard deviation (or standard error) is different from the acceptable standard deviation can be evaluated with an F test.

INTERPRETING ERROR SPECIFICATIONS

The first step in dealing with instrument error is to understand the manufacturer's specifications. In addition to the ambiguities of nomenclature mentioned earlier, a simple statement such as "accuracy is $\pm 2\%$ of full scale" really says little by itself. It does not give us a clue as to the proportion of measurements it applies to (is it a two- or three-sigma error or something else?). It is not clear whether the specification is a statement of total error or a tolerance interval. It may even be a nonparametric tolerance interval. Unfortunately, such information is usually not provided by manufacturers and it is often difficult to locate someone in a given manufacturing organization who can provide it or even understand the issues.

To confirm the manufacturer's error specifications, the user must conduct some rather detailed statistical analyses of data from device performance studies. One might expect that error specifications are originally generated in a similar manner. This, however, is usually not the case. Although the exact procedures differ, manufacturers typically use the following approach in creating error specifications for their products: First, in the design stage, a set of functional specifications is developed for a proposed product. These specifications are based on things like published error ratings for similar products, industry standards (e.g., those of the American Society for Testing and Materials or the International Standards Organization), perceived user needs, and an analysis of combined component tolerances (e.g., simple electrical resistors can be purchased with tolerances of ± 1, ± 5, or $\pm 10\%$).

The desired error specifications for the product might be stated as, for example, $\pm 2\%$ of full scale plus $\pm 1\%$ of reading, or simply $\pm 2\%$ of full scale. The usual implicit assumption is that the error bands will encompass 95% of the individual readings from repeated measurements of a given quantity (i.e., approximately two standard deviations of a normal distribution). A graph is made showing the ideal input versus the output performance (the line of identity). The desired performance is indicated as error or tolerance bands, or lines above and below the line of identity. The distance between these lines and the line of identity represents the error specifications. For example, the line of identity will have the mathematical form of: output = input. Assuming for simplicity that the scale reads from 0 to 100, error bands for a specification of $\pm 2\%$ of full scale would have the mathematical form of: output = true value ± 2. Thus, if the reading was 50, the true value would be between 48 and 52. Error bands for a specification of $\pm 2\%$ of full scale plus $\pm 1\%$ of reading would have the form of: output = true value $\pm 2 \pm (0.01 \times$ true value). If the reading was 50, the true value would lie somewhere between 47.5 and 52.5.

Next, a sample of product prototypes is made. The performance of these prototypes is evaluated by measuring their output for a set of known inputs (i.e., values measured with highly accurate instruments whose calibrations are certified by the National Institute of Standards and Technology). The data from all the prototypes are plotted on the previously drawn graph and a judgment is made as to whether or not the device performs within the allowable error specifications (i.e., all data points lie within the error bands). If not, either the prototype is redesigned or the allowable error is reevaluated. If the prototype operates as expected, a production run is started and the graph is used for quality control. Devices are then rejected or sold depending on their performance relative to specifications.

Note that the inaccuracy of a given device may be different from the manufacturer's specifications depending on how it is used. Instrument specifications do not, for instance, include the various types of random and systematic operator errors. Also, the inaccuracy specification applies to the entire range of the device's readout scale and may be better for a limited section. For example, oxygen analyzers typically have errors of less than $\pm 3\%$ of full scale. Suppose such a device is calibrated by the user to read 100% using a source of pure oxygen. If we then immediately measured the output of an air-oxygen blender set at $F_{IO_2} = 1.0$

and obtained a reading of 100%, we would expect the error to be negligible because we have reduced the systematic error to essentially zero and greatly reduced the possibility of random error factors. In fact, if we did not obtain a reading of 100% we would be inclined to suspect a faulty blender rather than an error of measurement.

The user must be aware of the implications of manufacturer's error specifications. Assume, for example, that an inaccuracy specification of $\pm 2\%$ refers to two standard deviations of a normal distribution for an individual reading. Because the error is specified in terms of the full-scale reading, the device will be more accurate when measuring quantities at the upper end of the scale than at the lower end. For a scale of 0 to 100 units, the expected error would be ± 2 scale units. If a known quantity having a value of 95 was measured, the instrument reading would probably be between 93 and 97, or 98 to 102% of the true value. However, if the true value were 5, the expected reading would range from 3 to 7, or 60 to 140% of the true value. This represents an inaccuracy, for that particular reading, of $\pm 40\%$, which might be unacceptable depending on the application.

Inverse Estimation. — In *creating* inaccuracy specifications, we estimate the degree to which measured values will deviate from the true values. However, in *using* error specifications the problem is reversed. For a given measured value we want to know the range of values in which the true value will lie with some level of certainty.

Using the information from regression analysis, the confidence interval for the estimated true value $\hat{X}_0$, given a measured value Y_0, is[14]:

$$\left.\begin{array}{r} X_{\text{upper}} \\ X_{\text{lower}} \end{array}\right\} = \hat{X}_0 \pm \frac{\alpha k_1 S}{b} \tag{5-15a}$$

where

$$\hat{X}_0 = \frac{Y_0 - a}{b} \tag{5-15b}$$

The constants a and b are the intercept and slope, respectively, from regression analysis, α and k_1 are from Table 5–2, and S is the estimate of the standard deviation of repeated measurements of X_0 (using only regression information this would be $S_{Y \cdot X}$). A more precise but considerably more complex equation is given in the text by Draper and Smith, who call the upper and lower values for X the inverse confidence limits or "fiducial limits."[41]

If the inaccuracy of a measurement system is given in terms of a percentage of full-scale specification, the problem is simplified. Such a specification lumps together systematic and random error into an equivalent systematic error of zero and a random error equal to the $\pm$ inaccuracy value (Fig 5–8, A). Thus, a and b in Equation (5–15b) reduce to 0 and 1, respectively, and the confidence interval is:

$$\left.\begin{array}{r} X_{\text{upper}} \\ X_{\text{lower}} \end{array}\right\} = Y_0 \pm \alpha k_1 S = Y_0 \pm \frac{\text{Inaccuracy (\%FS)} \times \text{Full-scale reading}}{100} \tag{5-16}$$

If the inaccuracy specification is given as a percentage of the measurement reading, the upper error band for repeated measurements of X has a slope equal to (100 + inaccuracy)/100 and the lower band has a slope of (100 − inaccuracy)/100. For example, given a specification of ±2% of reading, the upper error band would have a slope of 1.02 and the lower band would have intercepts of zero. As a consequence, the limits of the estimated true value $\hat{X}_0$ will not be symmetrical. In particular, X_{upper} will be closer to $\hat{X}_0$ than will be X_{lower}, as shown in Figure 5–8, B. From these observations and Equation (5–15a), the upper and lower limits of the estimated true value of X are thus:

$$\left.\begin{array}{r} X_{\text{upper}} \\ X_{\text{lower}} \end{array}\right\} = \frac{Y_0}{\left(\dfrac{100 \pm \text{Inaccuracy}\ (\%R)}{100}\right)} \qquad (5\text{–}17)$$

where inaccuracy is expressed as a percentage rather than a decimal.

EVALUATION OF AGREEMENT[39, 45]

A frequent clinical problem is the need to know whether or not some new measurement system will give results comparable to one that is currently in use. Often we would like to know if the new system can serve as a substitute for the old while preserving the quality of medical decisions based on the system's measurements. Typically, studies are designed in which both systems are used to measure some variable and the results are analyzed for agreement. The most frequently used statistical analyses are least-squares linear regression, the t test, the F test, and Pearson's product moment correlation coefficient. However, there are several reasons why these techniques are inappropriate for agreement studies.[23, 39, 40, 45] Altman and Bland[39, 45] have suggested an alternative approach that has become popular among current researchers.[49–52]

Incorrect Methods of Analysis

As mentioned above, least-squares regression minimizes the sum of squares of the vertical distance between the observed data and the regression line. This illustrates the underlying assumption that only the data plotted on the Y-axis show variability. The assumption is appropriate for studies of inaccuracy where the reference values, plotted on the X-axis, are assumed to be known with negligible imprecision. However, it is not appropriate in the comparison of two methods that both exhibit variability. It can be argued that variability in the X-axis data can be accounted for by using the method suggested by Deming, which minimizes both the Y residual and the X residual by minimizing the sum of the squares of the perpendicular distances from the data points to the line.[12, 40, 53] However, regression still suffers from sensitivity to nonlinearity of the data and will give misleading results if the range of the data is too narrow (i.e., the best fit line is more strongly influenced by the scatter of the data

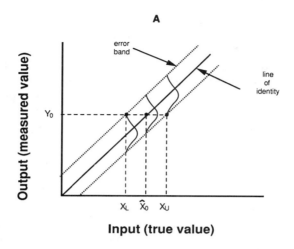

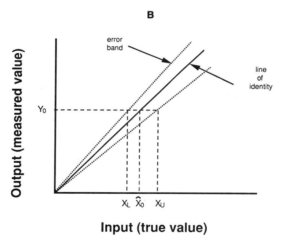

FIG 5–8.
Inverse estimation. **A,** Estimating the true value from a measured value when the inaccuracy is specified in the form ±% of full scale. Notice that the error bands around *X* are symmetrical and of the same magnitude as for *Y*. **B,** Estimating the true value from a measured value when the inaccuracy is specified in the form ±% of reading. The error bands around *X* are not symmetrical and are different than those for *Y*.

for narrow versus wide ranges).[11] Also, the approach suggested in the following is considerably easier to use.

Both the *t* test and the *F* test are sometimes used as indicators of agreement although they are only intended to tell whether the differences between two methods are significant. If the calculated value for the statistic is larger than some critical value, the performance of the measurement system in question is judged not acceptable. If the statistic is smaller, it is usually concluded that the methods agree and the new system is accepted. Such judgments may be erroneous for several reasons.

The *F* test is simply the ratio of the variances of the data from two measurement systems. It is a comparison of error levels, indicating the significance of any difference, and not an indicator of the acceptability of errors nor of their magnitude.[23]

The *t* test is a ratio of systematic and random errors,[11, 23]

$$ t = \frac{\text{Bias} \times \sqrt{n}}{S_d} $$

(where S_d is the standard deviation of the differences between paired measurements, see below) and therefore is not a measure of total error. This is analogous to the determination of blood pH by the ratio of bicarbonate to carbon dioxide tension.[23] A low pH does not tell whether the bicarbonate is low or the carbon dioxide is high. Treatment of acidosis requires assessment of both metabolic and respiratory factors. Similarly, interpretation of the *t* value requires assessment of both the systematic and random errors. There are at least four situations that that can cause erroneous judgments when using the *t* value[23]:

- The *t* value may be small when systematic error is small and random error is large. Thus, the more imprecision there is in the measurement data, the more likely we are to conclude that the methods agree!
- The *t* value may be small when both systematic and random errors are large.
- The *t* value may be large when both errors are small, in which case the more accurate the measurements are, the less likely we are to conclude that the methods agree!
- As shown in the preceding equation, *t* varies with the sample size *n*. Thus, even if systematic and random errors are acceptable, we might conclude that the methods do not agree if the sample size is large and vice versa.

A further limitation of the *t* test is that it is an indicator of the significant difference between *mean* values. It provides no information about the confidence we can place in *individual measurements* taken with the new method.

Perhaps the most widely misused indicator of agreement is the product moment correlation coefficient *r*. The fundamental problem with this statistic is that it is a measure of linear association, which is not the same as agreement. For example, suppose we plotted the data from two methods that gave exactly the same results when measuring a range of unknown values. The data would all lie on the line of identity. The *r* value would be 1.0 (perfect correlation) and it would be clear that the methods had perfect agreement. However, if one method gave exactly twice the value of the other or, say, twice the value plus 3 units, the data would still lie on a straight line with *r* = 1.0. However, it would be quite obvious that the two methods do not agree. The *r* value is an indicator of random error and is completely insensitive to systematic error.

There are other problems with the r statistic.[45] Correlation is sensitive to the range of the measurements and will be greater for wide ranges than for small ones. Because investigators usually compare methods over the whole range of values expected to be measured, a high correlation is almost guaranteed. Also, the test of a significance (i.e., that r is significantly different from zero) will undoubtedly show that the two methods are related because they are designed to measure the same quantity. The test of significance is therefore irrelevant to the question of agreement.

Suggested Method of Analysis

As with the assessment of inaccuracy, the first step is to plot the data generated when the two methods are used to measure the same quantity over a range of input levels. For each level of input, each method will give one data point, referred to hereafter as A and B. The best way to view the data is to plot the difference between methods $(A - B)$ on the Y-axis versus their mean value $[(A + B)/2]$ for each input value. The mean value for each level of input is used because it is the best estimate of the true value, which is not known. At this point it is important to assess whether or not the differences are related to the mean value. If they are, the estimate of random error may be overstated at one end of the range of measurements and understated at the other. The hypothesis of $r = 0$ can be tested statistically. If a significant relationship is found, a logarithmic transformation may be helpful.[45]

The next step is to calculate the mean difference between the two methods (i.e., the average of all $A - B$ values). Next, the "limits of agreement"[45] are calculated as the upper and lower values that encompass 95% of the observed differences:

$$\text{Limits of agreement} = \bar{d} \pm 1.96 S_d \approx \bar{d} \pm 2 S_d \qquad (5-18a)$$

where

$$\bar{d} = \text{Mean value of the differences}$$

and

$$S_d = \sqrt{\frac{\sum\limits_{i=1}^{n} (d_i - \bar{d})^2}{n - 1}} \qquad (5-18b)$$

where d represents the individual differences between measurements made with one method compared with the other $(A - B)$. The mean difference and the limits of agreement are included in the plot of the data. If the differences within the limits of agreement are judged to be clinically unimportant, then we conclude that the two methods may be used interchangeably.

The mean difference and the limits of agreement are point estimates. A confidence interval for the mean difference can be calculated by substituting $\bar{d}$ for $\hat{Y} - X_0$ in Equation (5–9). A confidence interval for the standard deviation of the differences can be calculated by substituting S_d for S into Equation (5–12). A confidence interval for the limit of agreement can be expressed as[32]:

$$\text{CI for limit} = \text{limit} \pm (t_{\alpha/2}) \cdot \sqrt{\left(\frac{1}{n} + \frac{2}{n-1}\right) S_d^2} \tag{5–19a}$$

where t is the two-tailed value for the desired significance level with $n - 1$ degrees of freedom. For large samples, the 95% confidence interval for the limit is approximately[32]:

$$\text{CI for limit} = \text{limit} \pm 1.96 \cdot \sqrt{\frac{3S_d^2}{n}} \tag{5–19b}$$

Assessing Repeatability.—In the preceding analysis, it was assumed that one data pair was used for each input level (one observation was made with each measurement system for each level of the measurand). However, it can be argued that estimates of imprecision based on this type of data suffer from a lack of information about repeatability (as mentioned above for the use of the standard error of the estimate). Poor repeatability leads to poor agreement. Even a new measurement system that is perfect will not agree with an old system that has a lot of variability. The problem is compounded if both methods have much variability.[45]

It is possible to include information about repeatability in the estimate of agreement using duplicate measurements by each of the two measurement systems on the same measured quantities. For each level of the measured quantity, the mean values of the repeated measurements are calculated for each system. This results in pairs of mean values (one for each measurement system) for each level of the measurand. If these pairs of means are then subjected to the analysis for assessing agreement described earlier, a problem arises. The average difference will be unaffected, but the estimate of the standard deviation of the differences will be too small because some of the random error has been removed by using mean values instead of the original data. However, this can be corrected by first calculating the standard deviations of the differences between repeated measurements for each method separately, S_1 and S_2, and the standard deviation of the differences between the means for each method S_d. The corrected standard deviation S_c is then[45]:

$$S_c = \sqrt{S_d^2 + \frac{S_1^2}{4} + \frac{S_2^2}{4}} \approx \sqrt{2S_d^2} \tag{5–20}$$

The repeatability of the two measurement systems may also be examined separately. Duplicate measurements are obtained for one system over the whole range of input levels.

Then, the differences between the duplicates are plotted against their mean value. The mean and standard deviation of the differences is calculated as before. As mentioned in the section on evaluation of inaccuracy, if the mean difference is significantly different from zero, the data cannot be used to assess repeatability because the first measurement is affecting the second. Also, when more than two repeated measurements are to be used, the calculations are more complex.[45] Next, a *coefficient of repeatability* can be calculated as[32]:

$$\text{Coefficient of repeatability} = 1.96 \sqrt{2S_{\text{dup}}^2} \approx 2.8\, S_{\text{dup}} \tag{5-21}$$

assuming a mean difference of zero. This coefficient (which has been adopted by the British Standards Institution) can be interpreted as the maximum difference between two measurements, with probability 0.95. This procedure can be repeated for the other measurement system and the coefficients of repeatability for the two measurement systems can be examined for comparability.

Another way is simply to compare the variances S_d^2 of each measurement system using an *F* test.

Using Agreement to Estimate Inaccuracy. — The method of determining the limits of agreement can be applied to the analysis of inaccuracy (of a single measurement system) instead of using the procedure based on linear regression described previously. Thus, instead of comparing data from two systems, measured values from one system are compared to the associated true values, (which are values measured with negligible error by methods traceable to the National Institute of Standards and Technology). The mean difference is taken as the bias, and the $\pm$ portion of the limits of agreement from Equation (5–18) is taken as the imprecision.

EXAMPLE ANALYSES

To demonstrate the use of the techniques described earlier, we will imagine a situation in which a manufacturer has provided a new model of oxygen analyzer for our evaluation and potential purchase. The manufacturer claims that the analyzer is accurate to $\pm 1\%$ of the full-scale reading (full scale is $F_{IO_2} = 1.0$), which is comparable to the specifications for the device that our department currently uses. Our evaluation could potentially address the following questions:

1. Can we believe the manufacturer's specifications?
   - What inaccuracy can we really expect from the device?
   - How much confidence can we place in individual measurements of F_{IO_2}?
2. If we purchase the new device, how will it affect our standard of care?
   - How well will measurements with the new device agree with the measurements we have been making?

Two simple experiments are designed to answer these two basic questions. Our general approach is to obtain some known concentrations of precise air-oxygen mixtures and then to measure these mixtures with both the new and the old analyzer. To assess inaccuracy, we will compare the measured values from the new analyzer with the known oxygen concentrations. To assess the potential impact on our standard of care, we will compare the measured values from the new analyzer with the old analyzer. This question may be academic if we discover that the new analyzer is actually less inaccurate. However, we will include it for the purpose of illustration. If we were evaluating measurements for which the true values were unknown (e.g., if we were using an air-oxygen blender with known inaccuracies rather than precision gas mixtures or if we were evaluating, say, end-tidal carbon dioxide tensions in human subjects), then inaccuracy studies would not be possible and agreement studies would have to suffice.

Frequently, clinical studies of the inaccuracy of a given measurement device are conducted only using one prototype. Repeated measurements with the device would give some information about the repeatability of the measurements. However, variability between devices is probably greater, in general, than variability between repeated measurements with the same device. For this reason, we ask the manufacturer to supply us with two new oxygen analyzers for our study. In addition, we will select two old (but perfectly functioning) devices from our own inventory. We will take one set of measurements, over the range of oxygen concentrations, with each device. The results of our experiments are shown in Table 5–4.

Because these experiments are only hypothetical, the results in Table 5–3 are simulated. The data for the new analyzers were selected at random from simulated normal distributions having mean values equal to the true oxygen concentration and an arbitrary standard deviation of 1.0. The data for the old analyzers were obtained similarly but from distributions having a standard deviation of 0.5, which is comparable to actual oxygen analyzer specifications. Knowing the characteristics of the sampling distributions will enable us to more objectively compare and evaluate the proposed analyses of inaccuracy and agreement. The simulated distributions were generated with a software spreadsheet using a simple yet elegant algorithm.[54] It makes use of the assumption (based on the central limit theorem) that the sum of a series of numbers will be normally distributed regardless of the underlying distribution from which the series of numbers is obtained. Specifically, it can be shown that the sum of 12 random numbers ranging in value between 0 and 1.0 is normally distributed with a mean value of 6.0 and a standard deviation of 1.0. From this observation, the following algorithm was derived for generating a random variable from a simulated normal distribution.

1. Take the sum of 12 random numbers ranging in value between 0 and 1.0.
2. Subtract 6 from the sum to get a z score (i.e., the difference between the observed value and the theoretical mean value divided by the standard deviation, which in this case is 1.0).
3. Multiply this z score times the standard deviation of the desired distribution.
4. Add the result of step 3 to the mean value of the desired distribution to generate a random value from the desired distribution.

TABLE 5–4.
Simulated Experimental Data from New Oxygen Analyzers*

| | Measured Values | | | | Calculated Values | | | |
| | New O_2 Analyzer A | New O_2 Analyzer B | Difference New A-True | Difference New (A-B) | Squared Difference | Mean New | Difference Mean New-True |
True Value							
20.0	19.9	21.2	−0.10	−1.35	1.83	20.5	0.55
40.0	39.0	39.0	1.00	−0.02	0.00	39.0	−1.03
60.0	60.8	59.1	0.80	1.70	2.90	60.0	−0.02
80.0	79.9	81.9	−0.10	−1.99	3.98	80.9	0.90
100.0	99.4	99.2	0.60	0.19	0.03	99.3	−0.71
			mean = 0.44	mean = −0.30	sum = 8.7		mean = −0.06
			S† = 0.51	S† = 1.44			S† = 0.81

* Calculations were performed with 14 significant figures but results are displayed with 3 significant figures.
† S = standard deviation with $n − 1$ degrees of freedom.

Evaluation of Inaccuracy (Linear Regression Method)

Method evaluation studies, in general, involve the comparison of two sets of data. Comparison analyses can be thought of as simply assessments of agreement. Thus, the evaluation of inaccuracy (i.e., bias and precision) of a measurement system can be seen as a special case in which measurement data are assessed for agreement with known or standard values. Therefore, we can use either linear regression techniques or the "limits of agreement" technique to determine the inaccuracy of an instrument or a population of instruments.

For the purpose of evaluating the inaccuracy of the new oxygen analyzer, we will include all the data from the two prototypes of the new device (data from the columns marked "New O_2 Analyzer A" and "New O_2 Analyzer B" in Table 5–4). Duplicate measurements are included because we want to include the between-device variability and to increase the sample size, which will improve the estimates of the population parameters. However, as mentioned before, we must validate the data by making sure that the mean difference between duplicate measurements is not significantly different from zero. The easiest approach using the data from Table 5–4 is to perform a paired *t* test. The value of *t* is:

$$t = \frac{\overline{d} - 0}{S_d/\sqrt{n}} = \frac{-0.3}{1.4/\sqrt{5}} = -0.48$$

where *d* is the mean difference between new analyzer A and new analyzer B measurements, S_d is the standard deviation of the differences (using Equation (5–2)], and *n* is the number of differences. The null hypothesis is that the mean difference equals zero. The alternate hypothesis is that the mean difference is not equal to zero. We will reject the null hypothesis if the calculated value for *t* exceeds the critical values found from a table. From a standard statistical table, we find the critical value for a two-tailed *t* test at the 0.05 significance level, $t_{0.975}$, with $n - 1 = 4$ degrees of freedom. This value is -2.8. Because -0.48 is not less than -2.8, we do not reject the null hypothesis and thus conclude that the duplicate measurements are valid (i.e., knowledge of the first measurement is not affecting the second and the process of measurement is not altering the quantity).

The first step after validation is to plot the data, judge the overall linearity, and fit a linear model to the data using least-squares analysis (Fig 5–9). The new analyzer data represent the dependent variable (plotted on the *Y*-axis) and the true oxygen concentration is the independent variable (plotted on the *X*-axis). The value of 0.997 for the slope of the regression line and the intercept of 0.120 indicate that there are negligible proportional and offset errors. The standard error of the estimate is 1.085 (which seems to be a very good estimate of the standard deviation of 1.0 used to generate the simulated data).

The final step is to calculate an estimate of inaccuracy using the regression results and Equation (5–14). Because a slight proportional error exists, the maximum value of $(\hat{Y} - X_0)$ will be about -0.2 when X_0 equals 100%. We would like a two-sigma tolerance interval so $\alpha = 1.96$. For a confidence level of 95% and a sample size of 10, k_1 from Table 5–2 is 1.72. Therefore, the inaccuracy is:

$$\text{Inaccuracy} = -0.2 \pm (1.96 \times 1.72 \times 1.085)$$
$$= -0.2 \pm 3.66$$

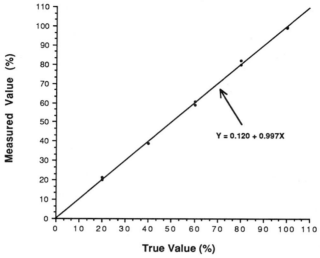

FIG 5–9.
Simulated data for evaluation of inaccuracy using linear regression.

and the maximum inaccuracy is $|-0.2 - 3.66| = |-3.86| \approx 3.9$ The bias (total systematic error) is low as expected because the mean values of the simulated data distributions were set equal to the true value. We can expect at least 95% of the measurements to be within 3.9% of the true F_{IO_2} and we make this assertion at a 95% confidence level.

When expressed as a percentage of full scale, our estimate of inaccuracy for the new oxygen analyzer is 3.9/100 or about ±3.9% FS. This does not seem to support the manufacturer's claim of ±1%. Note, however, that because we simulated the data, we know that 95% of the measurements will be within 2% of the correct F_{IO_2} with 100% confidence (because we specified the population mean and standard deviation). Our simulated experimental data indicated that the inaccuracy was larger simply as a function of the sample size and the presumed uncertainty in estimating the population mean and standard deviation with $\overline{X}$ and S, respectively. However, in a real experiment we would not know whether a discrepancy was due to the sample size, a larger standard deviation of the data, or both.

Evaluation of Inaccuracy (Limits of Agreement Method)

As with the previous method, we would like to pool all the data from the two new oxygen analyzers. However, for illustrative purposes, we will first evaluate agreement between measured and true values for a single analyzer and then use the modification based on duplicate measurements.

Analysis Based on Single Measurements.—The first step is to calculate the difference between the measured value and the true value for each datum. These data (Difference New

A − True from Table 5–4) are plotted as shown in Figure 5–10 and examined to make sure that the differences are not related to the true values.

The next step is to calculate some elementary statistics. The mean difference is 0.44 and the standard deviation of these values is 0.51. These statistics are used in Equation (5–18) to provide the limits of agreement between the measured and true values. In this case, the maximum value for a limit of agreement will be interpreted as the estimate of maximum inaccuracy. The limits of agreement are:

$$\text{Limits of agreement} = 0.44 \pm (1.96 \times 0.51)$$
$$= 0.44 \pm 1.00$$

Therefore, our estimate of maximum inaccuracy is $|0.44 + 1.00| = 1.44$. When expressed as a percentage of full scale, our estimate of inaccuracy for the new oxygen analyzer is 1.44/100 or about ±1% FS.

Analysis Based on Duplicate Measurements. — The first step is to calculate the mean value of each set of duplicate measurements (column "Mean New" in Table 5–4). Then the difference between the mean measured value and the true value is calculated for each level of oxygen concentration (column Mean New − True in Table 5–4). The average of these differences, −0.06, is our estimate of the bias of the new oxygen analyzer. As explained previously, we cannot simply take the standard deviation of the differences to calculate the limits of agreement because this would underestimate the true random error. Rather, we use Equation (5–20) to calculate a corrected standard deviation. To use this equation, we need the standard deviations of the differences between repeated measurements using two systems. However, in this application, there is only one measurement system and one set of true values. Thus, the standard deviation of the difference between repeated measurements using the new analyzer is 1.44 (from Table 5–4) and the other standard deviation is assumed to be zero. Finally, we need the standard deviation of the difference between the mean values of each system. Again, in this application we will take the standard deviation of the differences

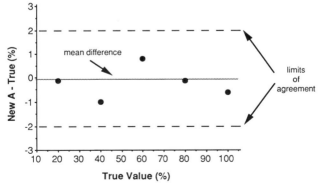

FIG 5–10.
Simulated data for evaluation of inaccuracy by calculating "limits of agreement."

between the mean values of repeated measurements and the true value, 0.81 (from Table 5–4). Substituting these values into Equation (5–20) yields:

$$S_c = \sqrt{0.81^2 + \frac{1.44^2}{4} + \frac{0^2}{4}} = 1.08$$

Using the mean difference the corrected standard deviation, and an appropriate t value ($t_{0.975}$ with $n - 1 = 9$ degrees of freedom is 2.26) with Equation (5–16) gives us:

$$\text{Limits of agreement} = -0.06 \pm (2.26 \times 1.08)$$
$$= -0.06 \pm 2.44$$

Therefore, our estimate of maximum inaccuracy is $|-0.06 - 2.44| = |-2.5| = 2.5$ (which is believable considering the parameters used to generate the simulated data and in light of the other estimates of inaccuracy). When expressed as a percentage of full scale, our estimate of inaccuracy for the new oxygen analyzer is 2.5/100 or about $\pm 3\%$ FS. Again, this value does not lead us to believe the manufacturer's specification of $\pm 1\%$ FS.

Evaluation of Agreement (Limits of Agreement)

Analysis Based on Single Measurements.—The purpose of assessing the agreement between the new oxygen analyzer and the old device is to determine whether or not the current standard of care (i.e., our ability to control F_{IO_2} accurately) will be maintained if the new analyzer is adopted. Beforehand, we arbitrarily decide that a difference in measured F_{IO_2} between the two systems as large as 1% is clinically significant because we frequently change F_{IO_2} in increments this small in premature infants prone to persistent pulmonary hypertension.

A plot of the difference between measured F_{IO_2} using the New O_2 Analyzer A and Old O_2 Analyzer A data from Table 5–5 shows that there is apparently no relation between the difference and the mean values (Fig 5–11). Table 5–5 shows that the mean difference between measurements from the new and the old analyzers is −0.14 with a standard deviation of 0.63. Using Equation (5–18) and $t_{0.975} = 2.78$ (with $n - 1 = 4$ degrees of freedom) we get:

$$\text{Limits of agreement} = -0.14 \pm (2.78 \times 0.63)$$
$$= -0.14 \pm 1.75$$

Our estimate of the maximum disagreement is therefore $|-0.14 - 1.75| = |-1.89| \approx 1.9$. Because this exceeds our arbitrary threshold of 1.0, we conclude that the new analyzer would not permit us to control F_{IO_2} as well as the currently used analyzers.

Analysis Based on Duplicate Measurements.—The mean difference between duplicate measurements made with the new analyzer and duplicate measurements made with the old

TABLE 5–5.
Simulated Experimental Data from Old Oxygen Analyzers*

	Measured Values		Calculated Values				
True Value	Old O_2 Analyzer A	Old O_2 Analyzer B	Difference Old (A-B)	Mean Old	Difference Mean New-Mean Old	Difference New A-Old A	Mean New A and Old A
20.0	19.8	20.6	−0.73	20.2	0.35	0.03	19.9
40.0	39.8	39.6	0.21	39.7	−0.77	−0.89	39.4
60.0	60.0	59.9	0.10	60.0	−0.01	0.79	60.4
80.0	80.0	80.2	−0.16	80.1	0.82	−0.10	80
100.0	99.9	100.1	−0.23	100.0	−0.73	−0.52	99.7
			S† = 0.36		mean = −0.07 S† = 0.69	mean = −0.14 S† = 0.63	

*Calculations were performed with 14 significant figures but results are displayed with 3 significant figures.
† S = standard deviation with $n - 1$ degrees of freedom.

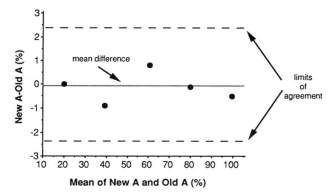

FIG 5–11.
Simulated data for evaluation of "agreement" between old and new oxygen analyzers.

analyzer is -0.07 (Table 5–5). The standard deviation of the mean differences is 0.69. The corrected standard deviation, using Equation (5–20) is:

$$S_c = \sqrt{0.69^2 + \frac{1.44^2}{4} + \frac{0.36^2}{4}} = 1.01$$

Using Equation (5–18) and $t_{0.975} = 2.78$ (with $n - 1 = 4$ degrees of freedom) we get:

$$\text{Limits of agreement} = -0.07 \pm (2.78 \times 1.01)$$
$$= -0.07 \pm 2.81$$

The estimate of maximum disagreement is therefore $|-0.07 - 2.81| = |-2.88| \approx 2.9$. This value exceeds the arbitrary threshold of 1.0, so we conclude that the new analyzer would not allow the same degree of control over F_{IO_2} as the currently used analyzers.

Evaluation of Repeatability

To calculate the coefficient of repeatability from Equation (5–21), we need the standard deviation of the differences between repeated measurements (from Table 5–4). The coefficient for the new analyzer is:

$$\text{Coefficient of repeatability} = 2.8 \times 1.44 = 4.03$$

This means that, 95% of the time, the difference between duplicate measurements will be less than about 4. For the old analyzer, the coefficient of repeatability is $2.8 \times 0.36 = 1.01$. The two analyzers seem to be clearly different in terms of repeatability.

REFERENCES

1. Weiss MD: *Biomedical Instrumentation*. Philadelphia, Chilton Book Co, 1973.
2. Bishop O: *Yardsticks of the Universe*. New York, Peter Bedrick Books, 1984; p. 114.
3. Syndeham PH: Standardization of measurement fundamentals and practices, in Sydenham PH (ed): *Handbook of Measurement Science*. Vol 1, *Theoretical Fundamentals*. New York, John Wiley & Sons, 1982, pp. 49–94.
4. Krebs DE: Measurement theory. *Phys Ther* 1987; 67:1834–1839.
5. Beckwith TG, Buck NL, Marangoni RD: *Mechanical Measurements*, ed 3. Reading, MA, Addison-Wesley Publishing Co, 1982.
6. Webster JG (ed): *Medical Instrumentation: Application and Design*. Boston, Houghton Mifflin, 1978.
7. Beers Y: *Introduction to the Theory of Error*. Reading, MA, Addison-Wesley Publishing Co, 1957.
8. Devore JL: *Probability and Statistics for Engineering and the Sciences*. Monterey, CA; Brooks/Cole, 1982, p. 199.
9. Rubin SA: *The Principles of Biomedical Instrumentation: A Beginner's Guide*. Chicago, Year Book Medical Publishers, 1987.
10. Miller WF, Scacci R, Gast LR: *Laboratory Evaluation of Pulmonary Function*. Philadelphia, J. B. Lippincott, 1987.
11. Lab management: Quality assurance for the clinical lag; method evaluation, 1989, Colorado Association for Continuing Medical Laboratory Education, Inc, 925 South Niagara Street, Suite 220, Denver, CO 80224.
12. Weisbrot IM: *Statistics for the Clinical Laboratory*. Philadelphia, J. B. Lippincott, 1985.
13. Cromwell L, Weibell FJ, Pfeiffer EA, et al: *Biomedical Instrumentation and Measurement*. Englewood Cliffs, NJ: Prentice-Hall, 1973.
14. Doebelin EO: *Measurement Systems: Application and Design*. New York, McGrall-Hill, 1966, pp. 38–209.
15. Baird, DC: *Experimentation: An Introduction to Measurement Theory and Experimental Design*. Englewood Cliffs, NJ: Prentice-Hall, 1962, p. 30.
16. Penny RK: *The Experimental Method*. London: Longman, 1974, pp. 73–79.
17. Bourke GJ, Daly LE, McGilvray J: *Interpretation and Uses of Medical Statistics*. Boston: Blackwell Scientific Publications, 1985, pp. 241–246.
18. Severinghaus JW, Naifeh KH: Accuracy of response of six pulse oximeters to profound hypoxia. *Anesthesiology* 1987; 67:551–558.
19. Severinghaus JW, Naifeh KH, Koh SO: Errors in 14 pulse oximeters during profound hypoxia. *J Clin Mon* 1989; 5:72–81.
20. Wedlock BD, Roberge JK: *Electronic components and measurements*. Englewood Cliffs, NJ: Prentice-Hall, 1969, p. 237.
21. Weber LJ, McLean DL: Electrical measurement systems for biologic and physical scientists. Reading, MA; Addison-Wesley, 1975; p. 119.
22. American Thoracic Society. Standardization of spirometry—1987 update. *Respir Care* 1987; 32:1039–1060.
23. Westgard JO, Hunt MR: Use and interpretation of common statistical tests in method-comparison studies. *Clin Chem* 1973; 19:49–57.
24. Chatburn RL, Primiano FP, Jr: Mathematical models of pulmonary mechanics, in Chatburn RL, Craig KD (eds): *Fundamentals of Respiratory Care Research*. Norwalk, Appleton & Lange 1988, pp. 59–100.
25. Ligas JR. Instrumentation, in: Chatburn RL, Craig KC (eds): *Fundamentals of Respiratory Care Research*. Norwalk, Appleton & Lange, 1988, pp. 281–303.

26. Gabe IT: Pressure measurement in experimental physiology, in Bergel DH (ed): *Cardiovascular Fluid Dynamics*. New York, Academic Press, 1972, pp. 11–50.

27. Chatburn RL, Carlo WA, Primiano FP, Jr: Airway-pressure measurement during high frequency ventilation. *Respir Care* 1985; 30:750–758.

28. Takai H: *Theory of Automatic Control*. London: Iliffe Books Ltd, 1966, pp. 87–107.

29. Funucane KE, Egan BA, Dawson SV: Linearity and frequency response of pneumotachographs. *J Appl Physiol* 1972; 32:121–126.

30. Jackson AC, Vinegar A: A technique for measuring frequency response of pressure, volume, and flow transducers. *J Appl Physiol* 1979; 47:462–467.

31. Klienman B: Understanding natural frequency and damping and how they relate to the measurement of blood pressure. *J Clin Monit* 1989; 5:137–147.

32. Bland M: *An Introduction to Medical Statistics*. New York, Oxford University Press, 1989, pp. 276–296.

33. Chatburn RL: Mathematical procedures, in Lough MD, Chatburn RL, Schrock WA (eds): *Handbook of Respiratory Care*. Chicago, Yearbook Medical Publishers, 1990, pp. 323–371.

34. Barford NC: *Experimental Measurements: Precision, Error, and Truth*. London, Addison-Wesley, 1967, pp. 37–40.

35. Truwit JD, Marini JJ: Evaluation of thoracic mechanics in the ventilated patient. Part 1: Primary measurements. *J Crit Care* 1988; 3:133–150.

36. Norton AC: Accuracy in pulmonary measurements. *Respir Care* 1979; 24:131–137.

37. Garner RM: Pulmonary function laboratory standards. *Respir Care* 1989; 34:651–660.

38. Hofmann D: Measurement errors, probability and information theory, in Sydenham PH (ed): *Handbook of Measurement Science*, Vol 1, *Theoretical Fundamentals*. New York, John Wiley & Sons, 1982, pp. 241–275.

39. Altman DG, Bland JM: Measurement in medicine: the analysis of method comparison studies. *Statistician* 1983; 32:307–317.

40. Cornbleet P, Gochman N: Incorrect least-squares regression coefficients in method comparison analysis. *Clin Chem* 1979; 25:432–438.

41. Draper NR, Smith H: Applied regression analysis, ed 2. New York, John Wiley & Sons, 1981.

42. Box GEP, Hunter WG, Hunter JS: *Statistics for Experimenters*. New York, John Wiley & Sons, 1978; p. 459.

43. Glantz SA. *Primer of Biostatistics*, ed 2. New York, McGraw-Hill, 1987, pp. 204–205.

44. Golish JA, Meden G: The physiologic basis for long-term oxygen therapy, in Lucas J, Golish JA, Sleeper G, O'Ryan JA (eds): *Home Respiratory Care*. Norwalk, Appleton & Lange, 1988, p. 13.

45. Bland JM, Altman DG: Statistical methods for assessing agreement between two methods of clinical measurement. *Lancet* 1986; 1:307–310.

46. Devore JL: *Probability and Statistics for Engineering and the Sciences*. Monterey, CA, Brooks/Cole, 1982.

47. Walpole RE, Myers RH: *Probability and Statistics for Engineers and Scientists*. New York, Macmillan, 1989, pp. 264–266, 242–244, 638–639.

48. Lindley DV, East DA, Hamilton PA: Tables for making inferences about the variance of a normal distribution. *Biometrika* 1960; 47:433–437.

49. Alexander CM, Teller LE, Gross JB: Principles of pulse oximetry: Theoretical and practical considerations. *Anesth Analg* 1989; 68:368–376.

50. Raurich JM, Ibañez J, Marse P: Validation of a new closed circuit indirect calorimetry method compared with open Douglas bag method. *Inten Care Med* 1989; 15:274–278.

51. Fuhrman BP, Smith-Wright DL, Venkataraman S, et al: Proximal mean airway pressure: A good estimator of mean alveolar pressure during continuous positive pressure breathing. *Crit Care Med* 1989; 17:666–670.

52. Praud JP, Carofilis A, Bridey F, et al: Accuracy of two wavelength pulse oximetry in neonates and infants. *Pediatric Pulmonology* 1989; 6:180–182.
53. Deming WE. *Statistical Adjustment of Data*. New York, John Wiley and Sons, 1943, p. 184.
54. McNitt LL. *Basic Computer Simulation*. Blue Ridge Summit, Tab, 1983, p. 80.
55. Chatburn RL, Craig KC: *Fundamentals of Respiratory Care*. Norwalk, Appleton & Lange, 1988.

Chapter 6

Quality Assessment and Maintenance of Respiratory Monitors

Gary Wiederhold

INTRODUCTION

Quality assessment (also called quality control or quality assurance) has become the main focus of almost every business in America. To compete successfully, a business must produce high-quality goods or services and maintain a reasonable price for their products. Quality assessment is equally important in health care, and a quality assessment program is necessary for hospital accreditation by the Joint Commission on Accreditation of Healthcare Organizations (JCAHO). The purpose of this chapter is to discuss quality assessment as it relates to monitors in respiratory care. The information presented in this chapter can be used to design a quality assessment program for monitors in hospitals. However, the specific aspects of a quality assurance program (e.g., choosing, evaluating, and reporting quality assurance monitors) are beyond the scope of this chapter. This chapter will cover the topic of quality assessment from the perspective of the monitors themselves and the persons using the monitors.

JCAHO REQUIREMENTS

Any hospital quality assessment program must meet or exceed the requirements of the JCAHO. Two sections of the JCAHO manual address the topic of quality assessment as it relates to monitors: (1) plant, technology, and safety management (PL) and (2) respiratory care services (RP). JCAHO standards provide a foundation for developing a quality assessment program that can be used for respiratory care monitors.

Plant, Technology, and Safety Management (PL)

Standards for equipment are described in JCAHO Standard PL.3. Meeting the requirements for this standard requires a program "designed to assess and control the clinical and physical risks"[1] of electrically powered equipment, including monitors.

An accurate inventory must be kept of all equipment, and written equipment testing procedures and user training programs must be documented. The training programs should be specifically designed to reduce clinical and physical risks. Testing is required on each piece of equipment prior to its initial use and annually, with the results of each test documented. Clinicians who either use or maintain the equipment should receive an initial orientation on the device and an annual refresher. The orientation and the refresher should be documented.

The quality assessment program should also have a system in place to "identify and document equipment failures and user errors."[2] Equipment failures, user errors, and published reports of equipment hazards should be reviewed. This will suggest potential problems that could cause an adverse effect on patient safety or the quality of care. This information can be used to avoid future problems and to set policy for the department.

Respiratory Care Services (RP)

Respiratory care is specifically covered in the RP section of the JCAHO manual. Guidelines RP.2 and RP.4 apply directly to the subject of this chapter. RP.2 states that "Personnel are prepared for their responsibilities in the provision of respiratory care services through appropriate training and education programs."[3] This standard includes in-service training. When monitors are involved, an in-service program should cover the monitor's proper use and also the routine maintenance that can be performed by the persons who will be using the monitor. Records should be made of the training received by each of the staff.

Of the standards mandated by the JCAHO accreditation manual, RP.4.3 most clearly describes what is required in relation to the equipment that is used in respiratory care: "All equipment is calibrated and operated according to the manufacturer's specifications and is periodically inspected and maintained according to an established schedule, as part of the hospital's preventive maintenance program."[4] The implication of this standard is that all clinicians who use a monitor must be familiar with the manufacturer's recommendations for use and maintenance. Further, a specific preventive maintenance program must be established for each monitor.

GOALS FOR QUALITY ASSESSMENT OF MONITORS

For a quality assessment program to be successful, it must have specific goals and standards. The three principal goals for a quality assessment program are listed in Table 6–1 and described following that table.

TABLE 6–1.
Goals of Quality Control

- Provide the best possible care for the patient
- Prevent problems rather than react to them
- Reduce the liability of the hospital and staff

Provide the Best Possible Care for the Patient.—This goal is the most important. If it is met, the other goals have been achieved as well. This is a very broad goal; in this chapter, we focus specifically on this goal in relation to monitors.

The best possible care for the patient can be attained by meeting the following criteria: maintaining patient safety, obtaining usable and accurate information from monitors, and controlling costs to the patient and hospital.

Patient safety can be affected in several ways. The monitor must be in good operating condition. Even a normally functioning monitor should be evaluated to determine that it is safe. This can be done by referring to records which indicate that electrical safety tests and preventive maintenance have been performed at the required intervals. Clinicians must appreciate that a normally operating monitor is not necessarily safe.

Usable and accurate information will also contribute to the quality of patient care. If a monitor is not calibrated, the data presented are of no value. In some cases, inaccurate data can actually be dangerous by causing steps to be taken or omitted based on questionable information from the monitor. Bad data are worse than no data at all!

Administrators, patients, and third-party payers are concerned about the costs of monitoring. Just because monitors are commercially available does not necessarily mean that they should be used; a valid indication of need should be assessed. This step can control the cost to both the patient and the hospital. Monitoring for the sake of monitoring increases the expense of caring for patients and increases the complexity of the care provided. On the other hand, occasions may occur when appropriate indications for the use of a monitor exist, but none is being used. This could have a negative impact on the patient. The highest priority is quality of patient care, and a monitor should be used when appropriately indicated, regardless of cost, to insure the best possible outcome for the patient.

Prevent Problems Rather than React to Them.—To prevent a problem is difficult, and may seem impossible at times. Preventing problems, rather than reacting to them, not only decreases their frequency, but also decreases their severity when they occur. Problem prevention can occur in several areas—patients, staff, or equipment.

Preventing a problem with the patient relates back to the first and highest priority—the best care for the patient. Monitors are specifically intended for this purpose. A properly functioning monitor will alert the clinician to changes that occur with the patient. The clinician can then take steps to correct the problem detected by the monitor.

The staff is a potential source of several types of problems. Prevention of problems in this area requires that all staff be properly trained in the use of the monitors. The JCAHO has outlined standards related to this in the quality assessment section of their manual. The specifics relate primarily to the clinical aspects of patient care. Any problem that develops through the use of a monitor should be recorded, reviewed by the staff, and the remedies discussed. This will raise the awareness of all the staff and avoid recurrence of the problem in the future. This is a valuable step in preventing problems, rather than reacting to them.

The equipment used is another potential source for problems. Specific decision-making before actually purchasing monitors can have a significant impact on the number and type of problems that are experienced with equipment. Getting the input of the clinical engineering (biomedical) department and staff clinicians is a very important step in selecting the best equipment for a specific application. The input from these persons can help clinicians avoid making the costly mistake of purchasing equipment that does not fit the clinical needs of the institution.

Before any monitor is purchased, it should have the approval of every department that will be affected by its use. The clinical engineering department is frequently consulted before a purchase. This department has a special area of expertise with equipment, and they are able to detect poor design and potential problems that could occur with the monitor. They also receive technical literature that discusses problems with equipment that is commercially available. By consulting the clinical engineering department, equipment with design flaws or high failure rates can be avoided.

Even though a monitor is acceptable to the clinical engineering department, the clinical staff that actually uses the equipment on a daily basis should also be consulted before purchase. These persons should be allowed to use the monitor in real clinical situations for a period of time. This will allow them to make evaluations of the monitor in its real environment. A piece of equipment that is difficult to use or causes clinical confusion should be avoided, and use of the monitor should be easy to learn.

The type of operator maintenance that is required should also be considered. If maintenance requires a lot of operator time or is complicated to perform, problems could arise. The clinician's time is better spent caring for patients. If routine maintenance is too complicated, it may be neglected, avoided, or performed improperly. When this occurs, the performance of the monitor could be adversely affected. This can have a cascading effect, and ultimately affect the quality of patient care.

An operator's manual is provided when a piece of equipment is purchased. This manual contains information about the monitor's use and maintenance. Anyone who uses the monitor, either clinical use or maintenance, should become familiar with the operator's manual. It explains proper clinical use of the monitor such as sensor placement, site preparation, and how to avoid some common problems that could cause erroneous results. Clinical situations that the monitor could "mask" or not be capable of detecting are explained. The operator's manual also explains how to set alarm thresholds and how to recognize an alarm condition when it occurs. The operator will also need to know how to display the desired data. Many of the commonly experienced problems with monitors are the result of an incomplete understanding of the use of the monitor. Reading the operator's manual will assist the clinician in understanding the equipment and will also make it easier to satisfy JCAHO criteria for quality assessment.

Maintenance of the monitor is also described in the operator's manual. The maintenance that needs to be performed and the time intervals for that maintenance are explained.

Some of this maintenance will be the responsibility of the operator, and some of it will be the responsibility of the clinical engineering staff. Maintenance of filters, probes, and sensors can usually be performed by the operator, as well as calibration of sensors. Internal calibration, replacement of circuit boards, and electrical safety testing are performed by the clinical engineering staff. To ensure that the monitor is operating at its peak performance, manufacturer-recommended maintenance schedules must be followed. This will decrease downtime and reduce overall costs for the monitor.

Reduce the Liability of the Hospital and Staff.—A quality assessment program should be designed to minimize the potential for litigation being brought against the hospital. As with the other goals, to accomplish this, the manufacturer's suggested maintenance must be observed. The equipment that is being used should be functioning as intended. The operator should also be knowledgeable of the operation of the equipment; a poorly trained user is a major potential for an adverse occurrence. If a reduction in litigation is realized, hospitals and their staff may realize savings in the form of lower insurance rates.

QUALITY ASSESSMENT FOR MONITORS IN RESPIRATORY CARE

The main focus of this part of the chapter will be directed at the quality assessment program itself. The concepts presented here are the result of many interviews with respiratory care practitioners. These individuals explained how their programs are designed to meet the goals and standards they have set. The beginning of this chapter was devoted to the standards set by the JCAHO and the goals set by the hospital. Using this information, a quality assessment program can be designed to meet the criteria that have been described.

Communication

The equipment quality assessment program should be a shared effort between the respiratory care department, the clinical engineering department, and, in some cases, a contracted outside service organization. The respiratory care and clinical engineering departments should be in close communication and should share information. Most problems that arise in any organization result from inadequate communication. Information exchange must be considered a key part of a quality assessment program. Both the respiratory care and the clinical engineering departments possess information that is unique to itself, but would benefit the other department. If this information is shared, the effectiveness of both departments will improve. Figure 6–1 shows the types of communication that would be useful to both departments.

Several ways exist to communicate this information from one department to another. Regularly scheduled meetings can be held either by phone or in person. A personal meeting is a good way to exchange information, but is not practical as an everyday practice. For as little as $1000, departments can share important information about monitors using a computer link. Such a computer system can provide up-to-date information about the status of the

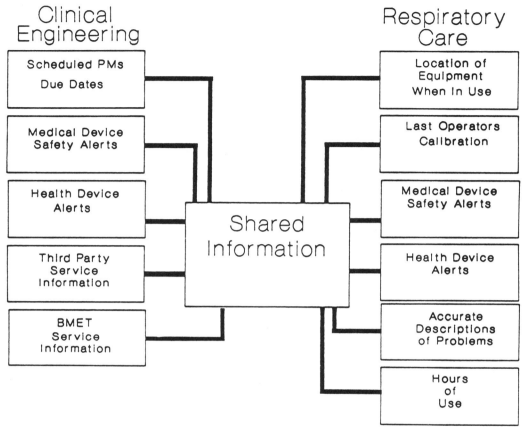

FIG 6–1.
Critical information to be shared between clinical engineering and respiratory care.

monitors. The computer data base can be accessed at any time, and thus provides the most current information.

Routine Daily Checks

For maximum performance of monitors, a planned procedure concerning their use should be in place. This procedure can be used to reduce downtime and increase the accuracy of the information obtained from the monitors. This section describes procedures that should be performed at least daily, or before the monitor is used on a patient. The flow chart in Figure 6–2 illustrates these steps.

One of the first steps that should be taken before putting the monitor into service is to determine if the monitor is due for any regularly scheduled maintenance. At regular intervals,

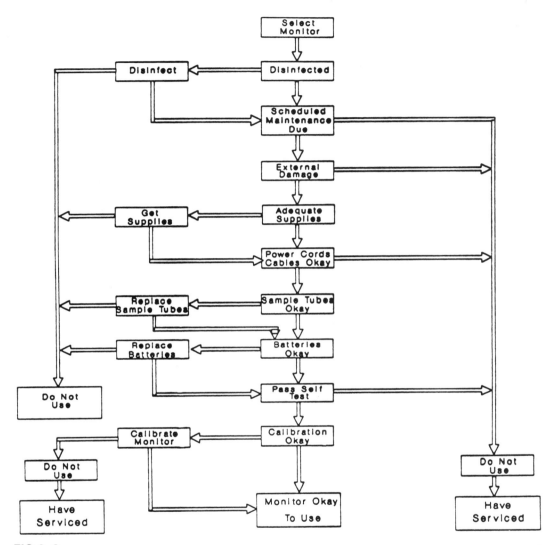

FIG 6–2.
Suggested procedure to be followed prior to placing a monitor into service.

monitors need preventive maintenance, internal calibration, and electrical safety tests. If records indicate that any of these tests needs to be performed, the monitor should be removed from service until they are completed. Regularly scheduled maintenance is the subject of the next section of this chapter.

Some monitors have the potential to transmit infection to the clinician or the patient. Prior to taking the following steps, it should be determined that the monitor has gone through proper disinfection procedures. The monitor and accessories should be disinfected or sterilized according to manufacturer's recommendations and hospital policy.

The operator's manual describes simple, routine checks that should be performed before a monitor is put into use. The operator should be familiar with the steps outlined in this manual. The exterior of the monitor should be visually checked for any obvious external damage. Dents, cracks, or anything broken could cause a problem with the monitor. Any type of liquid on the monitor should be considered external damage. If liquid is present, the monitor should not be used, and if it is in use, it should be immediately removed from service. Even though the monitor appears to be functioning normally, the liquid could penetrate the cabinet and cause severe internal damage. When any of the above conditions occur, the monitor should be inspected by qualified personnel before it is put back into use.

The next step is to make sure that all of the supplies necessary to use the monitor are available. Like the monitor itself, these supplies need to be checked to be certain that they are in proper operating condition. Power cords and cables that are cut or frayed present an unsafe condition for the operator and the patient. They should be repaired or replaced before the monitor is used.

Tubing should be inspected for leaks. If room air is entrained into the sample, or if the sample leaks out, this will cause the readings from the monitor to be inaccurate. This could also result in loss of gas that is intended for delivery to the patient. Leaky tubing can be a potential source for contamination of the patient environment, making other patients and operators susceptible to infection.

Batteries are a possible source of problems. Check the age of the batteries before using a monitor. If the expiration date has been reached, they should be replaced, even though the monitor appears to be operating correctly. As the batteries lose power, the accuracy of the monitor could be affected. This could also cause some difficulty if they went dead while in use on the patient. If this occurs and is undetected, it could produce an unsafe condition for the patient.

When the clinician has determined that the monitor and its supplies are safe to use, it needs to be checked for accuracy. The first step in doing this is to turn on the monitor. Many monitors perform a self-test when initiated. If this test fails, the monitor will produce an error code and cannot be used. Careful observation of the monitor while it is conducting its self-test can yield valuable information that can be used during troubleshooting. The error code that is produced and any other alarms or LEDs (light-emitting diodes) that are illuminated can be useful in determining the problem. Any error information should be relayed to those responsible for correcting the fault.

Although a monitor passes its self-test, the accuracy of the monitor is not guaranteed. To verify accuracy, a known signal must be used. For gas monitors, specially formulated calibration gases can be used. For other monitors, patient simulators such as the one in Figure 6–3 can be used. Both of these produce known signals. That is, the input to the monitor is a known value and the monitor, if calibrated, should display that value.

With the known signal applied, the monitor can be calibrated by the operator. Some monitors require a warm-up period before calibration, and calibration should not be attempted until the warm-up period has passed. The warm-up is required for the sensors to stabilize. A monitor that is calibrated before the warm-up is completed may not produce accurate readings

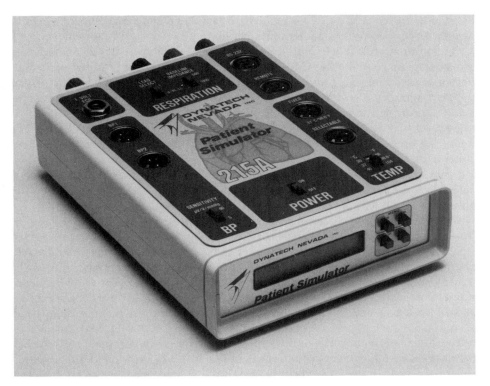

FIG 6–3.
Patient simulator.

after the warm-up. After calibration, the operator can use the monitor. A monitor that needs frequent calibrations, however, may need to be serviced because frequent calibrations could be an indicator of imminent failure.

Scheduled Maintenance

There are many reasons for sharing the information presented in Figure 6–1 between departments. One advantage to doing this involves preventive maintenance. A data base needs to be in effect to alert both the clinical engineering department and the respiratory care department of due dates for preventive maintenance. Preventive maintenance can be done on a calendar basis (e.g., every two months, every six months, every year) or based on the usage of the equipment. Usage information will be necessary to schedule preventive maintenance properly. The respiratory care department must make the equipment available when the preventive maintenance is due. When preventive maintenance is performed, parts are replaced, cleaned, or calibrated to prevent failures. This regularly scheduled maintenance should meet or exceed the manufacturer's recommendations and must not fall below such requirements.

Sharing information will help both the respiratory care and the clinical engineering departments to operate more smoothly. Clinical engineering will have the required parts to perform the preventive maintenance. This will result in less downtime for the respiratory care department. The respiratory care department can save time for the clinical engineering department by having the equipment ready and available for service.

If the preventive maintenance is not done internally, arrangements must be made with an outside service organization. A third-party service group can be contracted to make regularly scheduled visits or they can be contacted when necessary. As is the case with internal service, when a third party is contacted, it would be helpful if they knew exactly what type of equipment is to be serviced; also, the equipment should be made available when service is needed. Accomplishment of these steps requires good information and planning.

Another test that is done periodically is a series of electrical safety tests. These tests are done to verify that no excessive electrical current is leaking to the ground or to probes connected to the patient, that the unit is not drawing too much current, and that the ground is intact and functioning properly. Electrical safety tests will be discussed in detail later in this chapter.

An internal calibration may or may not be considered part of preventive maintenance. This calibration must be performed by qualified service personnel. It involves adjusting the circuit boards and sensors inside the monitor. The technician uses test points inside the monitor where equipment such as oscilloscopes or digital voltmeters are connected. Specific readings are expected at these points. When the expected reading is not obtained, the technician can make the necessary adjustments or replacements in order to attain the desired values.

The same data base used to schedule preventive maintenance can be used to record its completion. This will satisfy JCAHO requirements and document that the equipment is being properly maintained. This will also begin the cycle for the next maintenance schedule.

Record Keeping

One of the standards mandated by the JCAHO states that a system must be in place to track the equipment in each department. This can be accomplished by using the manufacturer's serial number, serial numbers assigned by the hospital, or by giving each monitor a unique name. These records can be used to coordinate all facets of the use of the monitor, which is why sharing information is important. Once this system is in place, accurate files must be maintained on each piece of equipment. This should be the foundation of the shared information mentioned earlier.

The location and the time of day when a monitor is used is information that can be kept by the respiratory care department, but is also very useful to the clinical engineering department. If there is a problem with intermittent failures of a monitor, this type of information is vital. The problem may be environmental (e.g., the monitor does not work in one room, but will work in another). By knowing where and when the failures occur, the biomedical technician can eliminate the problem.

Several monitors may be allocated to one area, such as the intensive care unit (ICU).

However, it is not enough to know that a pulse oximeter failed in the ICU. With only this information, much time could be wasted inspecting each pulse oximeter in the ICU. To save time, prevent further problems, and increase the efficiency of everyone involved, the biomedical technician needs to know specifically which monitor caused the problem. The monitor should then be taken out of use until it has been repaired.

The respiratory care department should also maintain records of the condition of the monitor before it was put into use. For example, a calibration performed on the monitor by the operator before it was put into use should be recorded. Records should be kept including readings before and after the calibration, and the frequency of the calibrations. This can provide valuable troubleshooting information for the clinical engineering department. Such information could produce a trend that would point toward a specific failure or a component that is about to fail. This will result in less time spent troubleshooting and less downtime for the monitor.

Another source of records that the respiratory care department should maintain is the service history of the monitor. Service history should be documented by the clinical engineering department or by a third-party service group. A trend could be observed that would point to problems with a particular monitor or manufacturer. From this information, a decision can be made to replace a monitor or to change manufacturers or suppliers.

Each time electrical safety tests are performed, the results should be recorded. These can be compared to previous readings to determine if there has been any deterioration in the operating condition of the monitor.

Any training on a specific monitor by the staff should also be recorded. Trained personnel are an asset because they have a better understanding of the equipment and its use. Trained staff can be used to remedy operator problems and machine failures. When there is a monitor failure, trained staff can provide more accurate information about the failure to the biomedical technicians.

Much of the record keeping suggested here may seem to be a burden on the hospital staff. This is usually only the case until a system is developed that is comfortable for everyone who uses it. Also, none of the records is of much value unless the people that need them have access to them. That is why it is strongly suggested that the records kept by each department are shared. The burden that may be created by keeping these records is far outweighed by the gains that can be realized by each department. Everyone involved profits from this sharing—including the respiratory care staff, the clinical engineering staff, and, most importantly, the patient.

Training

Another part of a quality assessment and maintenance program involves clinicians who are properly trained to operate the monitors. Although everyone who uses the monitor should be familiar with it, there are often a few key operators for each monitor. These persons should receive special training on a monitor and be a source of information for other staff.

Routine maintenance and calibration should be included in the training. The key operators could be assigned responsibility to perform these procedures or to oversee them when they are being done by others. This will assure that maintenance and calibrations are done properly.

Operators must be trained in the proper use of the monitor. Some examples of common problems that are experienced with the use of monitors include poor site preparation for transcutaneous electrodes, pulse oximeter probes exposed to ambient light or used with colored fingernails, and capnographs installed in such a way as to occlude the sample tubing with moisture and secretions. Other problems that can be avoided are operator misunderstandings about setting and recognizing alarms. Training will enable operators to recognize and avoid potential problems associated with improper use of the equipment.

Training is offered in many forms, and the type of training should be tailored to that which is most beneficial to the staff. Manufacturers offer classes that can be attended away from the hospital. This is probably the most expensive type of training, but also the most effective. By being out of the facility, staff avoid interruptions and can better concentrate on the training. Manufacturers also offer in-service training at the hospital. Having a manufacturer's representative conduct the training in the hospital allows more persons to become acquainted with the equipment. Additionally, real-life situations and applications can be explained to the people who need the information. This type of training is also more timely and less costly.

Refresher classes are also required by the JCAHO. Refresher classes have advantages over the other types of training described. These classes can occur when and where they are needed. They can be directed specifically to the people who need the training. Refresher classes should be offered at regular intervals. The objective of these classes is to keep important information about a monitor fresh in the minds of the staff that have already received training.

Equipment Replacement

One final issue affecting quality is determining when a piece of equipment should be replaced or its use discontinued. The driving force here is primarily cost, but other factors are also important (Table 6–2).

The maintenance expense for a monitor needs to be examined when determining whether or not it should be replaced. The costs of service contracts should also be considered. Here again, accurate records need to be kept to make a decision to discontinue the use of a monitor and purchase a new one. The person with responsibility for these expenses needs to set a limit. Once this limit has been reached it should be an indication that the monitor needs to be replaced.

Another consideration is downtime of the monitor. The monitor may be inexpensive to maintain, but is frequently not in service. This can have hidden expenses in the form of inconvenience. Another monitor or another technology may be needed to make the measure-

TABLE 6–2.
Reasons to Replace Equipment

- Cost of maintenance
- Amount of downtime
- Old technology
- Obsolescence
- Standard of care

ments that were required. A larger inventory of monitors may be needed to assure that a functioning monitor is available. In any case, the fact that the first choice of monitor was not functioning can cause additional expense by reducing the efficiency of the staff.

New technology could also produce a need to replace existing equipment. The new monitor could incorporate features that would improve patient care even though it is making the same measurements as an older model. A new monitor could make present units too expensive compared to the new model. Anything that makes the monitor easier for the operator to use could result in labor savings and reduce the risk of errors. An improvement in accuracy could also produce savings by making medical decisions more accurate. The result would be a reduction in the length of the patient's stay because treatment is improved.

At some point, it may become necessary for the manufacturer to declare a monitor obsolete. Obsolescence is not done to promote sales of newer products. It is done because a superior product has become available that can produce a better outcome for the patient. Many events in the market could prompt the manufacturer to discontinue support for one of their products. There may be a small population of a particular monitor in service, which would make it too costly for the manufacturer to support. Another monitor could have been designed to perform the same function as the older one but have significant advantages over the previous model. The new monitor could reduce the manufacturer's liability through better performance. Any of these events could prompt the manufacturer to take the older model out of service. Sales may fall for a monitor that once was a good selling unit, and at some point the manufacturer will have to discontinue its efforts in that particular market. Once the sales efforts are terminated, the manufacturer may withdraw the service support for that product. In any event, a product that has been declared obsolete will have a limited future. Once existing parts are exhausted, the monitor cannot be repaired properly and it should be removed from service. Obsolescence should signal the user that steps will need to be taken to replace the equipment.

To reduce the likelihood of successful litigation against the hospital, attention must be paid to procedures being used by other hospitals. A standard of care is developed through the use of common procedures. If it is standard practice for hospitals to use a particular monitor on all ventilator patients, then that becomes a standard of care. If an incident occurs that could have been detected by that monitor, the hospital could be found liable if a monitor was not being used. If use of a monitor has been established as a standard, then the hospital's failure to use this monitor could produce liability. The same could be true of monitors that are being phased out of use and replaced with more modern equipment.

Reporting Equipment Malfunctions

The US Pharmacopeial Convention (USPC) serves as the governmental agency for reporting medical equipment problems. This voluntary Product Problem Reporting Program is a clinician-oriented system used to communicate health hazards and product problems to government and industry. Equipment problems are reported to the USPC using a standard form. A copy of the report is forwarded by the USPC to the Food and Drug Adminstration (FDA) and the manufacturer of the device identified in the report, which should initiate corrective action.

The Safe Medical Devices Act of 1990 required the reporting of serious medical device problems to begin late in 1991. All incidents that suggest a probability that a medical device caused or contributed to the death, serious illness, or serious injury of a patient must be reported to the FDA. Facilities should report problems as soon as possible, but not later than 10 days after becoming aware of the incident. Reports should include information such as the identity of the reporting facility, product name, model, serial number, name of manufacturer, and description of the event. Patient deaths resulting from medical device problems should be reported to the FDA and the manufacturer. Serious illness and serious injury resulting from medical device problems should be reported to the manufacturer or the FDA.

ELECTRICAL SAFETY TESTS

Virtually all monitors are electrically powered. Electrical safety tests are included as a separate topic in this chapter because of their importance to the safety of both the patient and clinician. The purpose of electrical safety testing is to protect the patient and the operator from injury caused by an electromedical device. The JCAHO manual mandates in standard PL.3.2.1.1 that "Each piece of equipment is tested prior to initial use and at least annually thereafter; such testing is documented."[5] This section will discuss the electrical tests that are performed and the reasons for these tests.

The American National Standards Institute (ANSI) divides electromedical devices into four categories. These classifications are outlined in the ANSI standard, "Safe Current Limits for Electromedical Apparatus," Section ES1. Three classifications of monitors are affected by this standard. Each of these has different requirements for electrical safety. Equipment under discussion in this book falls into the three categories listed below:

> *Paragraph 2.1:* "Electromedical Apparatus with Isolated Connection: Electromedical apparatus intended to be connected to the patient and having a patient circuit that is isolated from ground, utility power systems, and other supporting circuitry to such a degree that the risk current at the patient connection(s) meets the limits set in this standard for isolated patient connections."

> *Paragraph 2.2:* "Electromedical Apparatus with Non-isolated Patient Connection: Electromedical apparatus intended to be connected to the patient and for which the risk current at the patient connection(s) meets the limits set in this standard for non-isolated patient connections."

> *Paragraph 2.3:* "Electromedical Apparatus Likely to Contact the Patient: Electromedical apparatus that does not have a patient connection, but which is intended for use in the patient vicinity."

The wall outlet for alternating current (ac) power has three receptacles that mate to three connectors on the plug of a piece of equipment (Fig 6–4). There is a U-shaped receptacle and two rectangular receptacles. The U-shape is the ground, the one rectangular shape is the "hot" incoming power (usually 120 V-120 VAC), and the other is the "neutral" power return (normally 0 V). With the ground receptacle at the top position, the neutral connector is on the right and the hot is on the left. The neutral rectangle is slightly larger than the hot, which will prevent the plug from being inserted backward. The ground pin that inserts into the U-shape is longer than the two inserts for the hot and neutral pins. Because it is longer, the

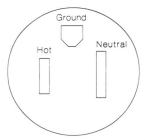

FIG 6–4.
Configuration of 120-VAC 60-Hz outlet.

ground will be the first connection made when plugging in a piece of equipment, and the last connection to be disconnected when unplugging a piece of equipment. Electrical safety testing of the plug will be described later in this section.

Normal current flow is from the hot terminal to the neutral terminal. The ground pin is installed for safety. The ground creates a second path for current to be carried safely away from the monitor should the normal (neutral) path fail. The ground also safely removes unwanted current potential that may exist between the machine and anyone who comes into contact with it. The electrical safety tests are designed to determine if this system is functioning properly.

Reference is made to a "chassis" when performing electrical safety testing. The chassis is considered to be the case of the equipment and any conductive surfaces of the monitor. An electrical connection exists between the chassis and ground on the plug (Fig 6–5).

The preceding text describes a normally insulated monitor. However, double-insulated pieces of equipment are also available. A double-insulated monitor can be viewed as the same device described above, but with an additional insulated shell or case built around it (Fig 6–6). The outside is insulated from conductivity with the inside box. The ground connection is made with the box on the inside.

Patient leads are electrical connections that come into direct contact with the patient. Some examples of these are ECG leads, transcutaneous sensors, and probes for pulse oximetry. Depending on the internal design of the machine, these leads can be either isolated or nonisolated. An isolated patient lead is one that has no electrical connection between the patient leads and the monitor. There is a patient side and a monitor side divided by the iolation line shown in Figure 6–7. Patient information and control from the monitor is passed back and forth across the isolation line using LEDs and photosensors, a transformer, or some similar device. This could be compared to someone sending signals using Morse code and a flashlight. Signals would be returned in the same manner, yet there is no physical connection between the persons communicating. The leads plug into the monitor, but the signals are not passed to the monitor over a wire. A nonisolated patient connection exists when there is a physical connection between the patient and the monitor. This means the signals to and from the leads are connected to the monitor through a wire (Fig 6–8).

To perform electrical safety testing, a safety analyzer (Fig 6–9) is required. Such devices

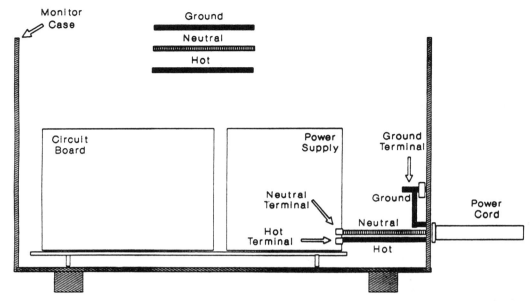

FIG 6–5.
Normally insulated monitor.

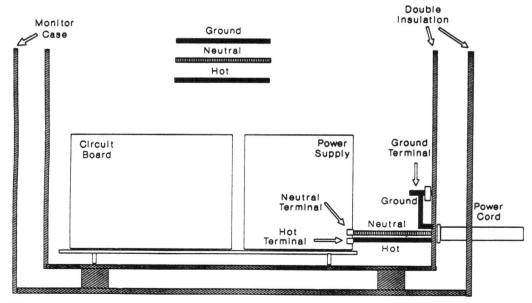

FIG 6–6.
Double-insulated monitor.

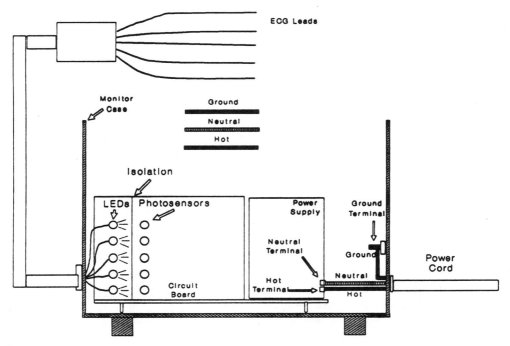

FIG 6–7.
Isolated patient connections.

are capable of performing all of the tests to be described. For the sake of simplicity, the pictures that accompany the following text shows the alterations being conducted inside the monitor. In reality, the alterations are created inside the safety analyzer. All of these tests are performed because these conditions have the potential to exist in the hospital. A disconnected ground could be caused by a broken ground wire in the power cord or the wall outlet. The wall outlet itself could be wired in reverse polarity. If the equipment fails any of these tests, it should not be used until it has been repaired. After it has passed the tests, there should be no danger from electrical shock from that piece of equipment.

When a biomedical technician performs the electrical safety tests, one of the things that is tested is current draw. Current draw is similar to the volume of water flowing through a hose in a given period of time. For electricity, this is the amount of current or amperage the monitor is using. The person performing the test creates the maximum current draw situation for the monitor. Referring to the service manual for that monitor allows the technician to know the amount of current that should be measured. Internal problems are indicated by a current draw that is too high.

Another electrical test involves the source current. This test measures the amount of current that could be experienced by the operator or patient under a number of conditions. The test will fail if more than $100\mu A$ rms (root-mean-square) is detected by the safety analyzer. This

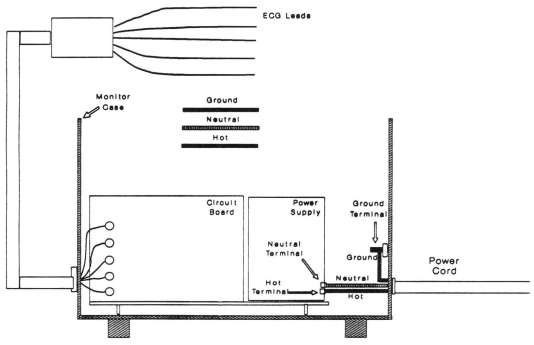

FIG 6–8.
Nonisolated patient connections.

is considered to be below the threshold of perception unless the area in contact with the equipment is less than 2 mm^2.

Source current measurements are made using a probe attached to the piece of equipment being tested. With the monitor plugged into the safety analyzer, the current potential is measured with the power switch on and off, with the electrical supply normal and reversed (Figs 6–10 and 6–11), and with the ground connected and open (Fig 6–12). The current measured is the current that would pass through the body of someone who comes into contact with the machine being tested.

Another test that is performed is case-to-ground line resistance. Current will flow through the path of least resistance. If a fault exists inside of a piece of equipment, the danger of electrical shock exists. Anyone who comes into contact with that piece of equipment could create a path to ground. The equipment has an internal path to ground designed to alleviate this problem. If the resistance to current flow in this internal ground is higher than the resistance through someone's body, the current will pass through the body instead of the internal ground. A wet hand has a resistance[6] of approximately 1000 Ω. When the case-to-ground line test is performed, it will fail if the resistance is greater than 0.1 Ω (Fig 6–10).

Patient source current is also evaluated during electrical safety testing. This test measures the current being applied to or received from the patient through the patient leads (Figs 6–13

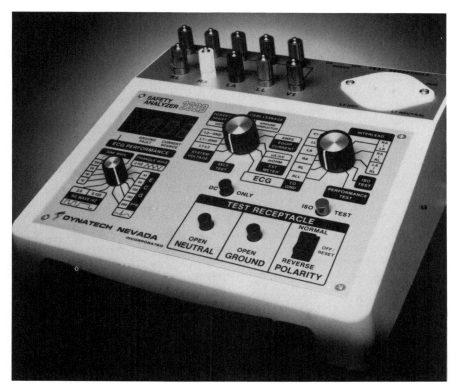

FIG 6–9.
Electrical safety analyzer.

and 6–14). The same conditions are created for this test that are used for source current testing. The measurements are made with the polarity of the current normal and reversed, power switch on and off, and the ground connected and disconnected. For machines with isolated patient connections, the test will fail if the current measured is above 10 μA, and for nonisolated patient connections if the fail point is current above 50 μA.

"Patient sink current" is the final test performed in the series of electrical safety tests. This test is not performed on equipment with nonisolated patient connections. Current is measured that travels into the monitor through patient leads when an external voltage is applied to the leads (Fig 6–15). Measurements are made with the monitor on and off, and properly connected to its power supply. The test is conducted by applying 120 VAC to the patient connection. When the cable is attached to the monitor, this current can be no greater than 20 μA rms at the patient end of the cable, and not greater than 10 μA rms at the input to the monitor. The patient sink current test is designed to protect the patient. If the current that could flow into the monitor is too high, patient injury could result. Such an event could cause discomfort, anxiety, burns, ventricular fibrillation, and possibly death.

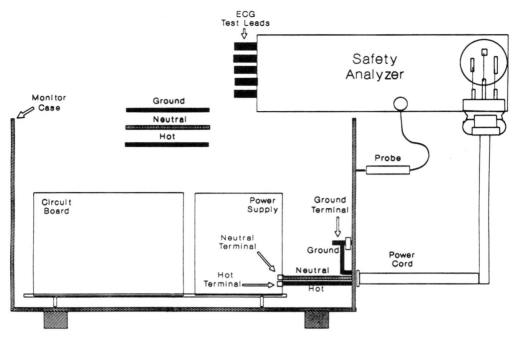

FIG 6–10.
Current leakage test being performed with normal polarity.

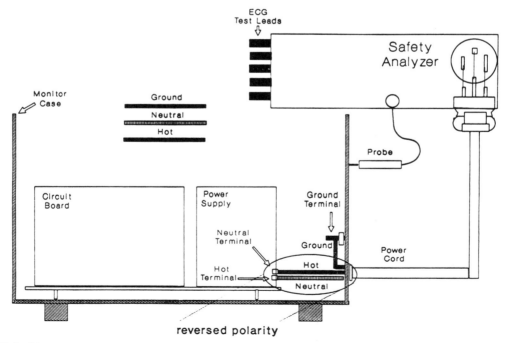

FIG 6–11.
Current leakage test being performed with reversed polarity.

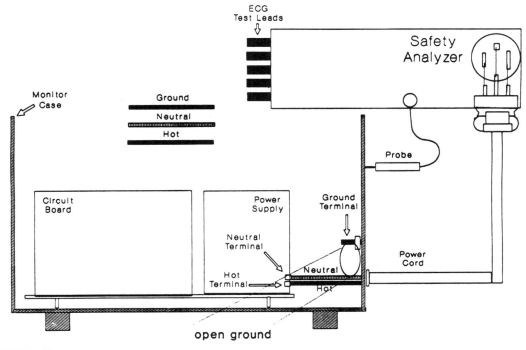

FIG 6–12.
Current leakage test being performed with an open ground.

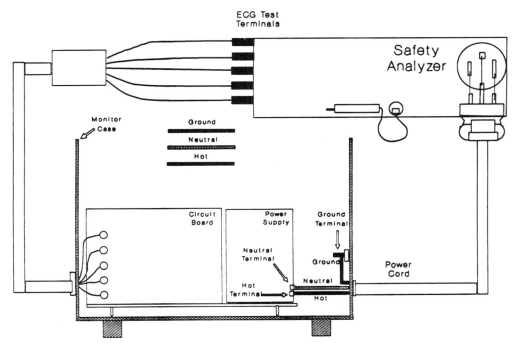

FIG 6–13.
ECG current leakage test with nonisolated leads.

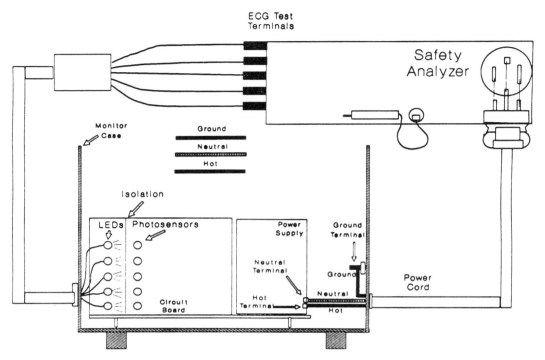

FIG 6–14.
Current leakage test being done through isolated ECG leads.

Electrical safety tests are designed to assure that the equipment is safe from the hazards of electrical shock. This series of tests evaluates the design and ability of the equipment to prevent an electrical shock. The pass/fail criteria for electrical safety that monitors are required to meet is chosen based on prior research in this area. If any of these tests fails, the machine should immediately be removed from service, and it should not be used until it has been repaired and can pass all of the tests described above.

SUMMARY

This chapter described the areas that a quality assessment program for monitors should encompass to meet the requirements of the JCAHO. Before a quality assessment program is initiated, goals for the program must be determined. The most important goal is the best possible care for the patient, the second goal is to prevent problems rather than react to them, and the final goal is to reduce the liability of the hospital and staff.

A quality assessment program will require a maintenance schedule for equipment and a training schedule for staff. This program should have provisions to guarantee that the equipment is maintained according to manufacturers' specifications, and that the maintenance is

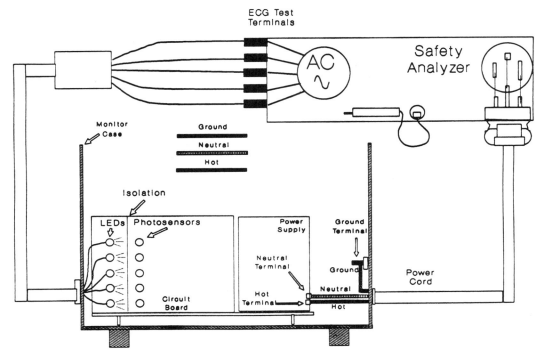

FIG 6–15.
Patient sink current test.

recorded. Personnel should receive refresher courses on equipment in their department at regular intervals. A quality assessment program will help to determine when to replace or retire monitors; knowledge of procedures in other facilities is a key factor in making this decision. A standard of care is established that the hospital should equal or exceed to protect it from litigation.

Cooperation between the respiratory care and clinical engineering departments, including the sharing of information, is necessary to the success of a quality assessment program for monitors. Electrical safety tests should be performed at their regularly scheduled intervals. These tests are designed to check a monitor's ability to protect patients, staff, and visitors from electrical shock in the event of a failure. Electrical safety tests are a critical part of the quality assessment program. No piece of equipment should be used if it fails these tests until it has been repaired by qualified individuals and meets all the criteria for the tests.

REFERENCES

1. *JCAHO 1990 Accreditation Manual.* PL.3, p. 200.
2. *JCAHO 1990 Accreditation Manual.* PL.3.3, p. 200.
3. *JCAHO 1990 Accreditation Manual.* RP.2, p. 228.

4. *JCAHO 1990 Accreditation Manual.* RP.4.3, p. 231.
5. *JCAHO 1990 Accreditation Manual.* PL.3.2.1.1, p. 200.
6. Stoner D, Smathers J, Hyman W, et al: *Engineering a Safe Hospital Environment.* New York, John Wiley and Sons, 1982, p. 8.

ADDITIONAL READING

Biloon F: Medical Equipment Service Manual Theory and Maintenance Procedures. Englewood Cliffs, NJ, Prentice-Hall, 1978, pp. 1–22.

Cromwell L, Weibell FJ, Pfeiffer EA: Biomedical Instrumentation and Measurement, ed. 2. Englewood Cliffs, NJ, Prentice-Hall, 1980, pp. 430–447.

Geddes LA, Baker LE: *Principles of Applied Biomedical Instrumentation*, ed 2. New York, John Wiley and Sons, 1975, pp. 549–550.

Cromwell L, Arditi M, Weibell FJ, et al: Medical Instrumentation for Health Care. Englewood Cliffs, NJ, Prentice-Hall, 1976, pp. 18,65, 325–347.

Bahill T. Bioengineering (Biomedical, Medical and Clinical Engineering). Englewood Cliffs, NJ, Prentice-Hall, 1981, pp. 255–294.

Webster JG. Medical Instrumentation Application and Design. Boston, Houghton Mifflin Co, 1978, pp. 667–707.

Chapter 7

Oxygen Transport from Lung to Tissue

Richard Teplick, M.D.

INTRODUCTION

This chapter is a survey of the processes involved in the transport of gases between the lung and tissue cells. The purpose is to integrate basic physiologic principles with clinical practice, so that a basis can be established to evaluate and critique the measurements used to assess the adequacy of each step in the processes of gas transport to and from tissues. We provide a brief overview of the features of the transport processes themselves, convection and diffusion. Next, the carriage by blood of inert gases, oxygen, and carbon dioxide is discussed. The following section focuses on the transfer of gases from the lung to the blood. This begins with the diffusion of gases between a single alveolus and blood, emphasizing the effects of the alveolar ventilation-perfusion ratio. Next, the genesis of alveolar-arterial partial pressure differences is considered, emphasizing the effects of alveoli with different ventilation-perfusion ratios, true shunt, and dead-space. This background is applied in another section to examine various indices of pulmonary gas exchange. The principles of gas diffusion to tissues are developed, emphasizing oxygen and the possible methods for compensating for increased tissue oxygen demand. These fundamentals are used in the next section to assess several proposed indices of tissue oxygenation, emphasizing limitations imposed by variations in local tissue metabolic rates and blood flow. The material from the preceding sections is then applied in the last section to examine the various methods that have been proposed for increasing tissue oxygenation without compromising the patient.

GAS TRANSPORT: GENERAL PRINCIPLES

The major goal in gas transport is to get sufficient oxygen (O_2) to tissues to meet their metabolic needs and to remove carbon dioxide (CO_2) at the rate that it is produced by tissues. Two physical processes are responsible for meeting these goals: convection and diffusion. Gases are transferred by convection if they are contained in a gas mixture or fluid that is in motion, usually driven by a pressure difference. For example, gases are transported in blood by convective flow driven by blood pressure differences throughout the circulation. In contrast, if the media containing the gas is not in motion, gas molecules may still move from one region to another by diffusion. The driving force is usually described as a concentration difference, but this is not necessarily true when the two regions have different properties (see the next section). For example, oxygen is transferred from alveoli to blood by diffusion.

Convection and diffusion are each dominant in different sites of gas transport to and from tissues. Convection is the major form of gas transport in the larger pulmonary airways. However, diffusion becomes progressively more important in the smaller airways so that by approximately the 16th generation of airways (the terminal bronchioles), the flows due to convection and diffusion are equal and diffusion dominates distal to the 17th division (the respiratory bronchioles). Gases diffuse from alveoli to blood but convective transport by blood brings the gases to tissues. Diffusion again conveys gases produced by cells into blood and blood convectively transports these gases back to the lung. Because these two modes of transport are so fundamental to gas exchange, the principles that govern them must be understood in some detail to analyze gas exchange and understand the bases and limitations of the measurements and indices used to evaluate the adequacy of gas transport between the lung and tissues.

Diffusion

The driving force for diffusion is usually related to concentration differences via Fick's first law of diffusion. This principle states that the flow of a material, in this case a gas, per unit area in a given time occurs from regions of higher to lower concentration at a rate that is proportional to the difference in concentration between the two regions. The constant of proportionality is called the diffusion coefficient or diffusivity of the gas. This implies that diffusion will continue until, at equilibrium, the concentrations are equal in the two regions. Yet clearly this cannot be true generally because, for example, when a gas mixture containing halothane is equilibrated with blood the concentration of halothane is approximately 2.3 times higher in the blood than in the gas phase. This apparent discrepancy arises because halothane is diffusing between two phases, gas and blood, and Fick's law, as stated above, applies only to diffusion within a single phase. Actually, Fick's law is a simplification. The driving force for diffusion is not truely concentration differences but rather the chemical potential difference of the substance in the two regions.[1] The regions can be in any phase—solid, liquid or gaseous.

The chemical potential is a quantitative way of describing the tendency of molecules to escape from whatever medium they are contained in, such as blood or a gas mixture. If the solute is sufficiently dilute to be considered ideal, meaning that it does not interact with other gases in the gas phase and all interactions are uniform in a solution, the change in potential can be related to the change in concentration. However, the chemical potential of a gas in a solution depends not only on its concentration, but also on its solubility. This seems reasonable because soluble gases have little tendency to escape from solution, whereas insoluble gases are difficult to keep in solution.

The partial vapor pressure of a gas is also a measure of the tendency of molecules to escape from the containing medium and thus is related to the chemical potential. Although the chemical potential of a given concentration may vary with solubility, the chemical potential at a given partial pressure is the same for any ideal gas. For example, although the ratio of the concentrations of halothane in the gas and blood phases at equilibrium is approximately 2.3, the partial pressures are equal in the two phases. For these reasons, although concentration differences are used to describe diffusion within a single phase, equilibrium between phases occurs when partial pressures and thus chemical potentials, not concentrations, are equal.

For nonideal gases a term called *fugacity* rather than partial pressure is related to the chemical potential. The term *activity*, which appears occasionally, refers to the ratio of the fugacity of a gas at a given temperature and pressure to the fugacity at the same temperature but at a standard pressure. Partial pressure for an ideal gas and fugacity or activity for a nonideal gas are all related to the escaping tendency of a gas from a solute and thus are important in the diffusion of gases. In this chapter, all gases will be considered ideal because any deviations from ideal are small and do not alter the principles of gas exchange.

Because the diffusivity coefficient usually is measured using concentration differences, it must be multiplied by the solubility of the gas in a liquid, usually blood, when partial pressures are used to describe diffusion. A reasonable approximation to Fick's law for diffusion across a membrane such as that separating alveoli and capillaries then is

$$R = D \cdot \lambda \cdot A \cdot \Delta P / H \tag{7-1}$$

where R is the rate of gas transfer across the membrane, D is the diffusion coefficient or diffusivity of the membrane, λ is the solubility of the gas in the membrane, A the surface area available for diffusion, ΔP the pressure difference across the membrane, and H is the thickness of the membrane. For most physiologic gases, the diffusion coefficient varies inversely with the square root of the molecular weight of the gas and increases about 2% per degree.

Convection (Blood Flow)

With the exception of the heart, organ blood flow is proportional to the difference in mean pressure between the arterial and venous blood vessels supplying and draining the organ and inversely related to the resistance of the vessels within the organ. Specifically:

$$Q = (BP_{art} - BP_{venous}) / \text{Resistance} \tag{7-2}$$

where Q is organ blood flow. In general, resistance is inversely proportional to the square of the cross-sectional area of the vessels. Thus, doubling the vessel area decreases resistance by one-fourth. Although this not precisely correct because it is true only for laminar flow and even then resistance depends on blood viscosity and velocity, it is an excellent approximation under most conditions.

Much confusion seems to exist about the role of cardiac output in determining organ blood flow. For example, it often is asserted that renal blood flow is reduced in hypovolemia because of the concomitant low cardiac output. Yet cardiac output is not part of Equation (7–2). Why then might renal flow decrease when a patient's intravascular volume is reduced? The answer is that the decrease in cardiac output resulting from reduced ventricular end-diastolic volumes decreases mean arterial pressure. In addition, the decreased stretch of the venous bed, the atria, and the arterial system increases sympathetic tone and probably other neurohumors that cause renal vasoconstriction and thus an increase in renal vascular resistance. It is important to note that these neurohumoral mechanisms are activated by stretch and are not directly sensitive to cardiac output. Thus, it is not the decrease in cardiac output *per se* that reduces renal blood flow, but rather the reduction in mean arterial pressure and stretch receptor mediated neurohumoral mechanisms. Conversely, many instances occur when cardiac output is increased greatly but renal and mesenteric blood flow are reduced. For example, in an athlete exercising to a oxygen consumption of 2 L/min, the cardiac output can be 25 L/min, a nearly fivefold increase.[2] However, this increase in flow is not uniformly distributed to all organs. In fact, renal and splanchnic flows drop to nearly one-fourth their basal rates, values lower than those found in patients with heart failure having reduced cardiac output.[3] Most of the enormous flow increase during maximal exercise goes to muscle. Thus, it is clear that one cannot make inferences about changes in organ blood flow from changes in cardiac output. In addition, even if total organ flow were known, the distribution of flow within the organ would not be known. Yet the distribution can profoundly affect organ function.

Most organs tend to maintain a relatively constant flow over a wide range of perfusion pressures (mean arterial minus venous). This phenomenon is termed *autoregulation*. As shown in Figure 7–1 and dictated by Equation (7–2), this is achieved by a change in resistance that is proportional to changes in perfusion pressure. Thus, if perfusion pressure decreases, organ vessels must dilate to maintain their blood flow. If perfusion pressure continues to fall, as shown in Figure 7–1, eventually a pressure is reached at which the vessels are maximally dilated. Any further decrease in pressure must then be accompanied by a decrease in organ flow. It is important to recognize that the ability to dilate, termed the *autoregulatory reserve*, varies enormously among organs. Although autoregulatory reserve can be defined as the pressure below which organ flow begins to fall, it is really a measure of the minimal resistance (maximal dilation) that the vessels in an organ bed can attain. Consequently, as shown in Figure 7–1, it may also be defined as the maximal increase in flow if pressure is held constant and the vessels are made to dilate maximally pharmacologically. If the maximum increase in flow is large, the vessels have a large capacity to dilate and therefore a large autoregulatory reserve. Equivalently, the knee of the autoregulatory curve of organs with large reserve is shifted to the left so that flow is preserved at low pressures.

The variation in autoregulatory reserve for different organs is shown in Table 7–1. It is noteworthy that, as shown in this table, the reserve of the kidney is the lowest in the body. It can increase its flow only by approximately 17%. Therefore, the knee of its autoregulatory curve is at relatively high pressures. This explains, in part, why the kidney is so readily damaged at low pressures whereas muscle survives.

Not only does the autoregulatory reserve vary widely among organs, but their responses to adrenergic stimulation also differ greatly. As shown in Table 7–2, the distribution of cardiac output to various organs differs markedly with different levels of exercise. With exercise, skeletal muscle flow increases enormously, reflecting both its large autoregulatory reserve and that its autoregulation is largely local. In contrast, renal flow falls by almost 75%. These data show that knowledge of cardiac output cannot be used to assess regional organ flow. However,

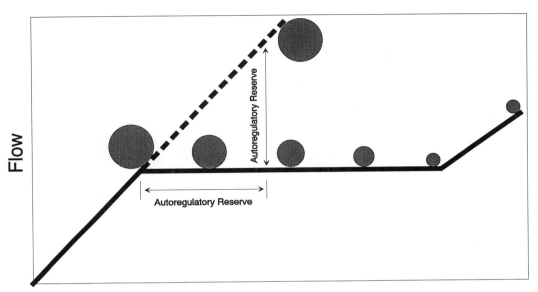

Pressure Difference

FIG 7–1.
Autoregulation and autoregulatory reserve. To maintain constant flow over a wide range of pressures (*horizontal solid line*), the vasculature in an organ must dilate as pressure falls. This is represented schematically by the hatched circles with increasing diameter as pressure falls. At some pressure, the vessels will be maximally dilated (*hatched circles on far left*). At this point, any subsequent decrease in pressure must be accompanied by a decrease in organ flow (*sloped solid line at left*). The autoregulatory reserve may be defined as the pressure difference below which organ flow begins to fall (*horizontal double-headed arrow*). Alternately, and more commonly, it is defined by causing maximum dilation of the organ vascular bed while holding pressure constant. This leads to an increase in flow that is proportional to the maximum dilation of the organ bed. This increase in flow (*vertical double-headed arrow*) also defines the autoregulatory reserve. If this maximum increase in flow is large, the "knee" of the autoregulatory curve is shifted to the left. In effect, reserve is a measurement of the maximum dilation that the organ vasculature can achieve. The sloped dashed line represents the relation between pressure and flow if maximum dilation were maintained. The solid sloped line at the right shows the relation between pressure and flow when the vasculature is maximally vasoconstricted.

understanding the differences in autoregulatory reserve helps explain the differences in organ tolerances to hypotension.

GAS TRANSPORT ACROSS THE LUNG

The diffusion of all gases between an alveolus and the surrounding capillaries or vice versa is so rapid that under almost all conditions the blood leaving the region of an alveolus has the same partial pressures as the alveolus. In other words, even if the time of contact were prolonged, there would be no further net transfer of gas because there would be no partial

TABLE 7–1.
Basal and Maximum Flows for Major Organs

	Heart	CNS	Muscle	GI	Liver	Skin	Kidney	Salivary	Fat
Basal flow/100 gm	70	50	2.5	35	29	9.5	400	40	8.0
Maximum flow/100 gm	400	140	60	275	176	181	467	500	30
Basal flow	210	750	750	700	500	200	1200	20	800
Maximum flow	1200	2100	18000	5500	3000	1400	1400	250	3000
Weight	0.3	1.5	30.0	2.0	1.7	2.1	0.3	0.05	10.0

Basal and maximum flows are in ml/min. Weight is in kg.
Adapted from Wade, O. L. and J. M. Bishop. *Cardiac Output and Regional Blood Flow*, Oxford: Blackwell Scientific Publications, 1962.

TABLE 7–2.
Change in Organ Flow during Exercise in Humans

Organ	Blood Flow (ml/min)			
	Rest	Light Exercise	Heavy Exercise	Maximal Exercise
Splanchnic	1400	1100	600	300
Renal	1100	900	600	250
Cerebral	750	750	750	750
Coronary	250	350	750	1000
Muscle	1200	4500	12500	22000
Skin	500	1500	1900	600
Other	600	400	400	100
Cardiac output (ml/min)	5800	9500	17500	2500
Oxygen uptake (ml/min)	140	400	1200	2000

From Wade, O. L., Bishop, J. M., Donald, K. W. *Cardiac Output and Regional Blood Flow,* Oxford: Blackwell Scientific Publications, 1962: 107.

pressure difference to drive gaseous diffusion. This phenomenon is termed *end-capillary equilibrium* because equilibrium occurs by the time blood reaches the end of the alveolar capillary. In fact, the time of contact required for end-capillary equilibrium under normal conditions is estimated to be less than one-quarter of a second, whereas the usual alveolar transit time is approximately three-quarters of a second. The rapid diffusion of gases across alveoli, which has been reviewed in depth by Wagner,[4] occurs because the rich capillary network provides a very large surface area for diffusion and the distance between an alveolus and its capillaries is very small. In fact, the transport of oxygen and carbon dioxide across alveoli is so rapid that the rate of diffusion would not limit their exchange even if the total alveolar surface area were reduced by nearly one-eighth or if the blood transit time was decreased fivefold as in extreme exercise. It is, however, possible that end-capillary equilibrium does not occur with exercise at high altitude. Data are insufficient to determine if this also is true in some disease states, but even if it does occur, it is certainly the exception rather than the rule.

The assertion that alveolar gas exchange is virtually never diffusion limited (i.e., that end-capillary equilibrium occurs) is somewhat confusing because diffusing capacity, measured clinically using carbon monoxide (D_{CO}), is reduced in many clinical conditions. The basis of the D_{CO} measurement is the inhalation of carbon monoxide in low concentrations and measurement of its rate of uptake by blood. Because carbon monoxide is almost totally bound to hemoglobin, the blood partial pressure is assumed to be zero. Therefore, because alveolar partial pressure and uptake can be measured, Equation (7–1) may be solved for $D \cdot A/H$. Consequently, the carbon monoxide diffusing capacity can be altered by changes in either surface area, such as atelectasis, alveolar-capillary membrane thickness, such as in interstitial fibrosis, or the diffusion coefficient, which probably changes rarely if ever. The uptake of carbon monoxide is also affected by the hemoglobin concentration. For these reasons, reductions in carbon monoxide diffusing capacity do not imply that gas exchange is diffusion limited but rather that there has been a change in the overall gas exchanging characteristics of the lung. Such changes do not necessarily imply that gas exchange is impaired because of the enormous reserve for diffusion.

Although the diffusion coefficient for oxygen is only one-twentieth that of carbon dioxide, the diffusion rates across the lung are similar for the two gases.[4] This occurs because hemoglobin serves as a "sink" for oxygen. That is, because oxygen binds to hemoglobin, the increase in oxygen partial pressure as venous blood takes up oxygen is relatively small, thereby maintaining a high partial pressure gradient. In contrast, the relation between carbon dioxide content and partial pressure in blood is almost linear and relatively flat so that the P_{CO_2} decreases comparatively rapidly as CO_2 is eliminated from blood by the lungs. Thus, the diffusion gradient for O_2 is well maintained as it diffuses into blood whereas that for CO_2 drops rapidly, thereby rapidly attenuating its rate of diffusion from blood to alveolar gas.

The importance of this very rapid diffusion is that the differences that always exist between mixed alveolar gas and systemic arterial blood are rarely, if ever, due to a diffusion limitation but rather to differences in the ventilation-perfusion ratios, V/Q, of alveoli. To understand how V/Q differences produce alveolar-arterial partial pressure differences, the carriage of gases in blood first must be understood.

Gas Carriage in Blood

Gases are carried in blood both bound to proteins and dissolved in plasma and red cells. Protein binding is negligible for some gases such as nitrogen or halothane, but it affects the carriage of carbon dioxide and is critical to the transport of oxygen. The transport in blood of inert gases, which are gases that are carried dissolved in blood but do not react appreciably with blood components, is important for several reasons. First, all gases dissolve in blood to some extent so that this aspect of carriage is relevant even to respiratory gases. Second, the analysis of the effects of V/Q on gas exchange across the lung is much simpler for inert gases than for protein-bound gases such as oxygen or carbon dioxide.

There are several confusing conventions used in describing gas transport. First, alveolar gas is expressed as body temperature and pressure, saturated, BTPS, whereas gas concentration in blood is standard temperature and pressure dry (STPD). To convert gas volumes in BTPS to SPTD, multiply by $[(P_B - 47)/P_B] \cdot [273/(273 + temp)]$ where P_B is barometric pressure, 47 is the vapor pressure of water in alveolar gas saturated with water vapor, 273 is 0°C expressed on the Kelvin temperature scale, and temp is body temperature in centigrade. A second point of confusion is that the sum of the venous partial pressures often is less than barometric pressure because the venous gases are not in equilibrium with atmospheric gases. In contrast, the sum of arterial partial pressures always equals alveolar pressure.

Inert gases

Inert gases, by definition do not react with blood components. Their carriage in blood is therefore solely dependent on how much is dissolved in the blood. The concentration dissolved in blood is proportional to the partial pressure of the gas. Specifically:

$$C_b = \lambda \cdot F_g = \lambda P_g/P_B \qquad (7-3)$$

where C_b is the blood concentration in mL gas/mL blood; λ is the constant of proportionality, termed the Ostwald partition coefficient or the blood-gas partition coefficient; Fg is the gas fraction in equilibrium with the blood, Pg is the gas partial pressure, and P_B is the barometric pressure. Because blood content is expressed in mL gas/100 mL of blood, Equation (7–3) is usually multiplied by 100. If this is done, Fg is expressed as a percentage rather than a fraction. For example, if the alveolar partial pressure were 7.1, Fg would be 7.1/713 = 0.01. The denominator is 713 because alveolar gases are usually expressed as fractions of dry gas volume, which equals the partial pressure divided by barometric pressure − water vapor pressure in the lung. The latter is usually 47 mm Hg. Therefore, assuming a barometric pressure of 760 mm Hg, the denominator is 760 − 47. Assuming λ for halothane is 2.3, then C_b would be 0.023 mL halothane/mL blood. Multiplying both concentrations by 100 would yield a blood content of halothane of 2.3 mL/100 mL of blood, which corresponds to 1 mL halothane/100 mL of gas, which is, in turn, 1% by volume. Thus 1% halothane in equilibrium with blood would yield a content of 2.3 mL/100 mL of blood.

It is evident from Equation (7–3), that for the same blood concentration, a very soluble gas, such as acetone (λ, approximately 330) will have a much lower partial pressure than a relatively insoluble gas such as halothane. For example, if the blood content of both gases were 5 mL/100 mL blood, then the alveolar percentage of acetone in equilibrium with the blood would be 5/330 = 0.015%, which yields a partial pressure of (0.0 · 15/100) · 713 = 0.11 mm Hg. For the same blood concentration, the partial pressure for halothane would be (5/2.3) · (713/100) = 15.5 mm Hg.

Oxygen is relatively insoluble in blood, the Ostwald coefficient being approximately 0.22 so that at a partial pressure of 100 mm Hg there is only 0.31 mL O_2/100 mL blood. However, the total content of oxygen in blood at this partial pressure is approximately 20.5 mL O_2/100 mL blood. This difference of more than 20 mL O_2/100 mL blood reflects the carriage of oxygen by hemoglobin.

Oxygen

The carriage of oxygen in blood is considerably more complex than inert gases because it is bound to hemoglobin as well as dissolved in plasma. Moreover, the amount of hemoglobin binding depends on the Po_2 as shown in Figure 7–2. Each molecule of hemoglobin can carry a maximum of four molecules of oxygen. This binding is termed *cooperative* because the presence of the first molecule of oxygen makes binding of the second molecule easier. If each hemoglobin molecule carries the maximum four oxygen molecules then 1 g of hemoglobin would carry 1.34 mL of oxygen. However, the number of oxygen molecules bound to each hemoglobin molecule depends on the Po_2. This dependence is quantified by the oxyhemoglobin dissociation curve (OHDC), which indicates the average number of oxygen molecules carried by hemoglobin at a given partial pressure. For normal adult hemoglobin with a Po_2 of 26 mm Hg, there are an average of two oxygen molecules per hemoglobin molecule. Therefore, hemoglobin is said to be 50% saturated and a Po_2 of 26 mm Hg is termed the P_{50}. Consequently, at the P_{50}, a gram of hemoglobin would only carry 0.5 × 1.34 = 0.67 mL O_2. For a Po_2 of approximately 40 mm Hg, which is the usual value for mixed venous blood, the average number of oxygen molecules per molecule of hemoglobin is three so that hemlglobin is 75%

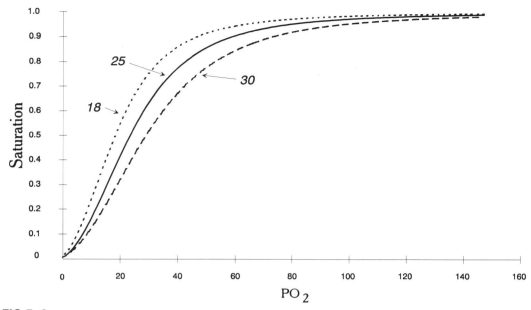

FIG 7–2.
The oxyhemoglobin dissociation curve (OHDC), which relates P_{O_2} to the saturation of hemoglobin. The solid line is the normal OHDC. The dashed line is an OHDC that is right-shifted. Typical causes of such a shift are hypercarbia, acidemia, hyperthermia, and excess 2-3 diphosphoglycerate. The dotted line is a left-shifted OHDC. A left-shift may be caused by hypocarbia, alkalemia, hypothermia, and diminished 2-3 diphosphoglycerate. These curves may be characterized by the P_{50} (numbers with arrows to the curves), which is the P_{O_2} at which 50% saturation occurs. The P_{50} for normal adult hemoglobin is approximately 26 mm Hg. Notice that regardless of the P_{50}, these curves converge to the same saturation at low and high P_{O_2}.

saturated and a gram of hemoglobin carries 1.0 mL O_2. Although each molecule of hemoglobin can carry only one, two, three, or four molecules of oxygen, the saturation can be any number between zero and one because at a given P_{O_2} not all hemoglobin molecules will carry the same number of oxygen molecules. For example, at a P_{O_2} of 90, the saturation is 96%. Although most hemoglobin molecules are carrying four oxygen molecules, some are carrying three, fewer are carrying two, and very few are carrying one or none so that on the average, each hemoglobin molecule carries $0.96 \times 4 = 3.84$ molecules of oxygen.

The total number of milliliters of oxygen in blood carried by hemoglobin equals the number of milliliters of O_2 per gram hemoglobin times the number of grams of hemoglobin per hundred milliliters of blood. For example, for a person with 15 g hemoglobin/100 mL blood and a saturation of 0.96, there are $1.34 \cdot 15 \cdot 0.96 = 19.3$ mL oxygen per 100 mL blood. As mentioned above, some oxygen also is carried dissolved in blood. Thus the total content of oxygen in blood is the amount carried by hemoglobin plus the amount dissolved. This is usually expressed as:

$$C_{O_2} = 1.34 \cdot Sat \cdot Hb + 0.0031 \cdot P_{O_2} \tag{7–4}$$

where the solubility is divided by 713 so that it may be multiplied by Po_2 rather than the fraction of O_2 [i.e., $0.0031 = 0.022 \cdot (Po_2/713) \cdot 100$, where the 100 in the right is to convert to mL O_2/100 mL blood].

The shape of the oxyhemoglobin saturation curve is altered by many factors (Fig 7–2). For example, low temperatures, alkalemia, and reduced 2,3-diphosphoglycerate all shift the curve to the left so that hemloglobin is less saturated for a given Po_2. The effects of such shifts on oxygen uptake by blood and delivery to tissue are discussed in later in this chapter.

Carbon dioxide

Between 5 and 15% of carbon dioxide is carried bound to blood proteins forming carbamino compounds. The amount carried by hemoglobin increases as hemoglobin-bound oxygen decreases (the Haldane effect). However, most of the carbon dioxide in blood reacts with water to form bicarbonate. Although relatively little is dissolved in plasma and red cells the sum of dissolved carbon dioxide and carbonic acid (H_2CO_3) behaves essentially like an inert gas with the concentration given approximately by $0.0301 \cdot Pco_2$.

Factors Affecting Gas Exchange

There is a difference between arterial blood partial pressure and average alveolar gas partial pressure for all gases that are taken up or eliminated via the lung. Given that the capillary blood leaving an alveolus has the same gas partial pressures as the alveolus that it perfuses, what is the genesis of these alveolar-arterial partial pressure differences and what determines their magnitude?

One possibility is the passage of venous blood into the arterial circulation without exposure to ventilated alveoli. This is termed *true shunt*. The widespread use of the "shunt equation" (see below) has fostered the belief that true shunt does generate the alveolar-arterial oxygen partial pressure differences, the $P(a - a)o_2$, in most individuals. However, this is probably not true. In fact, the genesis of alveolar-arterial partial pressure differences for all gases is due largely to inhomogeneity in the ratio of ventilation to perfusion, V/Q, among alveoli.

If there are two or more alveoli within a lung that have different V/Q, an arterial-alveolar partial pressure difference will result for every gas that has a net uptake or elimination (equivalently, any gas for which venous and alveolar partial pressures differ). For gases that are eliminated, such as CO_2, the average alveolar partial pressure (the term alveolar partial pressure will always mean average partial pressure for all alveoli when referring to the lung as a whole) is always less than arterial. The converse is true for gases that are taken up such as oxygen. To understand the genesis of this difference, the effect of the V/Q of an individual alveolus on the end-capillary and thus alveolar partial pressures must first be appreciated.

Gas Exchange in a Single Alveolus

Because all gases probably achieve end-capillary equilibrium within each alveolus, the effects of the V/Q on the equilibrium partial pressure for a gas can be studied by envisioning an alveolus and its surrounding capillary network statically; that is, as consisting of separate gas and blood chambers that are brought together in such a way that gases can diffuse freely between the two chambers. For the simplest case, begin with a small amount of an inert gas such as halothane or acetone in the alveolar chamber and none in the blood chamber and make the following assumptions: (1) The partial pressures of any other diffusible gases are equal in the blood and gas chambers so that no net diffusion occurs for these gases. (2) The initial concentration of halothane or acetone in the alveolar chamber is low enough so that the change in volume of the alveolus is negligible as halothane or acetone diffuses into blood.

Effects of Solubility.—As diffusion of the halothane or acetone from the alveolar to the blood chamber occurs, the concentration of these inert gases in the alveolus will decrease and that in blood will increase. This process will continue until the partial pressures in the blood and the alveolar chambers are equal. To determine what this equilibrium partial pressure will be and what factors affect it, consider first the effects of the volume of the alveolar and blood chambers. Suppose, as shown in Figure 7–3, A, that the blood volume is 200 mL and that the alveolar volume is 100 mL with an initial concentration of 1% halothane or 1% acetone. For both gases this corresponds to a partial pressure of 7.13 mm Hg. (0.01·713). As a given amount of gas, say one-tenth of 1 mL, diffuses into the blood the alveolar concentration will decrease (Fig 7–3, B). This new concentration will be the original amount (100 mL · 0.01 = 1 mL halothane) less the amount lost divided by the volume of the container [(1 mL − 0.1 mL)/ 100 mL = 0.009 = 0.9%]. For both gases this corresponds to a partial pressure of 0.009·713 =

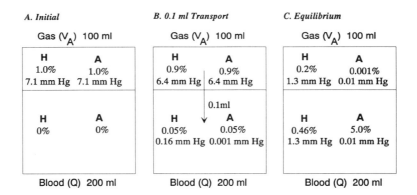

FIG 7–3.
The effects of solubility on gas exchange in a single alveolus. Panels **A, B,** and **C** represent a hypothetical alveolus with a gas volume of 100 mL and a blood volume of 200 mL (V/Q = 0.5). Initially, as shown in **A,** the concentrations of halothane (H) and acetone (A) are both 1% in the alveolus and zero in the blood **B,** The effect of 0.1 mL of either gas diffusing into the blood. This would decrease the alveolar concentrations by 0.1% and increase the blood content to 0.05% (.0005 mL gas/mL blood) for both gases. However, because of the difference in solubilities (2.3 for halothane and 330 for acetone), the partial pressures in blood differ. Because acetone is much more soluble than halothane, its partial pressure is much lower. Consequently, as a given amount of gas diffuses into blood, the rise in the partial pressure of acetone would be much less than for halothane despite equal decreases in alveolar partial pressures. As a result, the equilibrium partial pressure for acetone would be much lower than for halothane, **C.** Despite this, the equilibrium concentration of acetone in blood is much greater than for halothane, again becasue of its greater solubility. Thus, increasing the solubility of an inspired gas decreases its equilibrium partial pressure but increases its blood content (see the Appendix at the end of this chapter).

6.4 mm Hg. The concentration in blood after the one-tenth of 1 mL of gas diffuses into it will be 0.1/200 = 0.0005 mL gas/mL blood. The partial pressure that corresponds to this concentration depends on the gas solubility and may be calculated by asking what would the partial pressure in a gas phase be if blood with this concentration were in equilibrium with the gas phase? As described above, the concentration in the gas phase would then equal the concentration in blood divided by the blood-gas solubility. For example, for halothane, which has a solubility of approximately 2.3, the concentration of a gas phase in equilibrium with blood with a concentration of 0.0005 mL gas/mL blood would be 0.0005/2.3 = 0.00022. The corresponding partial pressure would be 0.00022·713 = 0.155 mm Hg. The same calculation for acetone, which has a solubility of approximately 330, yields a partial pressure of (0.0005/330) · 713 = 0.001 mm Hg.

It is evident from these calculations that for a given volume of gas diffusing from the alveolus to blood, the decrease in alveolar concentration and partial pressure is independent of the particular gas. Moreover, the resultant rise in blood concentration is also independent of the particular gas. However, the corresponding rise in blood partial pressure depends on the solubility of the gas in blood. A more soluble gas has a lower partial pressure for a given blood concentration. Consequently, as diffusion continues, the blood partial pressure rises much less for acetone than halothane. In other words, much more acetone than halothane will have to diffuse into blood to achieve a given rise in blood partial pressure. Because of this, the alveolar partial pressure of acetone will decrease much more than for halothane before the blood and gas partial pressures become equal. In this example, for which the initial partial pressures for both halothane and acetone were 7.13 (1%), the equilibrium partial pressures would be approximately 1.3 and 0.01 mm Hg, respectively (see the Appendix for calculations). As shown in Figure 7–3, C, although the equilibrium partial pressure for acetone is considerably lower than for halothane, the blood concentration is actually much higher because it is so soluble that even at a partial pressure of 0.001 mm Hg a considerable amount is dissolved in blood. This example illustrates two general principles. First, for equal initial alveolar concentrations, equilibration will occur more slowly and at a lower partial pressure for a more soluble gas. Second, for equal initial alveolar concentrations, at equilibration the blood concentration of a more soluble gas will be higher despite the lower partial pressure.

Effects of Ventilation-Perfusion Ratio (V/Q).—The other major factor that affects the equilibrium partial pressure within an alveolus is the ratio of ventilation to perfusion (V/Q). This may be understood by first considering the effects of reducing the alveolar gas container in the preceding example. If the alveolus were smaller but had the same initial concentration of gas, there would be a greater decrease in alveolar partial pressure for a given amount of gas transferred to the blood. For example, if the alveolar volume were only 50 mL but still contained 1% halothane (Fig 7–4, A), then loss of one-tenth of 1 mL of halothane would change the concentration to (0.01 · 50 − 0.1) / 50 = 0.008 mL gas/mL or 0.8%. That is, the concentration would decrease by 0.2% rather than the 0.1% illustrated above. However, the increase in blood partial pressure would be the same because 0.1 mL still entered the blood. Thus a smaller alveolus leads to a more rapid fall in alveolar partial pressure for a given amount of gas transferred to blood (Fig 7–4, B). At equilibrium, the partial pressures would be

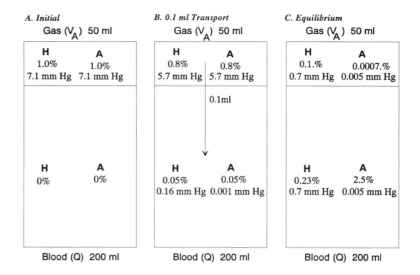

FIG 7–4.
The effects of decreasing the alveolar volume on gas exchange in a single alveolus. Compared with Figure 7–3, the alveolar volume has been decreased from 100 to 50 mL. As in Figure 7–3, **A,** shows the initial conditions, **B,** the effects of a 0.1-mL transfer of halothane or acetone into blood, and **C,** the equilibrium values. Because the alveolar volume has been halved, the loss of 0.1 mL doubles the percent decrease in alveolar concentration. However, because the blood volume is unchanged, the blood values are the same as in Figure 7–3, **B.** Because alveolar pressures drop more rapidly for a given volume of gas transferred into blood, the equilibrium partial pressures are lower for both gases as shown in **C.**

0.70 mm Hg for halothane and 0.005 mm Hg for acetone (Fig 7–4, C). Notice that the partial pressure for acetone is affected proportionally more than halothane. This is because, as indicated by Equation (7–20) in the Appendix, when the solubility is much larger than the V/Q, changes in equilibrium partial pressure are essentially linearly related to changes in V/Q, whereas as the solubility decreases, changes in the V/Q have progressively less effect on the equilibrium partial pressure.

Now consider doubling the blood volume to 400 mL without changing the alveolar volume (Fig 7–5). More alveolar gas would then have to diffuse into blood to achieve a given increase in blood concentration and therefore partial pressure. For example, if, as above, 0.1 mL of halothane diffused into blood, the blood concentration would only be 0.1/400 = 0.00025 mL halothane/mL blood. This corresponds to a partial pressure of 0.078 mm Hg, which is half that for a 200-mL blood volume. Because more gas must diffuse into blood to achieve a given increase in partial pressure, the equilibrium partial pressure will lowered. In this case, the equilibrium partial pressures for halothane and acetone are 0.70 and 0.005 mm Hg, respectively. Notice that these are the same pressures found with a 50-mL alveolar container and 200-mL blood container. In both cases the V/Q is 0.25. This illustrates the general rule, derived in the Appendix, that it is only the ratio of ventilation to perfusion that determines the equilibrium partial pressures, not the absolute values of each. This is true for both uptake and elimination of all gases regardless of the initial blood and gas concentrations (see the Appendix). However, whereas the equilibrium partial pressure increases as the V/Q

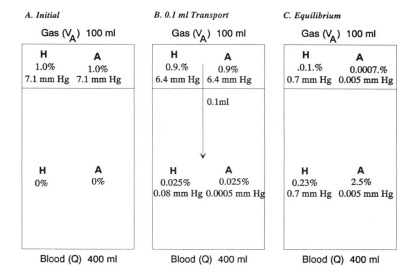

FIG 7–5.
The effects of doubling the blood volume on gas exchange in a single alveolus. Compared with Figure 7–3, the blood volume has been doubled to 400 mL while the alveolar volume remains at 100 mL. As in Figure 7–3, **A** represents the initial conditions, **B**, the effects of a 0.1-mL transfer of halothane or acetone into blood, **C**, the equilibrium values. Because blood concentrations rise less rapidly for a given volume of gas transferred into blood, the equilibrium partial pressures are lower for both gases as shown in **C**. Notice that these pressures and concentrations are the same as in Figure 7–4, **C**. This is because they depend only on the V/Q rather than the absolute gas or blood volumes.

becomes larger for gases that are transferred from alveolus to blood, the opposite is true for elimination. Thus, high equilibrium partial pressures for oxygen occur in high V/Q alveoli but the equilibrium partial pressures for carbon dioxide in such alveoli are relatively low.

Gas Exchange with Multiple Alveoli

True Pulmonary Shunt.—True pulmonary shunt occurs if systemic venous blood passes into the systemic arterial circulation without traversing any ventilated alveoli. That is, it results from alveoli with zero V/Q. Although the effects of true shunt on arterial oxygen partial pressures, Pao_2, are similar to those of low V/Q alveoli, they do differ in two respects. First, blood leaving even very low V/Q alveoli has a Po_2 slightly greater than venous blood and second, the Po_2 of such blood can be increased by raising the inspired oxygen tension.

Although true shunt is difficult to measure (see below) its effect on arterial oxygenation can be understood by considering the effects of an anatomic shunt such as that produced by right to left flow through a patent foramen ovale of 25% of the total cardiac output in a patient with normal pulmonary function. In this case, for every 100 mL of blood leaving the left ventricle, 75 mL comes from the normal lung. The Po_2 and oxygen content of this blood is normal. However, 25 mL comes from the right atrium and therefore has a relatively low Po_2 and content. If the Po_2 of blood leaving the lung were 95 mm Hg and that of the right atrium and thus the shunted blood were 40 mm Hg, if the hemoglobin were 15 g/100 mL, the respective contents would be about 19.8 and 15.2 mL $O_2/100$ mL blood. When the pulmonary and venous blood are mixed in a 3:1 ratio in the left ventricle, the resulting content would be 18.7 mL $O_2/100$ ml blood [$(0.75 \cdot 19.8 + 0.25 \cdot 15.2)/1.0$], which corresponds to a Po_2 of about 62 mm Hg. Thus the true shunt markedly decreases the arterial PO_2. It is interesting to note that increasing the FIO_2 will have relatively little effect on the Pao_2. For example, if the FIO_2 were increased so that the Po_2 of blood leaving the lung were 300 mm Hg, the Pao_2 leaving the left ventricle would increase to approximately 80/mm Hg. Increasing the FIO_2 further so that the Po_2 of blood leaving the lung were 400 mm Hg would only increase the arterial Po_2 to about 94 mm Hg. The reason these increments in Pao_2 are relatively small is because blood leaving the lung is nearly saturated. Thus the large increases in its Po_2 result in only small increments in content, due primarily to additional dissolved O_2.

True pulmonary shunt caused by blood that passes by unventilated alevoli often is invoked as a cause of hypoxemia. It frequently is assumed that the shunt fraction measured with oxygen indicates true shunt. However, as discussed later in this chapter, this index is affected by many factors other than true shunt, including low V/Q alveoli, and therefore is better termed *venous admixture*. Unfortunately, the measurement of true shunt is difficult and rarely performed. Theoretically, it could be measured by infusing a totally insoluble inert gas into the venous circulation. Such a gas would be completely eliminated from blood if it passed by any ventilated alveoli, no matter how low the V/Q. Therefore, the amount of gas detected in arterial blood would be proportional to the amount of blood that passed by unventilated alveoli, i.e., true shunt. Although such a gas does not exist, the calculation can be made by infusing inert gases of varying solubility, including some with very low solubility such as sulfur hexaflouride, and plotting the ratio of arterial to venous concentrations against their solubilities. Then by extrapolating back to zero solubility, true shunt can be estimated. Although the multiple inert gas method developed by Wagner, Saltzman, and West[5] does, in effect, perform this extrapolation, because of mathematical limitations in the methodology,[6, 7] the values obtained are generally overestimates of true shunt that include low V/Q alveoli. Nonetheless, studies using this methodology have demonstrated that true shunt accounts for a very variable amount of alveolar-arterial oxygen differences.[8-11] Using a nonlinear regression, we frequently found considerably lower true shunts than Dantzker et al.[8] using the published data for patients with adult respiratory distress. In fact, in some of these patients true shunt was nearly zero, despite relative hypoxemia breathing high oxygen concentrations. In these patients, the major reason for large alveolar-arterial oxygen tension differences is large differences in the V/Q of alveoli.

V_A/Q Mismatch.—As indicated above, knowledge of the V/Q of an individual alveolus and the initial concentrations and properties of the diffusible gas is sufficient to compute the equilibrium partial pressure for that gas. Although the partial pressures of gases in the blood leaving each alveolus are the same as in the alveolus (end-capillary equilibrium), if two or more alveoli with different V/Q are ventilated and perfused in parallel, an alveolar-arterial difference will elways exist for all gases for which there is net uptake or elimination. The magnitude of this difference will depend on the gas and the V/Q differences among the alveoli.

To illustrate the effects of two alveoli with different V/Q on the alveolar-arterial oxygen partial pressure difference, $P(A - a)_{O_2}$, and the arterial-alveolar carbon dioxide partial pressure difference, $P(a - A)_{CO_2}$, the results of simulations for three hypothetical lungs, each composed of two alveoli ventilated and perfused in parallel, are shown in Table 7–3. None of these lungs has any true shunt or dead-space. The total blood flow through each alveolus is fixed at 2.5 L/min. The total inspired alveolar ventilation is fixed at 4 L/min so that the average V_I/Q is 0.8 in all three lungs. However, the inspired ventilation is partitioned among the two alveoli to yield V_I/Q of 0.7 and 0.9 in lung 1, 0.4 and 1.2 in lung 2, and 0.1 and 1.5 in lung 3 (Figure 7–6). The expired alveolar ventilation (V_A) and thus V_A/Q depends on the net gas exchange in each alveolus. If more gas is taken up than is eliminated, the alveolar ventilation and V_A/Q will be lower than the inspired values and vice versa. For all three lungs, either the total oxygen consumption (V_{O_2}) and carbon dioxide production (V_{CO_2}) are fixed at 200 and 160 mL/min, respectively (respiratory quotient = 0.8), allowing the venous and arterial gas tensions to vary, or the venous gas tensions are fixed at 40 mm Hg for oxygen and 46 mm Hg for carbon dioxide, in which case V_{O_2} and V_{CO_2} vary. The inspired O_2 is 21%. To demonstrate the effects of anemia, the calculations for each lung are made for a hemoglobin of 13 and 6 gm/dL.

When the V_{O_2} and V_{CO_2} are fixed, the gas tensions shown for these lungs are computed by an iterative process that is based on Equation (7–24) in the Appendix. First a guess is made for the venous gas tensions. Next, the equilibrium alveolar partial pressures for each alveolus are computed. This is also an iterative process that depends on the venous and inspired gas tensions, as well as the V_I/Q and the blood flow to each alveolus. The basis of these alveolar calculations has been described by Olszowka and Farhi,[12] although some modification is needed to account for the difference between V_I and V_A. The alveolar partial pressures are then used to calculate the P_{aO_2} and P_{AO_2} which, in conjunction with the ventilation and perfusion to each alveolus, are used to calculate the V_{O_2} and V_{CO_2} and to ensure that the net uptake of nitrogen is zero. This process is repeated, adjusting the venous gas tensions until the specified V_{O_2} and V_{CO_2} are obtained. When the venous gas tensions are specified and V_{O_2} and V_{CO_2} allowed to vary, the calculation is much simpler. The equilibrium partial pressures for each alveolus are computed as above and used to calculate the P_{aO_2} and P_{AO_2} and V_{O_2} and V_{CO_2}.

Notice that for each lung in Table 7–2 a difference exists between the alveolar and arterial partial pressures both for CO_2 and for O_2. The magnitude of these differences is not the same for the two gases and increases as the V_I/Q of the two alveoli become more disparate. Notice also that the P_{AO_2} and P_{ACO_2} are unaffected by changes in the V_I/Q or hemoglobin when the V_{O_2} and V_{CO_2} are fixed. This occurs because

$$V_{O_2} = F_{IO_2} \cdot V_{IO_2} - F_{AO_2} \cdot V_{AO_2} \qquad (7-5)$$

Inasmuch as F_{IO_2}, V_I and V_A are fixed, F_{AO_2} also cannot vary. A similar argument holds for the P_{ACO_2}. The alveolar-arterial differences increase as the V_I/Q differences become greater because while alveolar gas concentrations remain constant, the P_{aO_2} progressively decreases whereas the P_{aCO_2} increases. The reason can be understood by examining the P_{O_2} data derived using fixed venous gas tensions, as shown in Table 7–3. Because the blood flow through each alveolus is the same, each contributes equally to the mixed arterial oxygen content (i.e., the blood leaving the two-alveolus lung). For example, for lung 3, the content leaving the alveolus

TABLE 7–3.
Effects of V_I/Q and F_{IO_2} on Gas Exchange and Indices of Pulmonary Function in a Two Alveoli Lung*

F_{IO_2}	V_I/Q_1	V_I/Q_2	Venous		Arterial		Alveolar		ΔO_2	Qs/Qt	Ratio	Vd/Vt
			Pv_{O_2}	Pv_{CO_2}	Pa_{O_2}	Pa_{CO_2}	PA_{O_2}	PA_{CO_2}				
0.21	0.7	0.9	41	28	114	29	115	29	1	0	546	0
0.50	0.7	0.9	45	33	324	29	324	29	0	0	648	0
0.80	0.7	0.9	50	33	540	29	540	29	0	0	675	0
0.21	0.4	1.2	40	34	101	30	115	29	14	3	482	4
0.50	0.4	1.2	45	34	317	30	324	29	7	1	634	4
0.80	0.4	1.2	50	35	537	30	540	29	3	0	670	4
0.21	0.1	1.5	32	36	49	32	108	29	58	38	247	10
0.50	0.1	1.5	44	38	243	34	324	29	81	7	486	14
0.80	0.1	1.5	49	38	512	34	540	29	28	2	640	14

* Oxygen consumption and carbon dioxide production are fixed at 200 mL/min and 160 mL/min, respectively. Blood flow is 2.5 L/min to each alveolus. The hematocrit is 39%. Venous and arterial gases are allowed to vary. Qs/Qt and Vd/Vt are percents. ΔO_2 is alveolar-arterial PO_2 difference. Ratio is ratio of arterial PO_2 to F_{IO_2}.

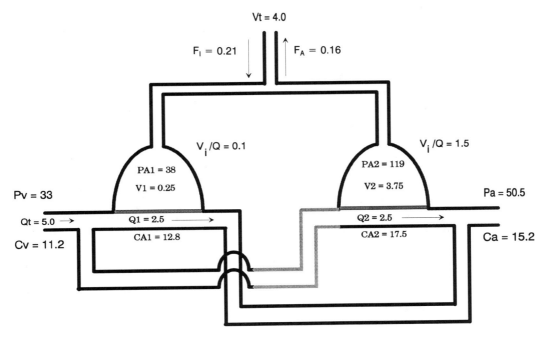

FIG 7–6.

Hypothetical two-alveoli lung ventilated and perfused in parallel (lung 3 used in calculations in Tables 7–2 and 3). Total ventilation is 4.0 L/min and total perfusion is 5.0 L/min. The perfusion to each alveoli is 2.5 L/min but the ventilation is partitioned so that the V_i/Q of the left and right alveoli are 0.1 and 1.5, respectively. The inspired Fio_2 is 0.21 and the Vo_2 and Vco_2 are fixed at 200 and 160 mL/min, respectively. PA_1 and PA_2 are the equilibrium O_2 partial pressures for each alveolus. CA_1 and CA_2 are the equilibrium O_2 contents assuming a hemoglobin of 13 g/100 mL. The arterial content (Ca) is the average of the two alveoli because they have equal blood flow. However, the average alveolar O_2 fraction (Fa) is weighted more towards alveolus 2 because its ventilation is much greater than that of alveolus 1. Although not shown, the expired ventilation for alveolus 1 is only 0.20 L/min because more O_2 is taken up than CO_2 eliminated in this alveolus. In contrast, the expired and inspired ventilations are virtually identical for alveolus 2.

with a V/Q of 0.1 is 12.8 and that leaving the alveolus with a V/Q of 1.5 is 17.5. Therefore, the mixed arterial content is $(25 \cdot 12.8 + 25 \cdot 17.5)/50 = 15.2$ mL O_2/100 mL blood, which corresponds to a Pao_2 of 51 mm Hg. In contrast, the two alveoli do not contribute equally to the PAo_2. Although the Po_2 of the alveolus with a VA/Q of 0.1 is only 38 mm Hg, its ventilation of 0.25 L/min contributes minimally to the total alveolar ventilation of 4L/min. In contrast, the other alveolus ($VA/Q = 1.5$) has a Po_2 of 119 mm Hg and contributes most of the alveolar ventilation (3.75 L/min). Therefore, the PAo_2 is weighted heavily toward the Po_2 of the high VI/Q alveolus as opposed to the equal contribution from both alveoli that occurs in the blood. However, as mentioned, the expired and inspired ventilations are not equal for each alveolus because there is a difference between the amount of O_2 taken up and CO_2 released from blood. As a result, the expired alveolar ventilation in the low V/Q alveoli is reduced from 0.25 L/min to approximately 0.21 L/min whereas that of the high V/Q alveolus is essentially equal to inspired ventilation. Consequently, the mixed alveolar Po_2 is $(38 \times 0.21 + 119 \times 3.75)/4.0 = 115$ mm Hg. This generates the observed alveolar-arterial partial pressure difference.

In summary, the two alveoli contribute equally to arterial content but the low V_I/Q alveolus, which has a low equilibrium Po_2, makes only a small contribution to the mixed alveolar Po_2. Consequently, the mixed arterial Po_2 is reduced more by the low Po_2 of the low V_I/Q alveolus than is the mixed alveolar Po_2. Qualitatively, similar results would be found for any inspired gas being taken up by the body. However, the magnitude of the partial pressure difference would depend on the properties of the gas. Similar alveolar-arterial partial pressure differences would also occur if the alveolar ventilations were equal and the perfusions differed. In this case, the low V_I/Q alveolus would contribute equally to the alveolar Po_2, but it would account for a relatively large percentage of the total blood flow. Because its content would also be low, it would reduce the mixed arterial content and thus Po_2. As shown in Table 7–3, as the difference in the V_I/Q of the two alveoli increases, the alveolar-arterial differences also increase. This occurs because the Po_2 of the low V_I/Q alveolus decreases while its contribution to the mixed alveolar gas increases but it still contributes equally to mixed arterial blood. Notice that the blood O_2 contents were used to compute the arterial content, which was then converted to Pao_2. In contrast, alveolar Po_2 was used to compute the PAo_2. Actually, concentrations are used in both calculations. However, partial pressures may be substituted for concentrations in the alveoli because gas concentrations are proportional to partial pressures. This is not true in blood except for inert gases.

Table 7–3 also shows that venous Po_2 always decreases with anemia but the decrease is greater if the difference in V_I/Q between the two alveoli is small. The effect of anemia on arterial Po_2 and thus the $P(A-a)o_2$ is variable. There is a noticeable decrease in Pao_2 with anemia only in the lung with the greatest difference in V_I/Q. Anemia affects arterial Po_2 in two ways. A decrease in hemoglobin effectively increases the V/Q of each alveolus because for a given amount of O_2 transported into blood the rise in O_2 content and thus Po_2 is greater if the hemoglobin is lower. As shown in Table 7–3, as the hematocrit drops from 39 to 18%, the equilibrium Po_2 for each alveolus is increased if the venous Po_2 remains constant. However, if Vo_2 is fixed, the venous Po_2 must decrease with anemia because even though the arterio-venous oxygen content difference is unchanged, the reduced oxygen-carrying capacity of blood causes marked venous desaturation. These two effects essentially offset each other in lungs 1 and 2 for which the V/Q of the two alveoli are relatively similar. However, in lung 3 the decrease in venous Po_2 predominates and the arterial Po_2 falls with a decrease in hematocrit. Thus in general, anemia has relatively little effect with normal lungs if cardiac output and Vo_2 remain constant. However, with respiratory failure, unless cardiac output increases markedly, anemia will lead to a decrease in arterial Po_2.

The most important feature of these simulations is that if there are at least two alveoli in a lung with different V/Q, an alveolar-arterial partial pressure difference will exist for every gas for which there is net uptake or elimination even in the absence of true shunt or dead-space. The magnitude of these differences depends on the gas but always increases as the V/Q difference becomes larger.

Describing gas exchange in a human lung is obviously much more complicated because there are approximately 300 million alveoli. However, the above principles still apply. That is, if the V/Q and blood flow to each of the 300 million alveoli could be known, then the alveolar, arterial, and venous partial pressures for any gas could be computed. To describe this graphically, a continuous distribution of V/Q may be drawn as shown in Figure 7–7. Although the exchange of any gas can be computed from such a distribution if the inspired and venous tensions are known and parallel ventilation and perfusion are assumed, even without such computations important information about gas exchange can be obtained from its shape. For example, the alveolar-arterial partial pressure differences for gases in a lung with a narrow distribution that peaks at the average Va/Q will be relatively small although, as described above, they will differ for different gases. As the distribution becomes wide and flat, the alveolar-arterial differences will increase for all gases. If the distribution is skewed so that there are large areas of low Va/Q regions, the alveolar-arterial differences for O_2 will increase but CO_2 will be relatively unaffected. Conversely, if the distribution includes large areas of high Va/Q but relatively little area in low Va/Q regions, there will be large arterial-alveolar differences for CO_2 but relatively little for inhaled gases such as O_2.

Although there is no doubt that in upright humans their V̄a/Q decreases from apex to base of the lung, there is no method of uniquely determining continuous Va/Q distributions such as that illustrated in Figure 7–7. The best attempts have made using the multiple inert gas technique.[5] However, the distributions recovered using this method are not unique. That is,

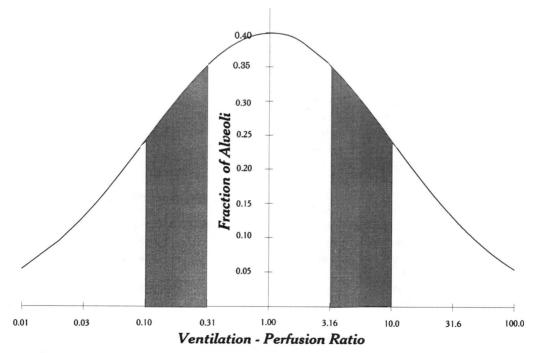

FIG 7–7.

Hypothetical log-normal distribution of ventilation-perfusion ratios within a lung. Notice that the V/Q are evenly spaced on a logarithmic scale so that there are as many alveoli with V/Q between 0.10 and 0.31 as between 3.16 and 10.0 (shaded regions). Notice also that most alveoli have V/Q in the range of 1.0.

a multitude of different-shaped distributions exist that can describe the data equally well.[6, 7] Nonetheless, a qualitative understanding of how changes in the shape of such distributions can effect gas exchange is important in understanding impaired gas exchange and the limitations of the indices used to assess it.

Adsorption Atelectasis

Many studies have shown that breathing pure O_2 can increase calculated shunt, as well as produce radiographic evidence of atelectasis and decreased functional residual capacity.[13–15] This phenomenon is termed *adsorption atelectasis*. Theoretically, if the uptake of alveolar gas by blood exceeds the ventilation of the alveolus, the conditions exist for adsorption atelectasis. Dantzker, Wagner, and West[16] showed that for any FiO_2, a critical V/Q could be determined below which these conditions do exist. This critical V/Q also depends on the venous gases because, as described above, they along with the FiO_2 determine the equilibrium partial pressures within the alveolus and thus the gas exchange across it. These authors also showed that the critical V/Q was approximately 0.001 with an FiO_2 of 0.21 and increased to approximately 0.05 with 100% inspired oxygen. Furthermore, the estimated minimum time till collapse of alveoli with V/Q below the critical value was more than 5 hours at an FiO_2 of 0.21, but decreased to approximately 10 minutes with 100% inspired O_2. Although the presence of the appropriate conditions does not ensure collapse because of hypoxic vasoconstriction, changes in venous gas tensions, collateral ventilation, and the support provided by adjacent structures, there is sufficient evidence from gas exchange data (see the on "Indices of Pulmonary Gas Exchange") and volume measurements to suggest that it does occur in some instances.

Shifts in the Oxyhemoglobin Dissociation Curve

The OHDC is generally characterized by the P_{50}, which is the oxygen partial pressure corresponding to a hemoglobin saturation of 50% (Fig 7–2). The P_{50} is right shifted (i.e., to higher values) in many acute situations. Probably the most common acute causes of a right shift are acidemia, hyperthermia, and an increase in 2,3-diphosphoglycerate. Shifts in the OHDC can theoretically affect both pulmonary and tissue O_2 exchange.

The theoretical effects of shifts in the P_{50} on pulmonary gas exchange are well summarized by Wagner.[17] Using simulations similar to those described above, he demonstrated that the effects of a shift in the OHDC depend on the V/Q distribution. For a single alveolus with the PvO_2 kept constant, a left shift in the OHDC (i.e., a reduction in the P_{50}) by 10 mm Hg could produce a maximum 30 mm Hg increase in alveolar PO_2. This occurred at a V/Q of 0.5 and decreased at higher or lower V/Q. This occurs essentially for the same reason that anemia increases PO_2 if venous PO_2 is kept constant. A left shift in the OHDC (Fig 7–2) in effect increases the V/Q of an alveolus because blood PO_2 will rise more rapidly for a given amount of O_2 transferred into the blood. However, because the OHDC converge at low and high PO_2 regardless of the P_{50} (Fig 7–2), this effect is observable only at PO_2 above the venous value and below the value producing 100% saturation. Specifically, for the reasons described in the section on the ventilation-perfusion ratio, regardless of the P_{50}, the end-capillary PO_2 must approach venous PO_2 as the V/Q approaches zero (i.e., true shunt). Because the PvO_2 was constrained to be the same regardless of the P_{50} in these simulations, and because a left shift in the OHDC results in a higher blood oxygen content for any $P_{V_{O_2}}$, the venous content was considerably greater at very low V/Q with a left-shifted OHDC. This led to an increase in end-capillary content. As the V/Q of the alveolus increased, the end-capillary content also increased. However, as the V/Q increases, differences in saturation of the end-capillary blood for OHDC with different P_{50} becomes negligible. Consequently, P_{O_2} differences diminish as V/Q increases. For these reasons, the maximal P_{O_2} differences occured at an intermediate V/Q (i.e., 0.5).

Similarly, for a normal lung, the effects of shifts in the OHDC would be expected to be detectable only in the P_{O_2}. This is because, regardless of the P_{50}, arterial blood will almost always be almost fully saturated. Therefore, the arterial content will be approximately the same regardless of the P_{50} if V_{O_2} and cardiac output do not change. This also constrains venous content to remain constant. However, a shift in the OHDC will produce a different $P_{V_{O_2}}$ for the same content. For example, a left shift in the OHDC would yield a lower $P_{V_{O_2}}$ for a fixed venous oxygen content. In contrast, for a lung with marked V/Q heterogeneity, a left shift in the OHDC would be expected to decrease both arterial and venous P_{O_2} while increasing their contents, again assuming a constant V_{O_2}, V_{CO_2}, and cardiac output. This occurs because the arteriovenous content difference must remain constant. However, the left shift in the OHDC has two effects. As mentioned, the effect on gas exchange is to increase the P_{O_2} of each alveolus for a given $P_{V_{O_2}}$. In contrast, although venous content must remain constant, the $P_{V_{O_2}}$ will decrease. In these simulations, the decrease in $P_{V_{O_2}}$ more than offset the increase in alveolar P_{O_2} that would occur at a fixed $P_{V_{O_2}}$. The net result is a decrease in the arterial P_{O_2}. These results are similar to those described earlier for anemia.

INDICES OF PULMONARY GAS EXCHANGE

Ultimately, the lung must supply enough O_2 to blood to meet total body oxygen requirements while eliminating the CO_2 produced by metabolic processes. Meeting oxygen demand not only requires that the amount of oxygen utilized by tissues be supplied but also that the P_{O_2} be high enough to deliver the oxygen to the tissues by diffusion, a process that will be discussed in the next section.

As discussed above, arterial P_{O_2} and P_{CO_2} depend not only on the intrinsic properties of the lung (e.g., the V/Q distribution, including true shunt and dead-space, which correspond to zero and infinite V/Q, respectively), but also on the factors extrinsic to the lung (e.g., venous and inspired patrial pressures). Consequently, inferences about changes in lung function cannot be made from changes in Pa_{O_2} or Pa_{CO_2} alone. To surmount this problem, many indices of gas exchange have been developed. Ideally, any change in such a gas exchange index would be due only to changes in intrinsic lung function. Such an index would have three important uses. First, changes in the index could, by definition, result only from changes in the V/Q distribution so that the effects of therapies and diseases on intrinsic lung function could be evaluated. Second, the index could be used to predict the Pa_{O_2} that would be obtained at different $F_{I_{O_2}}$ so that the inspired oxygen tension required to maintain an adequate Pa_{O_2} could be estimated. Third, the index could be used to compare lung function among patients receiving different FIO_2. Unfortunately, no clinically available index reliably meets any of these criteria. However, because many gas exchange indices are commonly used in clinical practice it is important to understand their bases and limitations. Therefore, they will be discussed in detail beginning with the shunt fraction (Qsp/Qt) which has been the "gold standard" among such indices.

Shunt Fraction

Classic Interpretation

The equation for deriving the shunt fraction is usually based on the simple lung model shown in Figure 7–8. In this model, the lung is assumed to be a perfect gas exchanger. That is, blood leaving the lung is assumed to have the same PO_2 as alveolar gas. In addition to the blood that perfuses the lung, it is assumed that some blood flow, Qsp, perfuses nonventilated alveoli, thus passing from the venous to the arterial side of the circulation without receiving any oxygen. This shunt corresponds to flow through zero V/Q alveoli. Its ratio to total cardiac output, Qt, is termed the shunt fraction (Qsp/Qt).

The equation for the shunt fraction in this model may be derived by noting that the total milliliters of oxygen leaving the left ventricle per minute must equal the number of milliliters per minute leaving the lung plus the number of milliliters per minute that passes through the shunt. That is:

$$CaO_2 \cdot Qt = CaO_2 \cdot Q\lambda + CvO_2 \cdot Qsp \qquad (7-6)$$

where $Q\lambda$ is blood flow through this "perfect" lung and CaO_2 (often termed $Cc'O_2$ for capillary content) is the oxygen content of blood leaving this lung. CaO_2 cannot actually be measured but instead is calculated from the alveolar PO_2 by assuming that the PO_2 of blood leaving this lung is the same as alveolar PO_2 (i.e., the lung is a perfect gas exchanger), using a Severinghaus slide rule, a table, or formulas easily implemented on a programmable calculator.[21] The alvoelar PO_2, in turn, is usually estimated as

$$PAO_2 = PIO_2 - PACO_2/R \qquad (7-7)$$

where R is the respiratory quotient, often assumed to be 0.8. More correctly, the rightmost term in this equation should be multiplied by $[1 - FIO_2 \cdot (1 - R)]$ to correct for the difference between inspired and expired alveolar volumes resulting from the inequality between oxygen consumption and carbon dioxide production. However, the magnitude of this correction usually is small and is generally ignored clinically. By noting that $Qt = Qsp + Q\lambda$ [Equation (7–6)] may be solved for Qsp/Qt to yield

$$Qsp/Qt = (CaO_2 - CaO_2)/(CaO_2 - CvO_2) \qquad (7-8)$$

These calculations are illustrated in Figure 7–8 assuming a hemoglobin of 15 g/100 mL. The total cardiac output of 5 L/min is divided into 3.9 L/min passing through the ideal lung and

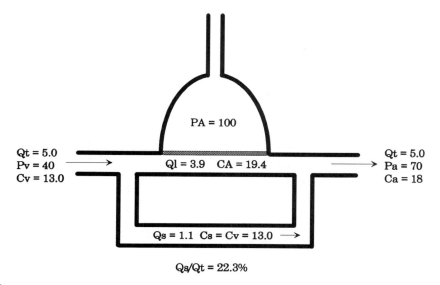

FIG 7–8.

Lung model used to derive the shunt equation. The lung is assumed to consist of a single alveolus so that there is no difference between the alveolar P_{O_2} and that of the blood leaving the lung. Any alveolar-arterial P_{O_2} difference is assumed to be due to a true shunt with blood flow Qs. In this example, the cardiac output (Qt) is 5.0 L/min. Of this, 3.9 L/min flows through the single-alveolus lung and 1.1 L/min through the shunt. The P_{O_2} and content of the shunted blood are the same as the mixed venous blood whereas the P_{O_2} of the blood leaving the lung has the same P_{O_2} as the alveolus (100 mm Hg), which corresponds to a content of 19.4 mL O_2/100 mL blood. The arterial content is $(3.9 \cdot 19.4 + 1.1 \cdot 13.0) / 5.0 = 18.0$. This content corresponds to a P_{O_2} of 70 mm Hg. Thus the alveolar-arterial difference is 30 mm Hg. In calculating the shunt fraction (Qs/Qt), usually venous and arterial P_{O_2} are measured and their corresponding contents calculated. The alveolar P_{O_2} is also calculated (see text), and the content that pulmonary venous blood would have if the P_{O_2} equaled alveolar is then computed. These values are then used to compute Qs/Qt as described in the text.

1.1 L/min passing through the shunt. The alveolar P_{O_2} is 100 mm Hg, which would yield a calculated content of 19.4 mL O_2/100 mL blood if blood leaving the lung also had a P_{O_2} equal to 100 mg Hg. The arterial and mixed venous contents would normally either be measured or calculated from the measured P_{O_2}. Substituting these values in Equation (7–8) yields a shunt fraction of 0.22, which corresponds to the fraction of cardiac output flowing through the shunt (1.1/5.0).

The limitation in this model lies mainly in the incorrect assumption that the P_{O_2} of blood leaving ventilated alveoli is the same as the average alveolar P_{O_2}. As discussed previously, this can be true only if all alveoli have the same V/Q, an assumption that is patently incorrect. The consequences of this assumption are that the shunt fraction computed using Equation (7–8) is affected by factors other than intrinsic changes in the lung. This is illustrated in Table 7–3. This table shows the effect of altering V/Q and $F_{I_{O_2}}$ on Qsp/Qt and several other often used indices of pulmonary function. Notice that for lungs 2 and 3 (V$_I$/Q of 0.4 and 1.2 for lung 2 and 0.1 and 1.5 for lung 3), Qsp/Qt decreases as $F_{I_{O_2}}$ increases. The effects of $F_{I_{O_2}}$ on

TABLE 7–4.
Effects of Changes in Hematocrit and Hemoglobin on Gas Exchange in Two Alveoli Lungs

	Hct	Venous		Alveolus #1			Aveolus #2			Arterial		Alveolar			
		PvO_2	$PvCO_2$	Vi/Q	PAO_2	$PACO_2$	Vi/Q	PAO_2	$PACO_2$	PaO_2	$PaCO_2$	PAO_2	$PACO_2$	ΔO_2	ΔCO_2
+	0.39	41	33	0.7	111	29	0.9	118	28	115	29	115	29	1	0
+	0.18	27	32	0.7	111	29	0.9	118	28	115	29	115	29	1	0
*	0.39	30	30	0.7	85	29	0.9	98	28	91	28	92	28	2	0
*	0.18	30	30	0.7	116	28	0.9	122	27	119	27	119	27	0	0
+	0.39	40	34	0.4	87	33	1.2	124	28	101	30	115	29	14	1
+	0.18	27	33	0.4	86	32	1.2	124	28	101	30	115	29	14	1
*	0.39	30	30	0.4	56	30	1.2	109	26	69	28	97	28	28	1
*	0.18	30	30	0.4	102	29	1.2	130	25	115	27	120	26	8	1
+	0.39	33	36	0.1	38	36	1.5	119	28	51	32	115	29	65	3
+	0.18	17	35	0.1	26	35	1.5	120	28	39	32	115	29	76	3
*	0.39	30	30	0.1	35	30	1.5	116	25	47	28	112	25	65	2
*	0.18	30	30	0.1	42	30	1.5	131	24	56	27	126	24	71	3

+ Oxygen consumption and carbon dioxide production fixed at 200 mL/min, respectively.
* Venous gases are fixed and oxygen consumption and carbon dioxide production vary. FiO_2 is 0.21. Total inspired alveolar ventilation is 4 L/min. Blood flow is 2.5 L/min to each alveolus. ΔO_2 is alveolar-arterial differences for oxygen. ΔCO_2 is arterial-alveolar difference for carbon dioxide.

Qsp/Qt and other indices to be discussed below are calculated for lung 3 are shown in more detail in Figure 7–9. This occurs because as the F_{IO_2} increases, the partial pressures in both alveoli increase to the point where hemoglobin is fully saturated. Beyond this point, increases in F_{IO_2} increase the oxygen content only by a small amount corresponding to the slight increase in dissolved oxygen. Consequently, at high F_{IO_2} the oxygen contents of blood leaving each alveolus will be nearly equal so that there can be little difference between the content of arterial blood and that of each alveolus. Therefore, the numerator of the shunt equation decreases, becoming nearly constant once the F_{IO_2} is high enough to saturate fully the hemoglobin in the blood leaving each alveolus. However, as shown in Table 7–3, at low F_{IO_2} the calculated shunt fraction can be quite large if the V/Q of the two alveoli differ widely even though there is no true shunt. Thus, not only can a literal interpretation of calculated shunt be misleading physiologically, but the value calculated also varies with F_{IO_2} despite the constancy of the lung itself. The other indices in this table are discussed in later sections.

Results from clinical studies in humans have been variable. Although a decrease in Qsp/Qt has been observed[22–24] with increasing F_{IO_2}, in some instances, Qsp/Qt increased as the F_{IO_2} approached 1.0. This probably occurred because of adsorption atelectasis of low V/Q alveoli or release of hypoxic pulmonay vasoconstriction.

Because the effects of V/Q inhomogeneity are diminished at high F_{IO_2}, the shunt fraction calculated at an F_{IO_2} of 1.0 has been used to estimate true shunt. However, in dogs this has been shown[25] generally to overestimate true shunt by as much as 10%, especially when the

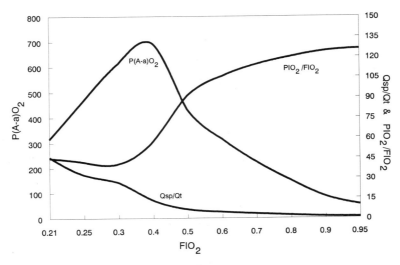

FIG 7–9.
Changes in three indices of gas pulmonary exchange with F_{IO_2} for a hypothetical two-alveoli lung. The V/Q of the alveoli are 0.1 and 1.5. Each alveolus has a blood flow of 2.5 L/min. Oxygen consumption and carbon dioxide production are fixed at 200 and 160 mL/min, respectively. There is no true shunt or dead-space. All of these indices vary markedly with F_{IO_2}. However, Qsp/Qt and P_{IO_2}/F_{IO_2} are both relatively stable for F_{IO_2} above approximately 0.5. Nonetheless, none of these indices is useful by the criteria described in the text.

true shunt fraction is less than 20%. This not unexpected because even when breathing pure oxygen, the alveolar CO_2 still prevents blood leaving each alveolus from equilibrating with pure oxygen. Consequently, very low V/Q alveoli can still have low equilibrium Po_2 leading to an alveolar-arterial oxygen difference, which violates the assumption in Equation (7–8) that blood leaving the lung has the same Po_2 as the alveoli. This leads to an error in the measurement of true shunt. Although the V/Q of such alveoli is so low that they can be considered effectively as true shunt, their response to therapeutic maneuvers such as positive end-expiratory pressure (PEEP) may make this distinction important. In addition, the calculation of Qsp/Qt at an Fio_2 of 1.0 can produce adsorption atelectasis by the mechanism described earlier. Wagner et al.[26] demonstrated this by showing the development of true shunt when patients breathed 100% oxygen. Thus, because the act of measuring true shunt may change its actual value, such measurements seem pointless.

Another Interpretation

The shunt fraction may be interpreted more realistically as a measure of inefficiency of oxygen transport across the lung into blood. Efficiency of a process is usually defined as the amount of work done by the process divided by the energy theoretically available to do the work. For example, the efficiency of muscle in lifting a weight is defined as the work done (the weight times the distance it is lifted) divided by the maximum energy that theoretically could be generated from the amount of oxygen used by the muscle. By analogy, admittedly imperfect, the efficiency of the lung in oxygenating blood could be loosely defined as the amount of oxygen transported from the alveoli into blood divided by the maximum amount that theoretically could be transported. The amount actually taken up, which equals total body oxygen consumption, Vo_2, is the number of milliliters per minute of O_2 entering the pulmonary circulation minus the number of milliliters per minute leaving it. That is,

$$Vo_2 = 10 \cdot Qt \cdot Cao_2 - 10 \cdot Qt \cdot Cvo_2 = 10 \cdot Qt \cdot (Cao_2 - Cvo_2) \qquad (7–9)$$

where the factor 10 is needed to correct for the fact that Qt is usually expressed in liters per minute and content is in mL O_2/100 mL blood.

The maximum amount of oxygen that theoretically could be taken up by blood, Vmo_2, would occur if arterial and alveolar Po_2 were equal so that

$$Vmo_2 = 10 \cdot Qt \cdot Cc'o_2 - 10 \cdot Qt \cdot Cvo_2 = 10 \cdot Qt \cdot (Cc'o_2 - Cvo_2) \qquad (7–10)$$

The efficiency of the lung then is calculated by dividing the Vo_2 by Equation (7–10) to yield

$$\text{Efficiency} = (Cao_2 - Cvo_2)/(Cc'o_2 - Cvo_2) \qquad (7–11)$$

The inefficiency of O_2 uptake across the lung is 1 − efficiency, which is exactly Equation (7–8), the shunt equation.

Recognition that the shunt equation is not really a measure of true shunt but rather of the inefficiency of oxygen transport into blood explains why even if the V/Q distribution of a lung doesn't change, Qsp/Qt is affected by alterations in Fio_2 and Pvo_2. For example, as shown in

Tables 7–3, increasing F_{IO_2} decreases Qsp/Qt because the difference in oxygen content of blood leaving alveoli even with very different V/Q is minimized so that the lung actually is more efficient. Because this calculation of shunt fraction, which is more appropriately referred to as *venous admixture*, varies with F_{IO_2} and P_{VO_2} it does not fulfill the criteria set out above for a useful index. Although Qsp/Qt may be useful in comparing lung function between patients or within a patient of F_{IO_2} and P_{VO_2} remain constant, it cannot be used to distinguish between changes in V/Q and true shunt nor can it be used to compare lung function at different F_{IO_2} because the change in Qsp/Qt with F_{IO_2} depends on the underlying V/Q distribution and therefore is unpredictable (Table 7–4). To use the shunt fraction to predict the P_{aO_2} that will result from changes in F_{IO_2}, both the change in Qsp/Qt and in P_{VO_2} would also have to be predictable. However, as shown in Tables 7–3 and 7–4, these values cannot be predicted unless the underlying V/Q distribution is known. In fact, when examined in this manner, Qsp/Qt does not seem to yield any more information than the P_{aO_2}, which is much simpler to obtain. Therefore, the shunt fraction does not appear to be a very helpful index of gas exchange despite its widespread use. Furthermore, it can be misleading if interpreted literally as true shunt because, for example, if a large true shunt were responsible for the low P_{aO_2} of patients with chronic lung disease, then, as discussed above, a very limited response to increasing the F_{IO_2} would be expected and supplemental oxygen might not be administered. However, many such patients have nearly normal P_{aO_2} at high F_{IO_2} because their hypoxemia while breathing room air is due primarily to very broad V/Q distributions and the true shunt usually is small. Finally, because of the possibility of adsorption atelectasis, increasing the F_{IO_2} to 1.0 to calculate Qsp/Qt is unwarranted. Also because the increase in F_{IO_2} may actually change the V/Q distribution and because the calculation does not fulfill the above criteria for a useful index, this practice makes little sense and should be avoided.

The Alveolar-Arterial Oxygen Difference

The difference between the PA_{O_2} calculated using Equation (7–7) and the P_{aO_2} measured in arterial blood, the $P(A-a)_{O_2}$, was developed as a simple approximation to the shunt equation. The relation to Qsp/Qt may be seen by rewriting Equation (7–8) as:

$$Qsp/Qt = (C_{AO_2} - Ca_{O_2})/(C_{AO_2} - Ca_{O_2} + Ca_{O_2} - Cv_{O_2}) \qquad (7-12)$$

If the alveolar and arterial P_{O_2} are high enough to saturate fully hemoglobin, then

$$C_{AO_2} - Ca_{O_2} = 0.0031 \cdot P(A-a)_{O_2}. \qquad (7-13)$$

Equation (7–12) then may be rewritten as

$$Qsp/Qt = 0.0031 \cdot P(A-a)_{O_2} / [0.0031 \times P(A-a)_{O_2} + a\text{-}v_{DO_2}] \qquad (7-14)$$

where $a\text{-}v_{DO_2}$ is the arteriovenous oxygen content difference. The magnitude of $0.0031 \cdot P(A-a)_{O_2}$ will be much smaller than $a\text{-}v_{DO_2}$. Therefore Equation (7–14) is approximately

$$Qsp/Qt = \text{P(A-a)o}_2 \, / \, \text{a-vDO}_2 \qquad (7-15)$$

Because Equation (7–15) implies that changes in P(A-a)o$_2$ approximate those in Qsp/Qt if a-vDO$_2$ remains constant the P(A-a)o$_2$ was proposed as an easily measurable index of pulmonary gas exchange. However, since it approximates Qsp/Qt, the P(A-a)o$_2$ will, at best, have all of the limitations of Qsp/Qt. Moreover, because a constant a-vDO$_2$ and fully saturated hemoglobin are assumed, the P(A-a)o$_2$ actually is even further from meeting the criteria set above for a useful index than Qsp/Qt.

For example, Farhi and Rahn[27] used simulations to study the effects of V/Q distributions and shunt on the P(A-a)o$_2$. Their results predicted that without true shunt, the P(A-a)o$_2$ would increase with F$_{IO_2}$ and then at some point decrease, reaching relatively low values at an F$_{IO_2}$ of 1.0. The addition of true shunt was predicted to result in a progressive increase in this index with increasing F$_{IO_2}$. Although this study suggested that this index would not be useful, they used, by necessity, some simplifying assumptions including fixed venous gases that could produce some quantitative errors. Table 7–3 shows the effects of F$_{IO_2}$ on P(A-a)o$_2$ determined for the three hypothetical two-alveoli lungs. Figure 7–9 depicts in detail the dependence of P(A-a)o$_2$ on F$_{IO_2}$ for lung 3, which has the most disparte V/Q. For this lung, P(A-a)o$_2$ more than doubles as F$_{IO_2}$ is increased from 0.21 to 0.35, and then it decreases markedly with further increases in F$_{IO_2}$ as also shown by Farhi and Rahn. However, the P(A-a)o$_2$ progressively decreases with increasing F$_{IO_2}$ for both lungs 1 and 2 rather than first reaching a maximum. Notice that Qsp/Qt decreases with increasing F$_{IO_2}$ in all three lungs.

Qualitatively similar results have been found in clinical studies. Shapiro, Virgilio, and Peters[28] found that a change in F$_{IO_2}$ from 0.21 to 1.0, resulted in directionally opposite changes in the P(A-a)o$_2$ and Qsp/Qt in 20% of the studies. Marked changes in the P(A-a)o$_2$ with increasing F$_{IO_2}$ also have been found by others.[29-33] However, in contrast to the simulations discussed above, in these clinical studies, the P(A-a)o$_2$ usually becomes larger with increasing F$_{IO_2}$.

Discrepancies between changes in Qsp/Qt and the P(A-a)o$_2$ would be expected to increase for larger Qsp/Qt. This can be shown by solving Equation (7–14) for the P(A-a)o$_2$ to yield

$$\text{P(A-a)o}_2 = Qsp/Qt \cdot \text{a-vDO}_2 \, / \, [0.0031 \cdot (1 - Qsp/Qt)] \qquad (7-16)$$

Which indicates that even if the a-vDO$_2$ were constant, changes in P(A-a)o$_2$ and Qsp/Qt would be proportional only if Qsp/Qt were very small. Otherwise, increases in Qsp/Qt would cause the denominator of Equation (7–16) to decrease. As a result, as Qsp/Qt increased, P(A-a)o$_2$ would increase by progressively greater increments rather than proportionally. Equation (7–16) also indicates that the P(A-a)o$_2$ could change in the opposite direction from Qsp/Qt as observed by Shapiro, Virgilio, and Peters[28] if Qsp/Qt and the a-vDO$_2$ change in opposite directions.

Thus, it would seem that changes in the P(A-a)o$_2$ reflect similar changes in Qsp/Qt only under very restricted circumstances. Unfortunately, these instances cannot be determined *a priori*. Consequently, clinical decisions based on the P(A-a)o$_2$ can be misleading. For example, suppose a patient arrives in a recovery room after 8 hours of surgery still anesthetized, paralyzed, and fully ventilated with a temperature of 34°C. Because the patient has a history of chronic lung disease, a blood gas is obtained on an F$_{IO_2}$ of 1.0. The Pao$_2$ is 500 mm Hg and the Pco$_2$ is 40 mm Hg. A few hours later, the patient is warm, awake, agitated, and ready for extubation. However, because of the history, another blood gas is obtained. The Pa_{O_2} is now 420 mm Hg and the P_{CO_2} is still 40 mm Hg. Thus the $P(A-a)_{O_2}$ has increased from approximately 173 mm Hg (713 − 40 −500) to 253 mm Hg · sp Physical exam is normal. Should the patient be extubated or should he remain intubated pending chest physiotherapy, a chest x-ray, and further evaluation?

This example demontrates the problem in trying to interpret the $P(A-a)_{O_2}$ when patients are not in a steady state. The full set of data for this patient are shown in Table 7–5. Despite the increase in the $P(A-a)_{O_2}$, Qsp/Qt has actually decreased from 15.4 to 11.9%, indicating that the lung has become more efficient rather than more abnormal as suggested by the marked rise in the $P(A-a)_{O_2}$. However, this change in shunt fraction does not imply any change in the lung for the reasons discussed above. The decrease in Qsp/Qt has occurred because as the patient warmed, the oxygen consumption increased from 150 to 300 mL/min. This led to a reduction of the venous P_{O_2}. Because the venous P_{O_2} is on the steep portion of the OHDC, there was a large decrease in the venous content. In contrast, because of the high arterial P_{O_2}, arterial content changed minimally. This violates the assumption used in approximating Qsp/Qt by the $P(A-a)_{O_2}$; that the a-vD_{O_2} remains constant with the result that the $P(A-a)_{O_2}$ increased when Qsp/Qt decreased.

In summary, the $P(A-a)_{O_2}$ can be misleading because its changes with F_{IO_2} are unpredictable and not only may not parallel those of Qsp/Qt but may be in the opposite direction. The $P(A-a)_{O_2}$ also is not helpful in predicting the P_{O_2} resulting from changes in F_{IO_2} because its relation to F_{IO_2} also depends on the underlying V/Q distribution. Consequently, the $P(A-a)_{O_2}$ is even further from fulfilling the criteria for a useful index of gas exchange than Qsp/Qt. The practice of placing a patient on 100% O_2 to evaluate the $P(A-a)_{O_2}$ should be avoided for the same reasons it should not be used in assessing Qsp/Qt. Therefore, the $P(A-a)_{O_2}$ should be abandoned as an index of gas exchange.

TABLE 7–5.
Patient Gas Exchange Cold and Asleep versus Awake, Warm, and Agitated

	Asleep	Awake
V_{O_2} (ml/min)	150	300
P_{IO_2} (mm Hg)	673	673
Ca_{O_2} (ml O_2/100 ml Blood)	22.18	22.17
Pa_{O_2} (mm Hg)	500	420
Ca_{O_2} (ml O_2/100 ml Blood)	21.63	21.36
Pv_{O_2} (mm Hg)	67.86	49.66
Cv_{O_2} (ml O_2/100 ml Blood)	19.63	15.36
Qsp/Qt (Percent)	15.4	11.9
$P(A-a)_{O_2}$ (mm Hg)	173	253

The PaO_2/FIO_2 and PaO_2/PaO_2 Ratios

The PaO_2/PaO_2 ratio, $P(a/A)O_2$, was proposed as a FIO_2 independent index of pulmonary function by Gilbert et al.[29, 30] because it equals $1 - P(A-a)O_2/PaO_2$ and therefore was thought to correct the $P(A-a)O_2$ for its dependence on FIO_2. For this to be true, the $P(A-a)O_2$ would have to be linearly related to the PaO_2 with an intercept of zero. That is, if $P(A-a)O_2 = K \cdot PaO_2$ then $P(a/A)O_2$ would equal $1 - K$ and would therefore be constant regardless of the PaO_2. Although Karetzky, Kieghley, and Mithoefer[32] did find such a linear relation in normals from an FIO_2 of 0.21 to 0.40, the intercept was not zero. Moreover, this linear relation is not a general finding in other studies. Therefore, because this requisite does not appear to be true, there are no experimental or theoretical reasons why this index should be independent of FIO_2. In fact, in the study in which Gilbert proposed this index,[29] in normal young adults the $P(a/A)O_2$ was relatively constant $(0.77 - 0.81)$ over an FIO_2 range of 0.21 to 1.0. However, for patients requiring ventilatory support, the ratio varied considerably with FIO_2 (approximately 0.4 to 0.7) with a minimum generally occurring at an FIO_2 of 0.40. Simulations performed later by Gilbert et al.[30] showed that the $P(a/A)O_2$ tends to decrease slightly and then increase markedly as FIO_2 is increased if true shunt was kept constant while the $P(a-A)O_2$ changes in almost the opposite direction. The clinical data also presented in this study indicate that the $P(a/A)O_2$ was relatively constant with changes in FIO_2 in patients thought to have large true shunts with relatively little V/Q imbalance, but they varied considerably in patients thought to have a large component of V/Q mismatch. The changes in the $P(A-a)O_2$ always were greater than in the $P(a/A)O_2$. The authors concluded that the $P(a/A)O_2$, i.e., the arterial-alveolar ratio, is relatively constant for FIO_2 greater than 0.4 in patients with large true shunts and otherwise varies considerably with FIO_2. Nonetheless, they considered it to be less sensitive to FIO_2 than the $P(A-a)O_2$ and to be superior to the ratio of PaO_2 to FIO_2 because the latter does not take into account the $PaCO_2$. Martyn et al.[33] found that overall only about 50% of the variation in Qsp/Qt could be accounted for by changes in the ratio of arterial oxygen tension to inspired oxygen fraction. The two alveoli lung simulation results shown in Table 7–3 and Figure 7–9 also show that this ratio generally increases with increasing FIO_2 in all three hypothetical lungs. The magnitude of this increase depends on the V/Q of the two alveoli.

Summary

If criteria for a useful index of gas exchange are accepted as those given in the beginning of this section, these clinical and theoretical data along with other clinical studies[34, 35] clearly show that currently no indices of gas exchange are useful in patients with markedly abnormal gas exchange. Consequently, simply following the PaO_2 is both simpler and provides at least as much information as any of the above-mentioned indices. This is important since clinical studies that stratify patients by these indices can be very misleading because none of these indices reflects the degree of gas exchange abnormality independently of FIO_2 and mixed venous PO_2. Therefore, we believe that the use of such indices should be abandoned and the quest for useful indices should begin with an understanding of the physiology of gas exchange.

OXYGEN TRANSPORT FROM BLOOD TO TISSUES

Oxygen delivery from blood to tissues differs from that to alveoli to blood because the source (blood) is moving and the tissues consume oxygen, thereby serving as an oxygen sink. In contrast to alveoli, oxygen must diffuse across relatively large distances to get to tissues and the surface area available for diffusion is relatively small. Because blood flow, oxygen consumption, and diffusion distances vary even within a tissue bed, the Po_2 of tissue also varies, ranging from nearly that of arterial blood to only a few mm Hg. The importance of the factors governing diffusion in producing differences between venous and tissue Po_2 and the unimportance of diffusion in generating alveolar-arterial Po_2 differences is crucial to the understanding of the factors important in determining and assessing oxygen transport from alveoli to tissues. In addition, because tissue consumes large amounts of oxygen relative to alveoli, even if diffusion were very rapid, the Po_2 of the blood perfusing a given region would still be higher than that of the region being perfused.

Although there is much interest in assessing the gas exchanging capabilities of the lung and the carriage of gases by blood, ultimately the role of these two functions is to meet tissue metabolic needs. Recent attempts to assess the adequacy of oxygen delivery to tissues have focused on oxygen delivery (mL/min of O_2 leaving the left ventricle) and mixed venous oxygen partial pressure or saturation. To assess the utility of these measurements and indices, the physiology and pathophysiology of tissue oxygen delivery must be explored and then the clinical data evaluated. The important physiologic questions are as follows: (1) At the individual capillary level, how do changes in blood flow, oxygen partial pressure, and content affect tissue oxygen delivery? (2) What mechanisms are available to supply more oxygen to tissues when their requirements increase?

Regional Blood Flow

Although increasing organ blood flow is an effective method for compensating for greater oxygen demands, unfortunately, increasing cardiac output through various interventions does not guarantee that the increased blood flow is directed to the desired tissues. As discussed previously, the autoregulatory reserve and response to sympathetic stimulation varies markedly in different organs. Thus, for example, as indicated in Table 7–2, exercise and therefore probably epinephrine increases cardiac output enormously and results in greatly increased muscle and cardiac blood flow, but a reduction in flow to all other visceral organs. Conversely, heart failure decreases renal blood flow much more than splanchnic or cardiac flow. Thus it is impossible to infer adequacy of organ flow or oxygenation from cardiac output unless the distribution can be assessed.

The mechanisms by which tissue beds autoregulate blood flow in response to various stimuli such as hypoxia or changes in blood pressure are not fully understood and may differ for different stimuli. For example, it seems likely that the increases in flow that occur with hypoxia are related to metabolic changes and that blood flow therefore would be selectively increased to regions with relatively high oxygen demands. Such changes in blood flow distribution with hypoxia have been observed[36] and are thought to be related, in part, to chemoreceptor mediated reflexes[37] although increases in cardiac output still occur with hypoxemia if all reflexes are ablated.[38] In contrast, the changes in blood flow distribution are different in anemia than in hypoxia.[39] Thus it cannot be assumed that increases in cardiac output will be equally distributed to all organs. In the heart, infusion of the vasodilator adenosine produced a drop in blood pressure without a change in total coronary flow.[40] However, subendocardial ischemia worsened, implying that flow was maldistributed. Similarly, Cain[41] demonstrated that with alpha receptor blockade the time to cardiovascular collapse is shortened in hypoxemic dogs despite the same cardiac output and oxygen delivery as nonblocked hypoxemic dogs. In addition, in this study the relation between Do_2 and Vo_2 changed with alpha receptor blockade so that Vo_2 generally was lower for any Do_2 in the blocked dogs. Although Cain believes that changes in oxygen delivery mediate the changes in blood flow that occur during hypoxia, data exist that show capillary recruitment is related to Pao_2 not content.[42] This seems likely as oxygen diffusion to tissues will not be the same for a given content attained with a high Po_2 and low hemoglobin concentration as with a low Po_2 and high hemoglobin concentration. Consequently, it seems unlikely that changes in Do_2 due to hypoxemia would have the same effects on blood flow and Vo_2 as comparable changes due to decreases in cardiac output. However, this has not been systematically studied.

Diffusion of Oxygen from Blood to Tissue

Although the above questions can be answered qualitatively, a precise quantitative analysis of the delivery of oxygen from blood to tissue is not yet possible for three reasons. First, the relations between the changes in Po_2 or content along a single capillary and that of surrounding tissue have not yet been measured and mathematical models give different results depending on their assumptions. Second, there is great heterogeneity in blood flow and Po_2 within a given tissue bed.[43] Third, there are enormous differences in the oxygen requirements, basal blood flow, and blood flow reserve among different organs.

Although the distribution of oxygen partial pressures over a small area of tissue can be measured,[43] measurement techniques are not yet refined enough to examine the region supplied by a single capillary. Therefore, understanding the dynamics of oxygen transfer at this level relies largely on mathematical models. While the principles are the same as for o_2 transport from alveoli to blood, the process differs in ways that have important ramifications in developing measures of tissue oxygenation. Unfortunately, some of these differences make such models very complex. First, tissues are an oxygen sink. That is, they consume oxygen. Most models assume first-order kinetics for oxygen utilization so that at very low Po_2 tissue oxygen consumption is proportional to the tissue Po_2 whereas at high tissue Po_2, tissue oxygen consumption is essentially constant. At an intermediate Po_2, tissue oxygen consumption depends on tissue Po_2 in a more complex manner. Second, the geometric relation of tissue beds to capillaries is uncertain. Usually, a single capillary is modeled as being surrounded by a cylinder of tissue that it alone oxygenates. This is called the *Krogh cylinder*. There is some anatomic evidence in skeletal muscle to support this geometry. Third, the nonlinear OHDC make solutions to the governing differential equations difficult even using current computer technology. In addition, diffusion to tissue differs from that from alveoli to blood in several other important ways that affect tissue oxygenation: (1) the distance that oxygen must traverse to get to tissues is generally much larger than from alveolus to blood; (2) the capillary surface area in tissue is much smaller than that surrounding alvoeli; and (3) the oxygen source (i.e., the blood) is moving while the sink (the tissues) are immobile. In this latter sense, the delivery of oxygen to tissues is almost the mirror image of the transfer of oxygen from alveoli to blood where the source (the alveoli) is static and the blood is moving. Despite these problems it is worthwhile to review some of the findings from solving mathematical models because they are helpful in evaluating clinical indices of tissue oxygenation.

Because tissues utilize oxygen, the Po_2 of blood leaving a given capillary is always greater than that of the immediately surrounding tissues. In general, as shown in Figure 7–10, the capillary Po_2 decreases nonlinearly from the proximal to the distal end. As tissue-capillary distance increases, tissue Po_2 also decreases nonlinearly. As a result, the lowest tissue Po_2 occurs at the outside of the distal end of the tissue cylinder. This is termed the *lethal corner*. Unlike the alveolus, this blood-tissue Po_2 difference does not necessarily mean that diffusion

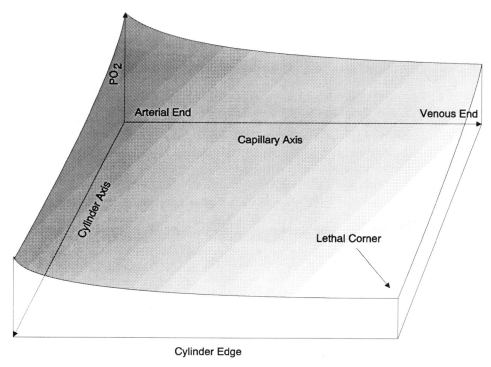

FIG 7–10.
Distribution of Po_2 within a Krogh cylinder. The height of the shaded area represents the Po_2. Also higher Po_2 is indicated by darker shading. The arterial end of the cylinder is on the left and the venous end on the right. Po_2 decreases both with distance from the capillary axis along the cylinder axis and with distance along the capillary axis. The lowest Po_2 is at the lethal corner because it is farthest from the arterial end of the cylinder.

is too slow to reach an equilibrium, but rather is the inevitable result of oxygen delivery to a sink. The difference between the proximal and distal tissue Po_2 is affected markedly by the rate of diffusion within the tissue at relatively low flow rates. As might be predicted intuitively, at low blood flow, diffusion within the tissue tends to minimize differences in tissue Po_2. That is, oxygen diffuses within the tissue tending to make the distribution of Po_2 more uniform. As expected, average tissue Po_2 tends to decrease with lower hemoglobin concentrations and increased oxygen consumption. These effects also are most marked at low flow rates. In summary, differences in tissue-capillary distances and perhaps local oxygen demand explain, qualitatively, the observations that tissue Po_2 may vary enormously over small regions. Such differences are affected markedly by blood flow and hemoglobin concentration. All of these factors alter the relationships between capillary and tissue Po_2.

Most of these findings have been confirmed qualitatively by experiments. In general, the Po_2 in tissues from most organs has a bell-shaped distribution[43] with a mode of 15 to 30 mm Hg, lower limits of 1 to 2 mm Hg, and upper limits of 60 to 90 mm Hg. The lung and outer cortex of the kidney are exceptions, having smaller spreads of Po_2 around the mode. In addition, the shape and modes of such distributions change considerably if oxygen demand or arterial Po_2 are changed.[44, 45] Studies performed on the cytochrome system[46] indicate that oxidative metabolism can proceed normally at Po_2 of a few mm Hg. Therefore, tissue regions other than those that are already at a very low Po_2 possess considerable Po_2 reserve.

Venous Po$_2$

Because the Po_2 of blood leaving a capillary must be greater than that of the immediately surrounding tissue, those tissues with high Po_2 must either be very close to the capillaries supplying them, near to the proximal ends of the capillaries, or have very low oxygen consumption. Tenney, using a simplified mathematical model of a cylinder of tissue supplied by a single capillary,[47] modeled the relation between the mean Po_2 of tissue and the Po_2 of the effluent blood from a capillary centered in the tissue. Although he found that under certain conditions the mean tissue Po_2 would be approximately the same as the capillary venous Po_2, in most cases (e.g., increased metabolic rate, anemia, and hypoxemia) the capillary effluent Po_2 was higher than mean tissue Po_2 by an amount that varied considerably depending on conditions. This model also depended on many unverified assumptions and ignored longitudinal oxygen diffusion within the tissue surrounding the capillary as well as potential disequilibrium between hemoglobin and plasma Po_2. The rate of diffusion within the tissue is important because if it is rapid enough to keep the Po_2 everywhere equal within a tissue region supplied by a single capillary, then the venous Po_2 would have to be higher than that of the tissue in all instances. Gutierrez[38] used a mathematical model to study the effects of the time required by red cells to release oxygen. He found that although end-capillary and venous Po_2 would be similar under basal conditions, during hypoxia the venous Po_2 would be expected to be higher than that in the portion of the capillary leaving the tissue because of insufficient time for oxygen to diffuse from the red cell to plasma to match the tissue uptake of oxygen from plasma.

Even if capillary venous Po_2 were equal to the average of the tissue region that it supplied, for the venous Po_2 leaving an organ to equal that of all of the organ tissue, the rate at which oxygen leaves regions with Po_2 higher than the overall organ venous value (i.e., the product of the content and the blood flow summed over all capillaries) would have to be offset exactly by the rate from capillaries from regions with Po_2 lower than the venous value. This proposition seems very unlikely. Finally, even if this were true, some tissues would deviate far from such a mean and this deviation would vary considerably when there are changes in demand, flow, or arterial Po_2. The deviation toward low Po_2 would potentially be important because such tissues might be at risk for hypoxia. However, their presence could not be detected from mixed organ venous Po_2. For example, the venous Po_2 of the kidney is approximately 60 mm Hg, which is considerably higher than that of mixed venous blood. However, because it generally accounts for at most 20% of cardiac output, changes in its venous Po_2 would be very hard to detect, especially if other organ flow increased (e.g., exercise).

In summary, both theoretical and experimental data indicate that venous Po_2 from even a single capillary will have a variable relation to the Po_2 of the surrounding tissue, and that the Po_2 of blood draining an organ not only will not reflect the adequacy of oxygenation of that organ but also that changes in venous Po_2 cannot be interpreted as changes in the adequacy of organ oxygenation. Furthermore, when the heterogeneity of organ blood flow and oxygenation is considered it seems extremely farfetched to think that the mixed venous Po_2 could in any way reflect the overall adequacy of organ oxygenation. This is even more evident when the methods for compensating for inadequate oxygenation are considered.

Effects of Shifts in the Oxyhemoglobin Dissociation Curve

Theoretically, a right shift in the OHDC should be advantageous in supplying O_2 to tissues because the partial pressure of O_2 in blood would be maintained at relatively high levels as O_2 is unloaded to tissues (Fig 7–2). However, some animals indigenous to high altitudes have left-shifted dissociation curves[18, 19] which suggests that such shifts may be beneficial. Shumacker et al.[20] studied the effects of an acute left shift in the OHDC on exercise tolerance in dogs exposed to 21, 12, and 10% inspired O_2. They were unable to show any change in exercise performance with a decrease in the P_{50} to an average of 19.5 mm Hg from a normal average value of 28.8 mm Hg. As predicted from the above discussion, the left shift in the OHDC led to an elevation in arterial O_2 content at all levels of exercise. Interestingly, the left shift in the OHDC caused Pvo_2 to decrease at all levels of exercise with 21% and 12% inspired O_2 as predicted. However, there was no effect on Pvo_2 at 10% inspired O_2, probably because of the marked increase in arterial content. A redistribution of pulmonary blood flow altering the V/Q distribution also could have occurred. There was no evidence of anaerobic metabolism under any conditions.

In balance, these and other studies suggest that tissue blood flow is redistributed with decreases in F_{IO} so that tissue diffusion remains adequate. Shumacker et al.[20] also suggest that a left shift in the OHDC may be beneficial with extreme hypoxia because the resultant increase in arterial content might allow capillary Po_2 to be maintained at higher levels, thereby facilitating diffusion to tissues.

Physiologic Methods for Increasing Oxygen Delivery to Tissue

The mechanisms generally available to meet increases in tissue oxygen consumption are (1) extracting more oxygen from the capillaries, (2) increasing the diffusion rate, (3) increasing the amount of oxygen in blood, and (4) increasing capillary blood flow. The effects of these mechanisms on the oxygen content of venous blood can be estimated from the equation

$$V_{TO_2} = 10 \cdot Q_t \cdot (C_{aO_2} - C_{v TO_2}) \qquad (7-17)$$

where V_{TO_2} is tissue oxygen consumption, Q_t is tissue blood flow, and $C_{v TO_2}$ is the oxygen content of blood leaving the tissue.

Increasing Extraction

The amount of additional oxygen that could be extracted from a capillary if blood flow and tissue distances were constant is markedly limited for those tissues that already have a very low P_{O_2}. Equation (7–17) implies that any increase in tissue demand would have to result in a drop in effluent blood content and thus P_{O_2} at all points along the capillary supplying that tissue region. Regions that already have a P_{O_2} in the range of a few mm Hg would be unable to increase extraction because the tissue P_{O_2} could not decrease enough to increase the diffusion gradient appreciably. In contrast, those regions that had a relatively high P_{O_2} could increase their oxygen delivery by reducing their P_{O_2} secondary to increased consumption. This would result in a lower P_{O_2} of the blood leaving such a region to values that are too low to supply adequate oxygen to more distal regions that already had very low P_{O_2}. Thus, one would expect that if tissue demands increased but capillaries could not be recruited and flow could not rise, then the venous P_{O_2} would decrease and some regions of the tissue could become hypoxic or a supply-limited decrease in oxygen consumption of these tissues could ensue. Such decreases have been observed experimentally and clinically with hypoxemia.

Increasing Diffusion

Fortunately, tissues can decrease tissue-capillary distance and increase the cross-sectional area available for diffusion if precapillary sphincters, which are occluded in the basal state, dilate, thereby increasing the capillary density. As a result, for a given partial pressure, the flux of oxygen to tissues would increase. Consequently, if tissue oxygen demands remained constant, the P_{O_2} at each point along the capillary would increase, resulting in a higher P_{O_2} in the effluent blood. This follows from Equation (7–17) because V_{TO_2} would decrease since each capillary would supply a smaller tissue mass. However, if tissue demands increased, the capillary P_{O_2} profile would depend on which effect dominated—capillary recruitment or the increased consumption. Specifically, Equation (7–17) indicates that if tissue consumption increased to the point where V_{TO_2} was greater than the prerecruitment value despite the reduced mass per capillary, then $C_{v TO_2}$ would decrease. Moreover, the decrease in venous P_{O_2} would not imply that tissue oxygenation was inadequate because the reduced diffusion distances could permit adequate oxygenation of all tissues even with the reduced P_{O_2} in the capillary. However, the profile of P_{O_2} along the capillary would differ considerably from that produced by increasing extraction without recruitment. This compensatory mechanism is used by patients with heart failure who cannot increase cardiac output by normal amounts when metabolic needs increase. Clearly, then, venous Po_2 cannot be used, even if it could be measured regionally, to make inferences about the adequacy of tissue oxygenation.

Increasing Blood Oxygen Content

The concentration of oxygen in blood can be augmented either by increasing the Po_2 or by raising the hemoglobin concentration. However, the role of Po_2 and hemoglobin in supplying oxygen to tissues is quite different. An adequate Po_2 is required to create a sufficient partial pressure gradient to deliver the oxygen to tissues. However, were it not for hemoglobin, the Po_2 would fall precipitously along the capillary, rapidly reaching values that would be too low to drive diffusion adequately. In this sense, hemoglobin is a reservoir of oxygen that permits the Po_2 to remain high while oxygen is unloaded to tissues. Consequently, rightward shifts in the oxyhemoglobin dissociation curve such as that caused by acidemia, hyperthermia, or hypercarbia (Fig 7–2) can be advantageous for tissue oxygenation because as oxygen is unloaded, the Po_2 will remain relatively high.

The different roles of Po_2 and hemoglobin in supplying oxygen to tissue suggest that adequate tissue oxygenation is not assured if the oxygen content is normal because acceptable oxygenation requires that both Po_2 and hemoglobin be sufficient. However, over the physiologic range of hemoglobin, it is unlikely that adequate content can be achieved without both the Po_2 and hemoglobin being within an acceptable range. Nonetheless, physiologically, it makes more sense to consider Po_2 and hemoglobin separately in assessing tissue oxygenation as they are the important factors, not content.

Increasing Blood Flow

Probably the most important compensatory mechanism for increases in tissue oxygen demands is to increase blood flow to such tissues. If oxygen consumption were constant, an increse in blood flow through already recruited capillaries would increase the diffusion rate of oxygen to tissues because the Po_2 at each point along the capillary would be increased. In this case the tissue Po_2 would rise and, as indicated by Equation (7–17), the venous Po_2 would also increase. However, if tissue oxygen requirements were raised, an increase in blood flow would allow for greater oxygen extraction without lowering the capillary Po_2 to levels too low to deliver adequate oxygen. Equation (7–17) indicates that the effect of this process on the venous Po_2 depends on the ratio of the demand to blood flow. If the increase in oxygen consumption exceeds the increase in flow, the venous Po_2 would drop, whereas otherwise it would rise.

GLOBAL TISSUE OXYGENATION INDICES

Although, potentially, all of the above mechanisms can be used to deliver enough oxygen to meet both normal and abnormal tissue oxygen needs, only crude clinical methods exist for assessing the adequacy of tissue oxygenation because measurements at the tissue level are generally not available. Therefore, more global measures have been sought. Two that have enjoyed considerable clinical popularity are oxygen delivery, Do_2, defined as the number of milliliters of oxygen leaving the left ventricle per minute, and the mixed venous Po_2 or saturation, Svo_2. This has occurred partly because with a pulmonary artery catheter, Svo_2 can be measured directly and Do_2 can be calculated from the cardiac output and the Pao_2. The Svo_2 has been advocated as a measure of tissue oxygenation despite the theory and data presented above that indicate that a decrease in Svo_2 may indicate better tissue oxygenation and vice versa. Oxygen delivery has received particular interest because of clinical observations that increasing Do_2 to supranormal levels may be accompanied by progressive increases in Vo_2 (see below). This phenomenon, often termed *supply-dependent oxygen consumption* (SDOC), has led some investigators to assume that oxygen delivery to tissues is inadequate until Do_2 is increased to a point where Vo_2 no longer rises. The experimental data are reviewed below and the possible clinical applications are discussed.

Supply-Dependent Oxygen Consumption

There have been many studies asserting that as oxygen delivery (Do_2) is progressively increased to supranormal levels in some critically ill patients, oxygen consumption (Vo_2) rises in a parallel fashion (Fig 7–11). Interest in SDOC is considerable in critically ill patients because many clinicians and investigators have assumed that the increase in Vo_2 is indicative of an oxygen

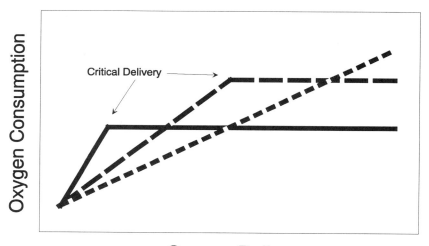

FIG 7–11.
Possible relations of oxygen consumption (Vo_2) to oxygen delivery (Do_2). It is thought that in normal individuals, as Do_2 drops below a critical value, Vo_2 falls in a parallel manner (*solid line*). This critical Do_2 is presumably well below the normal values. However, in some critically ill patients, Vo_2 seems to rise with increases in Do_2 well above the normal range (*dotted line*). This is termed supply-dependent oxygen consumption (SDOC). It is thought, without substantial evidence, that if Do_2 rises sufficiently in such patients that a plateau is reached at a critical Do_2 that is greater than the normal Do_2 (*dashed line*). SDOC is used as an argument for increasing Do_2, usually by increasing cardiac output, in critically ill patients.

debt and that, consequently, increasing Do_2 should be beneficial to patients because the consequent increase in Vo_2 should lessen this debt and therefore improve outcome. Although there seems to be little doubt that as the perfusion to at least some tissues drops below certain critical values, Vo_2 falls, there are substantial discrepancies and methodologic problems in patient studies. Moreover, many studies have failed to demonstrate SDOC in patients. The important questions then are as follows: (1) Does SDOC actually exist as Do_2 is elevated above normal levels? (2) If it does exist, does it reflect an oxygen debt? (3) Do clinical studies show any benefit in increasing Do_2? In this section, these issues will be examined. However, to answer these questions and account for the substantial discrepancies in the medical literature, important methodologic limitations in the design and analysis of these studies will first be considered.

Methodologic Problems

Snyder and Carrol[48] suggest that SDOC may be an artifact because cardiac output often is used both to calculate oxygen delivery and consumption. If, for example, cardiac output were spuriously increased because of measurement error, the values calculated for Do_2 and Vo_2 would also increase. Consequently, an increase in Do_2 would be associated with an increase in Vo_2. This potential artifact was demonstrated by Snyder and Carrol in 10 patients in whom Vo_2 was measured using respiratory gas exchange rather than the product of cardiac output and the arteriovenous oxygen content. SDOC was found in only two patients, whereas all 10 demonstrated this relation if Vo_2 was calculated from blood contents and cardiac output. Similarly, in a study of 13 septic patients, Vermeij, Feenstra, and Bruining[49] found that one patient had SDOC when Vo_2 was measured using respiratory gases, whereas three patients showed SDOC using Vo_2 calculated from blood measurements. None of these three patients showed SDOC when Vo_2 was calculated using respiratory gases. Thus measurement errors can lead to a spurious relation between Do_2 and Vo_2. However, it probably is not the cause of SDOC demonstrated in all studies because some studies using cardiac output to calculate Do_2 sometimes find SDOC in one group of patients but not in another. For example, Danek et al.[50] did not find any relationship in patients without respiratory failure. Moreover, SDOC was demonstrated by Pepe and Culver[51] by applying PEEP or venous obstruction to anesthetized dogs both with and without oleic acid-induced pulmonary edema and by measuring Vo_2 from inspired gases. Nonetheless, studies using cardiac output to calculate both Do_2 and Vo_2 that demonstrate SDOC should be interpreted with great caution.

A second problem with most studies demonstrating SDOC is that marked spontaneous variations in Vo_2 can occur over the duration of the study. A spontaneous increase in Vo_2 could easily result in an increase in Do_2, which if undetected could be incorrectly interpreted as SDOC. In a group of critically ill patients, Villar, Slutsky, and Hew[52] found a 7% to 147% (mean 38%) variation in Vo_2 and a 9% to 189% (mean 42%) variation in Do_2 over a 2-hour period. Kaufman, Rackow, and Falk[53] found that Vo_2 increased from normal or slightly subnormal levels with increases in cardiac output during fluid resuscitation of patients with hypovolemic or septic shock. However, the study took more than 1.5 hours to complete so that spontaneous changes in Vo_2 resulting in changes in Do_2 are likely. This duration is actually relatively short—other studies actually spanned days. Clearly, a control group without interventions is needed, but this is impractical in studies where measurements are made during resuscitation. However, control groups would be possible in studies where interventions are used in stable patients to raise Do_2 to supranormal levels.

A third related problem is that most studies do not systematically attempt to change Do_2 and then measure Vo_2. Instead, measurements are often made randomly. Moreover, even if Do_2 is systematically changed, it virtually never changed randomly. For example, if drugs such as dobutamine are used to increase Do_2, measurements are not made after discontinuation of the drug to determine if patients return to control values. Thus it is possible that the order of interventions affects the results. That is, results could differ if cardiac output were first decreased and then increased rather than vice versa. These design problems make cause and effect difficult to establish.

A fourth common problem is matching severity of disease. Although the commonly studied patients are those with sepsis and adult respiratory distress syndrome (ARDS), the definitions of these conditions vary widely among studies as does the severity of hemodynamic aberration. Such differences in patient groups may account for some of the variability in results, and whether or not lactate levels are increased.

Does Supply-Dependent Oxygen Consumption Exist?

As discussed above, theoretical descriptions of tissue oxygen consumption usually assume first-order kinetics, implying that oxygen is consumed by combining, reversibly, with a substrate. If this is true, when tissue oxygen concentration is high, oxygen consumption should be independent of concentration, whereas when oxygen concentration is very low, consumption should be approximately proportional to concentration. A critical Po_2 in a muscle sheet, below which oxygen consumption decreases nonlinearly, has been demonstrated experimentally.[44] A decrease in Vo_2 also was found by Shepherd et al.[54] in areflexic dogs made hypoxic. This concept was extended by Cain[55] who found a relatively linear relation between oxygen delivery and Vo_2 consumption in dogs made anemic euvolumically or made hypoxic. Notably, in Cain's study, mixed venous Po_2 was not highly correlated with oxygen consumption in either group but was higher for any given oxygen consumption in the anemic than the hypoxic group. Although difficult to discern from the data presented, it does appear that in both groups, the changes in oxygen delivery were largely due to progressive decrements in cardiac output terminating in cardiovascular collapse. In contrast, in Shepherd's studies,[54] the decrease in Vo_2 with hypoxia appeared independent of cardiac output and decreases in output with normoxia did not effect Vo_2. However, no attempt was made to relate Vo_2 to Do_2, and the decrease in cardiac output with normoxia may not have been sufficient to decrease Vo_2. A dependence of intestinal oxygen uptake on blood flow below approximately 30 ml/min/100 g also has been shown.[56]

Many studies in humans have demonstrated a linear relation between Do_2 and Vo_2 (SDOC) in various disease states. However, it is important to recognize that most human studies alter Do_2 by changing only cardiac output, not oxygen content. Therefore, although such studies try to relate Vo_2 to Do_2, they are actually relating Vo_2 to cardiac output. Consequently changes in Do_2 could just as well be termed changes in carbon dioxide or even sodium delivery.

Both Rhodes et al.[57] and Danek et al.[50] reported SDOC in patients with ARDS. Rhodes et al.[57] used mannitol to increase cardiac output and found overall an increase in Vo_2. Unfortunately, the relation between Do_2 and Vo_2 in the 11 patients studied was not quantitated and individual data are not presented. However, although Vo_2 increased in 10 patients, the patient with the decrease in Vo_2 had an increase in Do_2, whereas 2 of the patients with increases in Do_2 had decreases in Vo_2. Thus changes in Vo_2 may not have been related to Do_2, but rather to elapsed time or mannitol. The study by Danek et al.,[50] which used PEEP to decrease Do_2 is more convincing in that they did demonstrate a linear relation between Do_2 and Vo_2 in patients with respiratory failure but not in a control group of critically ill patients without respiratory failure. It appears that changes in oxygen delivery were largely a result of decreases in cardiac output due to PEEP although Danek did not present the Po_2 or oxygen content data. Interestingly, in this study, Pvo_2 did not change appreciably as cardiac output decreased and Vo_2 was generally normal or supranormal. Many newer studies (see Lorente et al.[58] for references) have demonstrated SDOC in patients with a variety of pathologic conditions although most commonly it has been demonstrated in patients with sepsis or ARDS.

Not all studies have found SDOC. For example, Annat et al.[59] did not find a relation between Do_2 and Vo_2 in patients with respiratory failure when cardiac output was decreased with PEEP or restored with volume infusions. Oxygen consumption also was unrelated to Do_2 in patients with respiratory failure who received progressive increases in PEEP.[60] In these patients, Vo_2 was surprisingly low (approximately 145 ml/min on average) and the decreases in Do_2 were a result of decreases in cardiac output. Oxygen consumption also was found to be independent of Do_2 in patients with either chronic heart failure or pulmonary hypertension treated with vasodilators.[61] In one of the few studies where Do_2 was increased by raising the oxygen-carrying capacity of blood, Ronco et al.[42] transfused 17 patients with ARDS with 600 ml of packed red blood cells plus 200 ml of normal saline over a 1-hour period. They measured Vo_2 from respiratory gases and did not find SDOC in these patients despite an average increase in Do_2 of 207 ml/min.

Does Supply-Dependent Oxygen Consumption Reflect a Tissue Oxygen Debt?

Two lines of evidence, discussed in detail in the next sections, have been used to support the contention that SDOC reflects a tissue oxygen debt: (1) the existence of a plateau in Vo_2 as Do_2 is increased to supranormal levels and (2) the assertion that SDOC is generally associated with increased lactate levels and therefore reflects tissue hypoxia. This view was also reinforced by Bihari's study[62] in which prostacyclin infusions produced an increase in cardiac output. There was a concomitant increase in Vo_2 and the oxygen extraction ratio in critically ill patients who did not survive but not in survivors. Bihari's interpretation of these findings was that the increase in Vo_2 reflected inadequate tissue oxygenation although a metabolic acidemia was present in only 5 of the 13 patients who died. However, as discussed by Cain and Curtis,[63] even if SDOC does occur in certain classes of patients, it is not evident that the increases in VO_2 reflect tissue hypoxia or would be beneficial if sustained. Cain speculates that this relation may be found in patients with respiratory failure but not in other critically ill patients both because flow is redistributed secondary to leukocyte plugs and because non–ATP-producing oxidase systems may be responsible for much of the increment of Vo_2. Were this true, attempts to increase Vo_2 by increasing Do_2 could theoretically be harmful. Although studies in isolated animal muscles have shown decreases in high-energy phosphates and performance along with increases in lactate when Po_2 was decreased to low levels in a hemoglobin free perfusate,[64] studies in humans have not generally reported evidence of anaerobic metabolism or tissue hypoxia with changes in Do_2 or Vo_2.

Does Oxygen Consumption Plateau with Increasing Delivery?

Finally, there is the question of whether Vo_2 plateaus at a sufficiently high value of Do_2 and if the appropriate independent variable is Do_2 or cardiac output. The former question is important because it is frequently assumed that such a Vo_2 plateau reflects Do_2 values that are sufficient to meet tissue oxygen demands and that below this plateau tissues are incurring an oxygen debt. However, there are several problems in analyzing data for a Vo_2 plateau. First, individual rather than pooled data should be analyzed because pooled data may spuriously suggest a plateau where individual data does not. This problem is illustrated in Figure 7–12, where all patients are shown to have SDOC based on two different Do_2, but the slope of the SDOC line varies among patients. There is no indication of a plateau in any patient. However, if the data are indiscriminately pooled, there appears to be a plateau due to the patients who have a relatively small increase in Vo_2 with increases in Do_2. Thus to demonstrate a plateau, there must be sufficient data points to analyze each patient separately. A second problem lies in the statistical methods used to determine a plateau. Statistical methods exist for determining

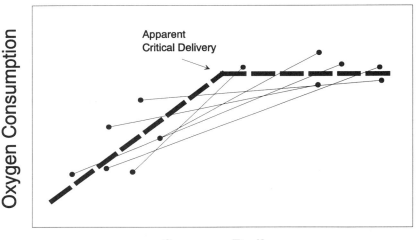

FIG 7–12.
Spurious plateau in oxygen delivery–consumption data due to improper data analysis. Each pair of dots connected by a thin line represents SDOC for an individual patient. The basal Vo_2 and the increase with an increase in Do_2 varies among patients. When the data are analyzed as an aggregate, Vo_2 appears to rise and then become constant, suggesting a plateau at the apparent critical delivery. However, this plateau is clearly an artifact resulting from pooling the data from all patients. To test reliably for a plateau, each patient must have enough data points to demonstrate individual plateaus.

if a set of data is better described by one or two lines and where the data should be divided to determine the two lines. Arbitrary cutoffs based on visual inspection do not suffice.

In animal experiments, a critical Do_2 can often be demonstrated that is below the normal range of Do_2. In Cain's original dog study,[55] the critical Do_2 was approximately 10 ml/min/kg although individual dog data were not presented. In humans, Shibutani et al.[65] performed a seminal study of patients undergoing cardiopulmonary bypass. They described a critical Do_2 of 330 ml/min (8.2 ml/min/kg). However, examination of their individual data indicates that the plateau is probably an artifact from the analyses problems described earlier. The method for determining the two lines is not described and their Figure 2 shows a flatter Vo_2-Do_2 slope for patients at higher baseline Do_2 and a decline in Vo_2 in some patients and does not suggest a plateau. Finally, a plateau is not demonstrated for any patient. Tuchshhmidt et al.[62] assert that based on a study by Mohsenifar et al.[61] the critical Do_2 in patients with ARDS appears to be about 21 ml/min/kg, and based on their own data,[62] above 15 ml/min/kg in septic patients. However, this assessment of Mohsenifar's data is also based on examination of pooled data. Examination of individual data (their Figure 1) indicates that this conclusion is based on pooling the data from two patients both of whom showed little or no SDOC. Therefore, this analysis also suffers from the problems stated above. Individual data points are not presented in Tuchschmidt's study[62] and the data are retrospective so that the time span for data collection cannot be determined. In addition it is not clear from their methodology how the two line segments were determined. Because of these severe methodological limitations in these studies, it can be concluded that none of them convincingly demonstrate a Vo_2 plateau. Moreover, many studies showing SDOC have done so at values of Do_2 well in excess of the critical values reported above and most human studies have failed to find a critical Do_2 despite achieving supranormal values.

Is There a Relation Between Supply-Dependent Oxygen Consumption and Lactate Levels?

It has been suggested that SDOC occurs in more severe disease and especially if lactate is increased. In a study[66] of fluid loading in 20 septic patients, 14 had an increase in Do_2 and 8 of these also increased Vo_2. Those 8 patients had higher initial lactate levels than the 6 who didn't increase their Vo_2, but lactate did not decrease in any of these 14 patients.

Gilbert et al.[67] found that infusion of colloid or blood led to SDOC only in patients with elevated lactate levels although, contrary to the interpretation provided by Tuchschmidt, Obletas, and Fried,[68] lactate levels did not decrease. However, in Gilbert's study SDOC was observed in a group given catecholamine regardless of lactate levels. Although these data were obtained within approximately 1.5 hours and the therapies were administered according to common clinical criteria, there are several serious methodologic flaws. First, both Do_2 and Vo_2 were computed from thermodilution cardiac output (see above). Second, eight patients who had decreases in Do_2 were excluded from analysis as were an unspecified number in the blood and catecholamine groups. Third, individual patient data were not presented. Nonetheless, this study is important because it is one of several cited as implying that the increase in Vo_2 with an increase in Do_2 should be beneficial because it occurred mostly in patients with elevated lactate, suggesting inadequate tissue oxygenation.

As reviewed by Weg,[64] not all studies have found a relation between lactate levels and SDOC. This would seem sensible because increases in lactate do not necessarily indicate increased anaerobic metabolism. As suggested by Cain and Curtis,[63] lactate may be increased by a number of other mechanisms. Examples are (1) reduced lactate clearance due to hepatic dysfunction; (2) a block in the conversion of pyruvate to acetyl Coenzyme A (i.e., inactivation of pyruvate dehydrogenase), which may be caused by endotoxin; and (3) an increase in glucose utilization. Conversely, if clearance were high enough, lactate could be normal despite the presence of significant anaerobic metabolism.

Summary

Although these data are not all consistent, it seems, in balance, that increasing Do_2 above normal values can result in an increase in Vo_2 under some conditions that have not been precisely defined. In addition, in general, Vo_2, Do_2, and cardiac output are not uniquely related or in some cases related at all to mixed Pvo_2. Somewhat more controversial is whether or not Vo_2 plateaus if Do_2 is raised far enough.

In summary, there are several problems in extrapolating the data showing changes in Vo_2 with Do_2 to guide therapeutic interventions. First, it must be shown that increasing Do_2 increases Vo_2 and that increasing Do_2 by increasing cardiac output, Pao_2, or hemoglobin are equivalent, a proposition that is very unlikely. In fact, most of the human studies have altered cardiac output rather than oxygen content. Thus these studies could have just as well discussed altered carbon dioxide or sodium transport. Second, it must be shown that such increases are beneficial because it is possible, as Cain speculates, that a decrease in non–ATP-producing oxygen-consuming processes may be beneficial in that it could reduce oxygen radical formation.

Mixed Venous Oxygen Tension

As discussed above, the oxygen partial pressure or saturation of the venous blood from individual organs does not reflect either the adequacy or level of oxygenation of the tissues within that organ. Furthermore, even if this were the case, because of the enormous heterogeneity of the ratio of organ oxygen consumption to blood flow (Table 7–2), Pvo_2 or Svo_2 could not possibly indicate the overall adequacy of tissue oxygenation. This is because organs having high ratios of consumption to flow, such as the heart, have low venous Po_2 and vice versa. Because Pvo_2 reflects a weighted average of the venous contents from each organ where the weight is the organ blood flow, changes in Pvo_2 will be dominated by organs that have large changes in blood flow. Consequently, in a condition such as septic shock where muscle and skin blood flow are probably high (no other organs can dilate enough to have such high flows), changes in the Pvo_2 of vital organs would be essentially undetectable. Similarly, increasing cardiac output using vasoactive or cardioactive drugs is likely to alter flow distribution, again rendering changes in Pvo_2 uninterpretable. Similar conclusions were reached in the oxygen delivery studies cited above because neither Pvo_2 nor Svo_2 were related to oxygen consumption, cardiac output, or oxygen delivery. In fact, in Cain's study,[55] the venous Pvo_2 below which Vo_2 began to fall varied depending on the method used to decrease delivery. In the study of Danek et al.,[50] Pvo_2 was unrelated to Vo_2 or cardiac output. Thus, althogh Svo_2 is readily measured using pulmonary artery catheters with fiber-optic sensors, both theoretical considerations and clinical studies confirm its inadequacy in assessing tissue oxygenation.

THERAPEUTIC STRATEGIES

It has been known for many years that although high levels of PEEP can improve Pao_2, the price paid may be a reduction in cardiac output and barotrauma. In addition, beyond a certain level, PEEP can decrease lung compliance and even Pao_2. Calculated indices such as Qsp/Qt, dead-space, and oxygen delivery also have variable relations to PEEP. Although it has been proposed that PEEP can be used prophylactically to prevent lung damage, no data exist to support this claim. Therefore, the most reasonable goal in applying PEEP seems to be to provide adequate oxygenation to tissues without damaging the lungs. To this end, the measurements that have been proposed to guide the adjustment of PEEP center around the following: (1) maximize oxygen delivery, (2) minimize the "shunt fraction" (3) minimize the arterial-alveolar carbon dioxide difference, $P(a-A)co_2$, and (4) maintain an adequate arterial Po_2 while keeping the inspired oxygen concentration below toxic levels.

Maximize Oxygen Delivery

Outcome Studies

Numerous studies [69–72] have shown that critically ill patients who survive tend to have higher cardiac outputs and Vo_2 than nonsurvivors. This has led Shoemaker, Appel, and Kram[73] to postulate that attempting to alter hemodynamics prophylactically so that patients have the hemodynamic patterns associated with survival will improve outcome. The underlying principle apparently is that in various forms of shock "maldistributed flow results in tissue oxygen debt that produces organ failure and death."[73] This concept is based largely on the concept that the SDOC observed in some of these patients indicates a tissue oxygen debt. However, as discussed above, it is not at all certain that SDOC actually reflects tissue oxygen debt or that the increase in Vo_2 is salutary. The major support for Shoemaker's postulate comes from a single study in which 88 patients were randomized into three groups.[74] Group A was monitored with a central venous catheter (CVP) using normal parameters as a therapeutic goal. Group B was monitored with pulmonary artery (PA) catheters using normal parameters available with PA monitoring as a therapeutic goal. Group C was monitored with PA catheters but had previously established supranormal hemodynamic and "oxygen-transport" values as a therapeutic goal.

Of the 88 patients in this study, 30 were randomized to group A, 30 to group B, and 28 to group C. The number of postoperative deaths was significantly lower for group C than group B, but was not significantly different between groups A and C or A and B. The authors interpret this as indicating that the achievement of supranormal values led to a reduction in mortality. However, numerous problems arise with this interpretation. First, the CVP control group (group A) did not have a significantly different mortality than the PA group with supranormal goal-directed therapy (group C). Thus, at best, this study indicates that if a PA catheter is placed, supranormal goals should be sought. Otherwise, a CVP catheter without such goals is equally efficacious. Put differently, the results imply that a PA catheter might be detrimental unless such goals are sought. However, the methods for seeking the supranormal values are not systematically described, and, in fact, these goals were not achieved on average for cardiac index or Vo_2.

The study is also confusing because an unspecified number of patients were considered separately because of a high cardiac index preoperatively. Which group they randomized to and their mortality rates are unreported. Moreover, 76 patients who were eligible for this study were not randomized. Their outcomes are not reported. Finally, the patients do not appear to be well matched between the groups. For example, 16 patients in group A and 13 patients in group B had an "acute abdominal catostrophe," whereas there were only 8 such patients in group C. There were 6 patients in group A and 5 patients in group C with "age over 70 and limited physiologic reserve," whereas there was only 1 such patient in group B. If these preexisting conditions are important in determining outcome, these inequalities could easily account for any differences among groups. For all of these reasons, this study must be viewed as inconclusive. Thus, to date, there are no prospective randomized studies indicating that the achievement of supranormal hemodynamics improves outcome. This coupled with the uncertainty about the physiology and cardiac consequences of increasing cardiac output strongly suggests that such therapy should not be applied pending further studies.

Best PEEP

Although Pao_2 may decrease at high levels of PEEP, it usually increases as PEEP is raised. However, this increase in Pao_2 is often accompanied by a decrease in cardiac output. If the Pao_2 were high enough to saturate hemoglobin before the PEEP was increased, any concomitant decrease in cardiac output could decrease Do_2. However, if hemoglobin were not fully saturated, the increase in content might offset any decrease in cardiac output so that the Do_2 might increase. The opposing effect of PEEP on cardiac output and oxygen content was the basis of a study performed by Suter, Fairley, and Isenberg[75] to test the hypothesis that the maximum compliance produced by adjusting the level of PEEP should correspond to the maximum Do_2. They studied 15 patients with acute respiratory failure with "adequate" intravascular fluid volume judged by normal central venous and pulmonary capillary wedge pressures. PEEP was applied to each patient in 3-cm H_2O increments until cardiac output was "markedly decreased." Do_2 reached a maximum in 13 of the patients at a level of PEEP that coincided with the maximum compliance, calculated from the ventilator plateau pressure. Moreover, the physiologic dead-space was minimized at this level of PEEP although Qsp/Qt fell progressively with increasing PEEP. The highest level of PEEP used in this study was 18 cm H_2O. The authors concluded that a "best PEEP" could be attained by adjusting the PEEP level until the static compliance reached a minimum.

Although this study was important in helping to define the cardiopulmonary effects of PEEP, it has numerous design problems that markedly restrict its utility. An important conceptual problem with this study is that the maximum compliance depends on tidal volume as well as the PEEP. This was clearly demonstrated in a later study by Suter, Fairley, and

Isenberg,[76] in which they showed that for 12 patients requiring ventilatory therapy for various reasons (the magnitude of respiratory failure was not described), as the PEEP was raised at low tidal volumes compliance increased progressively, but at higher levels of PEEP, as tidal volume was increased (above approximately 10 ml/kg), compliance did reach a maximum. Thus, at low tidal volumes, a "best PEEP" could not be found because the compliance never reached a peak. Moreover, as might be anticipated, at larger tidal volumes the PEEP yielding the maximum compliance varied with the tidal volume. It seems unlikely that the different levels of PEEP required to achieve this maximum at different tidal volumes would each correspond to the maximum oxygen transport.

There are also several design problems in Suter's first "best PEEP" study.[75] First, the Pao_2 without PEEP averaged 78 mm Hg with very little variation and increased to 99 mm Hg at a PEEP of 6 cm H_2O above the "best PEEP." Thus, the Pao_2 probably was adequate even without PEEP. Second, the order in which PEEP was applied was not randomized. Finally, the decrease in cardiac output, which never dropped below 6 L/min, that occurred beyond the "best PEEP" could easily have been prevented by fluids or inotropes—therapies that are not more likely to maldistribute blood flow than PEEP. Such support of the cardiovascular system while increasing PEEP has been advocated by a number of investigators.[77–80]

For all of these reasons, although the concept of "best PEEP" is intriguing it does not seem likely, either experimentally or theoretically, to be an optimum way to adjust PEEP to prevent tissue hypoxia even assuming that Do_2 is an adequate index of tissue oxygenation which, as already discussed, seems unlikely. However, a relation between changes in Do_2 with the application of PEEP and Vo_2 has been observed in patients with respiratory failure. Several investigators have advocated adjusting PEEP and expanding intravascular volume in such patients until Vo_2 and usually Do_2 are maximal.[81, 82] However, the theoretical and clinical value of such therapy remains unproven.

Minimize Q*sp*/Q*t*

Gallagher, Civetta, and Kirby[83] proposed that the level of PEEP becomes optimal when Q*sp*/Q*t* is less than 15% with an Fio_2 of 0.35 to 0.45. They applied this criterion to 480 patients, 421 of whom required less than 10 cm H_2O of PEEP to meet this criterion. However, their report is descriptive and does not in any way indicate that this criterion was beneficial. The report also is peculiar in that the authors state that the reduction of Q*sp*/Q*t* to 15% or less is considered by most clinicians to be consistent with adequate ventilatory function (unreferenced) and yet also state that PEEP is used with the sole intention of reducing inspired oxygen concentration to nontoxic levels (their Ref. 8). If the latter goal is used, there is no reason to even measure Q*sp*/Q*t*, especially since, as discussed above, it is not a measure of intrinsic lung function and varies with Fio_2. Conversely, the achievement of a specified value for Q*sp*/Q*t* does not always mandate that Pao_2 is adequate. Moreover, there is no obvious clinical or physiologic reason for choosing 15% (or any other number). Finally, although not specifically stated, the authors imply that this criterion was applied before either oxygenation became inadequate or the chest x-ray became grossly abnormal because they assert that "delay until radiographic changes or hypoxemia have occurred may compromise markedly the outcome," an assertion that has never been validated. Thus, although increasing PEEP until Qsp/Qt has decreased below some critical value has been advocated by some physicians, it seems devoid of any scientific merit. However, this and other studies[78, 84, 85] were important in demonstrating that PEEP could be increased to high levels without major deleterious effects if care was taken to support the cardiovascular system with volume or drug infusions.

Minimize Arterial Minus End-Tidal Carbon Dioxide Difference

This criterion is motivated by Suter's observation that the "best PEEP" not only maximized oxygen delivery and compliance but also minimized dead-space.[75] Murray et al.[86] reasoned that the arterial-alveolar CO_2 difference, $P(a\text{-}A)co_2$, should be minimal when there is maximal recruitment of perfused alveoli without overdistention. They assumed that this would occur when the alveolar dead-space, reflected by the $P(a\text{-}A)co_2$, was minimal. They tested this hypothesis in 10 dogs with oleic acid-induced respiratory failure and found that the minimum $P(a\text{-}A)co_2$ occurred at a PEEP near the value that produced the lowest Qsp/Qt. Furthermore, Qsp/Qt did not increase and Pao_2 did not decrease with further increases in PEEP. Although, the maximum compliance was found at a lower PEEP, oxygen delivery decreased progressively as PEEP was added. The authors concluded that minimizing the $P(a\text{-}A)co_2$ provided a relatively noninvasive method to adjust PEEP to obtain a small Qsp/Qt.

Unfortunately, several problems accompany attempts to extrapolate this study to humans or to compare it with other studies. First, the mean Pao_2 before the addition of PEEP was 109 mm Hg. Consequently, oxygen delivery would be affected only by cardiac output since hemoglobin always was fully saturated. Furthermore, a Pao_2 of 109 mm Hg on 50% inhaled oxygen indicates relatively mild respiratory dysfunction and would hardly warrant high levels of PEEP. Second, the application of PEEP was not randomized so that the effects of time alone on the $P(a\text{-}A)co_2$ cannot be determined. In addition, the assumptions that the $P(a\text{-}A)co_2$ would be minimized by recruiting perfused but unventilated alveoli without overdistending already ventilated alveoli is incorrect. As discussed earlier, the alveolar-arterial (or arterial-alveolar) partial pressure difference for any gas is determined primarily by the inhomogeneity of ventilation-perfusion ratios. If, for example, all alveoli were overdistended but had the same V/Q, the $P(a\text{-}A)co_2$ would be zero.

Thus, although there may be useful information in the $P(a\text{-}A)co_2$, it is not evident from this study that it is useful for titrating PEEP because its relation to oxygenation in severe respiratory failure is not defined and there is no reason to believe that minimizing Qsp/Qt is beneficial.

Reduce Inspired Oxygen Concentration to Nontoxic Levels

This method consists of increasing the PEEP until the Pao_2 is high enough to allow the inspired oxygen concentration to be decreased to nontoxic levels. Other variables, such as blood pressure or cardiac output may be observed and supported if necessary. It is important to remember that oxygen toxicity takes longer to occur at lower concentrations. Thus although 100% oxygen may be toxic within a few hours, it may take days of 70% oxygen to cause toxicity. Therefore, the need to increase PEEP to reduce the inspired oxygen concentration depends on both the concentration itself and the duration of exposure. In this sense, it is probably unimportant to increase PEEP to drop the FIO_2 to 0.6 from 1.0 within the first few hours of therapy. A reduction to 0.9 may suffice.

This technique is predicated on the fact that goals such as a reduction in Qsp/Qt or maximizing oxygen delivery are, as discussed, without any sound physiologic basis and may be misleading. However, because it is known that if the Pao_2 becomes too low oxygen cannot be delivered to some tissues and high inspired concentrations may cause toxicity, this method of adjusting PEEP seems the simplest in the face of ignorance of the effects on specific organ blood flow or oxygen delivery.

Maximize Mixed Venous Oxygen Partial Pressure or Saturation

Mixed venous Po_2 or oxygen saturation has been proposed as a useful predictor of outcome and therefore also useful for titrating PEEP.[87] Although low Pvo_2 or Svo_2 may be associated with death in critically ill patients, it remains to be shown that increasing these values via therapeutic interventions affects the outcome. Nonetheless, the measurement of Svo_2 has become quite popular because it can be obtained from specially equipped pulmonary artery catheters.

The reasons usually cited for measuring Svo_2 are (1) changes in Svo_2 provide an early warning of patient instability, (2) changes in Svo_2 reflect changes in cardiac output, and (3) Svo_2 is indicative of tissue oxygenation. The first premise may be true but has not been rigorously tested. The second premise is true only if Vo_2 and Cao_2 are constant, an unlikely occurrence in many critically ill patients. In addition, not only may changes in cardiac output reflect appropriate autoregulatory adjustments, but is also seems likely that any such change should be manifest in either central pressures, peripheral blood pressure, or heart rate changes, all of which are also measured on line. The third premise is, as discussed in an earlier section, clearly incorrect. However, this misconception has so permeated the clinical literature that it often is assumed without even considering its potential and actual limitations.[88] Nonetheless, the studies relating Do_2 to Vo_2 consistently fail to find relations between Do_2 or Vo_2 and Svo_2 or Pvo_2. In fact, as illustrated by Cain,[55] the critical level of Pvo_2, below which Vo_2 began to fall, varies according to whether Do_2 was reduced by hypoxemia or anemia. Thus although the utility of altering Do_2 is unproven, if it is important, Svo_2 cannot be.

SUMMARY

Although many indices have been proposed to assess the adequacy of tissue oxygenation and to assist in setting appropriate PEEP levels, a careful consideration of the underlying physics and physiology suggests that most, if not all, such indices are physiologically unsound or, at best, of unproven efficacy. Nonetheless, by developing an intimate grasp of the basic scientific principles of pulmonary gas exchange, gas transport, and tissue gas exchange, it is hoped that the ability to evaluate critically new modes of therapy will be enhanced, and that these principles can be applied to advance therapeutic techniques as well as to improve clinical care.

APPENDIX

For inert gases, the mathematical description of equilibrium in a single alveolus is relatively straightforward. First consider the uptake of an inert gas from alveolus to blood. Assume that the initial blood concentration is zero and that by the time the blood leaves the alveolus, the partial pressures in the blood and in the aveolus are equal. Then by mass balance, the amount lost from the alveolus must equal the amount that diffused into blood so that

$$V_I \cdot F_I - V_A \cdot F_A = Q \cdot Ca \tag{7-18}$$

where Q is the alveolar blood flow, Ca is the end-capillary gas concentration, F_I and F_A are the inspired and alveolar gas concentration and V_I and V_A are the inspired and expired alveolar ventilations. Because when the uptake and elimination of multiple gases are considered simultaneously, the amount of gas taken up and eliminated from blood may not be equal, the inspired and expired alveolar ventilations need not be equal. For example, commonly, the total uptake of O_2 is greater than the amount of CO_2 eliminated (if the respiratory quotient is less than unity).

Because the gas concentration in blood equals the solubility λ times the blood partial pressure divided by barometric pressure P_B, and the alveolar gas fraction equals the corresponding partial pressure divided by barometric pressure, Equation (7–18) can be rewritten as

$$(V_I \cdot P_I - V_A \cdot P_A)/P_B = Q \cdot \lambda \cdot Pa/P_B \tag{7-19}$$

By assuming end-capillary equilibrium, $P_A = Pa$, this equation may be solved for P_A to yield

$$Pa = P_A = P_I \cdot (V_I/Q)/(\lambda + V_A/Q) \tag{7-20}$$

which shows that the equilibrium partial pressure depends only on the inspired and expired V/Q rather than the absolute values of ventilation or perfusion.

Equation (7–20) shows that as solubility increases, the equilibrium pressure decreases. Conversely, as the V/Q increases, the equilibrium partial pressure increases. This equation also indicates that for very insoluble gases ($\lambda << V/Q$), changes in V/Q have virtually no effect on the equilibrium partial pressure.

A second relatively simple situation is when the initial alveolar gas concentration is zero and gas diffuses from the entering venous blood into the alveolus. The mass balance is then

$$V_A \cdot F_A = Q \cdot Cv - Q \cdot Ca \tag{7-21}$$

where Cv is the venous gas concentration. By using partial pressues as above, Equation (17–21) can be rewritten as

$$V_A \cdot P_A/P_B = Q \cdot \lambda \cdot (P_V - P_A)/PB \qquad (7-22)$$

Again assuming end-capillary equilibrium and solving for P_A yields

$$P_a = P_A = \lambda \cdot P_V/(\lambda + V_A/Q) \qquad (7-23)$$

This shows that if the V/Q is high relative to the solubility, exhaled gases are almost totally eliminated from blood. Conversely, very soluble gases are very difficult to eliminate. That is, arterial and alveolar partial pressures are nearly equal to the venous partial pressure so that very little gas is lost from the lung. This tends to be confusing because according to Equation (7–21), if F_A is high, the amount of gas eliminated by the lung should also be large. This is, in fact, true. However, because the gas is so soluble, the amount in blood is very large so that even though the alveolar elimination is large, it is still only a small fraction of the amount in blood.

The derivation for an inhaled gas where the initial blood concentration is nonzero is similar except the mass balance now indicates that the difference between inhaled and alveolar concentrations must equal the amount taken up by blood. Therefore,

$$F_I \cdot V_I - F_A \cdot V_A = Q \cdot Ca - Q \cdot Cv \qquad (7-24)$$

Replacing concentrations by solubilities and partial pressures as above yields

$$(P_I \cdot V_I - P_A \cdot V_A)/P_B = Q \cdot \lambda \cdot (P_a - P_V)/P_B \qquad (7-25)$$

which may be solved for $P_A = P_a$ to yield

$$P_a = P_A = (P_I \cdot V_I/Q)/(\lambda + V_A/Q) - P_V \cdot \lambda/(\lambda + V_A/Q) \qquad (7-26)$$

Notice that the terms associated with P_I and P_V are the same as in Equation (7–23). They reflect the amount of gas gained from the alveoli and lost from venous blood to the alveolus respectively. The term associated with P_I reflects the uptake of inhaled gas. As the V/Q becomes large relative to the solubility, P_A and P_a approach P_I. Thus, as the V/Q increases, so does the equilibrium partial pressure. However, for a very soluble gas, $P_a = P_A$ aproaches the lowest possible value, P_V. This indicates that the behavior of alveoli for inspired gases is basically a mirror image of that for expired gases.

The mass balance equations may also be used to solve for the equilibrium partial pressures of CO_2 and O_2. However, this is more complicated because of their nonlinear dissociation curves, partial pressures are not proportional to blood concentrations. Nonetheless, such solutions are readily obtainable using computers.

REFERENCES

1. Moore WJ: Physical Chemistry, ed 3. Englewood Cliffs, NJ, Prentice-Hall Inc, 1964.
2. Finch CA, Lenfant C: Oxygen transport in man. *N Engl J Med* 1972; 286:407–415.
3. Wade OL, Bishop JM, Donald KW: *Cardiac Output and Regional Blood Flow.* Oxford, Blackwell Scientific Publications, 1962.
4. Wagner PD: Diffusion and chemical reaction in pulmonary gas exchange. *Physiol Rev* 1977; 57:257–312.
5. Wagner PD, Saltzman HA, West JB: Measurement of continuous distributions of ventilation-perfusion ratios: theory. *J Appl Physiol* 1974; 36:588–599.
6. Teplick R, Snider MT, Gilbert JF: A comparison of continuous and discrete foreign gas Va/Q distributions. *J Appl Physiol* 1980; 48:684–692.
7. Olszowka AJ: Can Va/Q distributions in the lung be recovered from inert gas retention data? *Resp Physiol* 1975; 25:191–198.
8. Dantzker DR, Brook CJ, Dehart P, et al: Ventilation-perfusion distributions in the adult respiratory distress syndrome. *Am Rev Respir Dis* 1979; 120:1039–1052.
9. Dantzker DR, Patten GA, Bower JS: Gas exchange at rest and during exercise in adults with cystic fibrosis. *Am Rev Respir Dis* 1982; 125:400–405.
10. Schumacker PT, Rhodes GR, Newell JC, et al: Ventilation-perfusion imbalance after head trauma. *Am Rev Respir Dis* 1979; 119:33–43.
11. Matamis D, Lemaire F, Harf A, et al: Redistribution of pulmonary blood flow induced by positive end-expiratory pressure and dopamine infusion in acute respiratory failure. *Am Rev Resp Dis* 1984; 129:39–44.
12. Olszowka AJ, Farhi LE: A digital computer program for constructing ventilation-perfusion lines. *J Appl Physiol* 1969; 26:141–146.
13. Burger EJ, Macklem PT: Airway closure: demonstration by breathing 100% O_2 at low lung volumes and by N2 washout. *J Appl Physiol* 1968; 25:139–148.
14. Hedley-White J, Laver M, Bendixen H: Effect of changes in tidal ventilation on physiologic shunting. *Am J Physiol* 1964; 206:891–897.
15. Briscoe WA, Cree AEM, Filler S, et al: Lung volume, alveolar ventilation and perfusion inter-relationships in chronic pulmonary emphysema. *J Appl Physiol* 1960; 15:785–795.
16. Dantzker DR, Wagner PD, West JB: Instability of lung units with low Va/Q ratios during O_2 breathing. *J Appl Physiol* 1975; 38:886–895.
17. Wagner PD: The oxyhemoglobin dissociation curve and pulmonary gas exchange. *Sem Hematol* 1974; 11:405–421.
18. Banchero N, Grover RF: Effect of different levels of simulated altitude on O_2 transport in llama and sheep. *Am J Physiol* 1972; 222:1239–1245.
19. Bullard RW, Broumand WC, Meyer FR: Blood characteristics and volume in two rodents native to high altitude. *J Appl Physiol* 1966; 21:994–998.
20. Shumacker PT, Suggett AJ, Wagner PD, et al: Role of hemoglobin P_{50} in O_2 transport during normoxic and hypoxic exercise in the dog. *J Appl Physiol* 1985; 59:749–757.
21. Kelman GR: Digital computer subroutine for the conversion of oxygen tension into saturation. *J Appl Physiol* 1966; 21:1375–1376.
22. Douglas ME, Downs JB, Dannemiller FJ, et al: Changes in pulmonary venous admixture with varying inspired oxygen. *Anesth Analg* 1976; 55:688–695.
23. Oliven A, Adinader E, Bursztein S: Influence of varying inspired oxygen tensions on the pulmonary venous admixture (shunt) of mechanically ventilated patients. *Crit Care Med* 1980; 8:99–101.

24. Shapiro BA, Cane RD, Harrison RA, et al: Changes in intrapulmonary shunting with administration of 100 percent oxygen. *Chest* 1980; 77:138–141.
25. Hlastala MP, Colley PS, Cheney FW: Pulmonary shunt: a comparison between oxygen and inert gas methods. *J Appl Physiol* 1975; 39:1048–1051.
26. Wagner PD, Laravuso RB, Uhl RR, et al: Continuous distributions of ventilation-perfusion ratios in normal subjects breathing air and 100% O_2. *J Clin Invest* 1974; 54:54–58.
27. Farhi LE, Rahn H: Theoretical analysis of the alveolar-arterial O_2 difference with special reference to the distribution effect. *J Appl Physiol* 1955; 7:699–703.
28. Shapiro AR, Virgilio RW, Peters RM: Interpretation of alveolar-aterial oxygen tension difference. *Surg Gynecol Obstet* 1977; 144:547–552.
29. Gilbert R, Keighley JF: The arterial/alveolar oxygen tension ratio. An index of gas exchange applicable to varying inspired oxygen concentrations. *Am Rev Respir Dis* 1974; 109:142–145.
30. Gilbert R, Auchincloss JH, Kuppinger M, et al: Stability of the arterial/alveolar oxygen partial pressure ratio. *Crit Care Med* 1979; 7:267–272.
31. Kanber GJ, King FW, Eschar YR, et al: The alveolar-arterial oxygen gradient in young and elderly men during air and oxygen breathing. *Am Rev Respir Dis* 1968; 97:376–381.
32. Karetzky MS, Keighley JF, Mithoefer JC: The effect of oxygen administration on gas exchange and cardiopulmonary function in normal subjects. *Resp Physiol* 1971; 12:361–370.
33. Martyn JAJ, Aikawa N, Wilson RS, et al: Extrapulmonary factors influencing the ratio of arterial oxygen tension to inspired oxygen concentration in burn patients. *Crit Care Med* 1979; 7:492–496.
34. Cane RD, Shapiro BA, Templin R, et al: Unreliability of oxygen tension based indices in reflecting intrapulmonary shunting in critically ill patients. *Crit Care Med* 1988; 16:1243–1245.
35. Herrick IA, Champion LK, Froese AB: A clinical comparison of indices of pulmonary gas exchange with changes in inspired oxygen concentration. *Can J Anesth* 1990; 37:69–76.
36. Adachi H, Strauss W, Ochi H, et al: The effect of hypoxia on the regional distribution of cardiac output in the dog. *Circ Res* 1976; 39:314–319.
37. Abboud FM, Heistad DD, Mark AL, et al: Reflex control of the peripheral circulation. *Prog Cardiovasc Dis* 1976; 18:371–403.
38. Gutierrez G: The rate of oxygen release and its effect on capillary O_2 tension: a mathematical analysis. *Resp Physiol* 1986; 63:79–96.
39. Chapler CK, Cain SM: The physiologic reserve in oxygen carrying capacity: Studies in experimental hemodilution. *Can J Pharmacol* 1985; 64:7–12.
40. McFalls EO, Pantely GA, Anselone CG, et al: The importance of vasomotor tone to myocardial function and regional metabolism during constant flow in ischemia in swine. *Cardiovasc Res* 1990; 24:813–820.
41. Cain SM: Effects of time and vasoconstrictor tone on O_2 extraction during hypoxic hypoxia. *J Appl Physiol* 1978; 45:219–224.
42. Ronco JJ, Phang PT, Walley KR, et al: Oxygen consumption is independent of changes in oxygen delivery in severe adult respiratory distress syndrome. *Am Rev Respir Dis* 1991; 143:1267–1273.
43. Kessler M, Hoper J, Harrison DK, et al: Tissue O_2 supply under normal and pathological conditions. *Adv Exp Med Biol* 1984; 169:69–80.
44. Kawashiro T, Scheid P: Dependence of O_2 uptake on tissue PO_2: Experiments in intact excised rat skeletal muscle. *Adv Exp Med Biol* 1984; 169:497–505.
45. Harrison DK, Höper H, Günther H, et al: Microcirculation and PO_2 in skeletal muscle during respiratory hypoxia and stimulation. *Adv Exp Med Biol* 1984; 169:477–485.
46. Chance B, Oshino N, Sugano T, et al: Basic principles of oxygen determination from mitochondrial signals. *Adv Exp Med Biol* 1973; 37a:277–292.

47. Tenney SM: A theoretical analysis of the relationship between venous blood and mean tissue oxygen pressures. *Resp Physiol* 1974; 20:283–296.
48. Snyder JV, Carrol GC: Tissue oxygenation: A physiological approach to a clinical problem. Part I. *Current Problems in Surgery* 1982; 19:650–719.
49. Vermeij CG, Feenstra WA, Bruining HA: Oxygen delivery and oxygen uptake in postoperative and septic patients. *Chest* 1990; 98:415–520.
50. Danek SJ, Lynch JP, Weg JG, et al: The dependence of oxygen uptake on oxygen delivery in the adult respiratory distress syndrome. *Am Rev Respir Dis* 1980; 122:387–395.
51. Pepe PE, Culver BH: Independently measured oxygen consumption during reduction of oxygen delivery by positive end-expiratory pressure. *Am Rev Respir Dis* 1985; 132:788–792.
52. Villar J, Slutsky AS, Hew E: Oxygen transport and oxygen consumption in critically ill patients. *Chest* 1990; 98:687–692.
53. Kaufman BS, Rackow EC, Falk JL: The relationship between oxygen delivery and consumption during fluid resuscitation of hypovolemic and septic shock. *Chest* 1984; 85:336–340.
54. Shepherd AP, Granger HJ, Smith EE, et al: Local control of tissue oxygen delivery and its contribution to the regulation of cardiac output. *Am J Physiol* 1973; 225:747–755.
55. Cain SM: Oxygen delivery and uptake in dogs during anemic and hypoxic hypoxia. *J Appl Physiol* 1977; 42:228–234.
56. Kvietys PR, Granger DN: Relation between intestinal blood flow and oxygen uptake. *Am J Physiol* (*Gastrointest Liver Physiol*) 1982; 242:G202–G208.
57. Rhodes GR, Newell JC, Shah D, et al: Increased oxygen consumption accompanying increased oxygen delivery with hypertonic mannitol in adult respiratory distress syndrome. *Surg* 1978; 84:490–497.
58. Lorente JA, Renes E, Gomez-Aguinaga MA, et al: Oxygen delivery dependent oxygen consumption in acute respiratory failure. *Crit Care Med* 1991; 19:770–775.
59. Annat G, Viale JP, Pervival C, et al: Oxygen delivery and uptake in the adult respiratory distress syndrome. *Am Rev Respir Dis* 1986; 133:999–1001.
60. Sugimoto H, Ohashi N, Sawada T, et al: Effects of positive end-expiratory pressure on tissue gas tensions and oxygen transport. *Crit Care Med* 1984; 12:661–663.
61. Chappell TR, Rubin IJ, Markham RV, et al: Independence of oxygen consumption and systemic oxygen transport in patients with either stable pulmonary hypertension or refractory left ventricular failure. *Am Rev Respir Dis* 1983; 128:30–33.
62. Tuchschmidt J, Fried J, Swinney R, et al: Early hemodynamic correlates of survival in patients with septic shock. *Crit Care Med* 1989; 17:719–723.
63. Cain SM, Curtis SE: Experimental models of pathologic oxygen supply dependency. *Crit Care Med* 1991; 19:603–612.
64. Weg JG: Oxygen transport in adult respiratory distress syndrome and other acute circulatory problems: Relationship of oxygen delivery and oxygen consumption. *Crit Care Med* 1991; 19:650–657.
65. Shibutani K, Toru K, Kubal K, et al: Critical level of oxygen delivery in anesthetized man. *Crit Care Med* 1983; 11:640–643.
66. Haupt MT, Gilbert EM, Carlson RW: Fluid loading increases oxygen consumption in septic patients with lactic acidosis. *Am Rev Respir Dis* 1985; 131:912–916.
67. Gilbert EM, Haupt MT, Mandanas RY, et al: The effect of fluid loading, blood transfusion, and catecholamine infusion on oxygen delivery and consumption in patients with sepsis. *Am Rev Respir Dis* 1989; 134:873–878.
68. Tuchschmidt J, Obletas D, Fried JC: Oxygen consumption in sepsis and septic shock. *Crit Care Med* 1991; 19:664–671.

69. Abraham E, Bland RD, Cobo JC, et al: Sequential cardiorespiratory patterns associated with outcome in septic shock. *Chest* 1984; 85:75–80.
70. Bland RS, Shoemaker WC: Probability of survival as a prognostic and severity of illness score in critically ill surgical patients. *Crit Care Med* 1985; 13:91–95.
71. Hankeln KB, Senker R, Schwarten JU, et al: Evaluation of prognostic indices based on hemodynamic and oxygen tranpsort variables in patients with ARDS. *Crit Care Med* 1987; 15:1–7.
72. Edwards JD, Brown CGS, Nightingale P, et al: Use of survivors' cardiorespiratory patterns as therapeutic goals in septic shock. *Crit Care Med* 1989; 17:1098–1103.
73. Shoemaker WC, Appel PL, Kram HB: Oxygen transport measurements to evaluate tissue perfusion and titrate therapy: dobutamine and dopamine effects. *Crit Care Med* 1991; 19:672–688.
74. Shoemaker WC, Appel PL, Kram HB, et al: Prospective trial of supranormal values of survivors as therapeutic goals in high risk surgical patients. *Chest* 1988; 94:1176–1178.
75. Suter PM, Fairley HB, Isenberg MD: Optimum end-expiratory airway pressure in patients with acute pulmonary failure. *N Engl J Med* 1975; 292:284–289.
76. Suter PM, Fairley HB, Isenberg MD: Effect of tidal volume and positive end-expiratory pressure on compliance during mechanical ventilation. *Chest* 1978; 73:158–162.
77. Tenaillon A, Labrousse J, Gateau O, et al: Optimal positive end-expiratory pressure and static lung complaince. *N Engl J Med* 1978; 299:774–775.
78. Kirby RR, Perry JC, Calderwood HW, et al: Cardiorespiratory effects of high positive end-expiratory pressure. *Anesthesiol* 1975; 43:533–539.
79. Jardin F, Desfond P, Bazin M, et al: Controlled ventilation with best positive end-expiratory pressure (PEEP) and high level PEEP in acute respiratory failure (ARF). *Intensive Care Med* 1981; 7:171–176.
80. Greenbaum DN: Positive end-expiratory pressure, constant positive airway pressure, and cardiac performance. *Chest* 1979; 76:248–249.
81. Nelson LD, Houtchens BA, Westenskow DR: Oxygen consumption and optimal PEEP in acute respiratory failure. *Crit Care Med* 1982; 10:857–862.
82. Walkinshaw M, Shoemaker WC: Use of volume loading to obtain preferred levels of PEEP. *Crit Care Med* 1980; 8:81–86.
83. Gallagher TJ, Civetta JM, Kirby RR: Terminology update: optimal PEEP. *Crit Care Med* 1978; 6:323–326.
84. Venus B, Jacobs HK, Lim L: Treatment of the adult respiratory distress syndrome with continuous positive airway pressure. *Chest* 1979; 76:257–261.
85. Kirby RR, Downs JB, Civetta JM, et al: High level positive end expiratory pressure (PEEP) in acute respiratory insufficiency. *Chest* 1975; 67:156–163.
86. Murray IP, Modell JH, Gallagher TJ, et al: Titration of PEEP by arterial minus end-tidal carbon dioxide gradient. *Chest* 1984; 85:100–104.
87. Kasnitz P, Druger GL, Yorra F, et al: Mixed venous oxygen tension and hyperlactatemia. Survival in severe cardiopulmonary disease. *J Am Med Assoc* 1976; 236:570–574.
88. Heiselman D, Jones J, Cannon L. Continuous monitoring of mixed venous saturation in septic shock. *J Clin Mon* 1986; 2:237–245.

Chapter 8

Hemodynamic Monitoring

Alfred F. Connors, Jr., M.D.

INTRODUCTION

Invasive hemodynamic monitoring includes direct measurement of either arterial pressure via an arterial cannula, central venous pressure via a central venous catheter, intracardiac pressures and flows via a pulmonary artery catheter, or some combination of these three. Noninvasive measurements of cardiac function are obtained using a variety of techniques discussed in detail elsewhere (Chapter 14).

The indications for using each of the modalities available for invasive monitoring of cardiac status are determined by balancing the likelihood of obtaining useful information from a specific monitoring technique against the risks and discomfort of that technique. Perhaps the greatest value of hemodynamic monitoring is that it allows improved understanding of the pathophysiology of the patient's current disorder[1-4] and often allows a specific diagnosis to be made.[5] This information then guides the choice of initial therapy. After therapy is started, hemodynamic monitoring can alert caregivers to changes in the status of the patient and measure the effect of therapeutic interventions. Finally, measurements obtained by hemodynamic monitoring can be useful in predicting prognoses.[1]

SPECIFIC METHODS OF MONITORING HEMODYNAMICS

Arterial Pressure Monitoring

Arterial blood pressure, when considered alone, is, at best, a crude indicator of the hemodynamic state of the patient. The cardiac output, systemic vascular resistance, aortic impedance, and diastolic arterial blood volume all interact to determine arterial blood pressure. In addition, the sympathetic motor tone of the blood vessel walls, which is regulated by the autonomic nervous system, adjusts for changes in body position, blood volume, and cardiac output. The interactions among these many factors are complex. The regulation of arterial blood pressure is such that substantial hemodynamic abnormalities can occur while the arterial blood pressure is maintained within normal values. Consequently, the clinician should not depend on arterial pressure monitoring alone to assess hemodynamic status. In a patient where hemodynamic dysfunction is suspected or anticipated, the clinician should employ other means to assess cardiac function. Physical examination, chest roentgenography, or electrocardiographic monitoring may reveal signs of cardiac dysfunction while the arterial blood pressure remains normal. When hypotension is identified, however, prompt initial therapy and further assessment is needed.

Indications for Arterial Pressure Monitoring

Arterial pressure monitoring via an indwelling peripheral arterial catheter is the most commonly used mode of invasive hemodynamic monitoring. The two most common reasons for inserting an arterial catheter are to measure arterial pressure and to draw blood samples. Arterial pressure monitoring is indicated when rapid fluctuations of blood pressure are expected, when abrupt shifts in antihypertensive, vasodilator, or vasopressor therapy are anticipated, and in order to monitor response to drug therapy. Arterial catheterization is also appropriate in patients whose management requires frequent or repeated arterial or venous blood sampling. An indwelling arterial catheter can add considerably to the comfort of such a patient by avoiding the pain and local injury associated with frequent arterial or venous punctures. Of course, some authors have suggested that the very ease with which blood can be obtained through an arterial line may encourage excessive blood drawing.

Insertion Techniques

While arterial catheters can be placed by surgical cutdown, the percutaneous approach is much preferred. It is faster, simpler, and associated with fewer complications than surgical cutdown. Surgical cutdown is rarely necessary. The two popular percutaneous methods are transfixation and direct insertion (Fig 8–1). With *transfixation* the catheter completely penetrates the artery before the inner needle is withdrawn. The catheter is then withdrawn slowly until the free flow of arterial blood is seen. The catheter is then advanced slowly into the arterial lumen. With the *direct insertion* technique, the catheter, with the inner needle in place, is advanced into the arterial lumen until the free flow of arterial blood is seen and both the inner needle and the catheter are in the lumen. The catheter is then advanced into the lumen over the inner needle. With practice, either approach has a high rate of success and a low risk of complications.

Insertion Sites for Arterial Catheters

The radial artery is the most common site for the placement of a peripheral arterial catheter. This site seems to cause the least discomfort for patients since it allows considerable freedom of movement and does not require immobilization of the joint. Nurses also find this site to be convenient because it allows the patient relative freedom of motion while presenting little impediment to bathing the patient or changing dressings and gowns.

The risk of ischemic injury to the hand and digits associated with radial artery catheterization is low due to the presence of ample collateral circulation between the radial and ulnar arterial circulation. The circulation to the hand can be maintained through either of these arteries if

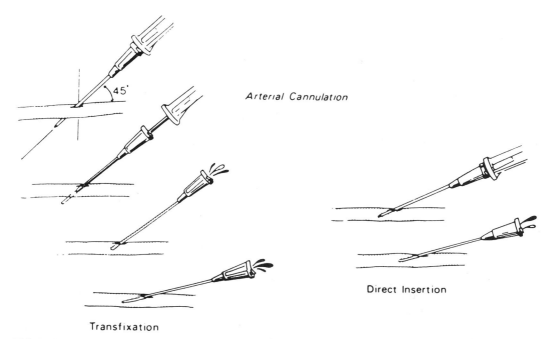

Arterial Cannulation

Direct Insertion

Transfixation

FIG 8–1.
Two methods of arterial cannulation: transfixation and direct insertion. For transfixation the cannula with its inner needle is first passed completely through the artery at a 45-degree angle. The inner needle is then removed and the catheter is slowly withdrawn until arterial blood flows from the catheter. Finally the catheter is carefully advanced into the arterial lumen. For direct insertion the inner needle and the tip of the cannula are advanced directly into the arterial lumen until arterial blood flows from the cannula. The catheter is then advanced into the arterial lumen over the inner needle. *(From Marini JJ:* Respiratory Medicine and Intensive Care for the House Officer. *Baltimore, William and Wilkins, 1981. Used by permission.)*

the other is occluded. The Allen test[6] can be performed to establish the presence of a patent ulnar artery. To perform the Allen test, occlude both the radial and ulnar artery until the palm blanches, then release the radial artery and assess the delay between release of the artery and blushing on the palm. The procedure is then repeated for the ulnar artery. A delayed capillary blush with either artery (greater than 5 seconds) or a substantial difference in the rate of capillary filling with either artery suggests occlusive vascular disease. Although the value of the Allen test as a predictor of ischemic complications has been questioned, most intensivists will avoid the radial artery in the presence of impaired or absent flow through the ulnar artery.

The dorsalis pedis artery may be used as an alternative to the radial artery. As in the hand, the dorsalis pedis and the posterior tibialis arteries provide collateral flow and reduce the risk of ischemia. However, about 20% of patients in one study had inadequate collateral flow to the toe when the dorsalis artery was compressed[7] and were judged to be poor candidates for arterial cannulation. This location is also convenient for the nurse and comfortable for the patient. The disadvantages of this artery are that cannulation can be difficult (80% success rate), thrombosis is common, and it is congenitally absent in as many as 12% of people.[7]

Some intensivists prefer the axillary artery for arterial cannulation. The reports on the use of this location[8] suggest that it is well tolerated by the patient and does not interfere with nursing care. The tendency for complications at this site appears to be low but few studies have been performed.

The femoral artery has both significant advantages and disadvantages, which makes it a controversial choice for routine arterial pressure monitoring. It is easily catheterized because of its large caliber and accessible location. The risk of thrombosis is low because of the large caliber and high flow.[8, 9] The disadvantage of this site is that the risk of infection has been reported to be increased in several studies.[10, 11] However, subsequent reports of the use of femoral artery catheterization[8, 9, 12, 13] have not shown an increased risk of infection compared to radial artery catheters. Clearly, this site should be avoided in the presence of incontinence, inguinal intertrigo, or other infectious or inflammatory disorders in the perineum or inguinal area. This site is also not suitable for patients who will be sitting in bed or in a chair.

Despite the disadvantages cited for chronic cannulation of the femoral artery, it is the preferred site for emergency arterial cannulation. This large central artery is ideal for arterial pressure monitoring during cardiac arrest and in severe shock states. However, in our unit if a femoral line is placed under emergency conditions, the catheter is removed within 24 hours and replaced in the radial artery.

The brachial artery should only be used for arterial cannulation only in emergencies. Since the cannulation occurs above the bifurcation of the radial and ulnar arteries, thrombosis of this artery risks ischemic injury to the hand and requires immediate surgical removal of the clot. In addition, brachial artery lines require immobilization of the elbow joint and interfere with nursing care as well as with patient comfort and mobility.

Benefits of Continuous Arterial Pressure Monitoring

The benefits of arterial pressure monitoring are (1) continuous, precise, reproducible measurements of systolic, diastolic, and mean blood pressure; (2) accurate diagnosis of hemodynamic disorders characterized by fluctuations in blood pressure; (3) guidance in the choice of therapy for hypotension or hypertension; and (4) continuous monitoring of the effect of therapy, allowing frequent adjustment of therapy for hypotension or hypertension. Another important benefit of a peripheral arterial cannula is that it allows painless blood drawing from seriously ill patients who would otherwise require multiple venous and arterial punctures. Often an arterial cannula is placed more to optimize patient comfort than to monitor arterial blood pressure. This benefit may be offset by the observation that critically ill patients with indwelling arterial lines have substantially more blood drawn than patients without arterial lines.[14]

Risks of Continuous Arterial Pressure Monitoring

Complications related to the percutaneous insertion of arterial catheters are usually the result of local trauma and are rarely serious. Ecchymosis, hematoma, and soreness at the site of insertion are common complications of arterial catheterization. Arterial laceration, A-V fistulas and false aneurysms have been reported but are rare.

The complications related to duration of catheterization are thrombosis, embolization, and infection. In early studies of radial artery catheterization, thrombosis was common, occurring in 30 to 38% of catheterizations.[15, 16] The size and type of the catheter is clearly a risk factor for thrombosis.[16-18] Thrombosis is most likely with large (18-gauge) polypropylene catheters and much less common with small (20-gauge) Teflon catheters. Studies[15-17] of radial artery cannulation with 20-gauge Teflon catheters revealed thrombosis in 0 to 8%. Other factors that increase the risk of thrombosis are small artery caliber, small wrist size, multiple punctures during cannulation, surgical cutdown, prolonged low cardiac output, hematoma formation at the insertion site, and prolonged duration of cannulation.[15-19] A persistently damped pressure tracing or difficulty withdrawing blood are signs of impending thrombosis and are an indication for removing the catheter.

Embolization appears to be common, occurring in 24% of radial artery cannulations in one study.[17] Ischemia at the insertion site or of digits or toes, however, occurs in only 0.2 to 0.6% of radial or dorsalis pedis artery catheterizations.[19, 20] Ischemia is more common in the presence of severe hypotension, severe peripheral vascular disease, or vasopressor drugs.[19] Use of the Allen test as described above is helpful in identifying patients at risk for ischemia.[17]

Contamination of the catheter by bacteria, usually skin flora, which grow along the surface of the catheter, occurs in 4 to 24% of catheterizations depending on duration of catheterization and attention to optimal care of the insertion site.[10-13, 20, 21] Catheter-induced sepsis (simultaneous positive cultures of the same organism from both the blood and catheter tip in a patient with clinical signs of sepsis) occurs in as many as 4% of catheterizations,[10] although several studies show that sepsis is exceedingly rare in the first 72 to 96 hours of catheterization.[10, 13, 20, 21] The risk of line sepsis is increased in the presence of surgical cutdown, catheter duration greater than 96 hours, and local inflammation. Sepsis has also been reported with contamination of infusion solutions, stopcocks, and transducer domes.[22-24] The risk of this can be minimized by the use of saline for all infusions, disposable transducer domes, and the shortest possible length of tubing from the transducer to the catheter. All lines and tubing should be changed every 48 hours.

Table 8–1 summarizes the optimal approach to minimizing the risk of complications with arterial cannulation.

Central Venous Pressure Monitoring

Benefits and Indications

Central venous pressure (CVP) monitoring provides a readily available measure of right ventricular filling pressures. As such, it is useful as an indicator of right ventricular function. Perhaps its most common use is to direct fluid therapy and monitor the effect of changes in fluid management.

Its use in this setting is somewhat limited. Forrester et al.[25] showed that central venous pressure does not strongly correlate with pulmonary capillary wedge pressure ($r = 0.45$) in patients with acute myocardial infarction or congestive heart failure. In patients with multiple organ system failure and/or sepsis, the correlation between central venous pressure and pulmonary capillary wedge pressure is much higher ($r = 0.72$).[26] Its relationship to left ventricular end-diastolic volume is probably even more tenuous but it has not been studied.

TABLE 8–1.

Minimizing the Risk of Complications from Arterial Catheters*

1. Use the radial artery whenever possible.
2. Perform an Allen's test prior to radial artery cannulation (palmar blush in less than 5 seconds).
3. Use *strict* aseptic technique (gloves, mask, drapes).
4. Use a 20-gauge Teflon catheter.
5. Use a heparinized saline flush system with a disposable transducer dome and very little tubing between the transducer and the flush valve.
6. Inspect the insertion site and distal extremity daily for inflammation or ischemia.
7. Change the dressing, transducer dome, tubing, and flush solution every 48 hours.
8. Catheters are removed and replaced at another site every 72 to 96 hours.
9. Remove the catheter promptly in the presence of:
   a. Generalized sepsis or bacteremia
   b. Insertion site infection or inflammation
   c. Distal ischemia
   d. Inability to withdraw blood through the catheter
   e. Persistently damped pressure tracing.

* This table is distilled from Ref. 6 through 24 and was inspired by a similar table in Ref. 25. It represents the current practice in our unit.

While CVP is certainly not a substitute for more direct measures of left ventricular filling pressures, it has the advantage of being readily available, its correlation with PCWP in many disease states is better than that reported for acute myocardial infarction,[26] a high CVP is rarely associated with a low PCWP,[25, 26] and the information it provides does allow insight into right ventricular function.[27] Thus, there are times when the measurement of CVP through an existing central venous catheter may give the clinician sufficient information to manage the patient without a pulmonary artery catheter.

Insertion Sites for Central Venous Catheters

The internal jugular and subclavian veins are most often used for placement of central venous catheters. The details of the insertion techniques have been described in detail.[28-30] Each route has advantages and disadvantages. The internal jugular vein has a low risk of pneumothorax[31, 32] (less than 0.5%) but, because it is more difficult to maintain a sterile dressing, the risk of infection may be greater.[21] The subclavian vein has a greater risk of pneumothorax. The reported range[33-36] of pneumothorax is from 0 to 6%, but experienced physicians usually are very close to the lower value. The risk of infection may be lower using the subclavian route, perhaps because it is easier to maintain a dry, sterile dressing.[21] However, a small prospective study[37] found that the rate of line sepsis was zero for both subclavian and internal jugular catheters when the catheters were all removed within 72 hours.

Risks of Central Venous Pressure Monitoring

The risks of central venous pressure monitoring can be divided into the risks associated with catheter insertion and those associated with prolonged catheter placement. At the time of insertion, pneumothorax, arterial puncture, pleural effusion, insertion site pain, ecchymosis, brachial plexus injury, thoracic duct injury, and air embolus have all been described. An analysis of 16 prospective and retrospective studies of over 10,000 central venous and pulmonary artery catheterizations revealed only four deaths due to catheter insertion complications.[32–46] Studies reporting the serious complications of central venous catheterization, i.e., those associated with a significant risk of morbidity or death, are summarized in Table 8–2. The complications associated with the insertion of a central venous catheter are summarized in Table 8–3.

When catheters are left in place for more than a few hours, the patient is exposed to the risk of catheter-induced thrombosis and catheter-related infections. Thrombosis has been reported in the superior vena cava, subclavian, innominate, and internal jugular veins.[47–50] Superior vena cava syndrome can occur. The exact incidence of venous thrombosis is unclear. In one study[47] in which venography was performed at the time of catheter removel, the prevalence of thrombosis was 17% in the first 3 to 7 days, 58% for 8 to 15 days, and 73% after 15 days. Chastre et al.[50] reported that 22 of 33 patients (66%) percent) had internal jugular thrombosis on venogram following a 2- to 6-day placement of a pulmonary artery catheter in the internal jugular vein.

I recommend a venogram when facial swelling or unilateral swelling of the hand, arm, or shoulder presents in a patient with a central venous catheter. Central venous thrombosis is commonly found in this setting. Therapy is controversial. It is our policy to remove the catheter, avoid central venous catheterization if possible, and give heparin for 10 to 14 days. However, it is not clear that catheter removal is mandatory. Patients with Hickman or Broviac catheters have done well following anticoagulant therapy without removal of the catheter.[49]

TABLE 8–2.
Complications Associated with Central Venous Catheter Insertion

Reference	N	Pneumothorax	Pleural Effusion	Arterial Injury	Other Serious	Deaths
31	6245	31	0	120	—	0
32	528	0	0	23	0	0
33	116	0	—	0	—	0
34	554	3	5	5	4	0
35	142	2	0	12	—	0
36	117	7	—	1	1	0
37	92	1	1	5	1	0
38	355	6	3	2	2	1
39	1438	18	—	29	4	3
40	263	6	—	10	—	0
41	294	4	—	11	—	0
42	85	2	—	—	—	0
43	80	1	—	6	1	0
44	75	2	—	2	—	0
45	470	8	—	29	4	0
46	292	1	0	38	0	0
TOTALS	11146	92 0.8%	9 0.08%	293 2.6%	17 0.15%	4 0.034%

TABLE 8–3.
Complications Associated with Inserting Central
Venous Catheters

I. Vascular Complications
    a. Arteries and veins
        1. Puncture
        2. Laceration
        3. Arteriovenous fistula
    b. Thoracic duct laceration
    c. Hematoma
        1. Subcutaneous
        2. Mediastinal
    d. Tissue infiltration with intravenous fluid
        1. Subcutaneous
        2. Mediastinal
    e. Persistent bleeding from insertion site
II. Pleural Complications
    a. Pneumothorax
    b. Subcutaneous emphysema
    c. Pleural effusions
        1. Hydrothorax
        2. Hemothorax
        3. Chylothorax
III. Cardiac Complications
    a. Myocardial puncture
    b. Ventricular arrhythmia
IV. Embolic Phenomena
    a. Air embolus
    b. Catheter or catheter fragment embolus
V. Neural Complications
    a. Brachial plexus injury
VI. Mechanical Complications
    a. Kinking, knotting, and plugging
    b. Malposition of the catheter

We need further study of this issue to determine the incidence, risk factors, consequences, and optimal therapy of thrombosis associated with central venous catheterization.

A great deal is known about the risk of catheter contamination and catheter-induced sepsis associated with central venous catheters. Catheter contamination, defined as positive quantitative cultures of the catheter, occurs commonly. Most catheters are sterile if cultured in the first 48 hours and have a low rate of contamination from 48 to 96 hours.[13, 20, 51–53] After that there is a steady, steep increase in the incidence of catheter contamination. Catheter-induced sepsis, defined as both a positive quantitative line culture and a positive blood culture with the same organism in a patient with clinical signs of sepsis, occurs less commonly and is clearly related to the duration of catheterization. Catheter-induced sepsis is unusual when lines are changed within 72 to 96 hours after insertion, occurring in less than 1% of cases.[20, 42, 52, 54, 55] Four prospective studies found only one episode of line sepsis when all catheters were removed within 96 hours (1 of 783 catheterizations; 0.01%)[20, 42, 52, 54]; no episodes of line sepsis occurred when the catheters were removed within 72 hours.[20, 42, 54] Line sepsis occurs in about 5% of patients whose lines are left in for 5 to 7 days.[41, 55–59] Since line sepsis increases mortality between 28 to 42%[60-65] and the risk of line changes is very low,[31-46] this clearly argues that changing lines frequently will save lives. In our unit we change central venous lines every 3 days unless there is a compelling reason not to.

Technology and practices to reduce the risk of line sepsis such as silver impregnated cuffs,[59] antibiotic bonding to catheters,[66] and changing lines over a guidewire[41, 56] may ultimately be proven to reduce the risk of sepsis to the point where longer catheterization is associated with lower risk of infection. Guidewire exchange avoids the risk of insertion complications. While this technique achieved rates of line sepsis similar to those seen with percutaneous insertion in some studies,[41, 42, 54] it was associated with a higher rate of clinical line infection in one study.[55] It is not clear how guidewire exchange influences the risk of thrombosis. Until the value of these approaches is established unequivocally, the practice of changing central venous lines every 72 to 96 hours, ideally at a new site, should yield a very low incidence of serious complications for your patient. A recent review on this subject[67] recommended the practice of changing catheters every 6 days, but in doing so, I believe the authors underestimated the increased mortality associated with line sepsis and exaggerated the risk to the patient from catheter insertion.

Table 8–4 summarizes the optimal approach to minimizing the risk of complications from central venous catherization.

Pulmonary Artery Catheterization

The pulmonary artery catheter was introduced by Swan and Ganz[68] in 1970. For the first time, physicians were able to assess pulmonary capillary pressures and the contractile state of the right and left ventricles outside of the cardiac catheterization laboratory. This catheter has revolutionized the care of hemodynamically unstable critically ill patients.

The pulmonary artery catheter is a balloon-tipped, flow-directed catheter that allows bed-

TABLE 8–4.
Minimizing the Risk of Complications from Central Venous Catheters

---

1. Either the internal jugular or subclavian approach is acceptable. The internal jugular route has lower risk complications in general, and specifically, reduced risk of pleural complications.
2. Use *strict* aseptic technique (gloves, mask, drapes).
3. Use a heparinized saline flush system with a disposable transducer dome and a minimum of tubing between the transducer and the catheter.
4. Inspect the insertion site daily for inflammation or tenderness.
5. Examine the patient daily for signs of congestion or swelling of the face, shoulder, or upper extremity. If these signs are present, perform a venogram promptly to evaluate for central vein thrombosis.
6. Change the dressing, transducer dome, tubing, and flush solution every 48 hours.
7. Catheters are removed and replaced at another site every 72 to 96 hours.
8. Remove the catheter promptly in the presence of:
   a. generalized sepsis or bacteremia
   b. insertion site infection or inflammation
   c. inability to withdraw blood through the catheter
   d. documented central vein thrombosis

side catheterization of the pulmonary artery. It has two ports, a proximal port 30 cm from the tip through which right atrial pressure can be measured and a distal port at the tip. The distal port allows measurement of pressures as the catheter is passed through the atrium and the ventricle into the pumonary artery. The catheter can be placed at the bedside by monitoring the pressure waveform as the catheter, with the balloon inflated, is pulled by bloodflow through the right atrium, the right ventricle and into the pulmonary artery (Fig 8–2). When fully advanced, the balloon occludes the pulmonary artery, stopping flow to a segment of the pulmonary vascular bed. The pressure in this static column of blood is equal to the pressure in the low-resistance pulmonary veins, which is equivalent to the left atrial pressure[69] (Fig 8–3). Blood flow is measured by the thermodilution technique. A known volume, usually 5 to 10 mL, of iced or room temperature saline is injected into the right atrium via the proximal port. This causes a fall in the blood temperature in the heart. A rapidly responding thermistor at the tip of the catheter records the magnitude of the fall in temperature in the pulmonary artery and the rate at which it returns to baseline values. Computer analysis of this information allows calculation of the cardiac output.[70] Finally, the catheter can be used to draw blood from the pulmonary artery to determine mixed venous blood gas concentrations.

Indications for Pulmonary Artery Catheterization

The best indication for pulmonary artery catheterization is significant uncertainty about a patient's hemodynamic status, which persists despite a thoughtful clinical evaluation and a

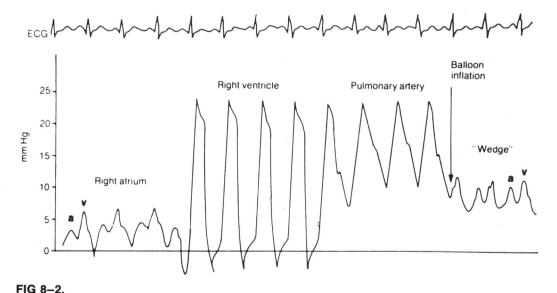

FIG 8–2.
Pressure waveforms seen during the passage of a pulmonary artery catheter. Typical waveforms for the right atrium, right ventricle, pulmonary artery, and the wedged catheter. The right atrial and wedge pressure tracings show the A and V waves typical of an atrial pressure waveform. *(From Matthay MA: Invasive hemodynamic monitoring in the critically ill patient. Clin Chest Med 1983; 4:233–239. Used by permission.)*

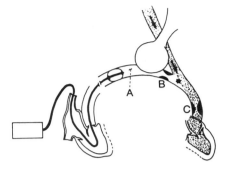

FIG 8–3.
Principle of the wedge pressure measurement. During balloon occlusion of the pulmonary artery, blood flow ceases between the catheter tip (point A) and the junction point for veins serving occluded and nonoccluded units (*). Narrowing of the static column (B) will not influence wedge pressure, whereas similar narrowing of the flowing column (C) will cause wedge pressure to overestimate left atrial pressure. *(From O'Quin R, Marini JJ: Pulmonary artery occlusion pressure: Clinical physiology, measurement, and interpretation.* Am Rev Respir Dis *1983; 128:319–326. Used by permission.)*

trial of therapy chosen on the basis of this evaluation. Pulmonary artery catheterization is especially useful in the following situations:

1. Determining the cause of a shock state
2. Differentiating cardiogenic and permeability pulmonary edema
3. Establishing left ventricular filling pressure
4. Assessment of pericardial tamponade or restriction
5. Guiding therapy in shock states
6. Guiding fluid therapy in critically ill patients, especially in the presence of impaired renal function
7. Postoperative management of cardiothoracic surgery patients or perioperative management of noncardiac surgery patients with unstable cardiac status.

Benefits of Pulmonary Artery Catheterization

Accurate Definition of Hemodynamic Status. — The clinical assessment of hemodynamic status is frequently inaccurate.[2–4, 71] Physician predictions of cardiac index and pulmonary capillary wedge pressure are accurate less than half the time.[2–4, 71] This is true regardless of the cause of the cardiac dysfunction.[71] The inaccuracy of physicians' estimates appears to be due, in part, to less than optimal use of the available information.[72] Pulmonary artery catheterization allows precise, repeated measurement of cardiac function. When this information is provided to physicians, it leads to significant changes in therapy in half of the patients.[2, 3, 71]

Choosing and Monitoring Therapy. — The information that we obtain through pulmonary artery catheterization gives us precise information about three key aspects of hemodynamic status: volume status or preload, the contractile state of the heart, and the afterload on the heart (the resistance of the systemic and pulmonary vascular systems). This information allows the physician to categorize the patient's cardiac status accurately and to choose optimal therapy. Later in this chapter the interpretation of hemodynamic data and their use in the care of the critically ill will be discussed.

Diagnosis of Pericardial and Intracardiac Disorders.—The pulmonary artery catheter can allow the physician to recognize specific clinical disorders based on the pattern of pressures and on variations from the normal waveforms. The best presentation of this topic was presented by Sharkey in an excellent review.[5]

Mitral insufficiency results in blood rushing into the left atrium during systole causing a sudden increase in left atrial pressure. This diagnosis is suggested by the presence of tall V waves on the pulmonary capillary wedge pressure tracing (Fig 8–4). These V waves are most likely to occur in the presence of acute mitral insufficiency when the left atrium is less compliant than in chronic mitral insufficiency, and the rise in pressure due to regurgitant flow is commensurately increased. The large V waves can be mistaken for the pulmonary artery waveform causing the clinician to think that the catheter is not wedging.

Right ventricular infarction is characterized by very high right atrial pressures, which equal or exceed the mean pulmonary capillary wedge pressure. The right atrial pressure waveform

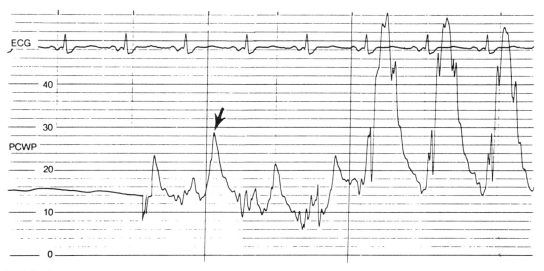

FIG 8–4.
Large V waves (*arrow*) are seen in this patient's pulmonary capillary wedge pressure tracing. The last three systoles on the tracing were recorded after the balloon was deflated to show the transition from the wedge pressure to the pulmonary artery pressure tracing. *(From Downes et al: Am J Cardiol 1987; 60:415–417. Used by permission.)*

demonstrates prominent X and Y descents. The pulmonary artery pulse pressure may be small due to a reduced cardiac output and stroke volume. This disorder should be suspected whenever signs of right-sided congestive heart failure present in a patient with acute inferior wall myocardial infarction.

Ventricular septal defect can be identified by the presence of a step increase in oxygen saturation (usually greater than 10%[5]) as the catheter passes through the right ventricle. The right atrial pressure is increased. Since a large percentage of left ventricular flow may be diverted to the right ventricle, systemic perfusion may be severely impaired in the presence of normal right-sided flows thermodilution cardiac output.

Pericardial tamponade is characterized by equalization of right atrial pressure, right ventricular end-diastolic pressure, and pulmonary capillary wedge pressure in the presence of a reduced cardiac output, hypotension, and a pericardial effusion.[5] The atrial pressures and ventricular end-diastolic pressures are equal to the increased intrapericardial pressure, which is usually elevated to 10 to 18 mm Hg by the time cardiac output and blood pressure are reduced.[73] Pulsus paradoxicus is usually present.

Pulmonary embolism cannot be diagnosed with certainty using a pulmonary artery catheter, but several hemodynamic findings may suggest this diagnosis. Pulmonary hypertension is seen with up to 70% of patients with pulmonary embolism.[74] The degree of hypertension is usually mild to moderate with mean pulmonary artery pressure remaining less than 40 mm Hg even with massive acute pulmonary embolus.[74] Greater levels of pulmonary hypertension suggest a more chronic process. The pulmonary artery diastolic pressure is usually substantially higher than the pulmonary capillary wedge pressure.[5] Occlusion of the tip of the catheter by contact with the clot[75] and failure to wedge the catheter due to a large central thrombus[76] have been reported.

Assessment of Prognosis.—Hemodynamic subsets based on wedge pressure and cardiac output are useful in predicting survival following acute myocardial infarction.[1] In patients with acute myocardial infarction, when the wedge pressure was less than 18 mm Hg and the cardiac output was greater than 2.2 L/min/m², mortality was only 3%. However, when the wedge pressure was more than 18 mm Hg and the cardiac index was less than 2.2 L/min/m², the mortality was 51%. Most studies looking at the relationship between cardiac function and survival in sepsis or multiple organ system failure have shown only a weak relation between initial hemodynamic status and survival.

Improvement of Overall Outcome.—The influence of a pulmonary artery catheter on outcome is hotly debated.[77-80] The pulmonary artery catheter has added greatly to our understanding of cardiovascular physiology in the critically ill patient. This knowledge has no doubt allowed improvement in the outcome of many patients.[80] While it is the judgment of most intensivists that, when employed appropriately by properly trained clinicians, the benefits of this procedure outweigh the risks, that has not been proven by a prospective, controlled trial. Such trials are needed to determine the balance between the risks and benefits of this procedure and its influence on the outcome of critically ill patients.

Risks of Pulmonary Artery Catheterization

The risks of inserting the pulmonary artery catheter are the same as those associated with central venous catheter placement with the addition of ventricular and atrial arrhythmias, right bundle branch block, valve injury, and pulmonary artery laceration.

The ventricular arrhythmias associated with the placement of pulmonary artery catheters usually occur during passage of the catheter tip through the ventricle. Elliot and colleagues[33] reported ventricular arrhythmias in 90 of 116 catheterizations (78%), while Boyd et al.[32] reported ventricular arrhythmias in only 66 of 528 catheterizations (13%). Several studies focussed only on advanced ventricular arrhythmias [salvos (3 to 5 consecutive premature ventricular contractions), ventricular tachycardia, and ventricular fibrillation[80-82]]. They occurred in 13 to 53% of catheterizations.[83, 81] Myocardial ischemia, myocardial infarction, hypoxemia, and acidosis were all significantly related to the incidence of advanced ventricular arrhythmias.[81] Perhaps the most important factor in reducing the risk of advanced ventricular arrhythmias is the catheterization time. Sprung et al.[81] showed that when the catheterization took less than 20 minutes only 37% of patients had advanced arrhythmias compared to 65% for more prolonged catheterizations.[81] Iberti and colleagues[83] studied 68 patients who were all catheterized in 20 minutes or less (mean = 176 seconds, SD = 263 seconds) and found advanced ventricular arrhythmias in only 7 patients (13%). Prophylactic lidocaine has been shown to reduce the incidence of arrhythmias,[82] but is probably not needed if the catheterization time is kept to a minimum.[83]

Ventricular arrhythmias are rarely serious if managed carefully. For safety, the patient should always be monitored during catheterization and someone should be assigned the job of watching the monitor. If advanced ventricular arrhythmias are seen as the catheter passes through the ventricle, one of two courses of action is appropriate: (1) advance the catheter rapidly into the pulmonary artery or (2) deflate the balloon and withdraw the catheter from the ventricle. Advanced arrhythmias are infrequent if the catheter is advanced rapidly through the ventricle. When ventricular tachycardia has been reported it is most often transient and self-limited.[83] If prolonged, it usually responds to precordial thump or lidocaine infusion.[32, 81, 82, 84] Rarely, cardioversion is needed.[32]

Right bundle branch block (RBBB) occurs in 3% of patients following pulmonary artery catheterization.[33, 85, 86] It is usually transient, lasting an average of 9 hours in one study,[86] and without symptoms. There has been some controversy over the years about the risk of RBBB from pulmonary artery catheterization in patients with left bundle branch block (LBBB). Several excellent studies have now clearly shown that the risk of RBBB is not increased in the presence of LBBB as had been thought.[86, 87] These studies recommend that pulmonary artery catheterization can be performed safely in patients with LBBB if an external transthoracic pacemaker is on standby and the equipment needed for transvenous pacemaker insertion is available at the bedside.[86, 87] Of course, the physician inserting the catheter must be trained in the use of this equipment.

Trauma to the tricuspid valve is most likely to occur if the catheter is withdrawn from the right ventricle without deflating the balloon. In one prospective study, 6% of catheters passed through the chordae tendineae of the tricuspid valve.[88]

Perforation of the pulmonary artery can occur due to overinflation of the balloon with laceration of the vessel wall or due to erosion of the tip through the vessel wall.[89, 90] Research in animals and in postmortem lungs strongly suggests that the former cause is more common.[89] Very high pressures can occur in the balloon, especially if it is inflated with liquid or if it is overinflated.[89] Pulmonary artery laceration can cause hemoptysis, hemothorax, intrapulmonary hemorrhage, and pseudoaneurysm of the pulmonary artery.[90-92] Of all the complications associated with pulmonary artery catheterization, this is the one most likely to result in a patient's death. Precautions that can reduce the risk of pulmonary artery laceration are listed in Table 8–5.

Risks of Indwelling Pulmonary Artery Catheters.—In addition to the risks associated with catheter placement, several serious complications can occur as a result of leaving the catheter in place over a period of time. The three most common categories of these complications are thrombosis, cardiovascular injury, and infections.

Thrombosis.—Thrombosis occurs commonly in association with pulmonary artery catheterization.[57, 88] The most likely mechanism for thrombosis is mechanical trauma to the venous endothelium as a result of repeated contact with the catheter as it moves due to cardiac contraction.[88, 93, 94] Platelets adhere to the damaged vessel wall and thrombogenesis occurs.[88, 94] Most of the premortem clots described are adherent to both the catheter and to damaged vessel endothelium.[88, 94] In one study, there were no cases of substantial clot, which were adherent only to the catheter.[88] These findings suggest that heparin-impregnated catheters[95-97] will not solve the problem of catheter-related thrombosis, since they do not prevent endocardial trauma, which is an important cause of thrombosis.

The most common site for catheter-induced thrombosis is the superior vena cava. Superior vena cava thrombosis is present in 33 to 61% of patients.[88, 94, 98] Thrombosis at the insertion site is also common.[50, 94] Intracardiac thrombosis, in the atrium, ventricle, and valves has been reported in 22% of patients who died with a pulmonary artery catheter in place.[88] Aseptic endocardial and valvular vegetations were also common. They have been reported in 14 to 53% of patients at autopsy.[88, 98-100] Thrombosis involving the pulmonary artery was seen in several prospective studies but was less common.[88, 100] These studies give convincing evidence that catheter-related thrombosis is a common complication of 2 pulmonary artery catheterization.

The risk of thrombosis increases with the duration of catheterization.[88, 94, 98, 99] The incidence of thrombosis was significantly lower in the first 36 to 48 hours of catheterization.[88, 99, 100]

TABLE 8–5.
Reducing the Risk of Pulmonary Artery Laceration*

1. Keep the tip of the deflated catheter in the large central vessels; do not allow the tip to extend beyond the hilar shadows on the chest roentgenogram.
2. Only use air to inflate the balloon, *never use liquids.*
3. Never exceed the recommended inflating volume of the balloon.
4. Inflate the balloon slowly while monitoring the pressure tracing.
5. If a wedge tracing is seen with less than the recommended volume, stop inflation and check catheter position since the catheter may have migrated peripherally.

* From Thompson IR, Dalton BC, Lappas DG, et al: *Anesthesiol* 1979; 51:359–362.

For example, Chastre et al.[50] reported a 66% prevalence of internal jugular vein thrombosis when most catheters were in place for 72 hours or longer; however, Perkins et al.[101] did not find internal jugular thrombosis when 80% of catheters were removed within 48 hours of insertion and all were removed within 72 hours. It is not clear how anticoagulation effects the risk of catheter-induced thrombosis, since one study reported a significant reduction of thrombosis when patients were anticoagulated[88] while another found no effect.[98]

The impact of catheter-related thrombosis on patient outcome is unclear. Superior vena cava syndrome has been described but is uncommon.[102–104] The risk of pulmonary embolism is also uncertain. In a small prospective autopsy study, 5 of 17 patients with catheter-related thrombosis had emboli visible in their pulmonary arteries, while none of the 16 patients without thrombosis had visible emboli.[88] Another, larger autopsy study looked for but did not find a significant relationship between catheter-induced thrombosis and pulmonary emboli.[94] There are several reports of well-documented pulmonary emboli due to pulmonary artery catheterization.[93, 105] There are also a number of reports of pulmonary infarcts due to pulmonary artery catheterization, but it is usually unclear whether the infarct is due to direct occlusion of the vessel by the catheter or due to emboli from a catheter-related thrombus.

Cardiovascular Injury.—Trauma to the chambers and valves of the heart can also occur as a result of pulmonary artery catheterization. While rare, ruptured chordae of the tricuspid valve can cause significant tricuspid insufficiency.[106] Erosions of the tricuspid and pulmonic valves,[88, 100, 107] subendocardial hemorrhage,[88, 98–100] and microscopic damage to the endothelium[88] have all been seen, but do not seem to cause any functional impairment. Some have speculated that the catheter itself might interfere with valve closure and cause insufficiency of the tricuspid and pulmonic valves. Doppler studies have shown that valvular insufficiency is too small to be clinically important.[108]

Infection.—The risk of infection due to the pulmonary artery catheter appears to be similar to the risk seen with central venous catheters.[11, 20, 32, 52, 53, 56, 58] The risk increases with the duration of catheterization.[20] Catheter contamination has been reported in 5 to 29% of catheters.[11, 20, 32, 52, 53, 56, 58] Catheter contamination occurs in less than 2.5% of patients in the first 48 hours of catheterization.[11, 20] Line sepsis is not reported in the first 72 hours and is rare before 96 hours of catheterization. The prevalence of line sepsis is between 0 and 6%.[11, 20, 32, 52, 53, 56, 58] This is a particular concern since line sepsis increases mortality 28 to 42% in critically ill patients.[60–65] Bacterial endocarditis was found in 4 to 8% of patients who either died with a catheter in place or died within one month of catheterization.[94, 99, 100] This may be due to the high incidence of aseptic vegetations found in the hearts of patients who die with catheters in place.[88, 98–100] Bacteremia in these patients might easily result in seeding of these vegetations, resulting in bacterial endocarditis.

The most serious complications of the pulmonary artery catheter are the infectious and thrombotic complications. Happily both of these complications are related to the duration of catheterization. Sepsis is rare in the first 72 hours of catheterization and most thrombotic complications seem to occur after 48 hours of catheterization. Clearly, the patient will be best served by avoiding prolonged catheterization. In our unit we try to remove catheters within

24 to 48 hours whenever possible. Usually optimal benefit from the catheter has been achieved by then and leaving it in longer increases the risk with little additional benefit.

Table 8–6 summarizes the best approach to minimizing the risk of complications from pulmonary artery catheterization.

ENSURING RELIABLE DATA

Physician Expertise

Maximum benefit from pulmonary artery catheterization is only possible if the physician who interprets and acts on the information provided by the procedure has a solid understanding of cardiovascular physiology and the risks and limitations of the procedure. A recent study by Iberti and colleagues[83a] demonstrated that physicians' knowledge of the risks and benefits of the pulmonary artery catheter was often lacking as was their grasp of cardiovascular physiology. Fewer than half of the physicians tested were able to interpret a straightforward pulmonary capillary wedge pressure tracing accurately. Performance on this test was highly correlated to level of training in the use of these catheters and direct experience with placing and interpreting information from pulmonary artery catheters. We can conclude from this paper that, if physicians have not had specific training in the use of the pulmonary artery catheter or if they use it infrequently, they should consult an intensivist for advice and assistance when performing pulmonary artery catheterization on their patients.

TABLE 8–6.
Minimizing the Risk of Complications from Pulmonary Artery Catheterization

1. Adhere to all the recommendations on Table 8–4 regarding central venous catheters.
2. Insert a pulmonary artery catheter only if the patient:
   a. Does not respond to a rational course of therapy chosen based on a careful clinical evaluation;
   b. Deteriorates before therapy can be evaluated; or
   c. If substantial uncertainty about the hemodynamic status persists after initial evaluation and therapy.
3. Monitor the electrocardiogram continuously during the passage of the catheter through the right ventricle. Remove the catheter at once if advanced ventricular arryhthmias are noted.
4. Always deflate the balloon prior to withdrawing the catheter.
5. Keep the duration of catheter insertion to a minimum. Three to 5 minutes is optimal; less than 20 minutes is satisfactory.
6. In patients with left bundle branch block, catheterization should only be performed with a transcutaneous pacemaker on standby and apparatus for the placement of a transvenous pacemaker at the bedside.
7. Adhere to the recommendations on Table 8–5 to reduce the risk of pulmonary artery laceration.
8. Once all measurements are taken, therapy is started or adjusted. The response to the new therapy is monitored to assure the desired response and the need for further pulmonary artery catheterization should be reassessed. Most of the benefit of pulmonary artery catheterization occurs in the first 24 hours. Removing the catheter within 24 to 48 hours will substantially reduce complications.

Transducer Calibration and Positioning

The next most common source of inaccuracy in the use of pulmonary artery catheters results from improper setup and calibration of the pressure monitoring devices. An excellent review of this subject was published by O'Quin and Marini.[69] The transducer must be positioned and fixed at the level of the left atrium. The left atrium is usually considered to be at a point 5 cm below the angle of Louis (the junction of the manubrium sternum and the body of the sternum). In our unit, the level of the left atrium is checked before each measurement using a 24-in. level. This eliminates the variation that occurs when people estimate the level of the left atrium. Once the transducer is leveled, it must then be balanced and the zero pressure set with the transducer open to atmospheric pressure. Once these steps have been completed, the transducer must not move relative to the left atrium until all pressures are measured. Next the transducer should be tested against a known pressure. This is usually accomplished using a mercury manometer. Extreme care must be taken to avoid forcing air into the patient causing an air embolus. Finally, the system should be carefully checked for bubbles, fibrin clots, and obstructions that will reduce the fidelity of the pressure signal.

Why must one know these technical details? Currently many monitoring systems have very simple and accurate procedures for balancing, zeroing, and electrically calibrating the transducer. These systems are generally accurate. However, when you question the accuracy of a measurement, you must know how to check for errors in the setup, placement, and calibration of the transducer that are likely to cause inaccurate measurements. Often the best and most direct check is to apply a known pressure to the transducer. If pressure measured by the transducer is more than 3% off the true value, you will need to find the cause or replace the transducer. Since a patient's therapy is directly influenced by these measurements, there must be no compromise in the level of accuracy we demand from these devices.

Respiratory Variation

Two further points are worth emphasis. First, all pressure readings must be taken at end-expiratory volume. The reason for this is simple. While we measure the intravascular pressure, we are really interested in the transmural pressure, the difference between the intraluminal and the pleural pressure. Since it is difficult to measure the pleural pressure, we get around this by measuring all pressures at the same lung volume and, thus, at the same pleural pressure. If this is done, we can then assume that changes in the intravascular pressure reflect equal changes in transmural pressure. Second, all measurements used for therapeutic decisions should be read from a strip chart recording, which also records ventilation and allows the end of expiration to be identified. These are the most reliable measurements. This practice also has the benefit of allowing review of the hardcopy when questions arise about the accuracy or interpretation of specific measurements.

Effect of Mechanical Ventilation and PEEP

At one time there were questions about whether positive pressure ventilation would interfere with the accurate measurement of PCWP. Several studies have shown that measurements of

PCWP obtained during mechanical ventilation accurately reflect left atrial pressure if they are taken at end-expiratory volume.[109, 110]

Positive end-expiratory pressure (PEEP) can influence measurement of PCWP. The addition of PEEP can increase the alveolar pressure above the pulmonary artery and venous pressure in portions of the lung. The portions of the lung so affected are equivalent to West Zones I and II (Fig 8–5.). If the catheter is wedged in this portion of the lung, the PCWP will reflect the alveolar pressure and not the left atrial pressure. If this is not recognized, errors in management can occur. Wedging of the catheter in a zone I or zone II portion of the lung can occur rarely when (1) the tip of the catheter is in a nondependent portion of the lung and (2) either the pulmonary artery pressure is low or the level of PEEP is high (greater than 10 cm H_2O).[111, 112] A summary of methods to determine whether a catheter may be wedging in zone I is presented in Table 8–7. If you suspect that the catheter is in a zone I or zone II portion of the lung, obtain a cross table lateral x-ray of the chest.[113] If the catheter tip is above the level of the left atrium, the catheter should be repositioned.

Since the pulmonary artery catheter is flow-directed, it is unusual for it to go to a nondependent portion of the lung.[113] It is also rare to find a catheter wedged in a zone I area of the lung. If the catheter tip is below the level of the left atrium, as it usually is, measurements of PCWP will accurately reflect LA pressure even with levels of PEEP up to 10 cm H_2O.[111, 112]

Positive end-expiratory pressure also affects PCWP by increasing the pleural pressure (P_{pl}). The degree to which the increased airway pressure (P_{aw}) is transmitted to the pleural space is determined by the compliance of the lung (C_l) and the compliance of the chest wall (C_{cw}). The relationship

$$\triangle P_{pl}/ \triangle P_{aw} = C_l/ (C_l + C_{cw})$$

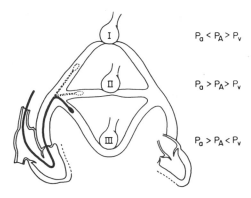

$P_a < P_A > P_v$

$P_a > P_A > P_v$

$P_a > P_A < P_v$

FIG 8–5.
Effect of catheter tip location and alveolar-vascular pressure relationships on wedge pressure. With increasing vertical distance above the left atrial plane, arterial (Pa) and venous pressure (Pv) decline relative to alveolar pressure (PA), which is similar in all three zones. In either zone I or zone II, PA exceeds Pv. Hence, during balloon occlusion of the pulmonary artery, alveolar capillaries collapse, causing wedge pressure to reflect PA rather than pulmonary venous pressure; wedge pressure estimates Pv accurately only in zone III. *(From O'Quin R, Marini JJ: Pulmonary artery occlusion pressure: Clinical physiology, measurement, and interpretation. Am Rev Respir Dis 1983; 128:319–326. Used by permission.)*

TABLE 8–7.
Evidence Suggesting that the Catheter Tip Is in a Zone I Portion of the Lung

1. In response to a trial of PEEP, the PCWP increases more than one-half of the increase in PEEP.
2. The pulmonary artery wedge pressure is greater than the pulmonary artery diastolic pressure.
3. When the airway pressure tracing is compared to the PCWP tracing, it is noted that for a given change in airway pressure the change in PCWP is more than one-half the change in airway pressure.
4. On a cross table lateral chest roentgenogram, the catheter tip is above the level of the left atrium.

describes how lung and chest wall influence the change on pleural pressure or any change in airway pressure.[69] Normally, lung and chest wall compliance are equal in the tidal volume range. Thus, the pleural pressure (and, consequently, the PCWP) will increase 0.5 cm H_2O for each 1 cm H_2O increase in airway pressure. In diseases that decrease lung compliance, the increment in pleural pressure will be less than one-half that of the airway pressure.[112, 114] This fact is the basis for one of the best ways to identify when the catheter is in a zone I portion of the lung. If the wedge pressure increases by more than half of an increment of PEEP, this strongly suggests that the catheter is in zone I.

Accurate Wedge Pressure

Morris, Chapman, and Gardner[115] recommended four criteria for assessing the validity of wedge pressure measurements. These criteria are shown in Table 8–8. Each of these criteria and the technical problems that cause them not to be satisfied will be described.

Criterion 1.—The mean pulmonary artery pressure must always be greater than the mean wedge pressure. A falsely high wedge pressure usually occurs if the catheter will not wedge (12% of measurements[111]) or if the balloon is overinflated.[115]

Criterion 2.—The phasic wedge pressure tracing should be consistent with an atrial waveform with identifiable a and v waves. When this does not occur it can be due to overdamping of the tracing or incomplete wedging, where characteristics of the pulmonary artery waveform are still identifiable on the "wedged" tracing.

TABLE 8–8.
Criteria for Assessing the Validity of Wedge Pressure Measurements*

1. The mean wedge pressure must be less than the mean pulmonary artery pressure.
2. The phasic wedge pressure recording must be consistent with an atrial pressure waveform.
3. Free flow through the catheter should be present with the catheter in the wedge position.
4. Blood aspirated through the wedged catheter should be highly oxygenated, "capillary" blood.
* From Morris AH, Chapman RH, Gardner RM: *Crit Care Med* 1984; 12:164–170.

Criterion 3.—Free flow through the catheter should be present with the catheter in the wedged position. This is, of course, essential if the wedge pressure is to truly represent left atrial pressure. In the old catheterization labs this was determined using the rate of emptying of a saline manometer through the wedged catheter. In the intensive care unit, this can be done by opening the flush valve, applying high pressure to the transducer and catheter, and then suddenly releasing the pressure. If flow from the tip of the catheter is unimpeded, the pressure tracing will fall abruptly, oscillate around the true pressure, and rapidly stabilize. If the pressure falls slowly, this suggests an obstruction to flow in the capillary bed or a catheter tip against the vessel wall. An overdamped system will not show the normal high-frequency components of the wedge tracing. This is usually due to bubbles or obstructions in the transducer or tubing. Another sign of catheter tip occlusion against the vessel wall is progressively increasing pressure when the catheter is wedged. This is called "overwedging" or "overinflation" and is well described by Morris.[115]

Criterion 4.—Blood aspirated through the wedged catheter should be highly oxygenated, "capillary" blood. This has been defined[116] as wedge $Po_2 > Pao_2$ and wedge $Pco_2 < Paco_2$. This criterion is met in about 50 to 60% of catheterizations.[115, 116] While not found in 55% of catheters that meet criteria 1 to 3,[115] meeting this criterion is the best evidence of a properly wedged catheter. After manipulation of the catheters, 84% of catheters were able to meet criterion 4 in one study.[117]

Morris et al.[115] found that 69% of wedge pressure measurement met criteria 1 to 3. In another study, this group showed that when these criteria were met, only 5% of the pressure measurements were more than 4 mm Hg from the true value.[117] Catheters that failed one or more of these criteria had a 33% prevalence of errors of more than 4 mm Hg in the wedge pressure.[117]

Accuracy of Thermodilution Cardiac Output

With proper attention to injection technique and timing, the thermodilution CO is a reliable measure of true cardiac output.[118-120] The technique[119] involves injection into the right atrium of a predetermined volume of saline at a known temperature. This results in cooling of the blood in the right atrium and ventricle. This cooled blood moves past a thermistor at the tip of the catheter in the pulmonary artery. The rate of rise of the temperature as the bolus of cool blood passes is a function of the cardiac output. The precise cardiac output is estimated by fitting an ideal curve to the observed temperature-time curve. When three cardiac output measurements are averaged, the standard error of measurement varied between 2 to 5% in nine studies reviewed by Stetz et al.[120] This means that the cardiac output has to change 6 to 15% to establish a significant change, i.e., a change greater than might occur due to measurement error alone.[120]

The measurement of cardiac output is influenced by the time within the respiratory cycle that the saline bolus is injected[121, 122] (Fig 8–6). This is especially true during mechanical ventilation. High airway pressures accentuate the variation in cardiac output during the respiratory cycle.[122] The cardiac output measurement varies from roughly 10 to 20% above

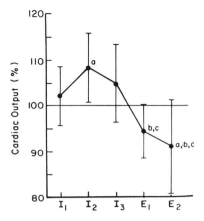

FIG 8–6.
Variation in thermodilution cardiac ouput during the ventilatory cycle in patients on mechanical ventilation. Thermodilution injections were performed at five points during the respiratory cycle. Points immediately before inspiration, at midinspiration and at end-inspiration are indicated by I_1, I_2, and I_3, respectively. Early and midexpiration are indicted by E_1 and E_2. *(From Okamoto K, Komatsu T, Kumar V, et al: Effects of intermittent positive-pressure ventilation on cardiac output measurements by thermodilution.* Crit Care Med *1986; 10:977–980. Used by permission.)*

the average value for injections given at midinspiration to about 10 to 20% below the average cardiac output for injections at midexpiration.[121, 122] Injections at end-expiration, immediately before the start of inspiration, will most closely approximate the true CO.[122] There is no consensus on how to minimize this artifact. Snyder and Powner[121] recommend sampling at three regularly spaced intervals in the respiratory cycle and averaging the three measurements. Okamoto and colleagues[122] suggest averaging paired measurements obtained at midinspiration and midexpiration.

INTERPRETING HEMODYNAMIC DATA

Hemodynamic monitoring provides the clinician with information about blood pressure, pulmonary capillary pressure, filling pressures of the left and right ventricles, ventricular contractility, vascular resistance, and oxygen metabolism. To gain optimal benefit from this information, the clinician must understand cardiovascular physiology and pathophysiology and be able to define accurately the patient's physiologic state and choose therapy appropriate for the patient's condition. An important step in that process is the evaluation of the contractile state of the left ventricle.

The contractile state of the ventricle is best determined by constructing a Starling curve for the heart as shown in Figure 8–7. In his initial description of the law of the heart, Starling related preload (ventricular end-diastolic volume or fiber length) to ventricular performance (e.g., cardiac index, stroke volume, or stroke work).[123] Patients can be categorized into one of

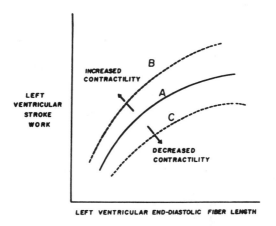

FIG 8–7.
The Starling relationship: the relationship between preload (left ventricular end-diastolic fiber length) and ventricular performance (left ventricular stroke work). Curve A is the normal function curve. Curve B is associated with increased contractility. Curve C is associated with reduced contractility. A function curve like this can be constructed for either ventricle. *(From Schlant RC: Normal physiology of the cardiovascular system. Chap 7 in Hurst JW, Logue RB, Schlant RC, Wenger NK (eds): The Heart. New York, McGraw-Hill Book Co, 1974, pp. 79–109. Used by permission.)*

several hemodynamic states based on their relation to a normal Starling curve. Patients with a high or low preload but a cardiac output appropriate for the preload have hemodynamic problems related to volume overload or volume depletion (Fig 8–7, curve A). They will respond to diuresis or fluid therapy, respectively. Decreased contractility is characterized by a cardiac output that is inappropriately low for a preload that is usually normal or elevated (Fig 8–7, curve C). Finally, elevated cardiac output in the face of a low preload is consistent with a hyperdynamic state (Fig 8–7, curve B) such as is seen with sepsis, arteriovenous shunting, and other forms of high-output failure.

The difficulty here is that the pulmonary artery catheter measures preload, the ventricular end-diastolic volume, indirectly as pulmonary capillary wedge pressure or right atrial pressure. The left ventricular end-diastolic volume that results from a given pulmonary capillary pressure can vary considerably depending on the compliance of the ventricle. Thus we must be cautious about judgments of hemodynamic status based on the assumption that the pulmonary capillary wedge pressure is a true representation of the left ventricular end-diastolic volume. Often it is not!

PCWP as a Measure of Left Atrial Pressure

PCWP is an accurate measure of LA pressure under most clinical conditions.[124, 125] However, discrepancies have been demonstrated[111, 112] at levels of PEEP above 10 cm H_2O in patients whose catheter tip is above the left atrium[111, 112] and in patients recovering from cardiac surgery.[126] In most patients it is safe to assume that the PCWP is an accurate reflection of the pressure in the left atrium.

PCWP as a Measure of Left Ventricular End-Diastolic Pressure

When we use PCWP as a proxy for left ventricular end-diastolic volume in the Starling relationship, we make a leap of faith that has very little support in the literature. We are assuming that ventricular compliance is the same from patient to patient and, thus, if we know the PCWP we can make some fairly accurate assumptions about the preload on the ventricle. Unfortunately, abnormalities of left ventricular compliance and pleural pressure can alter the relationship between left ventricular end-diastolic volume and PCWP. This has been observed clinically after acute myocardial infarction,[127] in the presence of chronic heart disease,[128, 129] after thoracic and cardiac surgery,[130, 131] and with sepsis.[132] Figure 8–8 shows wide variations in left ventricular compliance in actual patients and Figure 8–9 demonstrates how a single left ventricular end-diastolic volume can be associated with a wide range of PCWP. The PCWP is not a direct measure of preload and it cannot be assumed to reflect preload accurately.

This leaves us with the uncomfortable realization that pulmonary artery catheterization can only give us an approximation of the contractility of the left ventricle—in some situations, only a poor approximation. While most clinicians feel that it is appropriate to choose therapy based on the assumption that PCWP is a good indicator of left ventricular preload, the evidence to support this is mostly indirect. Several studies suggest that optimal preload of the left ventricle can be determined from the PCWP.[27, 133] Crexells et al.[133] demonstrated that a wedge pressure of 15 to 18 mm Hg is associated with the optimal cardiac output in patients with acute myocardial infarction. Packman and Rackow[27] showed that increasing the wedge pressure beyond 12 mm Hg did not significantly increase cardiac output in patients with sepsis. Differences in ventricular compliance between acute myocardial infarction and sepsis presumably account for the different results of these two very important studies.

A number of studies, however, demonstrate a poor relationship between PCWP and left ventricular end-diastolic volume in specific clinical states.[128–132, 134] One of the few controlled studies of the use of pulmonary artery catheters suggests that the postoperative cardiac surgery patients did about as well, and sometimes better, when managed with just central venous pressure monitoring.[135] In this study, 1094 consecutive patients undergoing coronary artery surgery were assigned to either one of four anesthesiologists who placed only central venous catheters preoperatively or one of five anesthesiologists who placed only pulmonary artery catheters preoperatively. There was no difference in survival or complications in the two groups of patients. Patients who received pulmonary artery catheters were more likely to receive vasopressors and stayed in the intensive care unit for more than a day longer.[135] The authors concluded that even high-risk cardiac surgery patients may be managed safely without routine pulmonary artery catheterization. They suggested delaying pulmonary artery catheterization until a clinical need develops.[135]

PCWP as a Measure of True Capillary Pressure

One of the real values of the measurement of PCWP is the information this measurement provides about the pressures in the pulmonary capillaries.[136–138] This is of critical interest when diffuse alveolar injury is suspected since mortality may be reduced by maintaining low pressures in the pulmonary capillary bed. It is also of importance in a patient without capillary

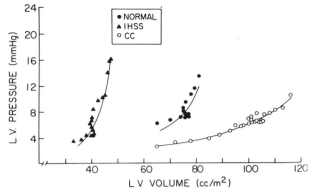

FIG 8–8.
The relationship between left ventricular (L.V.) pressure and left ventricular volume for three very different left ventricular compliances. In this example, the same left ventricular pressure is associated with three different left ventricular volumes. *(From Gaasch WH, Cole JS, Quinones MA, et al: Dynamic determinants of left ventricular diastolic pressure-volume relations in man. Circulation 1975; 51:317–323. Used by permission.)*

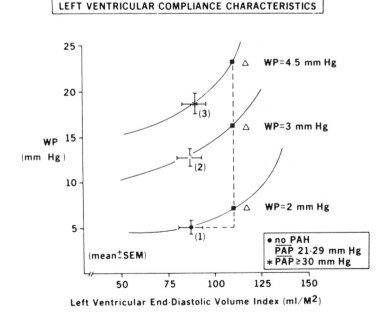

FIG 8–9.
The effect of different levels of right ventricular afterload on left ventricular compliance. Three levels of mean pulmonary artery pressure (PAP) are shown. Three different wedge pressures (WP) are associated with the same left ventricular end-diastolic volume index at the different levels of pulmonary hypertension. As compliance decreases, it takes a greater change in wedge pressure to achieve the same change in ventricular volume. *(From Sibbald WJ, Driedger AA: Right ventricular function in acute disease states: Pathophysiologic considerations. Crit Care Med 1983; 11:339–345. Used by permission.)*

injury since interstitial and alveolar edema will occur when the capillary pressure exceeds 18 to 24 mm Hg.

The PCWP is not a direct measure of true capillary pressure. However, it is closely related to the true capillary pressure. The true capillary pressure is somewhere between the mean pulmonary artery pressure and the left atrial pressure (PCWP). The difference between the true capillary pressure and the left atrial pressure is usually just a few cm H_2O except in the rare conditions that increase postcapillary resistance.[136-138]

Several papers have recently described conceptually simple methods of determining capillary pressures at the bedside from the trajectory of the fall in pressure from the mean pulmonary artery pressure to PCWP after balloon occlusion of the pulmonary artery[132-134] (Fig 8–10). This should ultimately be an excellent tool for guiding fluid therapy in the critically ill. In addition, it will be a valuable research tool since this technique allows the separation of precapillary resistance from postcapillary resistance. This will allow insights into diagnosis and treatment of venous occlusive disease in the lung and into the mechanisms and therapeutic application of vasoactive drugs on pulmonary capillaries.

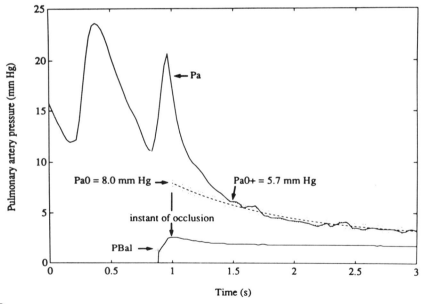

FIG 8–10.
Estimation of the pulmonary capillary pressure using the pulmonary artery occlusion technique. The instant of balloon occlusion is determined from the point of maximal balloon pressure (PBal). Starting 0.3 seconds after that point, a single exponential relationship is fitted over 2 seconds of data (*dashed line*). This line is extrapolated to the instant of occlusion to compute the postocclusion pressure (Pao). The Pao is highly correlated with the capillary pressure. The Pao+ is the point where the arterial pressure tracing crosses the fitted line. This value is less well correlated with the capillary pressure. (*From Hakim TS, Maaraek JMI, Chang HK: Estimation of pulmonary capillary pressure in intact dog lungs using the arterial occlusion technique. Am Rev Respir Dis 1989; 140:217–224. Used by permission.*)

Assessing Oxygen Delivery

One of the principal goals in the care of the critically ill patient is to assure sufficient delivery of oxygen to the tissues to support normal tissue metabolism and function. We do this by optimizing the cardiac output and arterial oxygen content. The pulmonary artery catheter is very useful in monitoring oxygen delivery and consumption (Table 8–9). The optimal value for oxygen delivery is unclear and may vary depending on the disease state. Studies in high risk postoperative patients suggest that a strategy which maintains supranormal levels of oxygen delivery was associated with improved outcome.[139] It is not clear, however, how these preliminary findings apply to other patient populations.

Despite this uncertainty, it seems prudent to monitor the patient to be sure that oxygen delivery is adequate for tissue needs. This can be done indirectly in two ways. The serum lactate can be monitored and cardiac output and oxygen content optimized until lactate levels are consistently normal. Serum lactate is a crude indicator of overall oxygen delivery. Normal values suggest that oxygen delivery is at least sufficient to suppress anaerobic metabolism. A second approach can be applied in low output states. In this setting, the mixed venous content or saturation may be an indicator of the adequacy of oxygen delivery, since if oxygen consumption and arterial oxygen content are constant, any reduction in cardiac output will reduce oxygen delivery and mixed venous oxygen content will fall. Thus, therapy can be aimed at maintaining a normal mixed venous oxygen content, which should be associated with adequate oxygen delivery. This may not be reliable in many critically ill patients. Oxygen consumption may vary with changes in cardiac output with unpredictable effects on mixed venous oxygen content.[140] In the distributive shock of sepsis there is poor tissue perfusion in the presence of elevated levels of mixed venous oxygen content due to precapillary shunting. In this setting the serum lactate may be a better guide to tissue oxygen delivery than mixed venous oxygen content or saturation.

Optimal Hemodynamic Profile

Once the arterial, central venous, or pulmonary artery catheters are in place, the patient has incurred most of the initial cost of hemodynamic monitoring. These costs include the discom-

---

TABLE 8–9.
Calculations Related to Oxygen Metabolism Made Possible by the Pulmonary Artery Catheter

1. The Fick Equation:
    Cardiac output = Oxygen consumption$/(CaO_2 - C\bar{v}O_2)$
2. Oxygen Delivery (DO2):
    DO_2 = Cardiac output $\times CaO_2$
3. Oxygen consumption ($\dot{V}O_2$):
    $\dot{V}O_2$ = Cardiac output $\times (CaO_2 - C\bar{v}O_2)$
4. Mixed Venous Oxygen Content ($C\bar{v}O_2$):
    If $\dot{V}O_2$ and CaO2 are constant then:
    Cardiac output $\propto C\bar{v}O_2$

fort, risks, and monetary cost associated with catheter placement and maintenance. To justify these costs, physicians are obliged to obtain optimal benefit for the patient from hemodynamic monitoring. We can do this by eliminating technical errors in the data collection, collecting all appropriate information, and then using this information intelligently to determine the patient's hemodynamic status, to choose therapy appropriate for the hemodynamic state, and to monitor the effect of that therapy.

The optimal hemodynamic profile includes blood pressure measurements, the measurements and calculations of Tables 8–10 and 8–11, and a measure of the adequacy of oxygen delivery (serum lactate or mixed venous oxygen saturation). This will allow an estimate of ventricular preload and cardiac contractility, measurement of cardiac output and afterload, and an estimate of the adequacy of oxygen delivery. With this information the patient can be categorized into one of several hemodynamic states (Table 8–12), which will guide the initial choice of therapy. Serial measurements of these values will allow the clinician to assess and adjust therapy to achieve more normal levels of cardiac function and, ideally, restore normal end-organ function.

SPECIALIZED CATHETERS

There are two types of specialized catheters currently in use in clinical practice. A catheter capable of measuring right ventricular ejection fraction (RVEF) and right ventricular end-diastolic and end-systolic volumes (RVESV and RVEDV) has recently been introduced. Another catheter capable of measuring the oxygen saturation of pulmonary artery (mixed venous) blood has been in use for many years. Both of these catheters are capable of making all the other measurements standard to pulmonary artery catheterization.

TABLE 8–10.
Measurements Available with a Pulmonary Artery Catheter

	Normal Values
Pulmonary vascular pressures[153]	
Pulmonary artery systolic pressure	15 to 28 mm Hg
Pulmonary artery diastolic pressure	5 to 16 mm Hg
Pulmonary artery mean pressure	10 to 22 mm Hg
Right ventricular function[153]	
Right atrial pressure	0 to 8 mm Hg
Right ventricular systolic pressure	15 to 28 mm Hg
Right ventricular diastolic pressure	0 to 8 mm Hg
Left atrial pressure[154]	
Pulmonary capillary wedge pressure	6 to 12 mm Hg
Cardiac output[154]	3.0 to 7.0 L/min

TABLE 8–11.

Calculations Possible with Measurements from Pulmonary Artery Catheterization

	Normal Values
Pulmonary vascular pressures[153]	
Pulmonary vascular resistance: [80 × (mean PAP − PCWP)/CO]	150 to 250 dynes × sec × cm^{-5}
Cardiac output[154]	
Cardiac index: (CO / BSA)	2.5 to 4.0 L/min/m^2
Stroke volume: (CO / HR)	70 to 130 mL/beat
Stroke index: (CI / HR)	40 to 50 mL/beat/m^2
Stroke work: (SI × MAP × 0.0144)	45 to 60 g × m/m^2
Systemic vascular pressures	
Systemic vascular resistance[154]: [80 × (MAP − CVP) / CO]	1100 to 1400 dynes × sec × cm^{-5}
Systemic vascular resistance index[139]: [80 × (MAP − CVP) / CI]	1800 to 2600 dynes × sec × cm^{-5}

Mixed Venous Oxygen Saturation Catheters

These catheters use reflectance oximetry to determine the oxygen saturation in the pulmonary artery. The oxygen content is measured continuously. The output can be monitored with alarms if a minimum level is reached or exceeded. The principal value of this catheter comes from the assumption that changes in cardiac output and oxygen delivery will be directly reflected in the measurements of mixed venous oxygen concentration. The Fick equation states that cardiac output is equal to the oxygen consumption divided by the arteriovenous oxygen content difference (Table 8–9). If oxygen consumption is constant, then cardiac output will be inversely proportional to the arteriovenous oxygen content difference. If arterial oxygen content is constant as well then increased cardiac output will increase oxygen delivery and mixed venous oxygen content will rise. If cardiac output falls, mixed venous oxygen content will fall. Thus, if these assumptions hold true, this catheter has the capability of giving the clinician an instantaneous index of cardiac output. The catheter could immediately alert caregivers to any alteration in cardiac output or oxygen delivery that results in a fall in mixed venous oxygen saturation.

While this catheter promised much when it was introduced, experience has revealed its limitations. In patients with multisystem dysfunction, oxygen consumption will often vary as cardiac output changes.[140] In this setting, studies show that a fall in cardiac output could be associated with a falling, rising, or constant mixed venous oxygen content.[140–142] Prospective studies of the impact of the oxygen saturation catheter on the management of critically ill patients showed that the changes in clinical status detected by the catheter were either not associated with significant changes in clinical status or were detected by other more standard monitoring techniques.[141–144] Monitoring with the mixed venous saturation catheter also tended to be more expensive overall than with the standard pulmonary artery catheter.[144, 145] This

TABLE 8–12.
Hemodynamic Measurements and Derived Values in Common Clinical States

| Diagnosis | Filling Pressures | | Cardiac Output | Contractility | Vascular Resistance | | Oxygen Metabolism | |
	RA	PCWP			PVR	SVR	Lactate	$C\bar{v}_{O_2}$
Hypovolemia	↓	↓	↓	Normal	↑	↑	NI, ↑	NI, ↓
Fluid overload	↑	↑	↑	Normal	↓	↓	NI, ↑	NI, ↓
Heart failure	↑	↑	↓	Decreased	↑	↑	NI, ↑	NI, ↓
Sepsis, early	↓	↓	↑	Increased	↓	↓	NI, ↑	↑, NI,
Sepsis, late	↑, NI, ↓	↑, NI, ↓	NI, ↓	NI, ↓	NI, ↑	NI, ↑	NI, ↑	↑, NI, ↓

catheter may be useful in monitoring patients with primary cardiac disease whose other organ systems are functioning normally. The catheter is commonly used in postcardiac surgery patients. Even in this group prospective, randomized, controlled trials are needed to prove that the oxygen saturation catheter truly improves management and leads to better outcomes.

Right Ventricular Ejection Fraction Catheters

In the last several years an exciting new catheter has been introduced that is capable of measuring RVEF and RVEDV.[146, 147] This catheter employs a rapid response thermistor to monitor temperature change following the saline injection to measure cardiac output. Because the thermistor has a very rapid response time, as it monitors the rise in temperature associated with the thermal washout curve, it can record the temperature rise associated with each systole. The ratio of the temperature change from two successive cardiac cycles is proportional to the residual fraction (RF) of blood left in the ventricle at end diastole.[146, 147] The RVEF is then determined by subtracting this residual fraction from one:

$$RVEF = 1 - RF$$

The RVEF can be measured at the same time as the cardiac output and stroke volume are determined (Fig 8–11). Once stroke volume is known, RVESV and RVEDV can be calculated as follows:

$$RVEDV = stroke\ volume/RVEF$$

$$RVESV = RVEDV - stroke\ volume$$

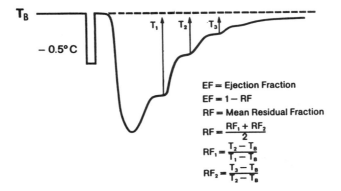

$$EF = Ejection\ Fraction$$
$$EF = 1 - RF$$
$$RF = Mean\ Residual\ Fraction$$
$$RF = \frac{RF_1 + RF_2}{2}$$
$$RF_1 = \frac{T_2 - T_B}{T_1 - T_B}$$
$$RF_2 = \frac{T_3 - T_B}{T_2 - T_B}$$

FIG 8–11.
The plateau method for calculating RVEF by thermodilution. The plateaus on the downslope portion of the thermodilution curve represent diastole, when there is little flow and, therefore, little change in temperature. The T_1, T_2, and T_3 represent the differences in temperature between baseline (T_B) and the respective diastoles. *(From Dhainaut JF, Brunet F, Monsallier JF, et al: Bedside evaluation of right ventricular performance using a rapid computerized thermodilution method.* Crit Care Med *1987; 15:148–152. Used by permission.)*

A number of reports on this catheter now suggest that the technique is comparable to 2-D echocardiography, biplane angiography, and radionuclide scanning in the measurement of RVEF and RVEDV.[148] The coefficient of variation is quite large, however, averaging about 12%.[148]

The main concern about this new technology is that it is uncertain that the knowledge of RVEF and RVEDV will have a meaningful clinical impact. It is not known whether patient management or outcomes will be enhanced beyond the value obtained with knowledge of wedge pressure, cardiac output, stroke volume, and vascular resistance. While the RVEF catheter has already made an impact on our understanding of right ventricular function,[149–152] it would seem most prudent to consider this catheter a research tool until it is clearly shown in a randomized controlled trial to yield improvements in management and patient outcomes that justify the expense of its use.

REFERENCES

1. Forrester JS, Diamond GA, Swan HJC: Correlative classification of clinical and hemodynamic function after acute myocardial infarction. *Am J Cardiol* 1977; 39:137–145.
2. Connors AF, McCaffree DR, Gray BA: Evaluation of right-heart catheterization in the critically ill patient without acute myocardial infarction. *N Engl J Med* 1983; 308:263–267.
3. Eisenberg PR, Jaffe AS, Schuster DP: Clinical evaluation compared to pulmonary artery catheterization in the hemodynamic assessment of critically ill patients. *Crit Care Med* 1984; 12:549–553.
4. Fein AM, Goldberg SK, Walkenstein MD, et al: Is pulmonary artery catheterization necessary for the diagnosis of pulmonary edema? *Am Rev Respir Dis* 1984; 129:1006–1009.
5. Sharkey WS. Beyond the wedge: Clinical physiology and the Swan-Ganz catheter. *Am J Med* 1987; 83:111–122.
6. Allen EV: Thromboangiitis obliterans: Methods of diagnosis of chronic occlusive arterial lesions distal to the wrist with illustrative cases. *Am J Med Sci* 1929; 178:237–244.
7. Husum B, Palm T, Eriksen J: Percutaneous cannulation of the dorsalis pedis artery: A prospective study. *Br J Anesth* 1979; 51:1055–1058.
8. Gurman GM, Kriemerman S: Cannulation of big arteries in critically ill patients. *Crit Care Med* 1985; 13:217–220.
9. Soderstrom CA, Wasserman DH, Dunham CM, et al: Superiority of the femoral artery for monitoring: A prospective study. *Am J Surg* 1982; 144:309–312.
10. Band JD, Maki DG: Infections caused by arterial catheters used for hemodynamic monitoring. *Am J Cardiol* 1979; 63:735–741.
11. Singh S, Nelson N, Acosta I, et al: Catheter colonization and bacteremia with pulmonary and arterial catheters. *Crit Care Med* 1982; 10:736–739.
12. Thomas F, Burke JP, Parker J, et al: The risk of infection related to radial vs femoral sites for arterial catheterization. *Crit Care Med* 1983; 11:807–812.
13. Norwood SH, Cormier B, McMahon NG, et al: Prospective study of catheter-related infection during prolonged arterial catheterization. *Crit Care Med* 1988; 16:836–839.
14. Smoller BR, Kruskall MS: Phlebotomy for diagnostic laboratory tests in adults: Pattern of use and effect on transfusion requirements. *N Engl J Med* 1986; 314:1233–1235.
15. Bedford RF, Wollman H: Complications of percutaneous radial-artery cannulation: An objective prospective study in man. *Anesthesiol* 1973; 38:228–236.

16. Davis FM, Stewart JM: Radial artery cannulation: A prospective study in patients undergoing cardiothoracic surgery. *Br J Anesth* 1980; 52:41–47.
17. Downs JB, Rackstein AD, Klein EF, et al: Hazards of radial-artery catheterization. *Anesthesiol* 1973; 38:283–286.
18. Bedford RF: Radial artery function following percutaneous cannulation with 18- and 20-gauge catheters. *Anesthesiol* 1977; 47:37–39.
19. Gardner RM, Schwartz R, Wong HC, et al: Percutaneous indwelling radial-artery catheters for monitoring cardiovascular function: Prospective study of the risk of thrombosis and infection. *New Engl J Med* 1974; 290:1227–1231.
20. Shapiro BA: Monitoring gas exchange in acute respiratory failure. *Respir Care* 1983; 28:605–607.
21. Damen J, Verhoef J, Bolton DT, et al: Microbiologic risk of invasive hemodynamic monitoring in patients undergoing open-heart operations. *Crit Care Med* 1985; 13:548–555.
22. Maki DG, Hassemer CA: Endemic rate of fluid contamination and related septicemia in arterial pressure monitoring. *Am J Med* 1981; 70:733–738.
23. Shinozaki T, Deane RS, Mazuzan JE, et al: Bacterial contamination of arterial lines: A prospective study. *JAMA* 1983; 249:223–225.
24. Weinstein RA, Emori TG, Anderson RL, et al: Pressure transducers as a source of bacteremia after open heart surgery. *Chest* 1976; 69:338–344.
25. Forrester JS, Diamond G, McHugh TJ, et al: Filling pressures in the right and left sides of the heart in acute myocardial infarction: A reappraisal of central-venous-pressure monitoring. *N Engl J Med* 1971; 285:190–193.
26. Rice CL, Hobelman CF, John DA, et al: Central venous pressure of pulmonary capillary pressure as the determinant of fluid replacement in aortic surgery. *Surgery* 1978; 84:437–440.
27. Packman MI, Rackow EC: Optimum left heart filling pressure during fluid resuscitation of patients with hypovolemic and septic shock. *Crit Care Med* 1983; 11:165–169.
28. Linos DA, Mucha P, van Heerden JA. Subclavian vein: A golden route. *Mayo Clin Proc* 1980; 55:315–321.
29. Belani KG, Buckley JJ, Gordon JR, et al: Percutaneous cervical central venous line placement: A comparison of the internal and external jugular vein routes. *Anesth Analg* 1980; 59:40–44.
30. Defalque RJ: Percutaneous catheterization of the internal jugular vein. *Anesth Analg* 1974; 53:116–120.
31. Shah KB, Rao TLK, Laughlin S, et al: A review of pulmonary artery catheterization. *Anesthesiol* 1984; 61:271–275.
32. Boyd KD, Thomas SJ, Gold J, et al: A prospective study of complications of pulmonary artery catheterizations in 500 consecutive patients. *Chest* 1983; 84:245–249.
33. Elliot CG, Zimmerman GA, Clemmer TP: Complications of pulmonary artery catheterization in the care of critically ill patients. *Chest* 1979; 76:647–652.
34. Eisenhauer ED, Derveloy RD, Hastings PR: Prospective evaluation of central venous pressure (CVP) catheters in a large city-county hospital. *Ann Surg* 1982; 96:560–564.
35. Patel C, Laboy V, Venus B, et al: Acute complications of pulmonary artery catheter insertion in critically ill patients. *Crit Care Med* 1986; 14:195–197.
36. Herbst CA: Indications, management, and complications of percutaneous subclavian catheters. *Arch Surg* 1978; 113:1421–1425.
37. Senagore A, Waller JD, Vonnell BW, et al: Pulmonary artery catheterizations: A prospective study of internal and subclavian approaches. *Crit Care Med* 1987; 15:35–37.
38. Ryan JA, Abel RM, Abbott WM, et al: Catheter complications in total parenteral nutrition. *N Engl J Med* 1974; 290:757–761.

39. Wolfe BM, Ryder MA, Nishikawa RA, et al: Complications of parenteral nutrition. *Am J Surg* 1986; 152:93–99.
40. Sitzmann JV, Townsend TR, Siler MC, et al: Septic and technical complications of central venous catheterization: A prospective study of 200 consecutive patients. *Ann Surg* 1985; 202:766–770.
41. Eyer S, Brummitt C, Crossley K, et al: Catheter-related sepsis: Prospective, randomized study of three methods of long-term catheter maintenance. *Crit Care Med* 1990; 18:1073–1079.
42. Snyder RH, Archer FJ, Endy T, et al: Catheter infection: A comparison of two catheter maintenance techniques. *Ann Surg* 1988; 208:651–658.
43. Puri VK, Carlson RW, Bander JJ, et al: Complications of vascular catheterization in the critically ill: A prospective study. *Crit Care Med* 1980; 8:495–499.
44. McCarthy MC, Shives JK, Robison RJ, et al: Prospective evaluation of single and triple lumen catheters in total parenteral nutrition. *JPEN* 1987; 11:259–262.
45. Bolinn GW, Anderson DJ, Anderson KC, et al: Percutaneous central venous catheterization performed by medical house officers: A prospective study. *Cath Cardio Diag* 1982; 8:23–29.
46. Katz JD, Cronau LH, Barash PG, et al: Pulmonary artery flow-guided catheters in the perioperative period: Indications and complications. *JAMA* 1977; 237:2832–2834.
47. Brismar B, Hardstedt C, Jacobson A: Diagnosis of thrombosis by catheter phlebography after prolonged central venous catheterization. *Ann Surg* 1981; 194:779–783.
48. Fritz T, Richeson JF, Fitzpatrick P, et al: Venous obstruction: A potential complication of transvenous pacemaker electrodes. *Chest* 1983; 83:534–539.
49. Anderson AJ, Krasnow SH, Boyer MW, et al: Thrombosis: The major Hickman catheter complication in patients with solid tumor. *Chest* 1989; 95:71–75.
50. Chastre J, Cornud F, Bouchama A, et al: Thrombosis as a complication of pulmonary-artery catheterization via the internal jugular vein. *N Engl J Med* 1982; 306:278–281.
51. Michel L, McMichan JC, Bachy JL: Microbial colonization of indwelling central venous catheters: Statistical evaluation of potential contaminating factors. *Am J Med* 1979; 137:745–748.
52. Pinilla JC, Ross DF, Martin T, et al: Study of the incidence of intravascular catheter infection and associated septicemia in critically ill patients. *Crit Care Med* 1983; 11:21–25.
53. Heard SO, Davis RF, Sherertz RJ, et al: Influence of sterile protective sleeves on the sterility of pulmonary artery catheters. *Crit Care Med* 1987; 15:499–502.
54. Civetta JM, Hudson-Civetta JA, Nelson LD, et al: Utility and efficacy of guidewire exchanges (abstract). *Crit Care Med* 1987; 15:380.
55. Gil RT, Kruse JA, Thill-Baharozian MC, et al: Triple- vs single-lumen central venous catheters: A prospective study in a critically ill population. *Arch Intern Med* 1989; 149:1139–1143.
56. Mogeson JV, Fredricksen W, Jensen JK: Subclavian vein catheterization and infection: A bacteriological study of 130 catheter insertions. *Scand J Infect Dis* 1972; 4:31–36.
57. Hilton E, Haslett TM, Borenstein MT, et al: Central catheter infections: Single-versus triple-lumen catheters: Influence of guidewires on infection rates when used for replacement of catheters. *Am J Med* 1988; 84:667–672.
58. Horowitz HW, Dworkin BM, Savino JF, et al: Central catheter related infections: Comparison of pulmonary artery catheters and triple lumen catheters for the delivery of hyperalimentation in a critical care setting. *JPEN* 1990; 14:588–592.
59. Maki DG, Cobb L, Garman JK, et al: An attachable silver-impregnated cuff for prevention of infection with central venous catheters: a prospective randomized multicenter trial. *Am J Med* 1988; 85:307–314.
60. Maki DG. Nosocomial bacteremia: An epidemiologic overview. *Am J Med* 1981; 70:719–732.
61. Smith RL, Meixler SM, Simberkoff MS: Excess mortality in critically ill patients with nosocomial bloodstream infections. *Chest* 1991; 100:164–167.

62. Spengler RF, Greenough WB: Hospital costs and mortality attributed to nosocomial bacteremias. *JAMA* 1978; 240:2455–2458.

63. Bryan CS, Hoernung CA, Reynolds KL, et al: Endemic bacteremia in Columbia, South Carolina. *Am J Epidemiol* 1986; 123:113–127.

64. Craven DE, Kunches LM, Lichtenberg DA, et al: Nosocomial infection and fatality in medical and surgical intensive care unit patients. *Arch Intern Med* 1988; 148:1161–1168.

65. Spengler RF, Greenough WB, Stolley PD: A descriptive study of nosocomial bacteremias at the Johns Hopkins Hospital, 1968–1974. *Johns Hopkins Med J* 1978; 142:77–84.

66. Kamal GD, Pfaller MA, Rempe LE, et al: Reduced intravascular catheter infection by antibiotic bonding: A prospective, randomized, controlled trial. *JAMA* 1991; 265:2364–2368.

67. Norwood S, Ruby A, Civetta J, Cortes V: Catheter-related infections and associated septicemia. *Chest* 1991; 99:968–975.

68. Swan HJC, Ganz W, Forrester O, et al: Catheterization of the heart in man with use of a flow-directed, balloon-tipped catheter. *N Engl J Med* 1970; 283:447–451.

69. O'Quin R, Marini JJ: Pulmonary artery occlusion pressure: Clinical physiology, measurement, and interpretation. *Am Rev Respir Dis* 1983; 128:319–326.

70. Stetz CW, Miller RG, Kelly GE, et al: Reliability of the thermodilution method in the determination of cardiac output in clinical practice. *Am Rev Respir Dis* 1982; 126:1001–1004.

71. Connors AF, Dawson NV, Shaw PK, et al: Accuracy of assessment of hemodynamic status in critically ill patients with and without acute heart disease. *Chest* 1990; 98:1200–1206.

72. Speroff T, Connors AF, Dawson NV: Lens model analysis of hemodynamic status in the critically ill. *Med Decision Making* 1989; 9:243–252.

73. Fowler NO: Pericardial disease, Chap 76 in Hurst JW, Logue RB, Schlant RC Wenger NK (eds): *The Heart.* New York, McGraw-Hill Book Co, 1974, pp. 1396–1400.

74. McIntyre KM, Sasahara AA: The hemodynamic response to pulmonary embolism in patients without prior cardiopulmonary disease. *Am J Cardiol* 1971; 28:288–294.

75. Fairfax WR, Thomas F, Orme JE: Pulmonary artery catheter occlusion as an indication of pulmonary embolus. *Chest* 1984; 86:270–271.

76. Traeger SM: "Failure to wedge" and pulmonary hypertension during pulmonary artery catheterization: A sign of totally occlusive pulmonary embolism. *Crit Care Med* 1985; 13:544–547.

77. Robin ED: The cult of the Swan-Ganz catheter: Overuse and abuse of pulmonary flow catheters. *Ann Intern Med* 1985; 103:445–449.

78. Robin ED: Death by pulmonary artery flow-directed catheter: Time for a moratorium (editorial). *Chest* 1987; 92:727–731.

79. Sibbald WJ, Sprung CL: The pulmonary artery catheter: The debate continues. *Chest* 1988, 94:899–901.

80. Matthay MA, Chatterjee K: Bedside catheterization of the pulmonary artery: Risks compared with benefits. *Ann Intern Med* 1988; 109:826–834.

81. Sprung CL, Pozen RG, Rozanski JJ, et al: Advanced ventricular arrhythmias during bedside pulmonary artery catheterization. *Am J Med* 1982; 72:203–208.

82. Sprung CL, Marcial EE, Garcia AA, et al: Prophylactic use of lidocaine to prevent advanced ventricular arrhythmias during pulmonary artery catheterization. *Am J Med* 1983; 75:906–910.

83. Iberti TJ, Benjamin E, Gruppi L, et al: Ventricular arrhythmias during pulmonary artery catheterization in the intensive care unit. *Am J Med* 1985; 78:451–454.

83a. Iberti TJ, Fischer EP, Leibowitz AB, et al: A multicenter study of physicians' knowledge of the pulmonary artery catheter. *JAMA* 1990; 264:2928–2932.

84. Sprung CL, Jacobs LJ, Caralis PV, et al: Ventricular arrhythmias during Swan-Ganz catheterization of the critically ill. *Chest* 1981; 79:413–415.

86. Sprung CL, Elser B, Schein MH, et al: Risk of right bundle-branch block and complete heart block during pulmonary artery catheterization. *Crit Care Med* 1989; 17:1–3.
87. Morris D, Mulvihill D, Lew WYW: Risk of developing complete heart block during bedside pulmonary artery catheterization in patients with left bundle-branch block. *Arch Intern Med* 1987; 147:2005–2010.
88. Connors AF, Castele RJ, Farhut N, et al: Complications of right heart catheterization: A prospective autopsy study. *Chest* 1985; 88:567–575.
89. Hardy JF, Morissette M, Taillefer J, et al: Pathophysiology of rupture of the pulmonary artery by pulmonary artery balloon-tipped catheters. *Anesth Analg* 1983; 62:925–930.
90. Barash PG, Nardi D, Hammond G, et al: Catheter-induced pulmonary artery perforation: Mechanisms, management, and modifications. *J Thorac Cardiovasc Surg* 1981; 82:5–12.
91. Dieden JD, Friloux LA, Renne JW: Pulmonary artery false aneurysms secondary to Swan-Ganz pulmonary artery catheters. *AJR* 1987; 149:901–906.
92. Fraser RS: Catheter-induced pulmonary artery perforation: Pathologic and pathogenic features. *Hum Pathol* 1987; 18:1246–1251.
93. Goodman DJ, Rider AK, Billingham ME, et al: Thromboembolic complications with the indwelling balloon-tipped pulmonary artery catheter. *N Engl J Med* 1974; 291:777.
94. Ducatman BS, McMichan JC, Edwards WD: Catheter-induced lesions of the right side of the heart; A one-year prospective study of 141 autopsies. *JAMA* 1985; 253:791–795.
95. Hoar PF, Wilson RM, Mangano DT, et al: Heparin bonding reduces thrombogenicity of pulmonary-artery catheters. *N Engl J Med* 1981; 305:993–995.
96. Mangano DT: Heparin bonding and long-term protection against thrombogenesis. *N Engl J Med* 1982; 307:894–895.
97. Nichols AB, Owen J, Grossman BA, et al: Effect of heparin bonding on catheter-induced fibrin formation and platelet activation. *Circulation* 1984; 70:843–850.
98. Lange HW, Galliani CA, Edwards JE: Local complications associated with indwelling Swan-Ganz catheters: Autopsy study of 36 cases. *Am J Cardiol* 1983; 52:1108–1111.
99. Ford SE, Manley PN: Indwelling cardiac catheters: An autopsy study of associated endocardial lesions. *Arch Pathol Lab Med* 1982; 106:314–317.
100. Rowley KM, Clubb KS, Smith GJW, et al: Right-sided infective endocarditis as a consequence of flow-directed pulmonary-artery catheterization. *N Engl J Med* 1984; 311:1152–1156.
101. Perkins NAK, Cail WS, Bedford RF, et al: Internal jugular vein function after Swan-Ganz catheterization. *Anesthesiol* 1984; 61:456–459.
102. Gore JM, Matsumoto AH, Layden JJ, et al: Superior vena cava syndrome: Its association with indwelling balloon-tipped pulmonary artery catheters. *Arch Intern Med* 1984; 144:506–508.
103. Dye LE, Segall PH, Russell RO, et al: Deep venous thrombosis of the upper extremity associated with use of the Swan-Ganz catheter. *Chest* 1978; 73:674–675.
104. Yorra FH, Oblath R, Jaffe, et al: Massive thrombosis associated with use of the Swan-Ganz catheter. *Chest* 1974; 65:682–684.
105. Bradway W, Biondi RJ, Kaufman JL, et al: Internal jugular thrombosis and pulmonary embolism. *Chest* 1981; 880:335–336.
106. Smith R, Glauser FL, Jemison P: Ruptured chordae of the tricuspid valve: The consequences of flow-directed Swan-Ganz catheterization. *Chest* 1976; 70:790–792.
107. Ettinghausen SE, Pearlman SH, Brandstetter RD: Tricuspid valve erosion from Swan-Ganz catheters. *Chest* 1981; 80:509–510.
108. Stewart D, Leman RB, Kaiser J, et al: Catheter-induced tricuspid regurgitation: Incidence and clinical significance. *Chest* 1991; 99:651–655.

109. Davidson R, Parker M, Harrison RA: The validity of determinations of pulmonary wedge pressure during mechanical ventilation. *Chest* 1978; 73:352–355.
110. Cengiz M, Crapo RO, Gardner RM: The effect of ventilation on the accuracy of pulmonary artery and wedge pressure measurements. *Crit Care Med* 1983; 11:502–507.
111. Berryhill RE, Benumof JL: PEEP-induced discrepancy between pulmonary arterial wedge pressure and left atrial pressure: The effects of controlled vs. spontaneous ventilation and compliant vs. noncompliant lungs in the dog. *Anesthesiol* 1979; 51:303–308.
112. Rajacich N, Burchard KW, Hasan FM, et al: Central venous pressure and pulmonary capillary wedge pressure as estimates of left atrial pressure: Effects of positive end-expiratory pressure and catheter tip manipulation. *Crit Care Med* 1989; 17:7–11.
113. Shasby DM, Dauber IM, Pfister S, et al: Swan-Ganz catheter location and left atrial pressure determine the accuracy of the wedge pressure when positive end-expiratory pressure is used. *Chest* 1981; 80:666–670.
114. O'Quin RJ, Marini JJ, Culver BH, et al: Transmission of airway pressure to the pleural space during lung edema and chest wall restriction. *J Appl Physiol* 1985; 59:1171–1177.
115. Morris AH, Chapman RH, Gardner RM: Frequency of technical problems encountered in the measurement of pulmonary artery wedge pressure. *Crit Care Med* 1984; 12:164–170.
116. Williams WH, Olsen GN, Allen WG, et al: Use of blood gas values to estimate the source of blood withdrawn from a wedged flow-directed catheter in critically ill patients. *Crit Care Med* 1982; 10:636–640.
117. Morris AH, Chapman RH, Gardner RM: Frequency of wedge pressure errors in the ICU. *Crit Care Med* 1985; 13:705–708.
118. Ganz W, Donoso R, Marcus HS, et al: A new technique for measurement of cardiac output by thermodilution in man. *Am J Cardiol* 1971; 27:392–396.
119. Weisel RD, Berger RL, Hechtman HB: Measurement of cardiac output by thermodilution. *N Engl J Med* 1975; 292:682–684.
120. Stetz CW, Miller RG, Kelly GE, et al: Reliability of the thermodilution method in the determination of cardiac output in clinical practice. *Am Rev Respir Dis* 1982; 126:1001–1004.
121. Snyder JV, Powner DJ: Effects of mechanical ventilation on the measurement of cardiac output by thermodilution. *Crit Care Med* 1982; 10:677–682.
122. Okamoto K, Komatsu T, Kumar V, et al: Effects of intermittent positive-pressure ventilation of cardiac output measurements by thermodilution. *Crit Care Med* 1986; 10:977–980.
123. Starling EH: The Linacre Lecture on the Law of the Heart. London, Longmans, Green & Co, Ltd, 1918.
124. Connolly DC, Kirklin JW, Wood EH: The relationship between pulmonary artery wedge pressure and left atrial pressure in man. *Circ Res* 1954; 2:434–440.
125. Lappas D, Lell WA, Gabel JC, et al: Indirect measurement of left-atrial pressure in surgical patients: Pulmonary-capillary wedge and pulmonary-artery diastolic pressures compared with left-atrial pressure. *Anesthesiol* 1978; 38:394–397.
126. Mammana RB, Hiro S, Levitsky S, et al: Inaccuracy of pulmonary capillary wedge pressure when compared to left atrial pressure in the early postsurgical period. *J Thorac Cardiovasc Surg* 1982; 84:420–425.
127. Orlando J, Vicario MD, Aronow WS, et al: Correlation of mean pulmonary artery wedge pressure, left atrial dimension, and PTF-V$_1$ in patients with acute myocardial infarction. *Circulation* 1977; 55:750–752.
128. Gaasch WH, Cole JS, Quinones MA, et al: Dynamic determinants of left ventricular diastolic pressure-volume relations in man. *Circulation* 1975; 51:317–323.

129. Sibbald WJ, Driedger AA: Right ventricular function in acute disease states: Pathophysiologic considerations. *Crit Care Med* 1983; 11:339–345.

130. Ellis RJ, Mangano DT, VanDyke DC: Relationship of wedge pressure to end-diastolic volume in patients undergoing myocardial revascularization. *J Thorac Cardiovasc Surg* 1979; 78:605–613.

131. Hansen RM, Viquerat CE, Matthay MA, et al: Poor correlation between pulmonary arterial wedge pressure and left ventricular end-diastolic volume after coronary artery bypass graft surgery. *Anesthesiol* 1986; 64:764–770.

132. Calvin JE, Driedger AA, Sibbald WJ: Does the pulmonary capillary wedge pressure predict left ventricular preload in critically ill patients? *Crit Care Med* 1981; 9:437–443.

133. Crexells C, Chatterjee K, Forrester JS, et al: Optimal filling pressure in the left side of the heart in acute myocardial infarction. *N Engl J Med* 1973; 289:1263–1266.

134. Raper R, Sibbald WJ: Misled by the wedge? The Swan-Ganz catheter and left ventricular preload. *Chest* 1986; 89:427–434.

135. Tuman KJ, McCarthy RJ, Spiess BD, et al: Effect of pulmonary artery catheterization on outcome in patients undergoing coronary artery surgery. *Anesthesiol* 1989; 70:199–206.

136. Cope DK, Allison RC, Parmentier JL, et al: Measurement of effective pulmonary capillary pressure using the pressure profile after pulmonary artery occlusion. *Crit Care Med* 1986; 14:16–22.

137. Cope DK, Parker JC, Taylor MD, et al: Pulmonary capillary pressures during hypoxia and hypoxemia: experimental and clinical studies. *Crit Care Med* 1989; 17:853–857.

138. Hakim TS, Maaraek JMI, Chang HK: Estimation of pulmonary capillary pressure in intact dog lungs using the arterial occlusion technique. *Am Rev Respir Dis* 1989; 140:217–224.

139. Shoemaker WC, Appel PL, Kram HB, et al: Prospective trial of supranormal values of survivors as therapeutic goals in high risk surgical patients. *Chest* 1988; 94:1176–1186.

140. Carlile PW, Gray BA: Effect of opposite changes in cardiac output and arterial PO_2 on the relationship between mixed venous PO_2 and oxygen transport. *Am Rev Respir Dis* 1989; 140:891–898.

141. Kuff JV, Vaughn S, Yang SC, et al: Continuous monitoring of mixed venous oxygen saturation in patients with acute myocardial infarction. *Chest* 1989; 95:607–611.

142. Vaughn S, Puri VK: Cardiac output changes and continuous mixed venous oxygen saturation measurements in the critically ill. *Crit Care Med* 1988; 16:495–498.

143. Boutros AR, Lee C: Value of continuous monitoring of mixed venous blood oxygen saturation in the management of critically ill patients. *Crit Care Med* 1986; 14:132–134.

144. Jastremski MS, Chelluri L, Beney KM, et al: Analysis of the effects of continuous on-line monitoring of mixed venous oxygen saturation on patient outcome and cost effectiveness. *Crit Care Med* 1989; 17:148—153.

145. Rajput MA, Richey HM, Bush BA, et al: A comparison between a conventional and a fiberoptic flow-directed thermal dilution pulmonary artery catheter in critically ill patients. *Arch Intern Med* 1989; 149:83–85.

146. Dhainaut JF, Brunet F, Monsallier JF, et al: Bedside evaluation of right ventricular performance using a rapid computerized thermodilution method. *Crit Care Med* 15; 1987:148–152.

147. Vincent JL, Thirion M, Brimioulle S, et al: Thermodilution measurement of right ventricular ejection fraction with a modified pulmonary artery catheter. *Intensive Care Med* 1986; 12:33–38.

148. Hurford WE, Zapol WM: The right ventricle and critical illness: A review of anatomy, physiology, and clinical evaluation of its function. *Intensive Care Med* 1988; 14:448–457.

149. Biondi JW, Schulman DS, Soufer R, et al: The effect of incremental positive end-expiratory pressure on right ventricular hemodynamics and ejection fraction. *Anesth Analg* 1988; 67:144–151.

150. Schulman DS, Biondi JW, Matthay RA, et al: Effect of positive end-expiratory pressure on right ventricular performance: Importance of baseline right ventricular function. *Am J Med* 1988; 84:57–67.

151. Eddy AC, Rice CL, Anardi DM: Right ventricular dysfunction in multiple trauma victims. *Am J Surg* 1988; 155:712–715.
152. Reuse C, Vincent JL, Pinsky MR: Measurements of right ventricular volumes during fluid challenge. *Chest* 1990; 98:1450–1454.
153. Schlant RC. Normal physiology of the cardiovascular system, Chap 7 in Hurst JW, Logue RB, Schlant RC, Wenger NK (eds): *The Heart*. New York, McGraw-Hill Book Co., 1974, pp. 79–109.
154. Voyce SJ, Urbach D, Rippe JM: Pulmonary artery catheters, Chap 4 in Rippe JM, Irwin RS, Alpert JS, Fink MP (eds): *Intensive Care Medicine*. Boston, Little, Brown, and Co, 1991, p. 62.

Work of Breathing and Respiratory Muscle Function*

M. Jeffrey Mador, M.D.

John M. Walsh, M.D., M.S.†

Martin J. Tobin, M.D.

INTRODUCTION

Critically ill patients commonly display increases in the work of breathing and abnormalities in respiratory muscle function. In this chapter, we review the following topics: work of breathing, transdiaphragmatic pressure, pressure-time product, pressure relaxation rate, and electromyographic assessment of respiratory muscle function.

WORK OF BREATHING

External work W is performed when a force moves its point of application through a distance. In the case of a fluid system, work is done when a pressure P changes the volume V of the system:

$$W = P \times V$$

* Supported in part by grants from the Research Service of Department of Veterans Affairs, American Heart Association of New York, American Lung Association of New York, and Chicago Lung Association.

† Recipient of a Parker B. Francis Research Fellowship award.

The units of the work of breathing are as follows:

> *Standard units of work:* kg · m or Joule
>   One joule equals 0.1 kg · m
> *Usually normalized to volume:* kg · m/L or joule/L
> *Power or work per unit time expressed as* kg · m/min or Joule/min

When a muscle contracts mechanical work is performed only if displacement takes place. During a miometric contraction, the muscle shortens and the work performed is called *positive* (i.e., the muscle does work on something). During a pliometric contraction, the muscle lengthens and the work performed is called *negative* (i.e., something does work on the muscle). During an isometric contraction, no displacement takes place and, therefore, no mechanical work is performed—there is, of course, a metabolic cost for exerting this force.

Components of Mechanical Work

The respiratory muscles perform work against the following types of forces:

1. Elastic forces that are developed in the tissue of the lungs and chest wall when a volume change occurs
2. Flow-resistive forces that depend on the resistance of the airways to the flow of gas and on the resistance offered by the nonelastic deformation of tissue
3. Inertial forces, which depend on the mass of the tissues and gases
4. Gravitational forces, which can be considered as part of the inertial forces, but in practice are included in the measurement of elastic forces
5. Distorting forces of the chest wall.

Inertial Work

The inertial forces of the respiratory system have been measured and are relatively small.[1, 2] Thus, inertial work has been considered to be negligibly small in comparison to the other components of work. Furthermore, most of the inertial work done during the accelerative phase of a breathing cycle is recovered during the decelerative phase. However, Sharp and colleagues have shown that respiratory system inertance is abnormally high in very obese subjects (predominantly the tissue component, which presumably results from the massive chest wall).[3] Since there are no experimental estimates of inertial work, it is possible that inertial work may be of some importance in such patients, especially at high levels of ventilation.

Elastic Work

At functional residual capacity (FRC), the elastic forces of the chest wall are equal and opposite to that of the lung. If the chest wall-lung system is displaced to any other volume, elastic forces that oppose the displacing force develop. If a subject is capable of completely relaxing his or her respiratory muscles, this displacement force can be measured as pressure, and a relaxation pressure-volume curve of the total respiratory system can be obtained (Fig 9–1).[4] With this curve the work required to overcome elastic forces can be estimated. In Figure 9–1, if inspiration involves a volume change from A to B, a pressure difference represented by BC has to be developed across the system by the inspiratory muscles. The elastic work required during inspiration equals the area ABCA. The work done during inspiration is stored in the elastic structures of the system and can be used during the subsequent expiration. If expiration involves a volume change from A to D, a pressure difference represented by DE has to be developed across the system by the expiratory muscles. The elastic work required equals the area ADEA. The energy stored during expiration is available for the subsequent inspiration.

If the pressure-volume relations of the lungs and chest wall are known, the elastic work of breathing may be examined in greater detail.[5] The lung static pressure can be measured in terms of the pressure applied to the lungs at a constant volume. The pressure applied to the lungs is the difference between alveolar (P_{alv}) and pleural pressure (P_{pl}), i.e., transpulmonary pressure (P_L) = $P_{alv} - P_{pl}$. Under static conditions with the glottis open, P_{alv} is equal to the pressure at the airway opening (P_{aw}). Pleural pressure P_{pl} is estimated by measurement of esophageal pressure (P_{es}). The pressure applied to the respiratory system (P_{rs}) is the difference between alveolar pressure and body surface pressure, i.e., $P_{rs} = P_{alv} - P_{bs}$. The pressure applied to the chest wall (with the respiratory muscles completely relaxed) is the difference between P_{pl} and P_{bs}, i.e., $P_{cw} = P_{pl} - P_{bs}$. The chest wall component can be obtained indirectly by subtracting the pressure applied to the lungs from that applied to the total respiratory system, i.e., $P_{cw} = P_{rs} - P_L = (P_{alv} - P_{bs}) - (P_{alv} - P_{pl}) = P_{pl} - P_{bs}$. The chest wall component can also be obtained directly, although this measurement is quite difficult to make.

In Figure 9–2, the relaxation-pressure curve of the total respiratory system and its components, the lung and chest wall, are shown. For tidal volume (AB), inspiratory elastic work of the total respiratory system is ABCA. The work required to increase lung volume is ABDEA,

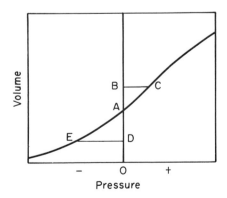

FIG 9–1.
Relaxation pressure-volume curve of the total respiratory system. *(Modified from Otis AB: The work of breathing, in Fenn WO, Rahn H (eds): Handbook of Physiology. Respiration. Washington, DC, American Physiological Society, 1964, Sec 3, Vol 1, Chap 17, pp. 463–478. Used by permission.)*

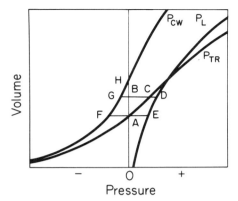

FIG 9–2.
Relaxation pressure-volume curve of the total respiratory system (P_{TR}) and its component parts, the lungs (P_L) and the chest wall (P_{CW}). *(From Otis AB: The work of breathing, in Fenn WO, Rahn H (eds):* Handbook of Physiology. Respiration. *Washington, DC, American Physiological Society, 1964, Sec 3, Vol 1, Chap 17, pp 463–478. Used by permission.)*

which is greater than the work required to inflate the entire system (ABCA). This is because at point A, force is applied to the chest wall (FA) to keep it at a volume lower than its equilibrium position (H). As the chest wall moves closer to its equilibrium position (F → G), energy is released (represented by AFGBA), which can be used to inflate the lungs (area AFGBA = area ACDEA). When the chest wall is inflated above point H, this counterspring effect is lost because the elastic forces of both the lung and chest wall act in the same direction.

Flow Resistive Work

During a breathing cycle, work must be performed to overcome flow-resistive forces in addition to elastic forces. During inspiration the pressure gradient required to overcome flow resistance is initially zero, increases to maximum at peak flow, and then falls back to zero. In Figure 9–3, A, inspiratory flow resistive work is equal to area AICA. Expiratory flow resistive work is equal to CEAC. In this example, CEAC lies completely within area ABCA, which represents the elastic energy stored during inspiration. Hence, in this example, there is ample stored energy to overcome expiratory flow resistance and no work is required of the expiratory muscles. The area ABCEA represents negative work performed by the inspiratory muscles, which lengthen during early expiration. If expiratory flow resistance had been larger, or expiratory flow more rapid, the work required during expiration would have exceeded that stored during inspiration and the expiratory muscles would be required to perform work (represented by area ABEA in Figure 9–3, B).

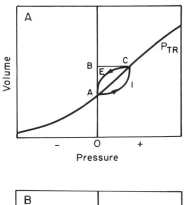

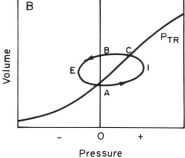

FIG 9–3.
Pressure-volume relations of the respiratory system during a breathing cycle. Inspiration starts at point A and ends at point C. Expiration starts at point C and ends at point A. The distance between the relaxation pressure-volume curve and the curved line AIC represents the pressure gradient required to overcome flow-resistive forces during an inspiration AB. *(From Otis AB: The work of breathing, in Fenn WO, Rahn H (eds):* Handbook of Physiology. Respiration. *Washington, DC, American Physiological Society, 1964, Sec 3, Vol 1, Chap 17, pp 463–478. Used by permission.)*

Work Due to Chest Wall Distortion

The chest wall consists of two compartments, the ribcage and abdomen. These compartments can move completely independently of one another.[6] When the respiratory muscles are completely relaxed, the relative displacements of the ribcage and abdomen are dependent on the compliance of the two compartments and the nature of the distending force. If the distribution of volume change between these two compartments differs from the pattern obtained during relaxation, extra work must be performed to overcome the elastic cost of this distortion.[7] At rest, such distortions are small. However, when ventilation is stimulated by CO_2 or exercise, the relative distribution of volume change can be preferential to one or another compartment (depending on the relative activation and coordination of the respiratory muscles) leading to the performance of extra work.[8]

In addition to changes in the degree of displacement of the ribcage and abdominal compartments relative to their relaxation characteristics, the two compartments can also move out of phase with each other (asynchrony) or in opposite directions (paradox). This is particularly important during resistive loading and in patients with severe respiratory disease when the degree of asychrony and/or paradox can be quite high. When there is asynchrony or paradoxical movement of the two compartments, the sum of the volume displacement of the ribcage and abdominal compartments will be greater than the change in lung volume; as a result, extra work is performed (the extent of which depends on the degree of asychrony and paradox).

In normal subjects at high levels of ventilation, the extra work due to chest wall distortion can be up to 25% of the total work[8] (Fig 9–4). In patients with respiratory disease or during respiratory loading, the degree of asychronous and/or paradoxical breathing is markedly higher than that seen in normal subjects.[9, 10] Thus, the extra work due to chest wall distortion is likely to be considerably higher in such patients than that observed in exercising normal subjects. Finally, the respiratory system can behave with more than two degrees of freedom, i.e., the shape of the ribcage or abdominal compartment can be distorted, and this will also increase

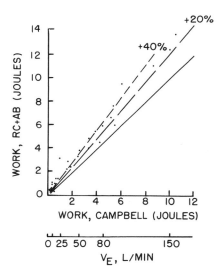

FIG 9–4.
Mechanical work measured for a breathing cycle (average of three to five consecutive breaths) in joules. Work estimated from measurements of areas on separate rib cage and abdominal pressure-volume tracings is plotted on vertical axis and estimate derived from Campbell diagram is plotted on horizontal axis. Difference between work estimated from separate rib cage and abdominal pressure-volume tracings and that from a Campbell diagram reflects work necessary to produce chest wall distortion. Average minute ventilations are shown on the lower horizontal axis. Data are shown for all subjects (*n* = 6) during exercise. *(From Goldman MD, Grimby G, Mead J: Mechanical work of breathing derived from rib cage and abdominal V-P partitioning. J Appl Physiol 1976; 41:752–763. Used by permission.)*

the amount of elastic work. Ribcage or abdominal distortion is negligible in normal subjects even during heavy exercise.[11] However, during resistive loading (or in patients with obstructive lung disease) this type of chest wall distortion becomes more prominent[12, 13] and may contribute significantly to the elastic work of breathing.

Measurement of the Mechanical Work of Breathing

At present, no method is capable of directly measuring the total mechanical work performed during spontaneous breathing. This is because the respiratory muscles, which perform the work, cannot be separated from the elastic and flow-resistive loads on which they are working. Thus, the total pressure gradient across the system cannot be measured. The total mechanical work of breathing may be estimated by measuring the differential pressure between the airway opening and the body surface ($P_{rs} = P_{aw} - P_{bs}$) and the resultant volume change during mechanical ventilation.[14] For this method to be accurate, the subject must be able to relax his or her respiratory muscles completely during mechanical ventilation, or the measurements must be made in the paralyzed state. Sharp and colleagues demonstrated that subjects can completely relax their intercostal and abdominal muscles during mechanical ventilation as reflected by the absence of measurable EMG activity from these muscles.[15] Unfortunately, these investigators did not measure diaphragmatic, parasternal, or scalene EMG activity during mechanical ventilation so that it is not clear that all of the inspiratory muscles were truly relaxed.

In addition to the problem of incomplete relaxation of the respiratory muscles, this method is based on the assumption that the work performed on the passive relaxed respiratory system (by an applied pressure difference) is identical to that accomplished by the respiratory muscles during spontaneous breathing. The ribcage contribution to tidal volume and the shape of the ribcage have been shown to differ between normal resting spontaneous breathing and during positive pressure breathing with the respiratory muscles paralyzed,[16, 17] suggesting that this assumption is not entirely correct. Furthermore, chest impedance may be somewhat higher during active compared with passive inflation.[18] Accepting these limitations, Sharp et al.[15] found that total respiratory work was 0.073 ± 0.014 (SD) kg · m/L in normal subjects breathing at 20 breaths/min with a fixed tidal volume of 1 L. Similar results have been obtained by other investigators.[14]

Measurement of the work performed on the lungs alone, rather than total mechanical work, can be obtained during spontaneous breathing by simultaneously measuring changes in lung volume and the difference between P_{es} and mouth pressure. Work is calculated from the area enclosed by the pressure-volume loop. This method allows measurement of the elastic work done on the lungs and flow-resistive work done in moving gas and lung tissue. It does not measure the flow-resistive work done on the thorax. This component of total work has been found by some authors to account for as much as 18 to 26% of total mechanical work in healthy subjects during quiet breathing.[19, 20] Furthermore, flow-resistive work done on the thorax accounted for 29% of total mechanical work in mechanically ventilated patients with complete muscle paralysis due to neuromuscular disease and 20 to 65% of total mechanical work in patients with kyphoscoliosis. However, because the flow resistance of the lung increases progressively as ventilation increases, whereas the flow resistance of the chest wall does not, this component becomes a progressively smaller fraction of the total work as ventilation increases.[21] This method also does not measure the elastic work done on the chest wall and the negative work performed by the inspiratory muscles during early expiration unless the compliance of the chest wall is also measured (which can be difficult to do). Finally, the work performed to distort the chest wall is not measured unless both esophageal and gastric pressure and the volume displacement of the ribcage and abdominal components are also measured; even with these additional measurements, the work done in distorting the shape of the ribcage or abdomen is not measured.

During quiet breathing through the nose, the work of breathing per minute (rate of work or power) is approximately 0.4 kg · m/min or 4 J/min[22] (when 1 L is moved across a pressure gradient of 10 cm H_2O, 0.1 kg · m/L of work is performed). Approximately 80% of this value represents positive work done during inspiration and 20% represents negative work done by the inspiratory muscles during expiration. Ballantine and colleagues[23] measured the work of breathing in 100 untrained healthy young men resting in the semirecumbent position and breathing through a mouthpiece with noseclips applied. Work per min was 0.442 ± 0.274 (SD) kg · m/min, and work per liter was 0.048 ± 0.022 (SD) kg · m/L.

Measurements of the work of breathing are considerably influenced by changes in breathing pattern.[24] Increases in tidal volume will increase elastic work, whereas increases in flow will increase flow-resistive work. The work of breathing per minute (also termed *power*) sharply increases with increases in minute ventilation. For a 15-fold increase in ventilation (from rest to maximal exercise), the mechanical power of breathing increases more than 150-fold.[25, 26]

Several disease states cause an increase in the work of breathing. Diseases that decrease lung or chest wall compliance produce an increase in elastic work,[15, 19, 27] while diseases that increase airflow resistance produce an increase in flow-resistive work.[28] With disease, the work of breathing is particularly affected by the breathing pattern adopted by the patient. Thus, an increase in tidal volume in a patient with interstitial lung disease (decreased lung compliance) increases the elastic work of breathing to a much greater extent than an equivalent increase in tidal volume in a normal subject. Accordingly, patients with decreased lung or chest wall compliance attempt to minimize their work of breathing by adopting a pattern of rapid shallow breathing. When the breathing pattern is measured in such patients at rest, minute ventilation and respiratory frequency are increased compared to healthy controls but tidal volume is not significantly different.[29] However, since minute ventilation is higher in patients with interstitial lung disease, the failure of tidal volume to increase commensurately may be indicative of relatively shallow breathing. Indeed when ventilation is carefully matched during CO_2 rebreathing or exercise, breathing is both rapid and shallow in patients with interstitial lung disease compared with healthy controls.[30] Similarly when normal subjects breathe against an external inspiratory resistive load, inspiratory flow decreases to reduce flow-resistive work and a slow, deep pattern of breathing is usually observed.[31] However, patients with chronic obstructive pulmonary disease (COPD) do not breathe slowly and deeply[29]; presumably, this is related to the fact that the load in patients with COPD is not simply flow resistive but is considerably more complex.[32]

Respiratory Muscle Efficiency

We must appreciate that measurements of mechanical work do not necessarily provide a good indication of the energy expended by the respiratory muscles. For example, during an isometric contraction, no displacement takes place and, therefore, no mechanical work is performed, yet the metabolic cost to generate this force may be substantial. The true energy cost is determined not only by the mechanical workload but also by the efficiency of the respiratory muscles in producing useful work. Measurement of respiratory muscle efficiency requires measurement of the mechanical work of breathing and the energy cost of this work (Vo_2 resp). The ratio of these two measurements yields efficiency. Unfortunately, the metabolic cost of breathing is difficult to measure, and estimates of efficiency range from 1 to 25% between different studies.[14, 33–36]

In addition to measurement difficulties, the efficiency of the respiratory muscles varies depending on the respiratory task. For instance, for the same degree of external work, the O_2 cost of breathing is much greater during resistive loading than during hyperventilation[37] (i.e., respiratory muscle efficiency is reduced during resistive breathing). With these caveats in mind, respiratory muscle efficiency during normal voluntary breathing is of the order of 8 to 10% in normal subjects,[33, 34] but can decrease to 1 to 2% in patients with respiratory disease.

Measurement of Esophageal Pressure

To measure mechanical work during spontaneous breathing an estimate of P_{pl} is required. Von Neergaard and Wirz[38] first suggested that P_{es} might adequately estimate P_{pl}. Subsequently, P_{es} measurements have been compared with direct measurements of P_{pl} in man.[39–41] In these studies, pleural pressure was assessed by producing a small pneumothorax and measuring the pressure within the pneumothorax. Whether these measurements of P_{pl} are truly representative of mean P_{pl} in the absence of a pneumothorax can be questioned. Nevertheless, there was good agreement between P_{es} and P_{pl} measurements provided that the supine posture was avoided. Esophageal pressure is more positive in the supine posture compared with other postures, presumably due to the weight of mediastinal structures compressing the esophagus.[42–44] Thus, P_{es} provides a poor reflection of absolute P_{pl} in the supine posture. However, changes in P_{pl} with respiration can be accurately represented by P_{es} swings in the supine posture.[45]

Esophageal pressure is usually measured with a flexible latex balloon connected to polyehylene tubing, which, in turn, is connected to a differential pressure transducer. Tubing enclosed by the balloon has multiple perforations to allow transmission of the pressure within the balloon. Milic-Emili and colleagues[46] have shown that balloons 10 cm in length, 3.5 cm in perimeter, and 0.06 mm in wall thickness are adequate for pressure measurements. By being long, the balloon allows air to move to the point of most negative pressure reducing artifactual distortions in pressure. The smaller the volume of air inserted into the balloon, the more accurate the absolute pressure measurements.[46] Indeed, Milic-Emili et al. recommend using a variety of balloon volumes and then deriving the true pressure by back extrapolating to zero volume. This method is cumbersome and rarely employed. Instead, a balloon volume of ≤0.5 ml is usually used. Larger volumes of air may be required to prevent collapse of the balloon (which distorts the pressure signal) when large positive pressures are generated during breathing.[47] The balloon should have an unstressed volume close to zero, and when distended to 6 mL, measurable back pressure should not exist. Esophageal pressure measurements are best obtained from the midesophagus.[44] When measurements are obtained from the upper third of the esophagus, artifactual changes in pressure occur with flexion and extension of the neck and with pressure over the trachea. When the balloon is placed in the lower third of the esophagus, greater changes in pressure occur with variations in body position.

Since the pressure within the esophagus and balloon is subatmospheric, the balloon tends to gain air when the pressure tap is open to atmosphere. This air can be removed by having the subject perform a Valsalva maneuver. When inflating the balloon, it is customary to first inject a larger volume (e.g., 8 mL) and then withdraw all but 0.5 mL.

Optimal location of the esophageal balloon can be tested using the occlusion test[45]. When subjects perform static voluntary efforts while maintaining an open glottis, changes in esophageal pressure (ΔP_{es}) should be equal to changes in mouth pressure (ΔP_{mo}). Since airway occlusion prevents airflow, there is no dissipation of pressure due to airflow resistance and, thus, no pressure gradient between the occluded airway opening and the pleural space (i.e., $P_{aw} = P_{pl}$). Therefore, concordance between ΔP_{es} and ΔP_{mo} measurements indicates that the esophageal balloon catheter is adequately positioned to provide a valid measure of changes in P_{pl}. With the occlusion test, the airway opening is occluded at end-expiration and the subject makes an inspiratory effort against the occluded airway. If the $\Delta P_{es}/\Delta P_{mo}$ ratio is close to unity (within 10%), the balloon catheter is adequately positioned in the esophagus. This test is particularly important when measurements are made in the supine posture.

For measurement of work of breathing, it is essential to avoid a phase lag between esophageal pressure and volumetric signals since esophageal pressure at points of zero flow is important for several calculations. Macklem[48] has described a simple method for balancing the two signals.

Measurement of Volume

Changes in lung volume are usually measured at the mouth. However, due to gas compressibility, the change in volume measured at the mouth will underestimate the actual volume displacement of the chest wall.[49] This difference is trivial in normal subjects, but can become quite important during resistive loading or when patients breathe at high lung volumes. Under these conditions, failure to account for gas compressibility results in a significant underestimation of the mechanical work of breathing. This error can be avoided by directly measuring changes in thoracic gas volume with a body plethysmograph or changes in chest wall displacement with a respiratory inductive plethysmograph or magnetometers. Alternatively, if changes in volume are measured at the airway opening, mathematical formulas exist to estimate the work due to gas compressibility.[50]

Measurement of Gastric Pressure

To measure transdiaphragmatic pressure, an estimate of intra-abdominal pressure is required. Traditionally, the abdomen has been likened to a distensible fluid-filled container.[51] A hydrostatic pressure gradient exists within the abdomen and the difference in pressure between any two levels is given by the difference in height multipled by the specific gravity of the liquid. Since pressure swings equilibrate very quickly in a freely communicating liquid, change in pressure will be the same throughout the abdominal cavity. Experimental evidence that the abdomen behaves in this fashion was provided by Duomarco and Rimini[52] many years ago. Recently, Decramer and associates[53] measured local intraabdominal pressure in anesthetized dogs and found marked intraregional differences suggesting that the mechanical behavior of the abdomen may be considerably more complex. This work was subsequently criticized on the basis that pressure catheters inserted directly into the abdominal cavity may be unduly influenced by contiguous solid viscera (which may compress the pressure catheter, thus inflating the measured pressure). In contrast, catheters located in hollow organs may provide a more accurate measure of intra-abdominal pressure since they are protected from the distorting influences of the solid viscera. Mead and colleagues[54] have recently demonstrated that pressure changes within the stomach and rectum are virtually the same in humans during various breathing maneuvers, supporting the view that the abdomen can be considered a single fluid-filled compartment.

In 1960, Agostoni and Rahn[55] measured gastric pressure (P_{ga}) with air-filled balloons and used these measurements to estimate intra-abdominal pressure. As discussed above, this approach is valid as long as the abdomen behaves as a single fluid-filled compartment. The balloon must be filled with sufficient air to float on the surface of the gastric contents (2 mL of air is generally used). Since the stomach moves up and down with the diaphragm, pressure in the gastric air bubble will parallel subdiaphragmatic pressure. Gastric pressure is slightly higher than subdiaphragmatic pressure due to gastric wall tone and a hydrostatic gradient related to the height of the gastric air bubble. This pressure difference can be estimated by assuming that P_{di} is zero at FRC (i.e., $P_{pl} = P_{ab}$). The difference between P_{ga} and P_{es} with the subject relaxed at FRC is subtracted from P_{ga} to obtain P_{ab}. Successful placement of the balloon catheter into the stomach is easily verified by observing positive pressure deflections during inspiratory efforts.

Work of Breathing During Mechanical Ventilation

A common assumption is that patient effort is minimal during mechanically assisted breathing. We now know that patients can perform substantial active inspiratory work during mechanical ventilation. The amount of work that the patient performs can be quantitated in the following fashion. If the patient's inspiratory muscles are totally relaxed, the ventilator will perform all the work required to inflate the lungs and chest wall. The work performed by the mechanical ventilator can be calculated from the area enclosed by a plot of airway pressure and inspired volume (Fig 9–5, A). If the inspiratory muscles are active, the area contained in the airway pressure-inspired volume curve still indicates the work performed by the ventilator but this is no longer the total work (Fig 9–5, B). The difference between these two areas yields the work done by the patient's inspiratory muscles on the lungs and chest wall (Fig 9–5, C). To compare the airway pressure-inspired volume curves during relaxed (Fig 9–5, A) and active inspiration (Fig 9–5, B), the two curves must be generated under identical conditions of inspiratory flow, tidal volume, and respiratory frequency. Furthermore, the assumption is made that the total work required to inflate the lungs and chest wall is the same for active and passive contractions

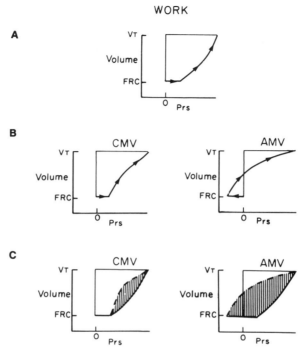

WORK

FIG 9–5.
Subtraction of the area subtended by the inflation pressure-volume curve in the presence of inspiratory muscle activity, **B,** from that recorded during passive inflation, **A,** yields the inspiratory work performed by the patient (*shaded areas,* **C**). CMV = controlled mechanical ventilation. AMV = assisted mechanical ventilation. *(From Ward ME, Corbail C, Gibbons W, et al: Optimization of respiratory muscle relaxation during mechanical ventilation. Anesthesiol 1988; 69:29–35. Used by permisison.)*

(an assumption that may not be entirely correct; see the section on measurement of mechanical work of breathing).

During controlled mechanical ventilation, inspiratory muscle activity can be virtually eliminated if inspiratory flow rates are adequate to meet patient demand and the patient is mildly hyperventilated[56–58] (i.e., a reduction in Pco_2 of 2 to 6 mm Hg). Examination of the airway pressure curve can be used to infer whether inspiratory muscle activity is present. In the absence of inspiratory muscle activity, airway pressure curves are characterized by a smooth rise and the curves are monotonously uniform from breath to breath. In contrast, when the inspiratory muscles are active, the curves lose their smooth contour and their shape varies from breath to breath. During assisted mechanical ventilation, the patient makes an inspiratory effort, which decreases airway pressure and, in turn, triggers the ventilator to deliver a mechanical breath (usually 1 to 2 cm H_2O at the most sensitive setting). Conceptually, if the inspiratory muscles are to be spared from performing substantial active work during assisted ventilation, inspiratory effort must cease with the onset of the machine-delivered breath. However, inspiratory effort typically continues following the onset of a machine-delivered breath. Marini and colleagues[59] have shown that the active work performed by the inspiratory muscle during assisted ventilation (at the most favorable ventilatory settings) averages 33 to 50% of total work in normal subjects[59] and 33 ±19% of total work in ventilator-dependent patients.[56] Furthermore, when calculated as a fraction of the total work performed during spontaneous breathing, the work performed by the inspiratory muscles during assisted ventilation was on average 63%, with a range 30 to 116%[56]; total work during spontaneous breathing was lower than total work during mechanical ventilation due to differences in minute ventilation and breathing pattern.

These measurements may underestimate the amount of patient work since this method does not measure work performed in distorting the chest wall. Reduced trigger sensitivity of the ventilator, inadequate inspiratory flow rates, and increased ventilatory requirements can all increase the amount of work performed by a patient during mechanical ventilation. Similarly, during intermittent mandatory ventilation (IMV), substantial patient work is performed during machine-assisted breaths at all levels of ventilatory support.[60] The effects of inspiratory pressure support, a relatively new mode of ventilatory assistance, on the work of breathing have been recently examined.[61] With pressure support, a constant preset positive airway pressure is maintained throughout inspiration. Respiratory rate, tidal volume and inspiratory time are regulated by the patient. Initial studies with pressure support suggest that both patient inspiratory work per liter of ventilation and patient work/min (i.e., power) progressively decrease with increasing levels of pressure support. Thus, this method of ventilatory support may allow the clinician to more easily titrate the degree of patient work; further studies are required to confirm this finding. Note that response times, algorithms for maintaining and terminating pressure support, and pressure/flow characteristics during pressure support vary with ventilator type—factors that affect the work of breathing.[62]

Work of Breathing During Weaning from Mechanical Ventilation

Fleury and coworkers[63] measured the work of breathing in patients with COPD in acute respiratory failure during a trial of spontaneous breathing. Total inspiratory work of breathing per minute was approximately twice that of normal subjects: 1.52 ± 0.36 and 0.76 ± 0.54 kg $\cdot$ m/min, respectively. Total inspiratory work per liter of ventilation was 0.19 ± 0.05 kg $\cdot$ m/L compared with 0.09 ± 0.02 kg $\cdot$ m/L in normal subjects. Inspiratory work per liter of ventilation was strongly correlated with measurements of pulmonary mechanics (compliance and resistance). Inspiratory work per minute, however, was not significantly correlated with measurements of pulmonary mechanics due to the fact that inspiratory power is disproportionately affected by a patient's minute ventilation. Both the severity of derangements in pulmonary mechanics and the patient's ventilatory requirements are important during weaning. Thus, both work per minute and work per liter of ventilation could have predictive value during weaning.

Fiastro and colleagues[64] measured the work of spontaneous breathing in patients successfully weaned from mechanical ventilation and in patients who were ventilator dependent. These authors recorded transpulmonary pressure ($P_{es} - P_{aw}$) and flow and, thus, they only measured work performed on the lungs; since all patients had parenchymal lung disease, increases in the work of breathing should be primarily due to increases in work performed on the lungs. The patients studied were a heterogenous group including patients with COPD and patients with decreased lung compliance (ARDS). Both work per minute and work per liter of ventilation were found to be important in predicting weaning outcome. Successful weaning was achieved when inspiratory work/min was ≤1.60 kg · m/min and inspiratory work per liter was ≤0.14 kg · m/L. These threshold values were achieved in all patients prior to successful weaning and were not present during unsuccessful weaning trials. Importantly, neither index, when taken on its own (work per minute, work per liter), was as good at predicting weaning outcome as the combination of the two factors.

Several studies have examined the value of work measurements in predicting weaning outcome in postoperative patients.[65-67] These studies measured work performed on the lungs only (i.e., measured transpulmonary pressure and flow). Henning and colleagues[65] reported that patients remain ventilator dependent when the work rate was >1.7 kg · m/min, whereas spontaneous ventilation could usually be resumed if the work rate was ≤1.0 kg · m/min. Peters and coworkers[66] found that patients generally required mechanical ventilation when the work rate was ≥1.8 kg · m/min or the work per liter was ≥0.180 kg · m/L. However, for each of the work indices, considerable overlap occurred between ventilator-dependent and ventilator-independent patients. Proctor and Woolson[67] measured work rate in a large number of postoperative patients (657 measurements in 168 patients). These authors found that a work rate of 1.34 kg · m/min provided the best separation of ventilator-dependent and ventilator-independent patients. However, this threshold work rate value was associated with a false-positive rate of 14% and a false-negative rate of 14%. Unfortunately, in these three studies, the combination of work rate and work per liter of ventilation as a predictor of weaning outcome was not assessed. It is obvious that the threshold values of work differ between the various studies. Furthermore, these threshold values were all determined on a *post hoc* basis, and the predictive value of work measurements has never been examined in a prospective fashion. We may conclude from these studies that the work of breathing is generally higher in ventilator-dependent than ventilator-independent patients. However, the predictive value of work of breathing measurements as an index of weaning outcome remains to be determined.

Measurement of the work of breathing during spontaneous breathing requires insertion of an esophageal balloon catheter and the ability to integrate the pressure-flow product or to measure the area enclosed by the relevant pressure-volume curve. Instrumentation to make these measurements is not routinely available at the bedside. However, measurements of the work required to inflate the respiratory system passively during mechanical ventilation can be more easily obtained[68] (see the section on work of breathing during mechanical ventilation). The limitations of measurements of work under passive conditions reflecting the amount of work performed when the inspiratory muscles are active have been discussed previously. Nevertheless, such measurements should reflect the severity of pulmonary mechanical derangement (and measurement of work rate should also reflect the patient's ventilatory requirements) and, thus, may be of some value in predicting weaning outcome. Hubmayr and colleagues[69] measured the work of breathing during passive inflation in five postoperative patients without significant cardiorespiratory disease who were easy to extubate and five patients who were ventilator-dependent with respiratory failure of diverse causes. Work rate and work per liter of ventilation (derived from Table 2, Ref. 69) were not significantly different between the two patient groups. Furthermore, the work rate did not predict weaning outcome. These results are discouraging, but further work in a larger number of patients is required to determine whether such measurements are of any value in predicting weaning outcome.

TRANSDIAPHRAGMATIC PRESSURE

Measurement of the pressures that can be generated during maximal inspiratory (PI_{max}) and expiratory (PE_{max}) efforts against an occluded airway provide a measure of the global strength of the repiratory muscles.[70] However, despite careful coaching, some subjects cannot perform PI_{max} and PE_{max} manuevers. In addition, these pressures do not directly reflect the function of the diaphragm, which is the single most important respiratory muscle, being responsible for about two-thirds of tidal volume during quiet breathing.[71]

In 1960, Agostoni and Rahn[72] described the technique of simultaneously measuring esophageal and gastric pressures (P_{es} and P_{ga}, respectively) as a method of investigating the contributions of different respiratory muscle groups. Balloon catheters can be placed in the esophagus and stomach (as described earlier), and the pressure across the diaphragm (transdiaphragmatic pressure, P_{di}) is calcualted as $P_{di} = P_{ga} - P_{es}$. Measurement of P_{di} has become a standard method of evaluating the force-generating capacity of the diaphragm in various experimental settings. In addition, measurement of P_{di} has been proposed as a clinical tool to diagnose severe weakness or paralysis of the diaphragm, since other diagnostic approaches such as fluoroscopy can be quite misleading[72] (Fig 9–6). However, considerable variability in the values of $P_{di,max}$ have been reported among normal subjects,[55, 73–77] making it important to pay particular attention to the method of making the measurement.

Methods of Measuring P_{di}

Slow Inspiration to Total Lung Capacity. — When using this method to measure P_{di}, the patient inspires slowly (0.1 to 0.2 L/sec, i.e., quasistatic maneuver) to total lung capacity (TLC). At TLC, the diaphragm is shortened to about 60% of its resting length, and since muscle strength decreases with reductions in muscle length, this method results in lower values of P_{di} than when measurements are obtained at functional residual capacity (FRC) or residual volume (RV).[74] Using this approach in 10 healthy men and 10 healthy women, De Troyer and Estenne[75] found Pi_{di} values of 48 $\pm$ 12 (SD) and 30 $\pm$ 11 cm H_2O, respectively. In a study of 15 patients with COPD, Fracchia et al.[78] reported P_{di} values of 79 $\pm$ 32 cm H_2O with this technique. In general, this is probably the least popular method of measuring P_{di}.

Maximal Static P_{di}.—Measuring P_{di} during a maximal static inspiratory effort against an occluded airway (a Mueller-type maneuver) is the usual method of measuring $P_{di,max}$. In a study of 20 untrained, healthy subjects, De Troyer and Estenne[75] noted enormous variability in maximal static measurements of P_{di} made at 60% of TLC following an inspiration from FRC (Table 9–1). The subjects were not given instructions as to how to perform the maneuver nor were they provided with a visual display of the tracings. The wide variability in P_{di} was due to differences in the pattern of recruiting different respiratory muscle groups. This was

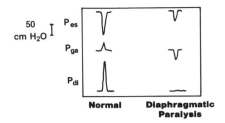

FIG 9–6.
Measurement of transdiaphragmatic pressure (P_{di}) in a normal subject and in a patient with bilateral diaphragmatic paralysis. P_{di} is measured by inserting balloon catheters into the esophagus and stomach; P_{di} is then electrically calculated by subtracting esophageal pressure (P_{es}) from gastric pressure (P_{ga}). When a patient with diaphragmatic paralysis makes a maximal inspiratory effort, the negative P_{es} generated by the other respiratory muscles pulls the flaccid diaphragm cephalad thereby resulting in a fall in P_{ga}. *(From Tobin MJ. Essentials of Critical Care Medicine. New York, Churchill Livingstone, 1989, p. 232. Used by permission.)*

reflected in particular by the large coefficient of variation (i.e., standard deviation divided by the mean and expressed as a percentage) in the P_{ga} values: half of the subjects developed a positive P_{ga} in association with a negative P_{pl}; 35% developed no change in P_{ga}; and the remaining 15% developed a fall in P_{ga}, indicating strong recruitment of the intercostal and accessory muscles with upward displacement of the diaphragm. In the subjects who developed a negative P_{ga}, a three- to six-fold increase in P_{di} was noted when the subjects were instructed to move their abdomen outward during inspiration (diaphragmatic Mueller maneuver).

Miller et al.[77] noted similar findings in 64 healthy subjects who performed maximal static inspiratory efforts at RV (Table 9–1). In this study, a visual display of the P_{es} tracing was provided to encourage the subject to make a maximal effort, and the subjects were requested to sustain the pressure for at least 1 sec. In addition, the maneuver was practiced a number of times, and a small leak was incorporated into the mouthpiece to keep the glottis open to ensure that action of the respiratory muscles was being measured rather than that of the buccinator muscles. As in the case of the study by De Troyer and Estenne,[75] wide variation in the P_{ga} measurements were noted and many of the values were negative (Table 9–1).

Laporta and Grassino[79] studied the measurement of $P_{di,max}$ in healthy untrained volunteers (nine men and one woman) using five different respiratory maneuvers. The measurements were made at FRC in the seated position, and great care was taken to maintain a fixed posture. The maneuvers consisted of:

1. PI_{max}, Mueller-type maneuver against closed airways
2. PI_{max}, Mueller-type maneuver with a mouthpiece containing a 1-mm hole to achieve a small leak
3. Abdominal expulsive maneuver (requested to "bear down")
4. Two-step maneuver consisting of first performing maneuver 3 and then adding maneuver 1
5. Feedback maneuver whereby P_{pl} and P_{ga} were displayed on a storage oscilloscope and the subject was allowed to combine an abdominal expulsive maneuver with a Mueller maneuver according to his or her choice.

TABLE 9–1.
Respiratory Pressures During Maximal Inspiratory Efforts

Author	Lung Volume		Mean (cm H_2O)	Range (cm H_2O)	CV %
DeTroyer[75]	FRC	Men	P_{es} −100	−64 to −126	20
		($n = 10$)	P_{ga} −1	−80 to 31	3927
			P_{di} 99	18 to 137	40
		Women	P_{es} −87	−68 to −123	20
		($n = 10$)	P_{ga} −3.6	−42 to 52	836
			P_{di} 83	36 to 120	37
		Total	P_{es} −93	−64 to −126	21
		($n = 20$)	P_{ga} −2	−80 to 52	1421
			P_{di} 91	18 to 137	39
Miller[77]	RV	Men	P_{es} −98	−38 to −164	28
		($n = 37$)	P_{ga} 10	−26 to 84	270
			P_{di} 108	52 to 164	27
		Women	P_{es} −62	−24 to −120	38
		($n = 27$)	P_{ga} 2	−22 to 88	942
			P_{di} 65	16 to 140	48
		Total	P_{es} −83	−24 to −164	38
		($n = 64$)	P_{ga} 7	−22 to 88	370
			P_{di} 90	16 to 164	41
Laporta[79]	FRC	Total	P_{es} −69	?	55
		($n = 10$)	P_{ga} 76	−8 to 148	70
			P_{di} 145	?	23
Laporta[79]	FRC	Total	P_{es} −70	?	34
	+Feedback	($n = 10$)	P_{ga} 110	63 to 143	20
			P_{di} 180	?	8

The $P_{di,max}$ values with the simple Mueller maneuver were higher than those recorded by De Troyer and Estenne[75] or Miller et al.,[77] although the marked variability in P_{ga} values was again noted (Table 9–1). The highest and most reproducible $P_{di,max}$ values were noted with the feedback maneuver (#5) (Table 9–1). Unlike the simple Mueller-type maneuver, which frequently resulted in negative P_{ga} values, the feedback maneuver resulted in higher and consistently positive P_{ga} values; it had no effect on P_{es} values. This suggests that visual feedback enhances the subject's control over the degree to which his or her diaphragm is activated.

Furthermore, even in well-trained subjects, the $P_{di,max}$ during a feedback maneuver is higher than that obtained during a Mueller manuever.[80] The mechanism for this difference is somewhat controversial. Although suboptimal activation of the diaphragm is likely to be a factor in untrained subjects, even in well-trained subjects, in whom maximal activation of the diaphragm has been clearly documented, the $P_{di,max}$ during a Mueller maneuver is still lower than that achieved during a feedback maneuver.[81, 82] Clearly other mechanisms must be important. During a feedback maneuver, the abdominal muscles are activated along with the diaphragm. Abdominal muscle activity may change diaphragmatic geometry (length and/or shape) and so alter the force it can generate.[83] In addition, abdominal muscle activity could produce stretching of the contracted diaphragm (pliometric contraction).[84] Compared with an isometric contraction, greater tension is generated if muscle length increases while it contracts.[85]

Evidence to support this latter mechanism has been provided recently.[84] Thus, measurement of $P_{di,max}$ during a feedback maneuver may overestimate the inspiratory pressure-generating capacity of the diaphragm. Furthermore, patients have considerable difficulty in performing this maneuver correctly.

Sniff P_{di}.—In the study of Laporta and Grassino,[79] the combined Mueller-abdominal explosive maneuver produced the highest and most reproducible results. However, many patients find it difficult to perform this maneuver. In contrast, most subjects and patients are able to perform a sniff, i.e., a short, sharp, voluntary inspiratory effort through the nostrils with the mouth closed. Miller et al.[77] measured P_{es}, P_{ga}, and Pi_{di} in 64 healthy subjects who performed maximal sniffs "free-style" through the nose at FRC without a mouthpiece or noseclips. The subjects could see their P_{di} tracings on an oscilloscope screen, and body movement was not restricted. Compared with the P_{di} values during a maximal static inspiratory maneuver (same subjects as in Table 9–1), the sniff P_{di} values were higher in 92% of the subjects and the normal range was narrower: 82 to 204 versus 16 to 164 cm H_2O, respectively (Table 9–2).

Reproducibility was assessed by repeating the measurements on three separate days in 8 subjects: the coefficient of variation was 7% for P_{di} during a sniff versus 13% for P_{di} during a PI_{max} manuever. The fact that P_{di} values were higher during a sniff compared with a PI_{max} maneuver is somewhat surprising. If both maneuvers were performed optimally, the P_{di} achieved during a PI_{max} maneuver should be higher than that during a sniff, since PI_{max} is a quasistatic maneuver while the sniff is a dynamic maneuver. The observation that P_{di} during a sniff was higher than P_{di} during a PI_{max} maneuver in 92% of subjects suggests that the PI_{max} maneuver was not performed optimally in the vast majority of subjects. Therefore, from a clinical perspective, measuring P_{di} during a sniff maneuver should be more useful in assessing diaphragmatic strength in patients.

In a study of 61 patients being evaluated for respiratory muscle dysfunction, Laroche et al.[86] compared esophageal pressure generated during a maximal sniff (sniff P_{es}) with mouth pressure during a maximal inspiration against a closed airway (PI_{max}). The sniff P_{es} values were

TABLE 9–2.
Respiratory Pressures During Maximal Sniffs*

Subjects	Mean (cm H_2O)	Range (cm H_2O)	CV %
Men	P_{es} −105	−52 to −150	16
($n = 37$)	P_{ga} 43	0 to 134	75
	P_{di} 148	112 to 204	16
Women	P_{es} −92	−52 to −140	21
($n = 27$)	P_{ga} 29	0 to 108	100
	P_{ga} 122	82 to 182	21
Total	P_{es} −100	−52 to −150	20
($n = 64$)	P_{ga} 37	0 to 134	85
	P_{ga} 137	82 to 204	20

* Based on data by Miller et al: *Clin Sci* 1985; 69:91–96.

higher than the $P_{I_{max}}$ values in 90% of the patients. Of importance, 11 patients (18%) had a low $P_{I_{max}}$ value and a normal sniff P_{es} value: P_{di} values were normal or only moderately reduced in these 11 patients. This indicates that many patients judged to have respiratory muscle weakness on the basis of $P_{I_{max}}$ measurements turn out to be normal when assessed by P_{es} sniff. Difficulties with the $P_{I_{max}}$ technique are likely to have been responsible for the falsely low values. Measurement of P_{es} is appealing since only a single balloon catheter is required, whereas two balloon catheters are needed to measure P_{di}.

More recently, Koulouris et al.[87] evaluated the relationship between P_{es} with nasopharyngeal pressure (P_{np}) and pressure within the mouth (P_{mo}) during maximal sniffs. In 10 healthy subjects and 12 patients with inspiratory muscle weakness, the sniff P_{np}/P_{es} ratio was 0.92 and 0.90, respectively, and the sniff P_{mo}/P_{es} ratio was 0.95 and 0.87, respectively. This indicates that these less invasive measurements were useful in the assessment of inspiratory muscle function. However, in patients with COPD, transmission of changes in alveolar pressure to the mouth is slower than normal[88] and, thus, may be incomplete during a sniff maneuver. Preliminary work suggests that sniff P_{np} underestimates sniff P_{es} in patients with COPD and the magnitude of this difference correlates with the abnormality in lung mechanics.[89] Thus, when using a sniff maneuver to evaluate respiratory muscle function in patients with COPD, it is preferable to use P_{es} measurements. In another study,[90] Koulouris et al. demonstrated the importance of standardizing posture when performing these measurements. Switching from the seated to the supine posture caused sniff P_{di} and shiff P_{es} to fall from 133 and 108 cm H_2O, respectively, to 109 and 99 cm H_2O, respectively.

Phrenic Nerve Stimulation

The most sophisticated method of studying respiratory muscle contractility is to measure the muscle force resulting from electrical stimulation. Transdiaphragmatic pressure (P_{di}) is substituted for diaphragmatic force, since the latter cannot be directly measured in humans. This technique has the added attraction of being independent of patient motivation.

The phrenic nerve is stimulated at the posterior border of the sternomastoid muscle at the level of the cricoid cartilage.[91–95] Surface, or less commonly needle, electrodes are used to deliver impulses to one or both phrenic nerves. A unidirectional square-wave impulse of 0.1 msec duration is applied. The diaphragmatic EMG is recorded to ensure constant phrenic nerve stimulation; the compound muscle action potential will fade if the stimulating electrode gets displaced.[93] The optimal position is determined by adjusting the stimulating electrode and increasing the voltage until no further increase in the muscle action potential is achieved[96–98]; the required voltage varies[94, 97–99] from 50 to 160 V. The voltage is then increased by 10 to 50% to ensure supramaximal stimulation.[96–100] A force-frequency or pressure-frequency curve of the diaphragm is generated by stimulating the phrenic nerve at various frequencies (10, 20, 50, and 100 Hz) and recording the resulting increase in P_{di}. To activate the diaphragm maximally, stimulation frequencies of 100 Hz are required.[93, 94] Such supramaximal tetanic stimulation of the phrenic nerve is very painful and also difficult to achieve because of electrode movement due to unavoidable costimulation of the neck muscles.[96] Consequently, phrenic nerve stimulation at a frequency of 1 Hz (twitch P_{di}) has become popular.[95, 97, 98] Like any other skeletal muscle, the pressure developed by the diaphragm depends on muscle length and geometry. Accordingly, measurements are usually made while the patient holds his or her glottis closed at FRC, and end-expiratory lung volume is monitored by inductive plethysmography or end-expiratory transpulmonary pressure recordings.[95, 96] To further ensure constancy of the chest wall configuration, a cast can be placed around the abdomen and the lower quarter of the rib cage.

Phrenic nerve conduction time is measured as the time from stimulus artifact to the onset of the diaphragm muscle action potential.[92] In a study of 50 normal subjects, Meir et al.[97] found that the conduction times were 6.94 ± 0.77 (SD) msec for the right and 6.61 ± 0.77 msec for the left phrenic nerve, with upper 99% confidence limits of 9.25 and 8.92 msec, respectively. Prolonged conduction times are observed with phrenic neuritis, mediastinal tumors, surgical trauma, and peripheral neuropathies. A normal conduction time does not exclude a pathologic process, since it can be normal in the presence of axonal degenerative neuropathy if some fast fibers are spared.

Meir et al.[98] also examined the usefulness of twitch P_{di} measurements in the routine evaluation of patients with respiratory muscle weakness. In 20 healthy subjects, twitch P_{di} during bilateral phrenic nerve sitmulation was 20.7 ± 5.3 (SD) cm H_2O, with a very wide range: 8.8 to 33.1 cm H_2O. These values showed considerable overlap with the values in 10 patients with diaphragmatic weakness, 15.1 ± 9.4 cm H_2O, range 3.1 to 26.8 cm H_2O. Only 4 patients had twitch P_{di} values that were below the values in the healthy subjects.

Clinical Usefulness of P_{di} Measurements

Newson-Davis et al.[72] were among the first investigators to recommend the use of P_{di} measurements in the clinical evaluation of patients with severe weakness or paralysis of the diaphragm. They studied eight patients with clinical features suggestive of diaphragmatic weakness. The change in P_{di} during the course of a maximum inspiration was zero in five patients and 2 to 6 cm H_2O in the remaining three patients, compared with >25 cm H_2O in healthy subjects. Fluoroscopy of the diaphragm was frequently misleading, since paradoxical movement (cephalad during inspiration) was observed in only one of the six patients in whom it was performed.

Mier-Jedrzejowicz et al.[101] studied 30 patients suspected of diaphragmatic weakness. They measured P_{di} during three voluntary maneuvers: maximal sniffs, slow smooth maximal inhalations to TLC, and maximal static inspiratory maneuvers (Table 9–3). Sniff P_{di} was abnormal in all patients, whereas P_{di} during a slow inspiration to TLC and during a maximal static maneuver was abnormal in 77 and 30% of the patients, respectively. Of importance, the presence of diaphragmatic weakness could not be predicted from pulmonary function tests [TLC, RV, vital capacity (VC), forced expiratory volume in 1 second (FEV_1)] or chest x ray in many of the patients.

In what clinical circumstances should P_{di} be measured? If diaphragmatic paralysis is suspected, other simpler tests should first be performed. Vital capacity should be measured in the standing and supine positions, and Allen et al.[102] have shown that a fall in vital capacity of >25% on switching to the supine position should arouse suspicion of significant diaphragmatic dysfunction. If unilateral diaphragmatic paralysis is suspected, fluoroscopy can be useful.

TABLE 9–3.
Measurements of P_{di} in Patients with Diaphragmatic Weakness*

Technique	Subjects	Mean (cm H$_2$O)	Range (cm H$_2$O)	Normal (cm H$_2$O)
Sniff	men (n = 18)	55	7 to 97	>98
	women (n = 12)	38	15 to 65	>70
Slow inspiration to TLC	total (n = 30)	19	0 to 50	>25
Maximal static maneuver	total (n = 30)	31	0 to 85	>18

* Data from Mier-Jedrejowicz et al: *Am Rev Respir Dis* 1988; 137:877–883.

Normally, the diaphragm descends during a sniff. With unilateral diaphragmatic paralysis, the affected hemidiaphragm paradoxically ascends during a sniff maneuver in the supine posture. There should be at least 2 cm of paradoxic motion of the entire hemidiaphragm for a study to be considered abnormal, and the abdominal muscles should be relaxed during the examination. Unfortunately, Alexander[103] observed paradoxic motion of one hemidiaphragm in 6% of normal subjects. Fluoroscopy is less helpful when the hemidiaphragm is weak but not completely paralyzed, and it can be particularly misleading when the diaphragm is affected bilaterally.[72] Diaphragmatic weakness produces a fall in PI_{max} (measured at the mouth), although PI_{max} may be near normal if other respiratory muscles are normal.[104] Thus, high values (>80 cm H$_2$O) of PI_{max} and PE_{max} virtually exclude clinically important respiratory muscle weakness.[104] While a low PI_{max} value may be due to severe respiratory muscle weakness, it may be also due to poor technique, and measurements of P_{di}, P_{es}, or P_{np} should be performed. In the clinical setting, measurement of these pressures during a sniff appears to be the simplest method of assessment.

Relative Changes in Esophageal and Gastric Pressures

Konno and Mead[105] proposed that the respiratory system can be considered to be a simple physical system with two moving parts, the rib cage and abdomen. These authors demonstrated that the respiratory system has two degrees of freedom of motion. By plotting motion of the rib cage and abdomen on an *XY* plot (the Konno-Mead plot), one can obtain useful information regarding the coordination and relative activity of different respiratory muscle groups.[70] Another way of studying respiratory muscle activity and coordination is by plotting delta P_{pl} against ΔP_{ga}. To calculate the $\Delta P_{ga}/\Delta P_{es}$ ratio, absolute end-expiratory and end-inspiratory gastric and esophageal pressures are measured at points of zero flow, and the delta values are defined as the pressure change between these two points. During normal inspiration, ΔP_{pl} becomes more negative while ΔP_{ga} becomes more positive (Fig 9–7). The magnitude of the increase in P_{ga} normally exceeds the magnitude of the decrease in P_{es}, with the result[106] that the $\Delta P_{ga}/\Delta P_{es}$ ratio is ≤ -1. In healthy seated subjects, Lisboa et al.[107] found an average $\Delta P_{ga}/\Delta P_{es}$ ratio of -1.95 ± 0.86 (SD). Although the $\Delta P_{ga}/\Delta P_{es}$ ratio was generally more negative than −1.0, the least negative value obtained during repetitive testing was −0.62. In general, the more negative the $\Delta P_{ga}/\Delta P_{es}$ ratio, the greater the contribution of the diaphragm.[108] In the presence of diaphragmatic weakness, increasing use of the intercostal and accessory muscles occurs during inspiration. As a result, a given decrease in P_{es} will be associated with a smaller than normal increase in P_{ga}, and the $\Delta P_{ga}/\Delta P_{es}$ ratio will be between −1 and zero.[109] With more severe diaphragmatic weakness, P_{ga} will usually decrease during inspiration, and the $\Delta P_{ga}/\Delta P_{es}$ ratio will exceed zero. In the presence of complete diaphragmatic paralysis, all of the negative intrathoracic pressure will be transmitted across the flaccid diaphragm, so that the swings in the $\Delta P_{ga}/\Delta P_{es}$ ratio will have a value of approximately +1 (Fig 9–7).

In a recent study of 18 patients with unilateral and bilateral diaphragmatic weakness, Hillman and Finucane[109] found a $\Delta P_{ga}/\Delta P_{es}$ ratio between −0.83 and 1.19, with a mean value of 0.28 ± 0.7 (SD), and a close correlation was observed between the $\Delta P_{ga}/\Delta P_{es}$ ratio and $P_{di,max}$ ($r = 0.89$). Similarly, Lisboa and colleagues[107] found a $\Delta P_{ga}/\Delta P_{es}$ ratio of 0.05 ± 0.80 (SD) in 15 patients with unilateral diaphragmatic paralysis. In this study, the $\Delta P_{ga}/\Delta P_{es}$ ratio was not significantly correlated with $P_{di,max}$. However, when one outlying patient was excluded from analysis, the correlation between the two variables became significant ($r = 0.74$). In the supine posture, a positive $\Delta P_{ga}/\Delta P_{es}$ ratio is associated with a pattern of paradoxic motion of the abdomen on a Konno-Mead plot. In the erect posture, however, abdominal muscle contraction during expiration with relaxation during the subsequent inspiration can lead to normal outward movement of the abdomen despite a decrease in P_{ga} during inspiration. Paradoxic abdominal motion may also result from abdominal muscle contraction during inspiration; this can be distinguished from diaphragmatic paralysis using a $\Delta P_{ga}/\Delta P_{es}$ plot, since P_{ga} will increase rather than decrease during inspiration. The $\Delta P_{ga}/\Delta P_{es}$ plots can help to evaluate diaphragmatic weakness, particularly in patients who have difficulty performing a maximal maneuver.

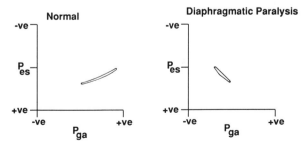

FIG 9–7.
Plot of esophageal pressure (P_{es}) versus gastric pressure (P_{ga}). During normal inspiration, P_{es} becomes progressively more negative as P_{ga} becomes more positive. In diaphragmatic paralysis, both P_{es} and P_{ga} become increasingly negative.

PRESSURE-TIME PRODUCT

Of the many factors that lead to muscle fatigue, the duration of a contraction and the tension developed by a muscle appear to be very important. Interest in tension and timing can be traced back to studies of myocardial energetics, where Sarnoff et al.[110] showed that myocardial O_2 utilization was closely related to a tension-time index, and that it showed little relationship to the heart's external work *per se*. Sarnoff et al.[110] calculated tension-time index as the product of mean systolic pressure and the duration of systole, and it was equivalent to the area under the systolic portion of the pressure curve. In studies of respiratory system energetics, the O_2 cost of breathing (V_{O_2} resp) is measured as the difference between the total body O_2 consumption when the respiratory muscles are at rest and total body O_2 consumption when the respiratory muscles are performing a certain task. In 1961, McGregor and Becklake[111] reported that V_{O_2} resp was more cloesly related to a force or tension-time index than to external mechanical work, similar to the findings in the isolated heart. Their index was calculated as the change in P_{es} from its end-expiratory level (irrespective of sign) integrated against time for the whole breath. In pointing out the poor relationship between external mechanical work and energy requirements, McGregor and Becklake[111] gave the example of how energy utilization will be very high when breathing against an obstructed airway, although mechanical work will be zero. A similar inspiratory pleural pressure-time index was shown by Rochester and Bettini[112] to be closely related to diaphragmatic energy expenditure in dogs. Martin et al.[113] also used a pressure-time product as a means of indirectly assessing energy utilization by the respiratory muscles in patients with asthma. This was derived by integrating the area between the curve of P_{es} and the corresponding relaxation pressure of the chest wall against time; a similar index was also calculated with P_{di} measurements.

In a highly influential paper, Bellemare and Grassino[114] described a different approach to tension and time. They reasoned that since the diaphragm contracts mainly during inspiration, the relative duration of inspiration (T_I) to the duration of the total respiratory cycle (T_{TOT}) should be an important determinant of diaphragmatic fatigue. In healthy subjects breathing against resistive loads of varying magnitude, they examined the relative importance of the mean transdiaphragmatic pressure swing developed during each inspiration (mean P_{di}) and T_I/T_{TOT} in determining the time that a target pressure could be sustained (T_{lim}). They found that the ratios of mean $P_{di}/P_{di,max}$ and T_I/T_{TOT} were equally important as determinants of diaphragmatic fatigue. They combined these factors into a tension time index of the diaphragm (TT_{di}), calculated as

$$TT_{di} = \text{mean } P_{di}/P_{di}\text{max} \times T_I/T_{TOT}$$

During inspiratory resistive loading, they observed a progressive fall in T_{lim} as TT_{di} was increased (Table 9–4), but that below a critical TT_{di} value of 0.15, breathing could be sustained indefinitely. Normal subjects breathing at rest have a TT_{di} value of 0.02, indicating approximately an eightfold reserve.[115]

In a subsequent study from that laboratory, Field et al.[115] reported that the O_2 cost of

TABLE 9–4.
Relationship Between Tension-Time Index of the
Diaphragm and Endurance Time*

TT_{di}	T_{lim}(min)
≤0.15	>45
0.24	25 to 35
0.32	7 to 15
0.42	1 to 3
0.60	0.5 to 1
0.75	0 to 0.5

* Based on data from Bellemare F, Grassino A: *J Appl Physiol* 1982; 53:1190–1195.

breathing (Vo_2 resp) in healthy subjects breathing against resistive loads could be better predicted by TT_{di} than by work of breathing (correlations of $r = 0.74$ and 0.31, respectively). This suggests that the development and maintenance of diaphragmatic muscle tension is the major determinant of Vo_2 resp, and that little O_2 is utilized by other factors such as the degree of muscle shortening or work performed. However, even in this study, the relationship between TT_{di} and Vo_2 resp varied with tidal volume. When the tidal volume was less than 1.25 L, the correlation between TT_{di} and Vo_2 resp was 0.86, whereas when the tidal volume was greater than 1.25 L, the correlation between TT_{di} and Vo_2 was only 0.58, suggesting that other factors may be important.

Collett et al.[116] reinvestigated this question in healthy subjects breathing against inspiratory resistive loads. They obtained a pressure-time *product* by electrically integrating negative mouth pressure with respect to time ($\int pdt$), which was equivalent to mean $P_m \times T_I$, and they also calculated a pressure-time *index* by relating each of these components to $P_{m,max}$ and T_{TOT}, respectively. They found that pressure-time product was an accurate index of Vo_2 resp only when inspiratory flow was constant; at a given pressure-time product, Vo_2 resp increased as inspiratory flow increased. The product of inspiratory flow and pressure-time product, which is equal to work rate, was a good predictor of Vo_2 resp. Subsequent studies by Clanton et al.[117] and McCool et al.[118] demonstrated that at a given pressure-time product, increases in inspiratory flow rate produced a decrease in respiratory muscle endurance. Inspiratory flow rate is thought to reflect the velocity of muscle shortening, which is known to affect directly the energy requirements of the respiratory muscles (the Fenn effect).[119] As a result of the force-velocity relationship, an increase in inspiratory flow leads to a decrease in P_{max}, and, thus, an increase in the mean P_m/P_{max} ratio at a given target pressure.

A problem in studies of respiratory muscle energetics is that many of the major determinants are interdependent on each other, which makes it difficult to sort out which of the factors is responsible for increases in Vo_2 resp. In a study where tidal volume, mean inspiratory mouth pressure, T_I/T_{TOT} and, hence, pressure-time product were kept constant, Dodd et al.[120] found that an increasing work rate produced a proportional decrease in endurance time (correlation, $r = 0.87$). Similarly, during inspiratory resistance loading, Cerny and colleagues[121] found that increases in work rate produced a proportional decrease in endurance time ($r = 0.62$)

when the TT_{di} and tidal volume were held constant. These studies suggest that work rate is an important independent determinant of Vo_2 resp. Theoretically, increases in respiratory frequency could increase Vo_2 resp since additional energy is required to initiate a contraction in muscle strips (activation heat).[122] However, a threefold increase in frequency, from 10.5 to 30.6 breaths/min, had no effect on Vo_2 resp when the pressure-time product and work rate were held constant.[123] Furthermore, changes in respiratory frequency had no effect on endurance time during threshold loading when the pressure-time index, work rate, and inspiratory flow rate were held constant.[117] These results suggests that frequency *per se* is unlikely to significantly affect Vo_2 resp.

As discussed above, increases in inspiratory flow produce a reduction in respiratory muscle endurance.[117, 118] However, in these studies inspiratory flow rate and work rate were coupled so that it is difficult to determine which factor was responsible for the decrease in endurance. Dodd and colleagues[123] have shown that a threefold increase in mean inspiratory flow rate had no effect on Vo_2 when the pressure-time product and work rate were held constant. In this study, however, mean inspiratory flow ranged from 0.40 to 1.02 L/sec. Thus, the possibility that inspiratory flow may affect Vo_2 resp at a higher flow rate cannot be excluded.

The importance of hyperinflation as a determinant of Vo_2 resp was examined by Collett and Engel,[124] who studied healthy subjects breathing against resistive loads at FRC and at a high lung volume (45 and 66% of vital capacity, respectively). Despite close matching of ventilation, inspiratory flow rate, pressure-time product, and work rate, Vo_2 resp was increased at the higher lung volume—an increase of about 1% in O_2 cost per unit work for each percent increase in VC. The authors speculated that the decrease in inspiratory muscle efficiency at high lung volume may be due to (1) changes in mechanical coupling, (2) changes in the pattern of recruitment of the respiratory muscles, or (3) changes in the instrinsic properties of the inspiratory muscles at a shorter length. In this study, increases in tidal volume at a constant end-expiratory lung volume, inspiratory flow rate, pressure-time index, and work rate had no effect on Vo_2 resp, suggesting that the degree of muscle shortening during inspiration does not significantly affect Vo_2 resp. In summary, these series of studies suggest that the major determinants of Vo_2 resp include pressure-time product, work rate, and lung volume.

Various methods have been used to calculate pressure-time indices, such as electrically integrating a pressure signal with respect to time or multiplying mean inspiratory pressure (mouth, esophageal, transdiaphragmatic) by T_I or by T_I/T_{TOT}. A further problem arises in that the time measurements can differ depending on whether they are derived from airflow or pressure recordings. In a study conducted in both healthy subjects and patients with COPD (at rest and during exercise), Barnard and Levine[125] showed that T_I, T_I/T_{TOT}, and TT_{di} were significantly higher when the latter indices were calculated from P_{di} recordings compared with airflow recordings (Table 9–5). In the normal subjects at rest, a very close temporal relationship was observed between flow and P_{di} at the onset of inspiration, but P_{di} remained elevated above the baseline level when flow had returned to zero at the end of inspiration. In the patients with COPD, a small increase in P_{di} was sometimes noted before the onset of inspiratory flow, and, as in the case of the normal subjects, P_{di} remained elevated above the baseline when flow had returned to zero at the end of inspiration. In both groups of subjects, these differences became more marked at the end of exercise. In a subgroup of subjects, Barnard and Levine obtained simultaneous diaphragmatic EMG measurements with an esophageal electrode. In the healthy

TABLE 9–5.
Time Indices Calculated from Airflow and Transdiaphragmatic Pressure Recordings*

		Normal Subjects		COPD Patients	
		Flow	Pressure	Flow	Pressure
TI (sec)	Rest	1.19	1.56	1.27	1.56
	Exercise	0.81	1.10	0.72	0.99
TI/T$_{TOT}$	Rest	0.40	0.53	0.40	0.50
	Exercise	0.46	0.63	0.41	0.56
TT$_{di}$	Rest	0.014	0.017	0.016	0.018
	Exercise	0.061	0.071	0.042	0.049

* Based on data of Barnard PA, Levine S: *J Appl Physiol* 1986; 60:1067–1072.

subjects, EMG activity was present throughout the interval in which P$_{di}$ was above the baseline, both at rest and during exercise. In the patients with COPD, at both rest and end-exercise, EMG activity usually commenced in synchrony with the increase in P$_{di}$ but it ended in synchrony with inspiratory flow and before P$_{di}$ had returned to baseline.

PRESSURE RELAXATION RATE

The lack of a reliable and easy-to-use method of making the diagnosis of respiratory muscle fatigue in a clinical setting continues to be a major problem. Recently, the use of the relaxation phase of various respiratory pressure signals has aroused considerable interest in this regard. Studies in various skeletal muscles have shown that, as a muscle fatigues, there is slowing of the rate at which the muscle relaxes from a stimulated or voluntary contraction. Based on the assumption that the decay portion of a respiratory pressure wave corresponds to the relaxation phase of respiratory muscle contraction, Esau et al.[126] studied this portion of P$_{di}$ tracings in four healthy subjects in whom they induced respiratory muscle fatigue.

They developed two indices to quantitate the rate of decay in P$_{di}$ swings. The first was the *maximum relaxation rate* (MRR), which was the peak rate of pressure decay. The MRR was calculated[126] as the slope of a tangent drawn to the steepest portion of the pressure curve, which invariably occurred early in the course of decay of P$_{di}$ (Fig 9–8). Alternatively, the pressure signal can be passed through a derivative computer, and the peak dP$_{di}$/dt taken as the MRR (Fig 9–9). Since MRR is pressure-dependent, it increases linearly with increases in the peak pressure of the contraction; thus, MRR should be normalized by dividing by peak pressure. In this way, contractions of varying intensity can be compared. The authors calculated a second index from the later portion of the pressure curve; this index was termed the *time constant* (τ). Tau was calculated by replotting the pressure signal on a semilog scale (Fig 9–10). This replotting yielded a straight line over the lower 50 to 70% of the decay curve, indicating that the pressure decay was monoexponential. The reciprocal of the slope of the

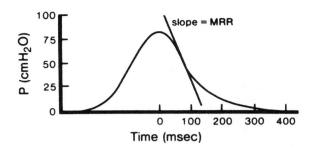

FIG 9–8.
Changes in transdiaphragmatic pressure during a sniff. The slope of a tangent drawn through the steepest portion of the pressure decline is the maximal relaxation rate (MRR). *(From Levy RD et al: Relaxation rate of mouth pressure with sniffs at rest and inspiratory muscle fatigue. Am Rev Respir Dis 1984; 130:38–41. Used by permission.)*

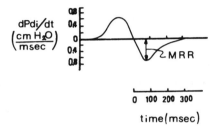

FIG 9–9.
The first derivation of transdiaphragmatic pressure (P_{di}) changes with a sniff. The peak dP_{di}/dt is equal to maximal relation rate. *(From Esau et al: Changes in rate of relaxation of sniffs with diaphragmatic fatigue in humans. J Appl Physiol 1983; 55:731–735. Used by permission.)*

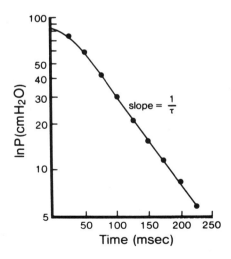

FIG 9–10.
A replot of pressure decline in transdiaphragmatic pressure on a semilog scale versus time. The linear portion indicates a monoexponential function with a time constant (τ) equal to 1/slope. *(From Levy et al: Relaxation rate of mouth pressure with sniffs at rest and inspiratory muscle fatigue. Am Rev Respir Dis 1984; 130:38–41. Used by permission.)*

lower portion of this line was taken as the time constant (based on the equation for an exponential function: $y=e^{-t}/\tau$). Before accepting a value of τ, the authors[126, 127] required that the correlation coefficient of the individual exponential regression be >0.96. Unlike MRR, tau was independent of peak pressure.

Esau et al.[126] studied healthy subjects who were generating P_{di} in a square-wave pattern while breathing against resistive loads. They calculated baseline MRR/P_{di} and τ from the first three breaths (i.e., before fatigue); these values are listed in Table 9–6. They induced respiratory muscle fatigue by having the subjects breathe against inspiratory resistive loads. When TT_{di} was in the nonfatiguing range during loading, there was no change in MRR or τ, but MRR decreased and τ increased when TT_{di} values exceeded 0.20 (i.e., a fatiguing pattern), with maximal changes at a TT_{di} of 0.40 (Table 9–7). Under fatiguing conditions, the time course of the change in MRR and τ correlated with that of the change in the high-to-low ratio of the diaphragmatic EMG (another index of fatigue, *vide infra*).

TABLE 9–6.
Relaxation Rate of Respiratory Pressures in Healthy, Nonfatigued Subjects

	MRR/P_{peak} (% pressure loss over 10 msec)	Time Constant (msec)	Author
P_{di} generated in square wave ($n = 4$)	10.0 ± 0.4 (SE)	53.2 ± 3.2 (SE)	Esau[126]
P_{di} sniff against occlusion ($n = 8$)	7.7 ± 0.3 (SE)	59 ± 2.4 (SE)	Esau[128]
P_{di} during unilat phrenic n. stim ($n = 4$)	7.8 ± 2.0 (SE)	57 ± 3.8 (SE)	Esau[128]
P_{mo} sniff against occlusion ($n = 27$)	7.8 ± 0.2 (SE)	51.5 ± 2.2 (SE)	Levy[130]
P_{di} sniff against occlusion ($n = 6$)	7.9 ± 0.5 (SE)	55.0 ± 1.7 (SE)	Levy[130]
P_{di} sniff against occlusion ($n = 5$)	6.4 ± 0.7 (SD)	57.2 ± 8.7 (SD)	Wilcox[127]
P_{di} during bilat phrenic n. stim ($n = 5$)	7.4 ± 1.8 (SD)	48.2 ± 7.4 (SD)	Wilcox[127]
P_{es} sniff unoccluded ($n = 10$)	8.9 ± 1.33 (SD)		Koulouris[139]
P_{np} sniff unoccluded ($n = 10$)	9.3 ± 1.19 (SD)		Koulouris[139]
P_{mo} sniff unoccluded ($n = 10$)	9.2 ± 1.21 (SD)		Koulouris[139]
P_{es} sniff against occlusion ($n = 5$)	8.8 ± 0.88 (SD)	51.3 ± 7.3 (SD)	Mador[141]
P_{es} sniff unoccluded ($n = 5$)	9.5 ± 0.88 (SD)	44.3 ± 5.5 (SD)	Mador[141]
P_{di} sniff against occlusion ($n = 5$)	8.6 ± 0.85 (SD)	56.7 ± 12.4 (SD)	Mador[141]
P_{di} sniff unoccluded ($n = 5$)	9.2 ± 1.0 (SD)	56.6 ± 14.6 (SD)	Mador[141]

TABLE 9–7.
Alteration in Relaxation Rate of Respiratory Pressures with Development of Respiratory Muscle Fatigue

Measurement	MRR/P_{peak} (% decrease)	Time Constant (% increase)	Author
P_{di} generated in square wave (TT_{di} = 0.40) (N = 4)	60 ± 9 (SE)	150 ± 13 (SE)	Esau[126]
P_{di} sniff against occlusion (*n* = 8)	18 ± 1.1 (SE)	41 ± 6.8 (SE)	Esau[128]
P_{di} sniff against occlusion (*n* = 6)	18	45	Levy[130]
P_{mo} sniff against occlusion (*n* = 6)	15	44	Levy[130]
P_{es} sniff unoccluded (*n* = 4)	33 (range, 20–42)		Koulouris[139]
P_{np} sniff unoccluded (*n* = 4)	32 (range, 18–43)		Koulouris[139]
P_{mo} sniff unoccluded (*n* = 4)	33 (range, 21–42)		Koulouris[139]
P_{es} sniff unoccluded (*n* = 5)	17 ± 8 (SD)	38 ± 20 (SD)	Mador[141]
P_{di} sniff unoccluded (*n* = 5)	16 ± 6 (SD)	38 ± 25 (SD)	Mador[141]
P_{es} sniff against occlusion (*n* = 5)	14 ± 12 (SD)	27 ± 25 (SD)	Mador[141]
P_{di} sniff against occlusion (*n* = 5)	11 ± 11 (SD)	27 ± 31 (SD)	Mador[141]

In a subsequent study,[128] these investigators reasoned that a short sharp sniff would approximate the diaphragmatic contraction produced by brief stimulation of the phrenic nerve. The MRR/P_{di} and τ_{di} values calculated from P_{di} tracings following sniffs against an occluded airway were similar to the values obtained from P_{di} tracings provided by unilateral phrenic nerve stimulation.[128] In contrast, Wilcox et al.[127] found that the MRR/P_{di} and τ_{di} were faster during bilateral supramaximal phrenic nerve stimulation than during a sniff maneuver. Inspiratory muscle relaxation rates increase with lung volume during bilateral supramaximal phrenic nerve stimulation.[129] The effect of lung volume on relaxation rates during sniff maneuvers is not so clear. At lung volumes below FRC, sniff relaxation rates do not appear to be substantially different from values obtained at FRC. However, at lung volumes above FRC, relaxation rates are faster than those obtained at FRC.[130] Thus, lung volume should be monitored during sniff maneuvers and efforts should be made to obtain sniffs at the same lung volume. During a sniff, both the diaphragm and the rib cage muscles contract. The relative contribution of each muscle group varies between subjects and between sniffs in a single subject. Esau and colleagues[128] have shown that the relative contribution of P_{ga} and P_{es} to P_{di} (an index of the pattern of respiratory muscle recruitment) does not affect diaphragmatic relaxation rates.

In vitro studies demonstrate that hypercapnia and/or hypoxia can slow relaxation in muscle strips.[131] However, recent *in vivo* studies suggest that hypercapnia and/or hypoxia do not affect the MRR of the quadriceps, adductor pollicis, or diaphragm in man. [132, 133] Relaxation rates can be also affected by metabolic factors such as temperature, and nutritional and thyroid status.[134-136] As expected, inspiratory muscle relaxation rates are abnormally slow in myotonic conditions.[138]

Following induction of fatigue, the MRR decreases and τ increases (Table 9–7). Both values return quickly to normal within 1 to 5 minutes.

To determine if relaxation rate could be measured in a less invasive way, Levy et al.[130] compared the relaxation rate of P_{di} measurements with that of mouth pressure (P_{mo}) generated during sniffs against an occluded airway. In 27 normal subjects, the values for MRR/P_{mo} and τ were similar to those reported for P_{di} (Table 9–6). Likewise, Koulouris et al.[139] found that MRR values were similar when measurements were obtained from P_{mo}, P_{np}, and P_{es} tracings in normal subjects. Also, fatigue caused changes in the relaxation rate of these less invasive pressures of similar magnitude to that observed with P_{di} (Table 9–7). However, in patients with COPD, MRR_{np} overestimated MRR_{es} in 7 of 10 subjects.[137] The MRR_{np}/MRR_{es} ratio varied from 0.87 to 1.56. Thus, these less invasive measures cannot be used in patients with obstructive lung disease.

In the course of these studies, a variable number of tracings have been considered unsuitable for analysis. Levy et al.[130] reported that 25% of their subjects were not able to perform a satisfactory sniff against an occluded airway, and among the remaining subjects there was a wide range in the number of acceptable tracings per subject (9 to 80%). Wilcox et al.[127] considered only 35% of sniff P_{di} tracings (performed against an occluded airway) suitable for analysis, with a wide range of acceptability (25 to 75%) between subjects. In contrast, Koulouris et al.[139] found that 94% of unoccluded sniff tracings (P_{es}, P_{mo}, and P_{np}) were acceptable, and Esau et al.[128] accepted 95% of P_{di} tracings obtained by sniffing against an occluded airway before the development of fatigue, 75% of post-fatigue sniffs, and 40% of phrenic stimulations. In general, the following criteria have been proposed for the acceptance of sniff tracings:

1. Rapid upstroke and smooth decay of pressure[130, 139]
2. Peak pressure maintained for <50 msec[130, 139]
3. Total sniff duration of <500 msec[139]
4. A clearly recognizable baseline, which should be FRC since MRR may vary with lung volume[129, 130, 140]
5. If a sniff is submaximal, the peak pressure should be at least 60% of maximum, because MRR slows when skeletal muscle is only partly activated during voluntary contractions.[139]

Within individual subjects, reproducibility of sniff maximal relaxation rates are reasonably good (coefficient of variation, 6 to 10%).[128, 130, 139] Variability of sniff τ can be somewhat higher (6 to 15%). It should be noted that these results were obtained in healthy young subjects. Greater variability may occur when sniff relaxation is measured in patients with pulmonary disease. There is a fairly wide range between subjects, and, unfortunately, considerable overlap exists between the values observed in the presence and absence of fatigue. Thus, isolated values cannot be used to diagnose fatigue, but serial measurements should be helpful.

ELECTROMYOGRAPHIC SIGNAL RECORDING AND ANALYSIS

The electromyographic signal (EMG) is the electrical signal emanating from an active muscle. It can be detected by a variety of electrodes, and it can be amplified, recorded, and analyzed in numerous ways. The EMG represents the temporal and spatial summation of individual action potentials of activated motor units as detected at the site of the recording electrodes. It is an alternating current (ac) signal that alternates above and below 0 V. Identifying the presence and quantifying the magnitude of the raw EMG signal is a useful way of evaluating the degree of muscle activation. In addition, characterization of the frequency content of the EMG signal can be used to predict and identify muscle fatigue.

While EMGs of numerous respiratory muscles have been examined, the diaphragm is the one most often studied. To record an EMG signal, surface or intramuscular (needle or fine wire) electrodes can be used. While surface electrodes are the simplest, the signal can be frequently contaminated by electrical activity of nearby muscles in addition to the muscle of interest. Detecting the presence of the EMG signal is frequently used to determine the onset and offset of the activation of various respiratory muscles. This is particularly useful in examining timing relationships between different respiratory muscle groups. For example, EMG recordings are frequently used to investigate the mechanism of airflow obstruction in sleep studies. In this application, diminished upper airway EMG activity associated with airflow obstruction implies that decreased muscle activation contributes to the development of airway obstruction.[142] The EMG can be also used to study the recruitment patterns of different respiratory muscle groups.[143]

In addition to inspecting the raw EMG tracing, the signal should be quantified since this is related to the degree of muscle activation. Quantification is usually accomplished by continuously averaging the rectified EMG [a process referred to as calculating a moving time average (MTA)] or by dividing the integrated rectified signal by the duration of integration. When employing these methods, a time interval of 100 to 300 msec is typically used to calculate the average. Another method of quantifying the EMG signal is calculation of the root-mean-square (rms) value, which is gaining in popularity. This consists of determining the square root of the sum of the squared voltages of the EMG signal within a given period and then dividing by that period. Some authors[144] recommend this approach above all other methods of EMG signal qualification. Quantification of the EMG signal is important because magnitude of the signal has been shown to correlate (at least in the absence of fatigue) with force generation of the muscle[145] as shown in Figure 9–11.

The relationship between the magnitude of the diaphragm EMG signal (E_{di}) and diaphragm force generation (quantified in terms of transdiaphragmatic pressure, P_{di}) is a useful way of studying the development of muscle fatigue; here we are referring to peripheral contractile fatigue, not to central or transmission fatigue. Contractile fatigue is associated with an increase in the E_{di}/P_{di} ratio, indicating a reduction in transdiaphragmatic pressure generation (P_{di}) for a given level of diaphragm activation (E_{di}). Figure 9–12 shows an example of progressive increases in E_{di} associated with simultaneous decreases in P_{di} in an experimental animal with cardiogenic shock.[146] A plot of sequential measurement of the E_{di}/P_{di} ratio in a group of animals

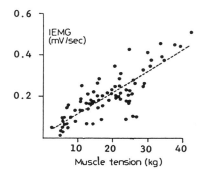

FIG 9–11.
The relationship between the integrated EMG and muscle tension produced in a limb muscle. Note that as muscle tension increases there is an associated linear increase in the integrated EMG signal. *(from Komi PV: Relationship between muscle tension, EMG and velocity of contraction under concentric and eccentric work, in Desmedt JE (ed):* New Developments in Electromyography and Clinical Neurophysiology. Basel, Karger, 1973, Vol 1, pp. 596–606. Used by permission.)

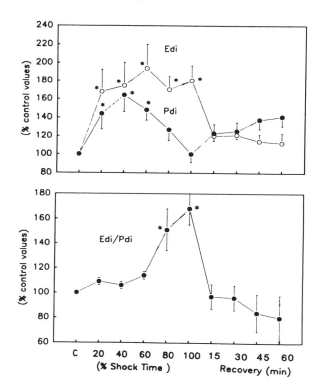

FIG 9–12.
The changes in E_{di}, P_{di}, and the ratio of E_{di}/P_{di} during the development and recovery of experimentally induced hypovolemic shock in a group of dogs. All values are displayed as percentages of control values, and data points represent the mean ± standard deviation. Note the decline in P_{di} that occurs with shock is associated with a rise in the E_{di}/P_{di} ratio, implying the development of contractile diaphragmatic fatigue. With recovery from shock this pattern is reversed representing the recovery from diaphragm fatigue. *(From Hussain, AN, Marcotte JE, Burnet H, et al: Relationship among EMG and contractile responses of the diaphragm elicited by hypotension. J Appl Physiol 1988; 65:649–656, Used by permission.)*

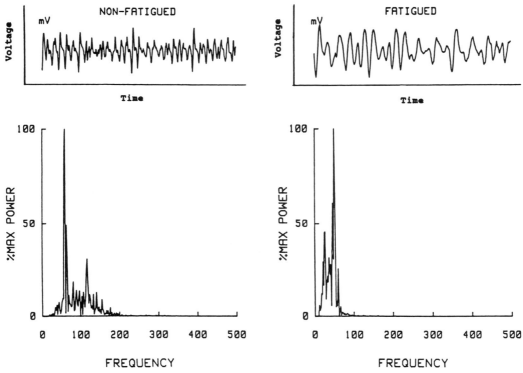

FIG 9–13.
The raw EMG and the corresponding frequency-power spectra obtained from a nonfatigued and fatigued muscle. Note the slowing of the raw EMG signal and the leftward shift of the power spectrum associated with the development of fatigue. *(From Barnes WS, Williams JH: Effects of ischemia on myo-electrical signal characteristics during rest and recovery from static work.* Am J Physical Med *1987; 66:249–263. Used by permission.)*

who developed contractile fatigue of the diaphragm as a result of cardiogenic shock is shown in Figure 9–12.[147]

In addition to the E_{di}/P_{di} ratio, the quality or characteristics of the EMG signal have been used as another means of investigating the development of respiratory muscle fatigue. The fundamental change in the character of the EMG is a shift toward low-frequency components within the EMG signal with the development of contractile fatigue. While first employed in limb muscle studies,[148] this method of fatigue detection has been applied to the respiratory muscles for the past 15 years, and over this time signal analysis technique has been refined. In early studies,[149] a shift in the frequency content was detected by calculating the high-low ratio (H/L), i.e., the ratio of power within a high-frequency range (150 to 350 Hz) relative to the power in a low-frequency range (20 to 47 Hz). A fall in the H/L ratio has been shown to occur in association with the development of contractile fatigue.

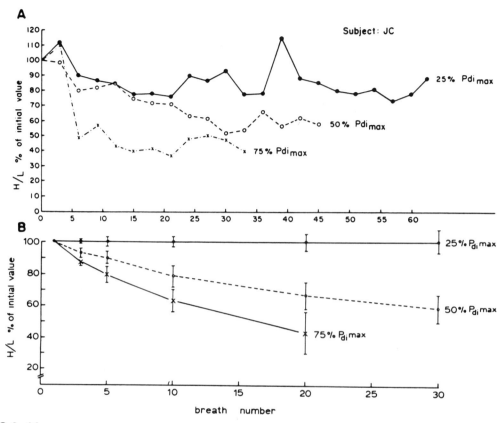

FIG 9–14.
Demonstration of a fall in the H/L ratio associated with the development of fatigue. The H/L ratio values expressed as percentage of initial (nonfatigued) value for three loads in one subject (**A**) and mean values for five subjects (**B**). Note that a nonfatiguing load (25% of maximal transdiaphragmatic pressure; $P_{di,max}$) produces no change in the H/L ratio, while the fatiguing loads (50 and 75% of $P_{di,max}$) are associated with a fall in the H/L ratio. *(from Gross D, Grassino A, Ross WRD, et al: Electromyogram pattern of diaphragmatic fatigue. J Appl Physiol 1979; 46:1–7. Used by permission.)*

Using the H/L ratio is a somewhat crude method of characterizing the EMG frequency components, and current methods are more sophisticated, such as the Fourier transform.[150] This method characterizes the frequency components of the EMG by generating a frequency-power spectrum, which is a plot of frequency versus magnitude (or quantity) of the EMG signal. Individual spectra can be compared by visual inspection, but calculation of the mean or median frequency of the spectrum facilitates more quantitative comparison.[151] The mean frequency represents the average frequency of the frequency-power spectrum, while the median frequency is that which divides the spectrum into two halves of equal power. Figure 9–13 shows an example of the raw EMG signal and the respective frequency-power spectra

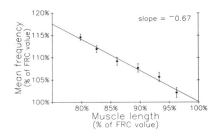

FIG 9–15.
The effect of diaphragm length on the frequency components of the EMG in the canine diaphragm. Diaphragm length is expressed as percentage of FRC (or resting length) and the frequency components of the EMG are represented by the mean frequency of the frequency-power spectrum. The data represent the mean values for 30 contractions of that diaphragm. Note that with a 20% shortening, an associated 15% increase is apparent in the mean frequency. *(from Walsh JM, Romano S, Grassino A: The effect of diaphragm length on the EMG power spectrum.* Clin Res *1990; 38:847A. Used by permission.)*

for both a nonfatigued and a fatigued limb muscle.[152] With the development of fatigue, the raw EMG becomes slower, and a leftward shift of the spectrum occurs, representing the shift toward lower frequencies within the raw EMG. Also in this example we can see a decrease in mean frequency with fatigue from 92.6 to 41.8 Hz. Changes in the frequency components of the EMG signal precede failure of the muscle to maintain a constant force (i.e., the development of mechanical failure). Consequently, EMG signal analysis has become an attractive method of predicting contractile fatigue.

Changes in the EMG frequency components associated with contractile fatigue of the diaphragm were first described in studies where normal subjects breathed through inspiratory resistances.[149] The H/L ratio was used to detect a shift in the EMG frequency components, and Figure 9–14 demonstrates the typical fall in H/L ratio that occurs when a subject breathes through a resistance that induces diaphragm fatigue. This method of detecting diaphragm fatigue has been applied to diaphragm training in quadriplegics[153], and to the detection of fatigue of the parasternal intercostal muscles.[154]

The use of EMG frequency component analysis to detect respiratory muscle fatigue has a number of limitations. One, it requires a baseline nonfatigued reference state for comparison in order to identify a shift in frequency components of the EMG. Two, current methods of EMG frequency component analysis are unable to detect intermittent episodes of fatigue that may occur when high fatiguing loads are applied intermittently. Three, muscle length may have an independent effect on the EMG power spectrum, as shown in Figure 9–15.[155] It may be possible to control for some of these factors, such as muscle length and, thus, be able to use EMG analysis more accurately in the study of respiratory muscle fatigue. In addition, it may be possible to modify EMG analysis so as to detect intermittent episodes of muscle fatigue.[156, 157]

In summary, EMG recordings of the respiratory muscles remain a valuable technique for determining muscle activation and EMG signal analysis may be usefully employed in the study of respiratory muscle fatigue.

REFERENCES

1. DuBois AB, Brody AW, Lewis DH, Burgess BF: Oscillation mechanics of lungs and chest in man. *J Appl Physiol* 1956; 8:587–594.
2. Mead J: Measurement of inertia of the lungs at increased ambient pressure. *J Appl Physiol* 1956; 9:208–212.
3. Sharp JT, Henry JP, Sweany SK, et al: Total respiratory inertance and its gas and tissue components in normal and obese man. *J Clin Invest* 1964; 43:503–509.
4. Rahn H, Otis AB, Chadwick LE, et al: The pressure-volume diagram of the thorax and lung. *Am J Physiol* 1946; 146:161–178.
5. Otis AB: The work of breathing, in Fenn WO, Rahn H (eds): *Handbook of Physiology Respiration.* Washington, DC, American Physiological Society 1964, Sec 3, Vol 1, Chap 17, p. 463–478.
6. Konno K, Mead J: Measurement of the separate volume changes of ribcage and abdomen during breathing. *J Appl Physiol* 1967; 22:407–422.
7. Konno K, Mead J: Static volume-pressure characteristics of the rib cage and abdomen. *J Appl Physiol* 1968; 24:544–548.
8. Goldman MD, Grimby G, Mead J: Mechanical work of breathing derived from rib cage and abdominal V-P partitioning. *J Appl Physiol* 1976; 41:752–763.
9. Tobin MJ, Perez W, Guenther SM, et al: Does ribcage-abdominal paradox signify respiratory muscle fatigue? *J Appl Physiol* 1987; 63:851–860.
10. Tobin MJ, Guenther SM, Perez W, et al: Konno-Mead analysis of ribcage-abdominal motion during successful and unsuccessful trials of weaning from mechanical ventilation. *Am Rev Respir Dis* 1987; 135:1320–1328.
11. Agostoni E, Torri G: An analysis of the chest wall motions at high levels of ventilation. *Respir Physiol* 1967; 3:318–322.
12. Agostoni E, Mognoni P: Deformation of the chest wall during breathing efforts. *J Appl Physiol* 1966; 21:1827–1832.
13. Agostoni E, Mognoni P, Torri G, et al: Forces deforming the rib cage. *Respir Physiol* 1966; 2:105–117.
14. Otis AB, Fenn WO, Rahn H: The mechanics of breathing in man. *J Appl Physiol* 1950; 2:592–607.
15. Sharp JT, Henry JP, Sweany SK, et al: The total work of breathing in normal and obese men. *J Clin Invest* 1964; 43:728–739.
16. Jones JG, Faithfull D, Jordon C, et al: Ribcage movement during halothane anesthesia in man. *Br J Anaesth* 1979; 51:399–407.
17. Vellody VPS, Nassery M, Balasaraswathi K, et al: Compliances of human rib cage and diaphragm-abdomen pathways in relaxed versus paralyzed states. *Am Rev Respir Dis* 1978; 118:479–491.
18. Behrakis PK, Higgs BD, Baydur A, et al: Active inspiratory impedance in halothane-anesthetized humans. *J Appl Physiol* 1982; 54:1477–1481.
19. Bergofsky EH, Turino GM, Fishman AP: Cardiorespiratory failure in kyphoscoliosis. *Medicine* 1959; 38:263–317.
20. Opie LH, Spalding JMK, Scott FD: Mechanical properties of the chest during intermittent positive-pressure respiration. *Lancet* 1959; 1:545–550.
21. Agostoni E, Campbell EJM, Freedman S. Energetics, in Campbell EJM, Agostoni E, Newsom-Davis J (eds): *The Respiratory Muscles:* Mechanics and Neural Control, Philadelphia, WB Saunders, 1970, Chap 5, pp. 115–142.
22. Roussos C, Campbell EJM: Respiratory muscle energetics, in Macklem PT, Mead J (eds): *Handbook of Physiology. The Respiratory System. Mechanics of Breathing.* Washington, DC, American Physiological Society, 1986, Sec 3, Vol 3, Part 2, Chap 28, pp. 481–509.

23. Ballantine TVN, Proctor HJ, Broussard ND, et al: The work of breathing: Potential for clinical application and the results of studies performed on 100 normal males. *Ann Surg* 1970; 171:590–594.
24. Otis AB: The work of breathing. *Physiol Rev* 1954; 34:449–458.
25. Milic-Emili J, Petit JM, Deroanne R: Mechanical work of breathing during exercise in trained and untrained subjects. *J Appl Physiol* 1962; 17:43–46.
26. Margaria R, Milic-Emili J, Petit JM, et al: Mechanical work of breathing during muscular exercise. *J Appl Physiol* 1960; 15:354–358.
27. West JR, Alexander JK: Studies on respiratory mechanics and the work of breathing in pulmonary fibrosis. *Am J Med* 1959; 27:529–544.
28. McIlroy MB, Christie RV: The work of breathing in emphysema. *Clin Sci* 1954; 13:147–154.
29. Tobin MJ, Chadha TS, Jenouri G, et al: Breathing patterns. Diseased subjects. *Chest* 1983; 84:286–294.
30. Dimarco AF, Kelsen SG, Cherniack NS, et al: Occlusion pressure and breathing pattern in patients with interstitial lung disease. *Am Rev Respir Dis* 1983; 127:425–430. See also Spiro SG, Dowdeswell IRG, Clark TJH: An analysis of submaximal exercise responses in patients with sarcoidosis and fibrosing alveolitis. *Br J Dis Chest* 1981; 75:169–180.
31. ImHof V, West P, Younes M: Steady state response of normal subjects to inspiratory resistive loads. *J Appl Physiol* 1986; 60:1471–1481.
32. Younes M: Load responses, dyspnea and respiratory failure. *Chest* 1990; 97:59S–68S.
33. Cain CC, Otis AB: Some physiological effects resulting from added resistance to respiration. *J Aviat Med* 1949; 20:149–160.
34. Campbell EJM, Westlake EK, Cherniack RM: The oxygen consumption and efficiency of the respiratory muscles of young male subjects. *Clin Sci* 1958; 18:55–64.
35. Fritts HN, Filler J, Fishman AP, et al: The efficiency of ventilation during voluntary hyperpnea. *J Clin Invest* 1959; 38:1339–1348.
36. Milic-Emili J, Petit JM: Mechanical efficiency of breathing. *J Appl Physiol* 1960; 15:359–362.
37. McGregor M, Becklake M: The relationship of oxygen cost of breathing to respiratory mechanical work and respiratory force. *J Clin Invest* 1961; 40:971–980.
38. Neergaard K Von, Wirz K: Uber eine methode zur messung der lungenalastizitat am lebenden menschen. insbesondere beim emphysem. *Z Klin Med* 1927; 105:35–50.
39. Cherniack RM, Farhi LE, Armstrong BW, et al: A comparison of esophageal and intrapleural pressure in man. *J Appl Physiol* 1955; 8:203–211.
40. Daly WJ, Bondurant S: Direct measurement of respiratory pleural changes in normal man. *J Appl Physiol* 1963; 18:513–518.
41. Mead J, Gaensler EA: Esophageal and pleural pressures in man, upright and supine. *J Appl Physiol* 1959; 14:81–83.
42. Knowles JH, Henry SK, Rahn H: Possible errors using esophageal balloon in determination of pressure volume characteristics of the lung and thoracic cage. *J Appl Physiol* 1959; 14:523–530.
43. Ferris BG, Mead J, Frank NR: Effect of body position on esophageal pressure and measurement of pulmonary compliance. *J Appl Physiol* 1950; 14:521–524.
44. Milic-Emili J, Mead J, Turner JM: Topography of esophageal pressure as a function of posture in man. *J Appl Physiol* 1964; 19:212–216.
45. Baydur A, Behrakis PK, Zin WA, et al: A simple method for assessing the validity of the esophageal balloon technique. *Am Rev Respir Dis* 1982; 126:788–791.
46. Milic-Emili J, Mead J, Turner JM, et al: Improved technique for estimating pleural pressure from esophageal balloons. *J Appl Physiol* 1964; 19:207–211.
47. Marini JJ: Monitoring during mechanical ventilation. *Clin Chest Medicine* 1988; 9:73–100.

48. Macklem PT: Procedures for standardized measurements of the lung mechanics. Bethesda, MD, National Heart Institute, Division of Lung Diseases, 1974.

49. Jaeger MJ, Otis AB: Effects of compressibility of alveolar gas on dynamics and work of breathing. *J Appl Physiol* 1964; 19:83–91.

50. McCool FD, Tzelepis GE, Leith DE, et al: Oxygen cost of breathing during fatiguing inspiratory resistive loads. *J Appl Physiol* 1989; 66:2045–2055.

51. Agostoni E, Mead J: Statics of the respiratory system, in: *Handbook of Physiology. Respiration.* Washington, DC, American Physiological Society. 1964, Sec 3, Vol 1, Chap 13, pp. 387–409.

52. Duomarco JL, Rimini R: La presion intra-abdominal en el hombre. Buenos Aires, El Ateneo, 1947.

53. Decramer M, DeTroyer A, Kelly S, et al: Regional differences in abdominal pressure swings in dogs. *J Appl Physiol* 1984; 57:1682–1687.

54. Mead J, Yoshino K, Kikuchi Y, et al: Abdominal pressure transmission in humans during slow breathing maneuvers. *J Appl Physiol* 1990; 68:1850–1853.

55. Agostoni E, Rahn H: Abdominal and thoracic pressures at different lung volumes. *J Appl Physiol* 1960; 15:1087–1092.

56. Marini JJ, Rodriguez RM, Lamb V: The inspiratory workload of patient-initiated mechanical ventilation. *Am Rev Respir Dis.* 1986; 134:902–909.

57. Ward ME, Corbeil C, Gibbons W, et al: Optimization of respiratory muscle relaxation during mechanical ventilation. *Anesthesiol* 1988; 69:29–35.

58. Altose MD, Castele RJ, Connors AF, et al: Effects of volume and frequency of mechanical ventilation on respiratory activity in humans. *Respir Physiol* 1986; 66:171–180.

59. Marini JJ, Capps J, Culver B: The inspiratory work of breathing during assisted mechanical ventilation. *Chest* 1985; 87:612–618.

60. Marini JJ, Smith TC, Lamb VJ: External work output and force generation during synchronized intermittent mechanical ventilation. Effect of machine assistance on breathing effort. *Am Rev Respir Dis* 1988; 138:1169–1179.

61. Brochard L, Harf A, Lorino H, Lemaire F: Inspiratory pressure support prevents diaphragmatic fatigue during weaning from mechanical ventilation. *Am Rev Respir Dis* 1989; 139:513–521.

62. Brochard L, Mollo JL, Mancebo J, et al: Comparison of the efficacy of inspiratory pressure support delivered by three ventilators. *Am Rev Respir Dis* 1989; 139:361A.

63. Fleury B, Murciano D, Talamo C, et al: Work of breathing in patients with chronic obstructive pulmonary disease in acute respiratory failure. *Am Rev Respir Dis* 1985; 131:822–827.

64. Fiastro JF, Habib MP, Shon BY, et al: Comparison of standard weaning parameters and the mechanical work of breathing in mechanically ventilated patients. *Chest* 1988; 94:232–238.

65. Henning RJ, Shubin H, Weil MH: The measurement of the work of breathing for the clinical assessment of ventilator dependence. *Crit Care Med* 1977; 5:264–268.

66. Peters RM, Hilberman M, Hogan JS, et al: Objective indications for respiratory therapy in post-trauma and post-operative patients. *Am J Surg* 1972; 124:262–269.

67. Proctor HJ, Woolson R: Prediction of respiratory muscle fatigue by measurements of the work of breathing. *Surg Gynecol Obstet* 1973; 136:367–370.

68. Marini JJ, Rodriguez M, Lamb V: Bedside estimation of the inspiratory work of breathing during mechanical ventilation. *Chest* 1986; 89:56–63.

69. Hubmayr RD, Loosbrock LM, Gillespie DJ, et al: Oxygen uptake during weaning from mechanical ventilation. *Chest* 1988; 94:1148–1155.

70. Tobin MJ: State of the art: Respiratory monitoring in the intensive care unit. *Am Rev Respir Dis* 1988; 138:1625–1642.

71. Agostoni E, Sant'Ambrogio G: The diaphragm, in: Campbell EJM, Agostoni E, Newson-Davis J

(eds): *The Respiratory Muscles: Mechanics and Neurological Control*, ed 2. London, Lloyd-Luke, 1970, pp. 145–160.

72. Newson-Davis J, Goldman M, Loh L, et al: Diaphragm function and alveolar hypoventilation. *Q J Med* 1976; 45:87–100.

73. Bellemare F, Grassino A: Effect of pressure and timing of contraction on human diaphragm fatigue. *J Appl Physiol* 1982; 53:1190–1195.

74. Braun NMT, Arora NS, Rochester DF: Force-length relations of the normal human diaphragm. *J Appl A Physiol* 1982; 53:405–412.

75. DeTroyer A, Estenne M: Limitations of measurement of transdiaphragmatic pressure in detecting diaphragmatic weakness. *Thorax* 1981; 36:169–174.

76. Gibson GJ, Clark E, Pride NB: Static transdiaphragmatic pressure in normal subjects and in patients with chronic hyperinflation. *Am Rev Respir Dis* 1981; 124:685–689.

77. Miller J, Moxham J, Green M: The maximal sniff in the assessment of diaphragm function in man. *Clin Sci* 1985; 69:91–96.

78. Fracchia C, Donner CF, Ioli F, et al: Transdiaphragmatic pressure and chest roentgenogram in diaphragmatic breathing assessment. *Bull Eur Physiopathol Respir* 1982; 18(Suppl 4):181–184.

79. Laporta D, Grassino A: Assessment of transdiaphragmatic pressure in humans. *J Appl Physiol* 1985; 58:1469–1476.

80. Hershenson MB, Kikucki Y, Loring SH: Relative strengths of the chest wall muscles. *J Appl Physiol* 1988; 65:852–862.

81. Gandevia SC, McKenzie DK: Activation of the human diaphragm during maximal static efforts. *J Physiol (Lond)* 1985; 367:45–56.

82. Gandevia SC, McKenzie DK, Plassman BL: Activation of the human respiratory muscles during different voluntary maneuvers. *J Physiol (Lond)* 1990; 428:387–403.

83. Grassino A, Goldman MD, Mead J, et al: Mechanics of the human diaphragm during voluntary contraction: Statics. *J Appl Physiol* 1978; 44:829–839.

84. Hillman DR, Markos J, Finucane KE: Effects of abdominal compression on maximum transdiaphragmatic pressure. *J Appl Physiol* 1990; 68:2296–2304.

85. Joyce GC, Rock PMH, Westbury DR: The mechanical properties of cat soleus muscles during controlled lengthening and shortening movements. *J Physiol (Lond)* 1969; 204:461–474.

86. Laroche CM, Mier AK, Moxham J, et al: The value of sniff esophageal pressures in the assessment of global inspiratory muscle strength. *Am Rev Respir Dis* 1988; 138:598–603.

87. Koulouris N, Mulvey DA, Laroche CM, et al: The measurement of inspiratory muscle strength by sniff esophageal, nasopharyngeal, and mouth pressures. *Am Rev Respir Dis* 1989; 139:641–646.

88. Murciano D, Aubier M, Bussi S, et al: Comparison of esophageal, tracheal and mouth occlusion pressure in patients with chronic obstructive pulmonary disease during acute respiratory failure. *Am Rev Respir Dis* 1982; 126:837–841.

89. Mulvey D, Elliott M, Goldstone J, et al: Relationship between sniff esophageal and nasopharyngeal pressures in patients with COPD. *Am Rev Respir Dis* 1990; 141:723A.

90. Koulouris N, Mulvey DA, Laroche CM, et al: The effect of posture and abdominal binding on respiratory pressures. *Eur Respir J* 1989; 2:961–965.

91. Sarnoff SJ, Sarnoff LC, Whittenberger J: Electrophrenic respiration. VII. The motor point of the phrenic nerve in relation to external stimulation. *Surg Gyncol Obstet* 1951; 93:190–196.

92. Markland ON, Kincaid JC, Pourmand RA, et al: Electrophysiologic evaluation of diaphragm by transcutaneous phrenic nerve stimulation. *Neurology (Cleveland)* 1984; 34:604–614.

93. Moxham J, Morris AJR, Spiro SG, et al: Contractile properties and fatigue of the diaphragm in man. *Thorax* 1981; 50:538–544.

94. Aubier M, Farkas G, DeTroyer A, et al: Detection of diaphragmatic fatigue in man by phrenic stimulation. *J Appl Physiol* 1981; 50:538–544.

95. Aubier M, Murciano D, Lecocguic Y, et al: Bilateral phrenic stimulation: A simple technique to assess diaphragmatic fatigue in humans. *J Appl Physiol* 1985; 58:58–64.

96. Bellemare F, Bigland-Ritchie B: Assessment of human diaphragm strength and activation using phrenic nerve stimulation. *Respir Physiol* 1984; 58:263–277.

97. Meir A, Brophy C, Moxham J, et al: Phrenic nerve stimulation in normal subjects and in patients with diaphragmatic weakness. *Thorax* 1987; 42:885–888.

98. Meir A, Brophy C, Moxham J, et al: Twitch pressures in the assessment of diaphragm weakness. *Thorax* 1989; 44:990–996.

99. Hubmayr R, Litchy WJ, Gay PG, et al: Transdiaphragmatic twitch pressure: Effects of lung volume and chest wall shape. *Am Rev Respir Dis* 1989; 139:647–652.

100. McKenzie DK, Gandevia SC: Phrenic nerve conduction times and twitch pressures of the human diaphragm. *J Appl Physiol* 1985; 58:1496–1504.

101. Mier-Jedrezejowicz AM, Brophy C, Moxham J, et al: Assessment of diaphragm weakness. *Am Rev Respir Dis* 1988; 137:877–883.

102. Allen SM, Hunt B, Green M: Fall in vital capacity with posture. *Br J Dis Chest* 1985; 79:267–271.

103. Alexander C: Diaphragmatic movements and the diagnosis of diaphragm paralysis. *Clin Radiol* 1966; 17:79–83.

104. Moxham J: Tests of respiratory muscle function, in Tobin MJ (ed): *The Respiratory Muscles.* Philadelphia, JB Lippincott Co, 1990; pp. 312–328.

105. Konno K, Mead J: Measurement of separate volume changes of rib cage and abdomen during breathing. *J Appl Physiol* 1967; 22:407–422.

106. Gibson GJ, Roussos C: Clinical assessment of thoracic function, in Roussos C, Macklem PT (eds): *The Thorax.* New York, Marcel Dekker, 1985, pp. 1281–1299.

107. Lisboa C, Pare PD, Pertuze J, et al: Inspiratory muscle function in unilateral diaphagmatic paralysis. *Am Rev Respir Dis* 1986; 134:488–492.

108. Martinez FJ, Couser JI, Celli BR: Factors influencing ventilatory muscle recruitment in patients with chronic airflow obstruction. *Am Rev Respir Dis* 1990; 142:276–282.

109. Hillman DR, Finucane KE: Respiratory pressure partitioning during quiet inspiration in unilateral and bilateral diaphragmatic weakness. *Am Rev Respir Dis* 1988; 137:1401–1405.

110. Sarnoff SJ, Braunwald E, Welch RB, et al: Hemodynamic determinants of oxygen consumptions of the heart with special reference to the tension-time index. *Am J Physiol* 1958; 191:148–156.

111. McGregor M, Becklake MR: The relationship of oxygen cost of breathing to respiratory mechanical work and respiratory force. *J Clin Invest* 1961; 40:971–980.

112. Rochester DF, Bettini G: Diaphragmatic blood flow and energy expenditure in the dog. *J Clin Invest* 1976; 57:661–672.

113. Martin JG, Shores S, Engel LA: Effect of continuous positive pressure on respiratory mechanics and pattern of breathing in induced asthma. *Am Rev Respir Dis* 1982; 126:812–817.

114. Bellemare F, Grassino A: Effect of pressure and timing of contraction on human diaphragm fatigue. *J Appl Physiol* 1982; 53:1190–1195.

115. Field S, Sanci S, Grassino A: Respiratory muscle oxygen consumption estimated by the diaphragm pressure-time index. *J Appl Physiol* 1984; 57:44–51.

116. Collett PW, Perry C, Engel LA: Pressure-time product, flow, and oxygen cost of resistive breathing in humans. *J Appl Physiol* 1984; 58:1263–1272.

117. Clanton TL, Dixon GF, Drake J, et al: Effects of breathing pattern on inspiratory muscle endurance in humans. *J Appl Physiol* 1985; 59:1834–1841.

118. McCool FD, McCann DR, Leith DE, et al: Pressure-flow effects on endurance of inspiratory muscles. *J Appl Physiol* 1986; 60:299–303.

119. Fenn WD: The relation between the work performed and the energy liberated in muscular contraction. *J Physiol (Lond)* 1923; 85:373–395.

120. Dodd DS, Kelly S, Collett PW, et al: Pressure-time product, work rate, and endurance during resistive breathing in humans. *J Appl Physiol* 1988; 64:1397–1404.

121. Cerny F, Lawler M, Mador MJ: Breathing frequency affects diaphragm fatigue. *Physiologist* 1988; 31:A37.

122. Hill AV: The heat of activation and the heat of shortening in a muscle twitch. *Proc R Soc London (Ser B)* 1948; 136:220–228.

123. Dodd DS, Collett PW, Engel LA: Influences of inspiratory flow rate and frequency on O_2 cost of resistive breathing in humans. *J Appl Physiol* 1986; 60:1067–1072.

124. Collett PW, Engel LA: Influence of lung volume on oxygen cost of resistive breathing. *J Appl Physiol* 1986; 61:16–24.

125. Barnard PA, Levine S: Critique on application of diaphragmatic time tension index to spontaneously breathing humans. *J Appl Physiol* 1986; 60:1067–1072.

126. Esau SA, Bellemare F, Grassino A, et al: Changes in relaxation rate with diaphragmatic fatigue in humans. *J Appl Physiol* 1983; 54:1353–1360.

127. Wilcox PG, Eisen A, Wiggs BJ, et al: Diaphragmatic relaxation rate after voluntary contractions and uni- and bilateral phrenic stimulation. *J Appl Physiol* 1988; 65:675–682.

128. Esau SA, Bye TP, Pardy RL: Changes in rate of relaxation of sniffs with diaphragmatic fatigue in humans. *J Appl Physiol* 1983; 55:731–735.

129. Smith J, Bellemare F: Effect of lung volume on in vivo contraction characteristics of human diaphragm. *J Appl Physiol* 1987; 62:1893–1900.

130. Levy RD, Esau SA, Bye TP, et al: Relaxation rate of mouth pressure with sniffs at rest and with inspiratory muscle fatigue. *Am Rev Respir Dis* 1984; 130:38–41.

131. Esau S: Hypoxic, hypercapnic acidosis decreases tension and increases fatigue in hamster diaphragm muscle in vitro. *Am Rev Respir Dis* 1989; 139:1410–1417.

132. Vianna LG, Koulouris N, Green M, et al: Effect of acute hypercapnia on limb muscle in humans. *J Appl Physiol* 1990; 69:1486–1493.

133. Vianna LG, Koulouris N, Green M, et al: Effect of acute hypoxia and hypercapnia on maximum relaxation rate of skeletal muscle in man. *Am Rev Respir Dis* 1988; 137:A73.

134. Wiles CM: The effect of temperature, ischemia and controlled activity on the relaxation rate of human muscle. *Clin Physiol* 1982; 2:485–497.

135. Wiles CM, Young A, Jones DA, et al: Muscle relaxation, fiber-type composition and energy turnover in hyper and hypothyroid patients. *Clin Sci* 1979; 57:375–384.

136. Lopez J, Russell DM, Whitehall J, et al: Skeletal muscle function in malnutrition. *Clin Sci* 1982; 36:602–610.

137. Mulvey DA, Elliott MW, Koulouris NG, et al: Sniff esophageal and nasopharyngeal pressures and maximal relaxation rates in patients with respiratory dysfunction. *Am Rev Respir Dis* 1991; 143:950–953.

138. Cole AT, Spence DPS, Hall H, et al: The relaxation time constant of sniff transdiaphragmatic pressure in myotonic dystrophy. *Thorax* 1990; 45:806–807.

139. Koulouris N, Vianna LG, Mulvey DA, et al: Maximal relaxation rates of esophageal, nose, and mouth pressures during a sniff reflect inspiratory muscle fatigue. *Am Rev Respir Dis* 1989; 139:1213–1217.

140. Griggs GA, Findley LJ, Suratt PM, et al: Prolonged relaxation rate of inspiratory muscles in patients with sleep apnea. *Am Rev Respir Dis* 1989; 140:706–710.

141. Mador MJ, Kufel TJ: Effect of inspiratory muscle fatigue on inspiratory muscle relaxation rates in healthy subjects (abstract). *Am Rev Respir Dis* 1991; 143:A365.

142. Hudgel DW, Harasick T: Fluctuation in timing of upper airway and chest wall inspiratory muscle activity in obstructive sleep apnea. *J Appl Physiol* 1990; 69:443–450.

143. Breslin EH, Garoutte BC, Kohlman-Carrieri V, et al: Correlations between dyspena, diaphragm and sternomastoid recruitment during inspiratory resistance breathing in normal subjects. *Chest* 1990; 98:298–302.

144. Bouisset S, Goubel F: Integrated electromyographic activity and muscle work. *J Appl Physiol* 1973; 35:695–702.

145. Komi PV: Relationship between muscle tension, EMG and velocity of contraction under concentric and eccentric work, in Desmedt JE (ed): *New Developments in Electromyography and Clinical Neurophysiology*. Basel, Karger, 1973, Vol 1, pp. 596–606.

146. Aubier M, Trippenbach T, Roussos C: Respiratory muscle fatigue during cardiogenic shock. *J Appl Physiol* 1981; 51:499–508.

147. Hussain AN, Marcotte JE, Burnet H, et al: Relationship among EMG and contractile responses of the diaphragm elicited by hypotension. *J Appl Physiol* 1988; 65:649–656.

148. Kadefors R, Kaiser E, Petersen I: Dynamic spectrum analysis of myo-potentials and with special reference to muscle fatigue. *Electromyography* 1968; 8:39–74.

149. Gross D, Grassino A, Ross WRD, et al: Electromyogram pattern of diaphragmatic fatigue. *J Appl Physiol* 1979; 46:1–7.

150. Bracewell RN. The Fourier transform. *Sci Am* 1989; June:86–95.

151. Schweitzer TW, Fitzgerald JW, Bowden JA, et al: Spectral analysis of human inspiratory diaphragmatic electromyograms. *J Appl Physiol* 1979; 46:152–165.

152. Barnes WS, Williams JH: Effects of ischemia on myo-electrical signal characteristics during rest and recovery from static work. *Am J Phys Med* 1987; 66:249–263.

153. Gross D, Ladd HW, Riley EJ, et al: The effect of training on strength and endurance of the diaphragm in quadriplegia. *Am J Med* 1980; 68:27–35.

154. Jardim J, Farkas G, Prefaut C, et al: The failing inspiratory muscles under normoxic and hypoxic conditions. *Am Rev Respir Dis* 1981; 124:274–279.

155. Walsh JM, Romano S, Grassino A: The effect of diaphragm length on the EMG power spectrum. *Clin Res* 1990; 38:847A.

156. Walsh JM, Ito T, Grassino A: A model to detect intermittent respiratory muscle fatigue. *Faseb J* 1990; 4:A291.

157. Walsh JM, Ito T, Grassino A: Detecting intermittent muscle fatigue by the variance of the median frequency. *Faseb J* 1991; 5:A1035.

Chapter 10 ———————————————————

Pulse Oximetry

Kevin McCarthy, R.C.P.T.

Michael J. Decker, C.R.T.T.

Kingman P. Strohl, M.D.

James K. Stoller, M.D.

INTRODUCTION

During the last decade, pulse oximeters, devices that provide continuous, noninvasive measurements of arterial oxygen saturation, have grown from relative obscurity to an almost indispensable patient monitoring modality. Because of its well-documented accuracy, ease of use, and good patient tolerance, pulse oximetry has become the preferred method for noninvasively monitoring arterial oxygen saturation in operating rooms, intensive care units (ICUs), exercise studies, and for outpatient assessment of oxygenation over time.

With such widespread application of pulse oximetry technology, the clinician who uses these devices must understand their operating principles and the practical limitations of their use. With this in mind, the goals of this chapter are to describe the fundamental operating principles used in pulse oximetry technology, acquaint clinicians with environmental and physiological conditions that may invalidate data from the pulse oximeter, and review the spectrum of clinical settings in which pulse oximetry is currently used and likely to be used in the future.

THE HISTORY OF PULSE OXIMETRY

Pulse oximeters rely on two primary principles of light transmission and reception, called *spectrophotometry* and *photoplethysmography*, to measure arterial oxygen saturation noninvasively. Spectrophotometry measures the percentage of oxygenated hemoglobin in the blood and photoplethysmography is used to differentiate arterial from venous blood.

Spectrophotometry is a technique that measures the concentration of a substance by the amount of light it absorbs. Spectrophotometric properties of hemoglobin were first elucidated in 1877, and by the early 1900s, *in vitro* spectrophotometry was used to determine the concentration of hemoglobin in the blood. During the following decades, reports of the absorption spectra of hemoglobin and its derivatives appeared in the literature.[1] Eventually, *in vitro* spectrophotometric techniques were used to measure the amount of oxygen bound to hemoglobin molecules.

Development of noninvasive spectrophotometric techniques to measure hemoglobin derivatives, and specifically oxygen saturation, were stimulated by World War II. With the development of high-altitude aircraft, monitoring techniques were needed to record physiological changes induced by extreme altitude. This demand for new technology generated research in the area of noninvasive physiologic monitoring. By 1940, Squire published "An Instrument for Measuring the Quantity of Blood and Its Degree of Oxygenation in the Web of the Hand."[2] While this device did not differentiate between oxygenated and deoxygenated hemoglobin, it was among the first to provide noninvasive *in vivo* measurements of total blood oxygenation. Then, in 1942, Glen Millikan developed the first functional noninvasive spectrophotometer, which used two optical filters to transmit light through the pinna of the ear.[3] Of these two filters, red and green, the red was responsible for measuring changes in the color of hemoglobin molecule while the green was considered a constant since it was only sensitive to the quantity of hemoglobin present, not its color. Unknown to Millikan at that time, the green filter did not transmit green light through the ear, but a light in the infrared region, similar to current pulse oximeters. Millikan named this new spectrophotometer the *oximeter*.

This new application of spectrophotometry, the ear oximeter, provided continuous *in vivo* measurements of hemoglobin oxygen saturation that were almost as accurate as invasive *in vitro* measurements. The major limitation of this early ear oximeter was that it could not compensate for intersubject variation in ear tissue thickness or skin pigmentation, both of which affect the Lambert-Beer laws of light transmission and absorption. This problem was addressed in 1949 by Wood et al.[4] who developed an inflatable bulb to be used with the ear oximeter. By placing the bulb on the ear and inflating it, the blood could be squeezed out and the blanched ear would be a reference measurement for pigmentation, tissue thickness, and nonblood tissue. This new ear oximeter equipped with a balloon was eventually manufactured by the Waters Company and became routinely used in research laboratories. Unfortunately, because of the rigorous calibration requirements before each application, it never received wide acceptance in clinical settings.

Following the introduction of the Waters ear oximeter, noninvasive oximetric technology remained essentially dormant until the introduction of the Hewlett-Packard ear oximeter in 1975. This oximeter was self-calibrating and used eight wavelengths of light, which were transmitted through fiber-optic cables to a housing strapped to the pinna of the ear. Hewlett-Packard's algorithm was based on a multicomponent model in which eight wavelengths of light were used to formulate a set of equations based on the Lambert-Beer laws. Each of the eight wavelengths was responsible for measuring particular variables such as tissue thickness and pigmentation, hemoglobin content, and oxygenated and deoxygenated hemoglobin, as well as dyshemoglobins.

The Hewlett-Packard device also had a heating element built into the earpiece housing to warm the ear and dilate nearby arterioles. This method of arterialization provided a maximally perfused arterial bed with minimal venous blood further increasing the oximeter's accuracy. Additionally, whereas earlier oximeters required the rigorous calibration procedure of squeezing blood from the ear to determine tissue thickness, as well as a two-point calibration to set the high and low limits of accuracy, the Hewlett-Packard ear oximeter had an internal calibrating slot with an automated calibration routine.

While the Hewlett-Packard ear oximeter received acclaim as a research tool, it never gained widespread acceptance in clinical applications due to its impractical size, cumbersome headgear, and costly retail price. These inhibiting factors eventually led to the discontinuation of the Hewlett-Packard ear oximeter in the late 1970s. Fortunately, since the time of the Hewlett-Packard device, advances in electronic engineering, such as light-emitting diodes (LEDs), photodetectors, and miniaturized amplifiers, have provided a means to refine oximetry technology to a low cost, state-of-the-art, noninvasive monitoring technique (Fig 10–1).

These advances in oximetry technology were brought about by innovative Japanese researchers who combined the principles of spectrophotometry with those of photoplethysmography to create the *pulse oximeter*.

FUNDAMENTALS OF SPECTROPHOTOMETRY AND PHOTOPLETHYSMOGRAPHY

Spectrophotometry measures oxygen bound to hemoglobin since the color and optical density of the hemoglobin molecule change with the amount of oxygen bound to it. Oxygenated hemoglobin (Hbo_2) is bright red while deoxygenated hemoglobin (Hb) is dark blue, so each species of hemoglobin has its own absorption characteristics.[5] By transmitting a constant

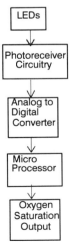

FIG 10–1.
Block diagram of a pulse oximeter.

amount of red light (in the region of 660 nm) through whole blood, the amount of red light absorbed is determined by the color of the hemoglobin, which is proportional to the amount of oxygen bound to it (Fig 10–2).

Spectrophotometric measurements of hemoglobin and its derivatives rely on the Lambert-Beer law of absorption. This law combines Lambert's law and Beer's law, both of which describe radiation transmitted through an absorbing substance. Briefly, Lambert's law states that the optical density of a homogeneous medium is directly proportional to the thickness of the medium.

Beer's law states that the optical density of a homogeneous absorbing substance is directly proportional to the concentration of the absorbing substance. The consolidated Lambert-Beer law specifies the relationship of the optical density to both path length and concentration of the absorbing substance. However, these laws can only be applied to blood if several conditions exist: (1) There can be no optical scattering of the medium; therefore, the blood sample must be hemolyzed. (2) No photochemical reaction can take place in the blood, such as fluorescence. (3) The optical radiation must be monochromatic and collimated.

Once these conditions are met, by employing the principles of the Lambert-Beer laws, spectrophotometry can be used to measure accurately hemoglobin and its derivatives. Since one condition to the Lambert-Beer laws is that the blood must be hemolyzed before analysis, it must be withdrawn from the subject. These *in vitro* measurements of hemolyzed blood by spectrophotometry are produced by devices called *co-oximeters* or *hemoximeters*. After placing a hemolyzed blood sample into the co-oximeter chamber, five wavelengths of light are transmitted through it to measure total hemoglobin, methemoglobin, carboxyhemoglobin, oxygen content, and oxygen saturation. Unfortunately, while hemoximetric measurements of hemoglobin and its derivatives are quite accurate and can be obtained very quickly, invasive arterial blood sampling is required, carrying an associated risk of morbidity. To avoid the risks of invasive blood sampling to measure arterial oxygen saturation, spectrophotometry was com-

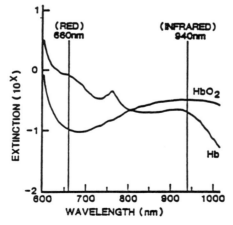

FIG 10–2.
The absorption (extinction) characteristics of oxyhemoglobin (HbO_2) and reduced hemoglobin (Hb) showing marked differences in absorption of red light (660 nm) and infrared light (940 nm). Courtesy of Ohmeda.

bined with photoplethysmography to produce a noninvasive monitoring device that could selectively measure arterial blood oxygenation.[6]

Photoplethysmography uses light reflectance or transmission through vascular tissue to measure arterial pressure waveforms generated by the cardiac cycle. The basic principle of photoplethysmography is that if a constant amount of light is transmitted through a pulsating vascular bed, more light is transmitted through the bed when the arterioles are nearly empty (cardiac diastole), and less light is transmitted through the bed when the arterioles are most full (cardiac systole). Therefore, if a constant beam of light is transmitted through a vascular bed, the intensity of the light that reaches the photodetector on the opposite side increases and decreases with the filling and emptying of the arterioles.

Photoplethysmography can be used to make noninvasive, relative measurements of arterial blood flow, blood pressure, and tissue perfusion. Since the majority of blood pulsing through a vascular bed is arterial, when photoplethysmography (to measure arterial pulsations) was combined with spectrophotometry (to measure the oxygen bound to hemoglobin), engineers were able to build a machine that could differentiate arterial from venous blood and therefore selectively measure arterial oxygen saturation. The application of this new pulse oximetric technology was a clinical tool that could effectively measure arterial oxygen saturation noninvasively.

PULSE OXIMETER SENSOR TECHNOLOGY

After the initial pulse oximeters were engineered, sensor technology played an important role in applying pulse oximetry technology to the clinical setting. With the previously mentioned advent of high-intensity LEDs, cumbersome fiber-optic cables for light transmission and photodetection were replaced with light gauge cables and miniaturized sensors to link the pulse oximeter to the subject.

The typical pulse oximeter sensor configuration is one or two red LEDs and an infrared LED, which are located on one side of the monitoring site. A photoreceiver is positioned on the opposite side of the monitoring site, directly opposite the LEDs (Fig 10–3). The function of the red and infrared LEDs is to transmit red and infrared light, while the photoreceiver measures their intensity on the opposite side of the monitoring site. Various sensors are available that utilize digits, noses, or ears as potential oxygen saturation monitoring sites, the only stipulation being that the site cannot be so thick as to prevent transmission of light through it.

As mentioned earlier, the intensity or proportion of transmitted red light to that which is received is primarily dependent on the color of the hemoglobin molecule, which is a function of the amount of the oxygen bound to it. In addition, pulse oximeters use a second light wavelength to measure oxygen saturation. This wavelength, which is in the infrared region, is called *isobestic*, that is to say, deoxygenated as well as oxygenated hemoglobin will absorb about the same amount of it.

One purpose of the infrared light is to provide a constant (a light intensity unaffected by the color of the hemoglobin). The oximeter microprocessor uses this constant as a value in its

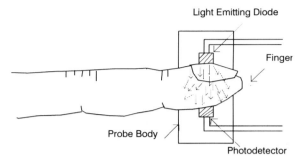

FIG 10–3.
Pulse oximeter finger probe.

calculation of oxygen saturation. As stated previously, red light transmission through a vascular bed is dependent on hemoglobin oxygen saturation, but the infrared light is not. Therefore, a ratio between the intensity of the transmitted and received red to infrared light can be calculated. It is this ratio of red to infrared light that the oximeter uses to derive a value of oxygen saturation (Fig 10–4).

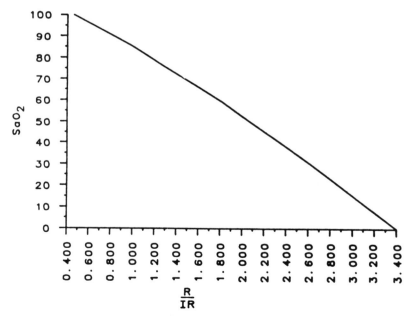

FIG 10–4.
Relationship of red (R)/infrared (IR) absorbance ratio to arterial oxygen saturation. (*From Wukitsch MW, Petterson MT, Tobler DR, et al: Pulse oximetery: Analysis of theory, technology and practice.* J Clin Monit 1988; 4:290–301. Used by permission.)

The basic operating principles of current pulse oximeters are important for an understanding of available devices. All currently available pulse oximeters use LEDs to transmit red and infrared light in the region of 660 and 960 nm, respectively. The light is transmitted through a vascular bed to a photoreceiver positioned opposite the LEDs. As the light passes through the vascular bed, its intensity is modulated by the filling and emptying of the arterioles, thus assuming an "ac" characteristic. The pulse oximeter only "looks" at the modulating light since it represents arterial blood. Both the red and the infrared light are modulated by the pulsating arterioles; however, the red light is further modulated by the color of the hemoglobin (the darker the hemoglobin molecule, the more red light it will absorb). The photoreceiver positioned opposite the LEDs measures the intensity of the red and infrared light that has passed through the vascular bed (Fig 10–3). The oximeter microprocessor then compares the intensity of the transmitted light to that which is received over the entire pulse waveform (Fig 10–7).

Most oximeters sample the red and infrared light modulation at 480 cycles per second (cps). Each cycle consists of three phases during which the red, infrared, and ambient light levels are measured. The intensity of ambient light levels measured when both LEDs are off is then subtracted from the measured red and infrared light (Fig 10–6).

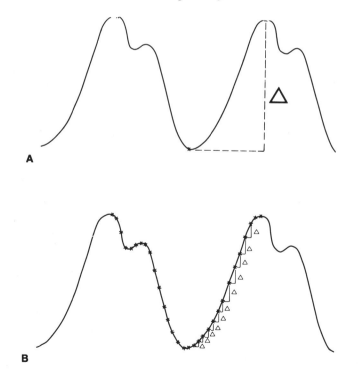

FIG 10–5.
Two schemes for measuring the changes in light absorption during a pulse. **A,** the change in light absorption from a "trough" to a "peak" value on the pulse waveform. **B,** the more common method of collecting multiple samples along the pulsatile waveform. These values are then subjected to various "weighting" maneuvers to help minimize displays of artifactual Spo$_2$. Courtesy of Ohmeda.

OXIMETER CALIBRATION METHODS

Calculation of oxygen saturation from the intensity of two light wavelengths transmitted through a vascular bed requires empirical calibration using healthy human subjects, the results of which are incorporated into the oximeter's algorithm for calculating hemoglobin saturation. To determine this calibration, subjects have an indwelling arterial catheter inserted, then the sensor of the pulse oximeter being tested is affixed to a well-perfused digit. The subjects are then ventilated with an isocapnic hypoxic gas mixture to lower their arterial oxygen saturation to predetermined levels.[7]

Once the desired level of hypoxemia is reached, the inspired oxygen is held constant to stabilize the subject at a specific arterial oxygen saturation, serial arterial blood samples are drawn from the indwelling catheter, and hemoximetry is used to measure oxygen saturation. The ratio of red to infrared light transmitted and received by the pulse oximeter is then measured and the corresponding value of oxygen saturation (as measured by the co-oximeter) is assigned to that ratio. This procedure is repeated at different levels of arterial oxygen saturation until a complete calibration curve is constructed. Then, the entire protocol is repeated in a series of subjects until the pulse oximeter and co-oximeter reproduce the same values of arterial oxygen saturation during both normoxic and hypoxic conditions.

PULSE OXIMETER ACCURACY AND RESPONSE TIMES

To validate the accuracy of pulse oximetry in clinical settings, investigators use the same protocol as the oximeter manufacturers to compare pulse oximetric values of oxygen saturation to invasive measurements. Early studies and, to some extent, current research use regression analysis and correlation coefficients to compare pulse oximetric values of oxygen saturation to invasive measurements. Unfortunately, the use of correlation coefficients is inappropriate when comparing pulse oximetry to co-oximetry. Analysis of correlation coefficients assumes a null hypothesis and since co-oximetry and pulse oximetry both use spectrophotometric means to estimate oxygen saturation, an inherently strong correlation exists. However, it has been suggested by Bland and Altman[8] that because pulse oximetry values of oxygen saturation (denoted Spo_2) "replace" invasive co-oximetric values of oxygen saturation (Sao_2), the two values should "agree" before one can replace the other. This method of agreement is used to determine statistically the mean of two values ($Sao_2 + Spo_2/2$) against their difference ($Sao_2 - Spo_2$). From these values, the pulse oximeter's bias and precision with respect to invasive measurements of oxygen saturation can be determined.

The bias of the pulse oximeter is the mean difference between simultaneous pulse oximetric and co-oximetric measurements of oxygen saturation. For example, if the pulse oximetry saturation is 97% while an arterial blood sample is obtained and the oxyhemoglobin by hemoximetry is 95%, the pulse oximeter demonstrates a bias of approximately 2%.

The precision of a pulse oximeter is the standard deviation of the mean bias. By multiplying the standard deviation of the mean bias by two, a 95% confidence interval can be determined. The 95% confidence interval is the predicted range into which 95% of random measurements would be expected to fall. Recent work[9] indicates that the 95% confidence limit of most pulse oximeters (compared to "gold standard" invasive measurements of oxygen saturation) range from 3 to 5%.

The response time of pulse oximeters depends on their data-averaging scheme (described earlier) as well as the patient's hemodynamic status. The circulation time between the lungs (where gas exchange occurs) and the fingertips (where pulmonary gas exchange is measured) will be influenced by heart rate and peripheral vasoconstriction due to hypoxic stress. It is also possible that during hypoxic events, a shunting of arterial blood to the vital organs decreases the flow of arterial blood to the extremities. Therefore, the location of the pulse oximeter probe will also affect the pulse oximeter's response time.

Severinghaus and Naifeh[10] found that the average response time to desaturation events was 10 to 20 seconds for oximeters with ear sensors and 24 to 35 seconds for oximeters with finger sensors. Warley, Mitchell, and Stradling[11] reported response times of 9.8 seconds for oximeters with ear sensors, 23.6 seconds for oximeters with finger sensors, and 56.8 seconds for oximeters equipped with toe sensors.

DATA AVERAGING AND ARTIFACT REJECTION SCHEMES

While small pulse-to-pulse variations do exist in measured values of oxygen saturation, displaying these variations could be distracting to the clinician. To help eliminate small variations in displayed oxygen saturation values, oximeter algorithms use data-smoothing schemes, which average values of oxygen saturation over several heart beats before they are displayed. Beside averaging pulse-to-pulse variations in oxygen saturation to provide a stable number to display, other advantages to signal smoothing exist. For instance, during infrequent episodes of motion, any sporadic artifactual readings are averaged together with the good readings to help avoid displaying erratic values of oxygen saturation. However, the pitfalls of lengthy signal-averaging routines include delayed machine response times during acute changes in oxygen saturation. Also, imprecise displays of high and low oxygen saturation values during hypoxic events can occur since normative values immediately preceding and following the events are averaged in with the lower values.

To help counter the possibility of the pulse oximeter's providing false values of oxygen saturation from artifactual pulse waveforms, and in an effort to keep data-averaging times to a minimum, the oximeter algorithm employs various artifact rejection schemes. Some oximeters employ predefined templates of arterial pulse waveforms to which all incoming pulse waveforms are fitted. If the incoming pulse waveform does not fit the template, one of several events will occur (dependent on the oximeter algorithm). Some algorithms will discard the pulse waveforms that do not fit within the template and, if a string of unusable waveforms appears, the oximeter displays an error message. Other oximeter algorithms (in the presence of unusable pulse waveforms) will freeze the last good oxygen saturation value. This value can be held in the display for several seconds until usable waveforms reappear.

Other techniques to filter out artifactual pulse waveforms are weighted pulse waveform averaging schemes. This strategy applies a "weight" or a measure of "how good" the incoming

TABLE 10–1.
Simplified Representation of Ten Spo$_2$ Values with Assigned Weights*

Variable	At 1/3 of 1 Second									
Spo$_2$	94	93	94	95	72	30	45	85	95	94
wt	10	10	10	9	5	1	1	7	9	10
Spo$_2$ × wt	940	930	940	855	360	30	45	595	855	940

Pulse oximetry saturation values showing assigned weights. Weights are assigned using several factors, including comparison of the current reading with the average value currently displayed. Readings that deviate greatly from the displayed value are assigned a low weight with a relatively small impact on the average value displayed.
* From Wukitsch MW, Petterson MT, Tobler DR, et al: Pulse oximetry: Analysis of theory, technology and practice. *J Clin Monit* 1988; 4:290–301. Used by permission.

pulse waveform looks. Values of oxygen saturation derived from waveforms weighted low in the averaging scheme contribute minimally to the overall calculation of oxygen saturation, whereas waveforms weighted highly contribute maximally to the calculation of oxygen saturation. When used in conjunction with pulse waveform templates, waveform weighting provides a fairly effective mechanism to discriminate artifactual from physiological pulse waveforms (Tables 10–1 and 10–2).

CONFUSION OVER FUNCTIONAL VERSUS FRACTIONAL SATURATIONS

Two different types of oxygen saturation, so-called "functional" saturation and "fractional" saturation have been specified to recognize that pulse oximeters using two wavelengths can mistake dysfunctional hemoglobins (like carboxy- and methemoglobin) for oxyhemoglobin. Fractional saturation can only be measured when oxyhemoglobin can be distinguished from carboxyhemoglobin and methemoglobin (e.g., with a hemoximeter) and divides oxyhemoglobin by the sum of reduced hemoglobin, oxygenoglobin, carboxyhemoglobin and methemoglobin, per Equation (10–1). In contrast, functional O_2 saturation differs from fractional saturation because dysfunctional hemoglobins are not considered per Equation (10–2).

TABLE 10–2.
Displayed Spo$_2$ Values Derived from 3-Second Averages*

	SECOND 1	SECOND 2	SECOND 3	SECOND 4
Processed Average	92 93 93	92 93 94	93 94 94	90 91 92

|——Displayed Value 1 = 93.1——|
|————Displayed Value 2 = 92.8————|
(Displayed Values are Rounded Up or Down)

Further processing of pulse oximetry values: data averaging.
* From Wukitsch MW, Petterson MT, Tobler DR, et al: Pulse oximetry: Analysis of theory, technology and practice. *J Clin Monit* 1988; 4:290–301. Used by permission.

$$Sao_2\% = \frac{Hbo_2}{(RHb + Hbo_2 + HbCO + MHb)} \times 100 \qquad (10-1)$$

where

RHb = reduced hemoglobin
Hbo_2 = oxyhemoglobin
$Hbco$ = carboxyhemoglobin
MHb = methemoglobin.

$$Spo_2\% = \frac{Hbo_2}{(RHb + Hbo_2)} \times 100 \qquad (10-2)$$

Although the difference between functional and fractional saturation is simple, the claim that two-wavelength pulse oximeters measure functional saturation is misleading. Two observations suggest that two-wavelength pulse oximeters do not actually measure functional saturation. First, such oximeters cannot distinguish oxyhemoglobin from carboxyhemoglobin, so the numerator of Equation (10–2) reflects both types of hemoglobin, not just oxyhemoglobin.

Further evidence that pulse oximeters do not really measure "functional" saturation lies in the fact that when the Fio_2 is 1.0 and significant concentrations of $Hbco$ and MHb are present, some pulse oximeters do not measure 100% saturation as would be expected if they were truly measuring "functional" saturation.[12, 13]

TECHNICAL LIMITATIONS OF PULSE OXIMETRY

Several technical factors can affect the accuracy of pulse oximetry measurements, including motion artifact, dysfunctional hemoglobins, fingernail polish, intravascular dyes, ambient light, and skin pigmentation. These factors are reviewed below.

Motion Artifact

When an oximeter sensor is on a digit subjected to excessive motion, the intermittent contact of the sensor with the skin can mechanically modulate the pathlength of the transmitted light as well as the amplitude and intensity of the received light. If the motion is repetitive or persistent, signals for similar amplitude will be received in both the red and infrared channels.

These mechanically induced variances in light transmission and reception through the monitoring site can produce false arterial pulse waveforms and the oximeter may not be able to differentiate the motion-induced waveforms from true arterial pulse waveforms. Thus, the pulse oximeter will present a spurious value for oxygen saturation.

The reason that pulse oximeters can calculate values of oxygen saturation from artifactually induced changes in light intensity is that the artifactual pulse waveform generates an ac signal larger in amplitude than the genuine arterial pulse-modulated ac signal. Then, during this period, because of their artificially heightened amplitude, the ratio of the red to infrared signals becomes almost entirely a function of the dc signal levels (Fig 10–7). Because of their large amplitude, the voltage of the two dc signals is similar and their ratio becomes 1. The calibration curve that most oximeters use to convert the ratio of absorbed red to infrared light defines[13] a ratio of 1 as an oxygen saturation of 84 to 88% (Fig 10–8).

Poor-quality pulse waveforms can also cause the oximeter to provide erroneous information. Poor-quality pulse waveforms commonly occur when the pulse pressure is low, so the amplitude of the pulse waveform may be so small that the oximeter cannot measure it accurately. To compensate for the small signal that it sees, the oximeter will increase the driving current of the LEDs as well as increase the gain of the photoreceiver to bring the measured amplitude of the pulse waveform into a workable range. This increase in LED driving current and increased photoreceiver gain concomitantly increases the noise-to-signal ratio. This makes the oximeter more susceptible to motion artifact and other mechanisms that could create false values of oxygen saturation. One such mechanism is sensor displacement.

In some older but still commonly used pulse oximeter models, the oximeter goes into a search mode if the sensor falls off the patient. As the oximeter searches for a nonexistent pulse

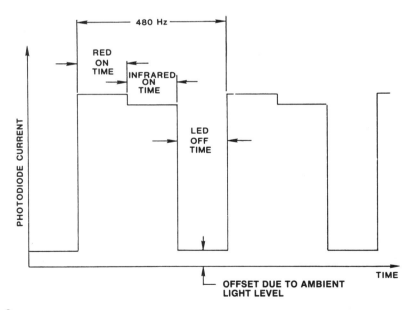

FIG 10–6.
Output of the pulse oximeter photodetector on the Ohmeda 3700 pulse oximeter demonstrating a sampling technique that allows for measurement of and compensation for ambient light. (*From Pologe JA: Pulse oximetry: Technical aspects of machine design.* Int Anesthesiol Clin *1987; 25:137–154. Used by permission.*)

PULSE OXIMETRY

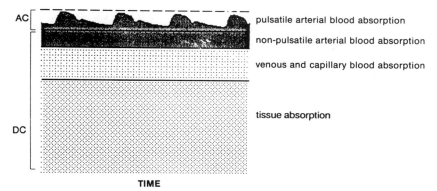

FIG 10–7.
The absorption signal of a pulse oximeter showing the pulsatile (ac) and nonpulsatile (dc) components of the signal. Courtesy of Ohmeda.

waveform, it increases the LEDs driving current and the photoreceiver gain. Then, if the conditions are right, the oximeter actually measures the fluctuating intensity of the LEDs and mistakes it for an arterial pulse waveform, from which the oximeter calculates a value of oxygen saturation. This phenomenon was particularly noticeable with some of the earlier pulse oximeters, which used small ear sensor attachments. These sensors were noted to provide values of oxygen saturation while clipped to newspapers.

Pulse oximeters will measure a small heartbeat-to-heartbeat variability in oxygen saturation. This variability can be caused by the initial arterial pulse pressure compressing and emptying the venous bed. As the arterial pressure decreases, the venous bed opens and fills, thus behaving like an artery. Because the venous and arterial pulsations occur simultaneously, a small amount of venous blood is seen and included in the calculation of oxygen saturation. The actual amount of blood remaining in the venous system can vary with heart rate, arterial blood pressure, or cardiac output, thereby creating these pulse-to-pulse variations in measured oxygen saturation.

Clinicians who wish to utilize pulse oximetric technology to its full potential must recognize the subtle signal processing limitations associated with noninvasive monitoring technology and certain physiological conditions that affect the machine's accuracy. Some acutely induced conditions (such as carbon monoxide poisoning or radiographic dyes) temporarily prohibit the use of pulse oximeters, while some chronic physiologic conditions warrant prudent use of pulse oximetry. The following section highlights specific physiologic conditions that affect pulse oximetry accuracy.

Carboxyhemoglobin

Carboxyhemoglobin is viewed by the pulse oximeter as if it were predominately oxyhemoglobin, although some of its absorption is attributed to reduced hemoglobin. Therefore, pulse oximeters will read approximately the sum of oxyhemoglobin and carboxyhemoglobin. This is not because pulse oximeters do not measure carboxyhemoglobin, but rather because two-wavelength pulse oximeters cannot discriminate between light absorption caused by the presence of oxyhemoglobin and absorption caused by the presence of carboxyhemoglobin. Thus, the pulse oximeter will overestimate the Sao_2 by an amount roughly equivalent to the amount of carboxyhemoglobin present.[12, 14] True distinction between oxyhemoglobin and carboxyhemoglobin, which is needed to calculate "fractional saturation" (see earlier discussion on confusion over functional versus fractional saturation), requires a hemoximeter.

Methemoglobin

Methemoglobin has significant absorption at both 660 and 940 nm (Fig 10–9). This tends to push the absorbance ratio at these two wavelengths to a value[13] close to 1.0. On the calibration curve used by pulse oximeters, an absorbance ratio of 1.0 corresponds to a saturation of 83 to 87%. As a result, increasing levels of methemoglobin cause the pulse oximeter reading to approach 85%. This could result in an underestimation or overestimation of O_2 saturation, depending on the patient's actual O_2 saturation (Fig 10–8).

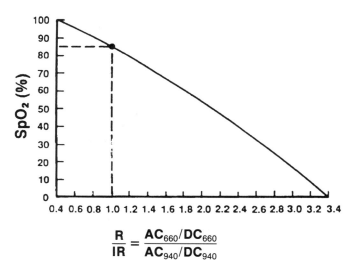

$$\frac{R}{IR} = \frac{AC_{660}/DC_{660}}{AC_{940}/DC_{940}}$$

FIG 10–8.
The absorbance ratio of red (R) to infrared (IR) showing a pulse oximeter saturation of 85% associated with a ratio of 1.0. This can occur in the presence of an elevated methemoglobin or low signal strenth coupled with motion artifact. (*From Welch JP, DeCesare R, Hess D: Pulse oximetry: Instrumentation and clinical application. Resp Care 1990; 35:584–597. Used by permission.*)

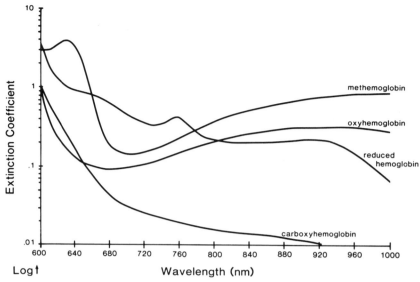

FIG 10–9.
The extinction coefficients of hemoglobin that can be measured in blood by hemoximetry. Methemoglobin exhibits significant absorption at both 660 and 940 nm, wavelengths commonly used for pulse oximetry. Courtesy of Ohmeda.

Intravascular Dyes

Radiographic dyes injected into a patient will also affect the accuracy of pulse oximeters. Since most radiographic dyes are either methyl blue or green, a prominent amount of blue dye in the arterial blood can be misinterpreted by the oximeter as being deoxygenated hemoglobin. This falsely low value has the potential of being misinterpreted by the unsuspecting clinician as true hypoxemia. Scheller, Unger, and Kelner[15] studied the effects of 5-mL injections of radiographic dyes in young healthy volunteers (Table 10–3). Six subjects received methylene blue injections, five received indocyanine green, and five received indigo carmine. Methylene blue produced the largest decreases in saturation, followed by indocyanine green. Indigo carmine had little or no effect on oximetric measurements of arterial oxygen saturation. When methylene blue or green was injected into the subject, pulse oximetric values of oxygen saturation were markedly decreased for several minutes. This study indicates that intravascular dyes transiently affect the pulse oximeter's ability to measure oxygen saturation. Therefore, these values may not reflect the true clinical condition of the patient.

Fingernail Polish

Several reports indicate that nail polish, particularly blue or black colors, will interfere with pulse oximetry measurements.[16, 17] This occurs since the color blue and, to a lesser degree, the color black can absorb the red light transmitted by the pulse oximeter. Also, these darker

TABLE 10-3.
Subject Characteristics and O_2 Saturation Reading Responses to IV Dyes*

Dye	Weight (kg)	Height (in.)	Latency (sec) Finger/Toe	Duration (sec) Finger/Toe	Nadir (O_2 Saturation) Finger/Toe
MeBl	75	70	80/65	70/90	91/80
	68	69	35/30	105/80	58/65
	79	72	40/40	65/50	76/59
	93	71	40/35	50/50	80/69
	46	64	35/30	115/80	1/32
InGr	83	74	35/45	10/40	96/96
	67	69	45/40	35/25	95/93
	70	70	45/35	45/70	93/84
	86	75	50/45	70/30	93/92
	70	69	NC/65	NC/60	99/88
InCa	83	74	NC/NC	NC/NC	NC/NC
	67	70	NC/40	NC/40	NC/93
	46	64	NC/25	NC/30	NC/92
	86	69	NC/NC	NC/NC	NC/NC
	65	68	NC/20	NC/20	NC/94

* From Scheller MS, Unger RJ, Kelner MJ: Effects of intravenously administered dyes on pulse oximetry readings. *Anesthesiol* 1986; 65:550–552. Used by permission.
MeBl = methylene blue; InGr = indocyanine green; InCa = indigo carmine; NC = no observed change; Latency = time to initial fall (sec); Duration = time from initial fall until return to baseline (ssec); Nadir = lowest Spo_2 reading observed.

colors can cause a degree of light shunting around the finger periphery. As discussed later, shunting of light has also been implicated as one of the mechanisms responsible for pulse oximeter inaccuracies in darkly pigmented people.[18]

Elevated Serum Bilirubin

The Hewlett-Packard (H-P) 3700 ear oximeter, which utilizes eight-wavelength spectrophotometry, displays erroneous oxygen saturations in patients with hyperbilirubinemia.[19] A study that examined eight-wavelength H-P ear oximeter saturations in 19 patients with varying degrees of jaundice found that ear oximetry saturation averaged 6% lower than actual measured oxygen saturations. The pulse oximeter, however, does not appear to be affected by high levels of bilirubin. Chelluri, Snyder, and Bird[20] compared pulse oximetry and hemoximetry measurements in 18 normal bilirubin and 21 hyperbilirubinemic critical care patients and found that the bias and precision levels for both groups were comparable. The mean bias and precision in patients with normal bilirubin were −0.055% and 1.87%, and were −0.667% and 1.96% in patients with hyperbilirubinemia. These authors included only patients with bilirubin >20 mg/dL in their hyperbilirubinemia group.

Low Perfusion States

Pulse oximeters depend on a clearly identifiable arterial pulse to operate properly. Their performance declines when peripheral pulses are weak or absent. When pulse amplitude is low as in hypovolemia, hypotension, hypothermia, vasoconstrictor infusions, or cardiac bypass surgery, Spo_2 readings are either intermittent or absent.

Some pulse oximeters may be better than others in processing weak signals. Vasodilating creams may increase the pulse amplitude in low perfusion states. The earlobe is less affected by vasoconstriction than the fingertip and may produce a sufficient signal to obtain a reading.[21] In low perfusion states, the signal-to-noise ratio is reduced and the oximeter will be more prone to display data caused by a motion artifact than when pulse amplitude is normal.

In routine clinical use, warming of the probe site by wrapping it in hot towels or rubbing with isopropyl alcohol may aid in obtaining a baseline reading, but it must be remembered that most pulse oximeter probes are unheated and the increase in peripheral circulation brought on by warming may only be temporary. This can be important when monitoring oxygen saturation trends over extended time periods.

Increased Venous Pressures

It has been suggested that the pulse of blood sensed by the pulse oximeter is arterial blood that has been shunted through cutaneous arteriovenous anastamoses to the veins.[22] While the pulse volume amplitude originates in the arteries and arterioles, the overall changes within arteriovenous anastamoses, capillaries, veins, and venules may contribute more to the total pulse volume amplitude. Therefore, admixing of venous and arterial blood in these vessels could conceivably lower values of oxygen saturation measured by pulse oximetry.

The concept of physiologic mixing of venous and arterial blood was explored by Graham, Paulus, and Caffee,[23] who looked at the use of pulse oximetry in replanted digits. By using a pulse oximeter to monitor values of oxygen saturation in the affected digit, they found that when a replanted digit developed venous obstruction (later confirmed by surgery), the disparity between pulse oximeter saturations and Sao_2 rose, and pulse oximeter values of oxygen saturation fell to approximately 85%.

Anemia

In anemic states, whether transiently induced during open heart surgery by thermodilution or pathologically induced by chronic renal failure, the chance of pulse oximeter error is increased. With anemia, pulse oximetry in the normoxic patient appears to be fairly accurate, but in the patient suspected of being hypoxic, pulse oximetry values should be validated by invasive arterial blood samples. The reason for this concern (which has been shown in theoretical models but not duplicated in a clinical setting) is that the oximeter algorithm is programmed to use a light intensity strong enough to transmit through a certain amount of red blood cells in any given area.

Theoretically, the oximeter can increase or decrease its light transmission intensity to compensate for tissue thickness. However, the scattering of the transmitted light by a certain amount of red blood cells is also factored into the oximeter algorithm, and if the light is not scattered to the degree that is expected (as with anemia), too much of the transmitted red light will reach the photoreceiver and potentially create a falsely high value of oxygen saturation.

As described earlier, during calibration trials in healthy subjects, specific ratios of red to infrared light are paired to actual arterial values of oxygen saturation. However, pulse oximeters are generally used in clinical settings in unhealthy patients. In other words, if only healthy subjects with normal blood chemistry are used to develop calibration curves for pulse oximeters, the possibility exists that the oximeter may respond differently if used on someone with abnormal blood chemistry.

Ambient Light and External Light Sources

As mentioned earlier, to some degree, ambient light is compensated for during the sampling of the pulse oximeter. The measurement strategy employed by most oximeters is rapid sampling (480 cps). Each cycle consists of three phases. During these three phases the red, infrared, and ambient light levels are measured. The first phase turns the red (660-nm) LED on, the second phase turns the red LED off and the infrared (940-nm) LED on, and both LEDs are off in the third phase. When both LEDs are off in the third phase, ambient light levels are measured.

The level of light measured when both LEDs are off is then subtracted from the red and infrared channels. By including this ambient light measuring phase, oximeters can compensate for changing lighting conditions (Fig 10–6).

However, high-intensity light from fluorescent lights, operating room lights, and infrared heat lamps have been reported to interfere with pulse oximeter performance. A xenon arc surgical lamp caused a Nellcor N-100 oximeter to display falsely an Spo_2 of 100% and a heart rate of 180 to 250 beats per minute.[24] Common fluorescent lights have been shown to cause pulse oximeters to display spurious results, again causing the pulse oximeter to display a pulse of approximately 190 beats per minute.[25]

Infrared light will increase the infrared signal to the oximeter probe's photodiode and has been reported[26] to lower both heart rate and Spo_2. Fiberoptic light sources may affect pulse oximeter readings and have been reported[27] to cause oximeter heart rate readings of 250 beats per minute.[27]

Direct sunlight has also been reported to cause inappropriately high pulse oximeter readings.[28] Pulse oximeter probes should be wrapped in some type of light barrier whenever interference from an external light source is suspected. Wrap the probe sight, exercising care to avoid compromising circulation to the probe site. Materials such as surgical towel drape, alcohol wipe packet, or other foil shield or gauze wrap have been suggested in the literature.[27, 29, 30] All light interference problems reported in the literature note a lack of correlation of the oximeter's displayed heart rate and the patient's actual heart rate.

SKIN PIGMENTATION

Skin pigmentation is associated with technical difficulties in pulse oximetry measurements. Ries, Prewitt, and Johnson[18] were unable to obtain a reading or obtained a warning message indicating poor signal strength in 18% of darkly pigmented patients compared to 1% of the rest of their study population using the earlobe as a probe site.

Jubran and Tobin[31] compared pulse oximetry measurements and simultaneously drawn arterial blood samples measured by hemoximetry in 25 stable white patients and 29 stable black patients in their medical ICU. They found that the bias and precision of the pulse oximetry saturations were greater in black patients than in white patients (average bias 3.3 + 2.7% in black patients versus 2.2 ± 1.8% in white patients). Their findings show that dark skin pigmentation does affect the accuracy of pulse oximetry saturation measurements. Also, the fact that different pulse oximeters can give different simultaneous readings on the same patient mandates that the target values suggested by Jubran and Tobin be validated before adopting the use of pulse oximetry alone for titrating F_{IO_2} levels.

Work by Cahan et al.[32] suggests that one possible mechanism of the measurement error in pulse oximetric values of oxygen saturation is a shunting of the red and infrared light around the periphery of the monitoring site. Since light follows the path of least resistance, in darkly pigmented people a portion of the transmitted light may travel subcutaneously from the LEDs to the photoreceiver. This subcutaneously shunted light is never exposed to a vascular bed so its intensity is not modulated by any deoxygenated hemoglobin that may be present deeper within the digit. When the shunted light reaches the photoreceiver, it may or may not have assumed low-grade ac characteristics. If the shunted light has assumed ac characteristics by coming in contact with less intense red and infrared light modulated by a vascular bed, it can potentially increase the overall intensity of that light. The oximeter then interprets this falsely bright red and infrared light as having passed through well-oxygenated bright red hemoglobin. Alternatively, if the shunted light did not develop ac characteristics, its presence is still noted by the photoreceiver as electrical noise. As described earlier, this increased noise-to-signal ratio also has the potential to cause erroneous values of oxygen saturation to be displayed.

ACCURACY AND PRECISION OF OXIMETRY MEASUREMENTS

Studies of the accuracy of pulse oximetry typically compare pulse oximetry measurements with simultaneously obtained arterial blood oximetry (hemoximetry).[8] Early studies typically reported regression analysis and excellent correlation coefficients between pulse oximetry and hemoximetry.[33, 34] While a high correlation coefficient r between two variables indicates that there is a strong relationship between them, it does not indicate how well the two methods agree. An instrument that consistently reads too high, for example, may still have an excellent correlation coefficient.

As described above, more useful descriptors of performance are termed *bias* and *precision*.[35] The accuracy of a pulse oximeter is also determined by the methodology used for calibration.

Some pulse oximeter manufacturers calibrate their instrument using functional saturation while others use fractional saturation (see earlier section for distinction). Pulse oximeters that are calibrated using functional saturation will typically report Spo_2 values that are a few percent higher than saturations measured by pulse oximeters calibrated using fractional saturations.

Interpreting manufacturers' reports of accuracy is further confounded by pulse oximeter manufacturers' tendency to revise the software used by the instrument to calculate Spo_2 frequently. Pulse oximetry users should understand the validity of methods for measuring oxygen saturation and decide for themselves which oximeter meets their needs best.

The gold standard used in pulse oximetry accuracy and precision evaluations is *in vitro* measurements made on multiple wavelength hemoximeters such as the IL Model 282 Co-oximeter or Radiometer OSM-3. These instruments will also have measurable accuracy and precision characteristics. Because arterial blood hemoximeters also have a measurement error, their use to provide a "gold standard" must be tempered by acknowledging that error. To compensate effectively for a gold standard that is not perfect, a statistical technique called "the comparison of two methods technique" has been used.[8] This technique compares the difference between two measurements to the mean of those measurements. The comparison of two methods technique describes the agreement between pulse oximetry measurements and arterial blood hemoximetry measurements.

Figure 10–10 shows the agreement between the Hewlett-Packard ear oximeter and the Instrumentation Laboratories Model 282 Co-oximeter in white patients (open squares) and black patients (closed squares), illustrating the "comparison of two methods" technique. The data in this figure were obtained from four normal subjects over the course of two hypoxic

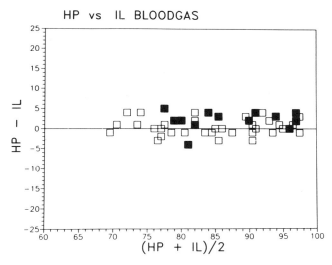

FIG 10–10.
Agreement of two means technique for comparing oximeter saturations (H-P ear oximeter) with oxygen saturation determined by hemoximetry in white patients (*open squares*) and black patients (*closed squares*). (*From Cahan C, Decker MJ: Agreement between noninvasive oximetric values for oxygen saturation.* Chest *1990; 97:814–819. Used by permission.*)

challenges.[32] This figure shows the 95% confidence limits of agreement between these two types of measurements to be approximately ±4%.

VARIABILITY OF ARTERIAL OXYGEN TENSION

When evaluating changes in pulse oximetry measurements, it is useful to know the expected variation of Pao_2 measurments. Even in stable patients, Pao_2 shows significant variation. Thorson et al.[36] studied serial, duplicate ABG measurements in 29 seriously ill but clinically stable ICU patients and found that the Pao_2 showed spontaneous variation of 16 ± 11 mm Hg (range of 1 to 45 mm Hg). The 95% confidence limit of expected variation over 10 minutes was 11%. This increased to 23% for samples obtained 50 minutes apart.

When considering the use of pulse oximetry monitoring, the relationship between the partial pressure of oxygen and hemoglobin should be remembered. This relationship is described by the oxyhemoglobin dissociation curve (Fig 10–11). The flat upper portion of this curve represents the range where relatively large changes in the partial pressure of oxygen (Pao_2) in the blood cause small changes in hemoglobin oxygen saturation. Increases in Pao_2 above 100 mm Hg cause very little change in hemoglobin oxygen saturation, which becomes relevant in clinical situations where hyperoxia is present (e.g., surgery). During general anesthesia, an

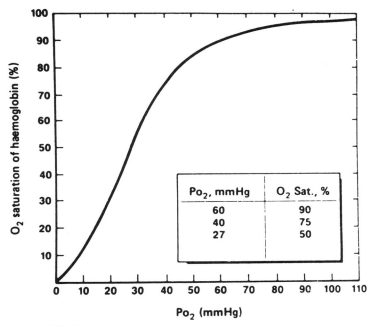

FIG 10–11.
Oxyhemoglobin dissociation curve. Courtesy of Ohmeda.

inspired oxygen concentration of 30% or more is common. In this case, healthy patients may achieve a Pao$_2$ of 200 mm Hg or more.

Subsequently, very large decreases in Pao$_2$ could occur without causing a fall in oxygen saturation. Therefore, pulse oximetry may not detect acute falls in Pao$_2$. Likewise, the typical 95% confidence limit of oximeters of ±4% renders pulse oximetry difficult to use as a monitoring device for hyperoxemia.

Knowledge of the expected intrasubject variability of repeat pulse oximetry measurements can aid interpretation of changes in repeat pulse oximetry measurements. Wagener and Hendricken[37] studied the reproducibility of repeated pulse oximetry measurements made on the same healthy individuals at different times, breathing both room air, hypoxic (15% O$_2$, 85% N$_2$), and hyperoxic (30% O$_2$, 70% N$_2$) mixtures. They found that while breathing room air, a change in Spo$_2$ of 2.1% can occur without indicating any change in pulmonary function. As the study subject's oxygen level decreased while breathing a hypoxic mixture, the variability of repeat measures increased to a high of 4.7%. This study evaluated measurements made on only one pulse oximeter and utilized only one operator. It is likely that measurements made on different units and different models of oximeters, using more than one operator, would show even greater intrasubject variability.

OXIMETER SAFETY

Although pulse oximetry measurements are considered by most to be risk-free, there have been several reports of patients' receiving burn injuries from pulse oximetry probes. Sloan[38] reported three patients who received burns on their fingertips after intraoperative pulse oximetry monitoring. These burns were attributed to a defective LED in the finger probe. More severe burns were reported by Murphy, Secunda, and Rockoff[39] (Fig 10–12). The burns on the fingers of these patients were attributed to using the finger probe from the wrong model of oximeter. The probe was connected to a different manufacturer's pulse oximeter of a different make without difficulty, and the oximeter sent an inappropriately high voltage to the probe. Within 3 minutes after connecting the probe to the oximeter, a temperature of 234°F was measured. In the future, manufacturers may key their connectors to prevent misconnection. Until this occurs, warning labels should be placed on both oximeters and probes to avoid this kind of mishap.

Burns associated with the use of pulse oximetry during magnetic resonance imaging have recently been reported.[40–42] These burns have been attributed to electrical currents in the conductive materials used in the probe and the cable induced by the radio-frequency magnetic field used during imaging. It has been suggested[41] that when using a pulse oximeter during magnetic resonance imaging, the following precautions should be followed: keep all unnecessary conductors out of the bore of the magnet, place the pulse oximeter sensor as far from the imaging site as possible, and do not allow any loops to form in wires or cables (such as ECG or oximetry cables) running into the bore of the magnet. The authors also advise making a braid of the slack portion of the wires connecting the individual electrocardiograph electrodes to the cable. It is also important to use adult-type ECG electrodes when performing imaging

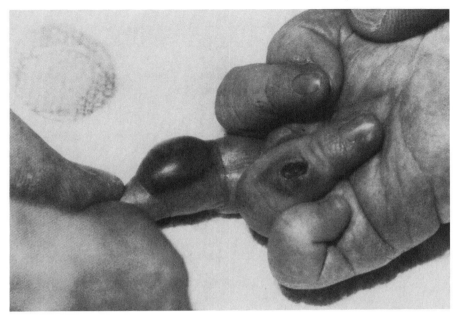

FIG 10–12.
Photograph of a burn injury caused by using a probe from one model of oximeter with another oximeter. The connection of the probe to the oximeter was made without difficulty. (*From Murphy KG, Secunda JA, Rockoff MA: Severe burns from a pulse oximeter. Anesthesiol 1990; 73:350–352. Used by permission.*)

in infants or children[43–45] and to place a thick layer of thermal insulation between any wires or cables and the patient's skin.

USING PULSE OXIMETRY IN CLINICAL SETTINGS

Spot Checks of Arterial Oxygen Saturation with Pulse Oximetry

Using pulse oximetry for purposes of "spot check" measurements of oxygen saturation invites errors in clinical management. Measurements should always be taken in duplicate or even triplicate to demonstrate reproducibility of the reading. Further, the heart rate displayed on the pulse oximeter should be compared to a manually palpated pulse measurement or heart rate by ECG. Agreement of the pulse oximeter heart rate display with the ECG heart rate display or the manually taken pulse within 5 beats/min indicates that the pulse oximeter is detecting an appropriate pulse waveform for every heartbeat and the results may be reliable.

Duplicate or triplicate measurements in series can further validate a reading. Duplicate measurements should agree within ±2%. Greater variation may indicate that the pulse oximeter reading should be considered unreliable. If a reading is shown to be reproducible, it may be reported. When using pulse oximetry to monitor oxygenation, documentation of the results should include a description of any and all variables that can affect oxygenation such as the patient's position, activity level, supplemental oxygen flow rate, and oxygen delivery device. Reporting indicators of the validity of the pulse oximetry measurements such as correlation of oximeter heart rate and ECG or radial pulse, stability of the Spo_2%, adequacy of signal strength, presence of low perfusion alarms, and the presence of absence of a typical plethysmographic waveform can aid the interpretation of the pulse oximetry saturation.

The American Association for Respiratory Care (AARC) has published guidelines for the use of pulse oximetry in clinical practice.[46] Those guidelines recommend thorough documentation and reporting of conditions relating to the measurement of pulse oximetry measurements. Table 10–4 lists information that should be provided with every clinical pulse oximetry measurement. If a disparity exists between pulse oximetry measurements and blood oximetry oxygen saturation measurements, possible technical causes should be explored before reporting pulse oximetry results. The guidelines also recommend that results not be reported if a disparity exists between oxygen saturation measured by pulse oximetry (Spo_2) and hemoximetry (Sao_2).

Spot Checks with Continuous Read Oximeters

The same principles used to validate "spot check" readings apply to pulse oximeters that display continuous readings. After the probe from a continuous-read pulse oximeter has been applied, the patient should be allowed to relax. A manual pulse should be measured, recorded, and compared to the heart rate display of the oximeter. Again, there should be a ±5 beats/min correlation between a manually taken pulse or ECG derived heart rate and the heart rate display on the oximeter. Record the manual (or ECG) pulse, the pulse display on the oximeter,

TABLE 10–4.
Documentation of Spo_2% results; reports should include the following:

Date and time of measurement
Patient position
Activity level
Location
Fio_2
Presence or absence of oxygen delivery device
Supplemental oxygen liter flow
Probe placement site and probe type
Manufacturer name and device model name
Subjective assessment of perfusion at the probe site
Heart rate from pulse oximeter
Heart rate from palpation or ECG (state which)
Relative strength of pulse amplitude signal or plethysmographic waveform
Comment on stability (or instability) of reading
Results of simultaneously obtained arterial blood gas and hemoximetry

If direct measurement was not simultaneously performed, an additional, one-time statement must be made explaining that the Spo_2 reading has not been validated by comparison to directly measured saturation.

---

and the Spo_2% reading. Wait another minute and record the oximeter heart rate and Spo_2% displayed values. This second Spo_2% reading should agree within ± 2% of the previous reading.

Exceptions to this agreement may occur when the patient's Pao_2 resides on the steep portion of the oxyhemoglobin dissociation curve. Such patients may show fluctuations greater than ± 2% during normal fluctuations associated with exertion such as coughing or simply talking. In such circumstances the comparisons should be made of readings taken during a relatively quiet state; the patient should be asked to sit quietly without talking. When variation greater than 2% exists between duplicate readings, every effort should be made to determine that peripheral circulation is optimized. If excessive variation still exists after warming the probe site, the range of the readings should be reported rather than a single reading. This range may represent the actual fluctuation of the patient's Sao_2%.

Pulse oximeters differ in the way they interpret the absorption signal, yielding different simultaneous Spo_2 values in the same patient. This makes reporting of the pulse oximeter manufacturer, model, probe type, and probe site useful when evaluating pulse oximetry data.

Use of Pulse Oximetry to Prescribe Oxygen for Hospitalized Patients and for Home Oxygen Therapy

Despite these precautions, judicious use of pulse oximetry is very valuable for titrating oxygen therapy. King and Simon[47] addressed the use of pulse oximetry for tapering supplemental oxygen levels in hospitalized patients recovering from acute respiratory insufficiency. They found that the use of pulse oximetry to titrate Spo_2 levels resulted in a significant reduction in the mean number of blood gases from 4.4 per patient in the control group to 1 per patient in the oximeter group. The protocol they used to reduce supplemental oxygen in the oximeter group used a target Spo_2 value of 90%. Pulse oximetry measurements were not used if the pulse oximeter heart rate display did not match the patient's radial pulse. Supplemental oxygen was then reduced in accordance with the physician's order. Twenty minutes later, the Spo_2 measurement was repeated. If the Spo_2 remained above 90%, the amount of supplemental oxygen was again reduced; this time by an amount considered appropriate by the therapist.

After another 20 minutes, saturation by oximetry was remeasured and the process was repeated until the patient was breathing room air or the Fio_2 was down to the prehospitalization level (for those receiving chronic home oxygen therapy) or the patient's saturation fell below 90%. If the latter occurred, the amount of oxygen was increased to a level that provided an Spo_2 of 90%.

The target Spo_2 value of 90% used in this protocol may not be sufficiently high enough to guarantee that every patient will have an arterial Po_2 above 55 mm Hg. Baseline correlation of Spo_2 and Sao_2 or Pao2 can aid in setting the most appropriate Spo2 target value.

Smoker et al.[48] describe a protocol in use at their institution that utilizes pulse oximetry to titrate oxygen therapy (Fig 10–13). This protocol is performed on every normocapnic patient that receives supplemental oxygen without having an arterial blood gas for evaluation of need. Their algorithm calls for titration of supplemental oxygen to provide an Spo_2 of 95%. Designating a conservative Spo_2 endpoint prevents underestimating oxygenation. The lower end of the 95% confidence range for an Spo_2 value of 95% is an Sao_2 of 91%, which will result

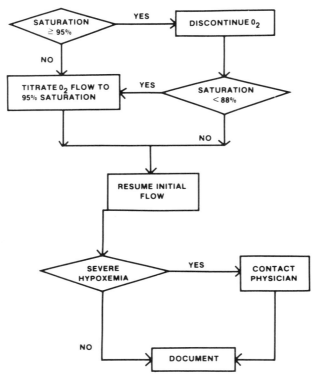

FIG 10–13.
Algorithm illustrating the oxygen-therapy-assessment protocol. (*From Smoker JM, Hess DR, Frey-Zeiler VL, et al: A protocol to assess oxygen therapy.* Respir Care *1986; 21:35–39. Used by permission.*)

in a Pao_2 well above the standard minimally acceptable Pao_2 of >55 mm Hg in most patients. Their protocol calls for a minimum of 5 minutes between changing the level of supplemental oxygen and remeasuring the Spo_2. Equilibration times of 10 minutes or more would ensure a more complete adjustment of Spo_2 in response to the change in the level of supplemental oxygen.

Difficulties in using pulse oximetry to determine the oxygen dose in hospitalized patients are also seen when prescribing oxygen for use at home. For example, Carlin, Clausen, and Ries[49] compared pulse oximetry measurements and simultaneously obtained arterial blood gases and hemoximetry saturations in 55 patients with chronic lung disease.

Oximetry measurements were made with a Hewlett-Packard 47201A multiple-wavelength ear oximeter and an Ohmeda Biox IIA two-wavelength pulse oximeter. Using a criterion of 88% Spo_2 as a threshold for requiring oxygen therapy, 24% of patients whose measurements were made with the Hewlett-Packard oximeter and 57% of the patients whose measurements were made with the Biox IIA would have been denied appropriate supplemental oxygen therapy (Fig 10–14).

Golish and McCarthy[50] reported similar findings when oxygen saturation values measured by a Nellcor N-100 were compared with simultaneously collected arterial blood samples. In

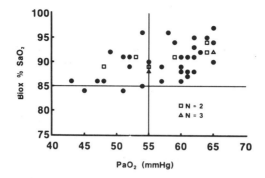

FIG 10–14.
The relationship between resting arterial oxygen tention (Pao$_2$) and pulse oximetry saturation measured by a Biox IIA ear oximeter. Points that fall in the quadrant bounded by a Spo$_2$ >88% and a Pao$_2$ <55 mm Hg demonstrate hypoxemia, yet would fail to qualify for Medicare reimbursement for oxygen therapy if pulse oximetry was the only means for assessing hypoxemia. (*From Carlin BW, Clausen JL, Ries AL: The use of cutaneous oximetry in the prescription of long-term oxygen therapy. Chest 1988; 94:239–241. Used by permission.*)

a subset of 16 patients with a Pao$_2$ less than or equal to 55 mm Hg, 5 patients (31%) would have been denied oxygen therapy on the basis of pulse oximetry measurements alone.

In this study of using pulse oximetry to establish the need for supplemental oxygen therapy, the positive predictive value of a pulse oximetry saturation below 88% was 69%. In the studies cited, a small number of patients with Pao$_2$ values ≤55 mm Hg demonstrated normal or near normal oximetry saturations of 93 to 95% (Fig 10–15). Both groups reported that most of their patients had normal values for carboxyhemoglobin and methemoglobin.

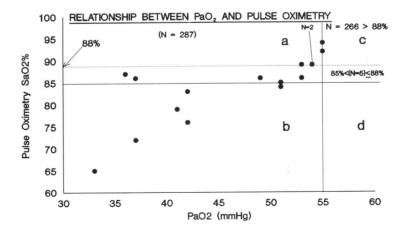

FIG 10–15.
The relationship between resting arterial oxygen tension (Pao$_2$) and pulse oximetry saturation measured by a Nellcor N-100 pulse oximeter. As in Figure 10–14, points that fall in the upper left quadrant demonstrate hypoxemia by arterial blood gas, but fail to meet the criteria established for demonstration of hypoxemia by pulse oximetry. (*From Golish JA, McCarthy K: Limitation of pulse oximetry in detecting hypoxemia. (abstract). Chest 1988; 94(suppl):50S. Used by permission.*)

When using pulse oximetry to justify the need for continuous supplemental home oxygen therapy, many patients having Pao_2 values of less than 55 mm Hg may fail to meet the existing criteria for reimbursable oxygen therapy. Because of the established benefits of home oxygen in patients whose Pao_2 is below 56 mm Hg, reliance on pulse oximetry means criteria should be lowered or, alternatively, only blood gases should be performed to establish the need for supplemental oxygen.

Use of Pulse Oximetry for Routine Screening of Pulmonary Patients

Loggan, Kerby, and Pingleton[51] attempted to determine whether routine outpatient assessment of Spo_2 was useful for detecting unsuspected severe desaturation, defined as a pulse oximetry saturation of less than 85%. Of 1675 measurements on pulmonary outpatients, only 18 measurements (1.1%) were less than 85%. Only two episodes of desaturation were not associated with changes in symptoms, spirometry, or both, which would have alerted the clinician to a possible problem. Bearing in mind that these findings would be affected by using a different Spo_2 threshold (i.e., 90 versus 85%), it seems that further evaluation is needed of the pulse oximeter as a screening tool for detecting unsuspected desaturation for pulmonary patients.

Use of Pulse Oximetry to Detect Desaturation During Exercise

Before widespread use of pulse oximetry, detecting desaturation during exercise was only possible with an indwelling arterial line or by sampling arterial blood within 20 seconds of stopping exercise. Currently, pulse oximeters have been shown to be very useful in detecting arterial oxygen desaturation during exercise. Ries, Prewitt, and Johnson[18] evaluated the Hewlett-Packard ear oximeter and the Biox IIA pulse oximeter by comparing pulse oximetry measurements made at rest and during exercise with arterial blood hemoximetry. They found that the Hewlett-Packard's 95% confidence limit for estimating arterial saturation was ±4.14% at rest and ±3.8% during exercise. The Biox IIA's 95% confidence limit was ±4.42% at rest and ±4.48% during exercise. Both instruments were more accurate for indicating a change in arterial saturation from a previous value than for measuring absolute values. They suggest that only changes in pulse oximetry readings greater than 3% be considered to represent true directional changes in measured arterial oxygen saturation.

In another study done by Escourrou, Delaparche, and Visseaux,[52] 101 patients were examined using one of three different pulse oximeters. They found that the mean difference between pulse oximetry saturation and measured oxygen saturation by hemoximetry was 1.1 ± 3%. The difference between pulse oximetry and hemoximetry saturations ranged from −9 to +16%. The pulse oximeter's 95% confidence limit range for predicting Sao_2 ranged from 4 to 6%. Most significantly, these investigators found that although the pulse oximetry values differed significantly from measured saturations at both rest and exercise, changes in measured arterial oxygen saturation between rest and exercise were significantly paralleled by changes in pulse oximetry saturation.

When using pulse oximetry to detect arterial oxygen desaturation overall, available data suggest that changes in Spo_2 from baseline of 4% or more can be considered significant. Given the wide range of the 95% confidence limits for Spo_2 measurements, a baseline correlation of Spo_2 with arterial blood hemoximetry or Pao_2 is strongly recommended when evaluating the need for oxygen during exercise.

Intraoperative Monitoring

The use of a continuous oxygen monitor during anesthesia was made a requirement by standards[53] put forth by the American Society of Anesthesiologists in 1986. These standards strongly recommend the use of pulse oximetry for intraoperative oxygen monitoring. In a study by Cooper et al.,[54] anesthesia personnel that were blinded to the pulse oximeter display were able to detect only 10 of 24 hypoxemic episodes in children undergoing surgery with general anesthesia. In all episodes detected by caregivers without benefit of pulse oximetry, the Spo_2 was less than 73%. Nine other episodes of desaturation below 73% went undetected. They also reported a lower frequency of major desaturations in children being monitored by pulse oximetry (14%) than those not being monitored (32%).

While pulse oximetry measurements are clearly more sensitive for detecting hypoxemia than clinical assessment, the high Fio_2 levels during surgery make early detection of desaturation difficult. These results indicate a twofold benefit of intraoperative Spo_2 monitoring: (1) an increase in the recognition of desaturations and (2) the prevention of major hypoxemic episodes. The value of pulse oximetry during transport of patients from the operating room to the recovery room has been very well documented. Transported patients are at increased risk for arterial desaturation, due to the effects of anesthetic agents, narcotics, and muscle relaxants. Preoxygenating patients prior to transport may not be sufficient to prevent desaturation, particularly in patients with preexisting lung disease.

Tyler et al.[55] studied the effects of transporting 95 ASA Status I or II patients that had undergone general anesthesia from the operating room to the recovery room. Thirty-five percent of their patients demonstrated desaturation below an Spo_2 of 90% and 12% showed desaturation below 85%. In spite of the fact that most patients studied by Elling and Hanning[56] had been preoxygenated prior to transport, 65% demonstrated a nadir Spo_2 of less than 91%. Blair et al.[57] found that 29% of patients they studied had Spo_2 values less than or equal to 90% during transport. Thus, desaturation is common during in-hospital transport, preoxygenation does not prevent desaturation, and close monitoring by oximetry may help to identify potentially dangerous circumstances during transport.

Use of Pulse Oximetry in Adult Critical Care

Niehoff et al.[58] studied the utility of using pulse oximetry and capnography in weaning patients from mechanical ventilation. Using definitions of a Pao_2 of <70 mm Hg and a pulse oximetry saturation of <95% to identify hypoxemic events, they reported that the pulse oximeter was 100% sensitive and 82% specific for detecting hypoxemia. By incorporating capnography and pulse oximetry into their criteria for obtaining arterial blood gases (ABG), they found that the mean number of ABG determinations was lower in the continuously monitored group (5.9 + 2.7) than the control group (10.5 + 1.8).

The use of pulse oximetry to titrate oxygen for ventilator-dependent patients has been studied. Jubran and Tobin[31] surveyed the medical directors of the ICUs in 25 hospitals across the United States and found that 88% of the ICU directors used pulse oximetry when titrating F_{IO_2} on ventilator patients. Of these, 77% always obtained an ABG to verify the level of oxygenation; the remaining 23% did so occasionally. Far less consensus was observed on an appropriate target for pulse oximetry saturation, with responses ranging from 85 to 95%; most used 90% as an oximetry target value for titration.

Jubran and Tobin[31] then examined the efficacy of various target value strategies to achieve a Pao_2 of >60 mm Hg while minimizing F_{IO_2}. As noted, the most appropriate target value was 92% for white patients and, because of a greater measurement error in their black patients, 95% for black patients. The target Spo_2 value of 92% for white patients resulted in a Pao_2 of >60 mm Hg in 13 of 14 patients and the remaining patient had a Pao_2 of 55 mm Hg. The target Spo_2 value of 95% for black patients resulted in 17 of 20 patients' having a $PaO2$ of >60 mm Hg; the remaining 3 had Pao_2 values between 55 and 60 mm Hg.

Rasanen, Downs, and DeHaven[59] have reported the use of real-time dual oximetry for titrating continuous positive airway pressure (CPAP). Dual oximetry combines pulse oximetry with pulmonary artery reflectance oximetry. This allows the calculation of the venous admixture and the oxygen utilization coefficient, which can be used for titrating CPAP. Dual oximetry was compared to a conventional method for titrating CPAP, which necessitates sampling of arterial and mixed venous blood gases and multiple measurements of thermodilution cardiac output. The two techniques yielded values for CPAP that were identical in 58% of the patients. Twenty-four percent of the values were within 2.5 cm H_2O and 18% were within 5 and 7.5 cm H_2O. When a difference between the two methods existed, the CPAP level determined by dual oximetry was consistently lower. Further study of the utility of dual oximetry in the critical care setting is needed.

Use of Pulse Oximetry in Neonatal Intensive Care

Perhaps because of their simplicity, pulse oximeters have found their niche as an oxygen monitor in the neonatal ICU. The ideal oxygen monitor in this setting would be one that would detect hypoxia and hyperoxia equally well; the limitations of the pulse oximeter in detecting hyperoxemia have been discussed.

Mok et al.[60] state that the pulse oximeter is superior to transcutaneous Po_2 monitors when hypoxia is present, but that a lack of sensitivity exists when Sao_2 values are over 90%. Bucher et al.[61] studied two different oximeters in the neonatal ICU and found that both correctly identified hyperoxemia (Pao_2 of >90 mm Hg) provided that the alarm limits were set appropriately. They found that the correct upper Spo_2 limit alarm for the Nellcor N-100 was 96% and the correct limit for the Ohmeda Biox 3700 was 88%. These settings gave the units a 95% sensitivity for detecting hyperoxemia, but the specificity was 38% for the Ohmeda and 57% for the Nellcor. Baeckert et al.[62] found that an upper limit for Spo_2 of 92% resulted in the best combination of sensitivity and specificity to hyperoxia (70% sensitivity and 62% specificity).

Hodgson et al.[63] found that the 95% confidence interval for an Spo_2 of 90% was an Sao_2 range of 85 to 98%. This range exceeds the currently recommended upper limit of Sao_2 for infants at risk for developing retrolental fibroplasia.

Blanchette, Dziodzio, and Harris[64] established pulse oximetry limits in their neonatal unit that resulted in Pao$_2$ values between 45 and 90 mm Hg. They obtained 353 paired measurements of Spo$_2$ and Pao$_2$ in 52 infants in their neonatal ICUs. As shown in Figure 10–16, using Nellcor N-100 and N-200 pulse oximeters, they found that Spo$_2$ values greater than or equal to 92% were associated with Pao$_2$ values of >45 mm Hg in 263 of 273 samples, yielding a positive predictive value of 96%. In establishing a safe upper Spo$_2$ value, they found that an Spo$_2$ of <96% was associated with Pao$_2$ values of less than or equal to 90 mm Hg in 239 of 246 samples.

The predictive value of an Spo$_2$ of <96% for detecting a Pao$_2$ of <90 mm Hg was 97%. They cautioned that their study group included many normoxemic patients whose Spo$_2$ values fell outside the range of 92 to 96% and occasional grossly aberrant Spo$_2$ values that occurred for no apparent reason. The large number of normoxemic patients demonstrating Spo$_2$ values outside the target range of 92 to 96% is a cause for concern (Fig 10–16). Presumably, oxygen therapy could be adjusted to bring the patient's Spo$_2$ within the desired range, possibly causing Pao$_2$ values outside the desired range.

These studies demonstrate that pulse oximetry can be useful in the neonatal ICU setting if and only if initial and periodic correlation with ABG measurements is incorporated in the monitoring strategy. Because different brands and even different models of pulse oximeters may display different Spo$_2$ values on the same patient (because of the different calibration data

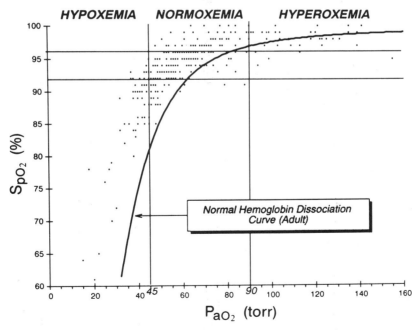

FIG 10–16.
Relationship of Spo$_2$ to Pao$_2$ in 347 neonatal measurements. (*From Blanchette T, Dziodzio J, Harris K: Pulse oximetry and normoxemia in neonatal intensive care. Respir Care 1991; 36:25–32. Used by permission.*)

and algorithms used by each model), it is important that the Spo$_2$ limits derived from any study be validated in the setting in which they will be used before adoption. Pulse oximetry should be considered a monitoring tool that can alert the clinician to unexpected hypoxemia during periods between regularly scheduled arterial blood sampling. Hyperoxemia is best detected by ABG monitoring.[65]

While pulse oximetry has a clear application as a tool for monitoring for hypoxemia, caution should be exercised when using it as a tool for hyperoxemia. As stated before, the current 95% confidence limit of pulse oximetry for predicting the Pao$_2$ is ±4%. The position of the safe upper limit of oxygen partial pressure (90 mm Hg) on the oxyhemoglobin dissociation curve causes relatively large changes of oxygen partial pressure to result in small changes in oxygen saturation. When these two facts are considered together, it is imprudent to place too great a reliance on pulse oximetry alone to detect hyperoxia.

Use of Pulse Oximetry in the Emergency Room

When properly used, pulse oximetry can be an extremely useful tool for health care practitioners working in an emergency room (ER). The pulse oximeter's value as a monitor of trends in oxygen saturation is seen clearly in the setting where rapid changes in a patient's status are common.

Though relatively little attention has been given to this issue, Jones et al.[66] described using the pulse oximeter as an aid in management of 40 consecutive patients presenting to their emergency department with respiratory distress. The mean duration of usage for the oximeter was 1.8 hours per patient. Baseline correlation with arterial blood hemoximetry was done in 29 patients. Validation of the Spo$_2$ measurement was accomplished by comparing the displayed heart rate on the pulse oximeter and the ECG heart rate. Correlation within five beats denoted an acceptable pulsatile signal. If a pulse oximetry measurement fell by 5% or more, an ABG was obtained. Overall, in this series, oximetry monitoring was extremely useful in assessing patient status, for titration of respiratory therapy (Fio$_2$ and PEEP optimization), and as an early warning of acute deterioration of respiratory status. Because of the tendency of the pulse oximeter to overstate oxygen saturation by an amount roughly equivalent to the level of carboxyhemoglobin, it is important to consider the pitfalls of using pulse oximetry data in ER patients who may have carbon monoxide poisoning and elevated carboxyhemoglobin saturations (e.g., fire victims, patients with attempted suicide).

Use of Pulse Oximetry for Monitoring Patients with Unilateral Lung Disease

While only a few studies exist, Brouwers[67] has reported on the utility of pulse oximetry monitoring in patients with unilateral lung disease on a rotating bed. In five patients with the diseased lung dependent, Spo$_2$ values dropped an average of 15.4 + 3.3%. Simultaneously obtained arterial oxygen saturations calculated from oxygen partial pressures fell 16.2 mm Hg ± 3.0 mm Hg. This report points out how position-dependent a single ABG value can be in a patient with unilateral lung disease. In such patients, pulse oximeters can be used to titrate changes in supplemental oxygen necessitated by positional changes. Baseline correlation of Spo_2 and Sao_2 or Pao_2 will aid the establishment of an appropriate target Spo_2.

Miscellaneous Proposed Uses for Pulse Oximetry

A variety of uses for pulse oximetry have been proposed that have unknown or unproven clinical utility currently. These are presented to stimulate the further clinical studies needed to establish the usefulness of pulse oximetry in these settings.

Cheng et al.[68] studied the utility of pulse oximetry to perform a variation of the modified Allen's test for collateral circulation. They examined 31 patients undergoing radial artery cannulation for intraoperative monitoring. The modified Allen's test was performed in the usual way and again using a pulse oximeter probe on the index finger. For the modified Allen's test, a "normal" response was defined as reperfusion of the palmar surface in <15 seconds; an "abnormal" response was defined as reperfusion in >15 seconds. The response was called "indeterminate" if no palmar color change occurred with occlusion or release of the arterial blood supply. When the pulse oximeter was used, detecting a pulse after release of the arterial blood supply was used as an indicator of reperfusion using the same time criteria as for the modified Allen's test.

The modified Allen's test identified 26 radial arteries as normal, 1 radial artery as abnormal, and 7 radial arteries as indeterminate. All of the radial arteries labeled as "indeterminate" by the modified Allen's test were judged to be "normal" using the pulse oximeter and were cannulated.

After cannulation, 8 patients were labeled "abnormal" by the modified Allen's test and 11 patients by the pulse oximetry technique. No clinically significant ischemic sequelae such as pain, numbness, or cyanosis resulted from arterial cannulation in any patient. Further study is needed to confirm the utility of the pulse oximeter for assessing collateral circulation prior to arterial cannulation or puncture.

Lawson et al.[69] demonstrated that pulse oximeters will still detect a sufficient signal to operate properly when total blood flow to the digit is between 4 and 8.6% of baseline flow. Further studies are needed addressing whether or not detecting a pulse by a pulse oximeter during an Allen's test identifies the presence of sufficient collateral blood flow to make radial artery cannulation a safe procedure.

Graham, Paulus, and Caffee[70] reported using the pulse oximeter to monitor postoperative vascular integrity of replanted digits. Of 16 patients, 9 successfully transplanted digits maintained Spo_2 values above 95%. Five patients demonstrated a fall in Spo_2 to 85% during the acute postoperative period. These patients were taken back to surgery and were found to have venous obstruction at the graft site. When Spo_2 values fell to zero, prompt exploration of the graft site revealed arterial obstruction. Rather than relying on the absolute accuracy of the pulse oximeter saturation reading, simultaneous demonstration of desaturation by pulse oximetry and a widening difference between pulse oximeter readings and simultaneous arterial blood hemoximetry saturations were used by Graham et al. as evidence of early subclinical ischemia during digit replantation. In contrast, these workers were unable to use pulse oximetry successfully to assess vascular integrity of replanted toes.

Narang[71] reported using the presence of a pulse signal from a pulse oximeter to confirm the adequacy of chest compressions in an infant who developed cardiac arrest while under general anesthesia.

Whether or not the presence of a pulse oximeter signal indicates adequate blood flow to the vital organs is unknown. Because the lack of a pulse signal at a digit or earlobe should not be taken as a sign of inadequate compression during cardiopulmonary resuscitation, further study is needed to evaluate the use of pulse oximetry during cardiopulmonary resuscitation.

Choi et al.[72] have reported using the pulse oximeter for long-term monitoring of changes in ventilation associated with treating pain by morphine. He studied 20 patients that were divided into two groups; one group received parenteral morphine and the other received epidural morphine. Members of both groups showed mild transient respiratory depression as demonstrated by an SpO_2 of <85%. Desaturation episodes in the parenteral morphine group occurred 2.7 + 1.9 hours after administration, while the epidural morphine group did not desaturate until an average of 13.7 + 5.9 hours after receiving the drug. The authors suggested that it would be useful to have oximetry information displayed at a centralized location, similar to electrocardiographic displays at nursing stations. Monitoring personnel would need to be trained formally in the proper use of oximetry and the frequency of motion artifact and disconnect alarms. Alarms that "cry wolf" too frequently eventually tend to get ignored. As in most oximetry applications, establishment of a baseline correlation of pulse oximetry with simultaneously drawn arterial blood gases and hemoximetry will maximize the utility of the pulse oximeter as an oxygen monitor.

Nocturnal pulse oximetry monitoring has been suggested as a means for screening patients suspected of having sleep apnea syndrome. Farney et al.[73] have recommended that pulse oximetry can be useful in screening patients with suspected sleep apnea syndrome to evaluate whether or not a full polysomnographic sleep study is indicated. In their study, pulse oximetry measurements recorded on a slow strip chart showed distinctive patterns that can distinguish onset of sleep, non-REM sleep, REM sleep, and apneas/hypopneas.

Studying 54 sequential hypersomnolent patients referred for polysomnography, they divided pulse oximeter saturation tracings into 3-minute epochs, and classified states of wakefulness, non-REM sleep, REM sleep, or apneas while blinded to all other data. Their results were compared with those of others who drew conclusions with the benefit of all of the polysomnographic data. Although sleep staging by oximetry alone underestimated the total sleep time, the sensitivity of oximetry alone in excluding or detecting sleep apnea was good in this study (sensitivity = 0.80, negative predictive value = 0.87). Apneas defined by pulse oximetry were also underestimated, which reduced the sensitivity to 0.71 and positive predictive value to 0.56.

While these results are fairly impressive, it must be noted that this study was conducted at an altitude of 1400 m where the average barometric pressure is 647 mm Hg. The mean baseline PaO_2 for the study group was 65 mm Hg, which resides on the steep portion of the oxyhemoglobin dissociation curve. It is likely that the sensitivity of the pulse oximeter in correctly identifying sleep stages would be greatly reduced at sea level, reducing the utility of the pulse oximeter as a screening tool for sleep apnea syndrome. Further study is needed.

Tiep et al.[74] have used pulse oximetry as a feedback device for COPD patients learning pursed lip breathing, which is taught routinely as a technique for improving the efficiency of breathing and controlling the anxiety caused by acute dyspnea. Their patients demonstrated a 3 to 5% increase in Spo_2 during pursed lip breathing. The instructor reported that the pulse oximeter aided in identifying patients performing the technique incorrectly. No comparison was made with a patient group learning pursed lip breathing using other techniques.

Actual Experience Using Pulse Oximetry in Clinical Practice

Two recent studies suggest that the enthusiasm for ordering pulse oximetry for clinical monitoring outstrips actual attention to pulse oximetry data or use of these data to guide clinical management.

In a study of 40 patients for whom continuous pulse oximetry data were ordered for monitoring on clinical wards, Bowton et al.[75] observed a striking inattention to oximetry data. Specifically, although at least one episode of desaturation (Spo_2 of <90%) occurred in 75% of patients, documentation of desaturation was evident in only 33% of nurses' notes and in only 7% of physicians' notes. More importantly, desaturation elicited a change in respiratory therapy in only 26% of patients, suggesting that pulse oximetry monitoring had infrequently affected patient respiratory care.

Observation in the Cleveland Clinic Post-Operative Care Unit[76] also suggest that oximetry is frequently ordered but underused for titrating oxygen therapy. In an audit of 20 consecutive low-risk patients in the Post-Operative Care Unit, Komara recorded standing orders for both oxygen therapy and twice daily pulse oximetry in all 20.

Although criteria for discontinuing oxygen were specified in all patients, these criteria were met in only 20% of patients. In the remainder of the patients, the Spo_2 value specified equaled or exceeded the preoperative Spo_2 value, and the target value was not met by the time the patient was discharged to the regular nursing unit. This suggested that the criteria for discontinuing oxygen were overly conservative.

After this audit, a standard criteria of an Spo_2 of 92% was established for discontinuing oxygen therapy for low-risk patients in the Post Anesthesia Care Unit.

These studies suggest that unfamiliarity with pulse oximetry principles may account for inattention to oximetry data, a situation that can be improved by increased educational efforts.

SUMMARY

Pulse oximetry measurements are easy to make but require careful interpretation to avoid misleading information. The list of established applications for pulse oximetry is large and still growing, while the appropriateness of using pulse oximetry for certain applications is still controversial. Certainly, available literature makes it clear that using a single pulse oximetry measurement for detecting hypoxemia will cause a significant underdetection of hypoxemia.

The strength of pulse oximetry lies in its ability to follow trends. A baseline correlation of Spo_2 and Sao_2 or Pao_2 strengthens any judgment made on the basis of pulse oximetry measurements. Decisions about instituting or removing oxygen therapy are best made when pulse oximetry measurements can be interpreted in conjunction with an arterial blood gas.

REFERENCES

1. Drabkin DL, Austin JH: A technique for the analysis of undiluted blood and concentrated hemoglobin solutions. *J Biol Chem* 1935; 112:105–115.
2. Squire JR: An instrument for measuring the quantity of blood and its degree of oxygenation in the web of the hand. *Clin Sci* 1940; 4:331–339.
3. Millikan GA: The oximeter, an instrument for measuring continuously the oxygen saturation of arterial blood in man. *Rev Sci Instr* 1942; 13:434–438.
4. Wood EH, Geraci JE: Photoelectric determination of arterial oxygenation in man. *J Lab Clin Med* 1949; 34:387–401.
5. Horecker BL: The absorption spectra of hemoglobin and its derivatives in the visible and near infrared regions. *J Biol Chem* 1943; 148:173–183.
6. Nakajimi S, Hirai S, Takase H, et al: New pulsed-type earpiece oximeter (close English translation). *Kokyo To Junkan* 1975; 23(8):709–713.
7. Saunders NA, Powles AC, Rebuck AS: Ear oximetry: Practicability in the assessment of arterial oxygenation. *Am Rev Respir Dis* 1976; 113:745–749.
8. Bland JM, Altman DG: Statistical methods for assessing agreement between two methods of clinical measurement. *Lancet* 1986; 1:307–310.
9. Ries AL, Farrow JT, Clausen JL: Accuracy of two pulse oximeters at rest and during exercise in pulmonary patients. *Am Rev Respir Dis* 1985; 132:685–689.
10. Severinghaus JW, Naifeh KH. Accuracy of response of six pulse oximeters to profound hypoxemia. *Anesthesiol* 1987; 67:551–558.
11. Warley MH, Mitchell JH, Stradling JR: Evaluation of the Ohmeda 3700 pulse oximeter. *Thorax* 1987; 42:892–896.
12. Barker SJ, Tremper KK: The effects of carbon monoxide inhalation on pulse oximeter signal detection. *Anesthesiol* 1987, 67:599–603.
13. Barker SJ, Tremper KK, Hyatt J, et al: Effects of methemoglobinemia on pulse oximetry and mixed venous oximetry (abstract). *Anesthesiol* 1987; 67:A171.
14. Eisenkraft JB: Carbon monoxide and pulse oximetry. *Anesthesiol* 1988; 68:300.
15. Scheller MS, Unger RJ, Kelner MJ: Effects of intravenously administered dyes on pulse oximetry readings. *Anesthesiol* 1986; 65:550–552.
16. Cote CJ, Goldstein EA, Fuchsman WH, et al: The effect of nail polish on pulse oximetry. *Anesth Analg* 1988, 67:683–686.
17. Rubin AS. Nail polish color can affect pulse oximeter saturation. *Anesthesiol* 1988; 68:825.
18. Ries AL, Prewitt LM, Johnson JJ: Skin color and ear oximetry. *Chest* 1989; 96:287–290.
19. Chaudhary BA, Burki NK: Ear oximetry in clinical practice. *Am Rev Respir Dis* 1978, 117:173–175.
20. Chelluri L, Snyder JV, Bird JR: Accuracy of pulse oximetry in patients with hyperbilirubinemia. *Respir Care* 1991; 36:1383–1386.
21. Evans ML, Geddes LA: An assessment of blood vessel vasoactivity using photoplethysmography. *Med Instr* 1988; 22:29–32.
22. Kim JM, Arakawa K, Benson KT, et al: Pulse oximetry and circulatory kinetics associated with pulse volume amplitude measured by photoelectric plethysmography. *Anesth Analg* 1986; 65:1333–1339.
23. Graham B, Paulus DA, Caffee HH: Pulse oximetry for vascular monitoring in upper extremity replantation surgery. *J Hand Surg* 1986; 11A:687–692.
24. Costarino AT, Davis DA, Keon TP: False normal saturation reading with the pulse oximeter. *Anesthesiol* 1987; 67:830–831.

25. Amar D, Neidswski J, Wald A, et al: Fluorescent light interferes with pulse oximetry. *J Clin Monit* 1989; 5:135–136.

26. Brooks TD, Paulus DA, Winkle WE: Infrared heat lamps interfere with pulse oximeters (letter). *Anesthesiol* 1984; 61:630.

27. Block FE: Interference in a pulse oximeter from a fiberoptic light source. *J Clin Monit* 1987; 3:210–211.

28. Abbott MA: Monitoring oxygen saturation levels in the early recovery phase of general anaesthesia, in Payne JP, Severinghaus JW, (eds): *Pulse Oximetry*. Dorchester, Springer-Verlag, 1986, pp. 165–172.

29. Siegel MN, Gravenstein N: Preventing ambient light from affecting pulse oximetry (letter). *Anesthesiol* 1987; 67:280.

30. Zablocki AD, Rasch DK: A simple method to prevent interference with pulse oximetry by infrared heating lamps (letter). *Anesth Analg* 1986; 66:915.

31. Jubran A, Tobin MJ: Reliability of pulse oximetry in titrating supplemental oxygen therapy in ventilator-dependent patients. *Chest* 1990; 97:1420–1425.

32. Cahan C, Decker MJ, Hockje PL, et al: Agreement between noninvasive oximetric values for oxygen saturation. *Chest* 1990; 97:814–819.

33. Chapman KR, Liu FLW, Watson RM, et al: Range of accuracy of two wavelength oximetry. *Chest* 1986; 89:540–542.

34. Cecil WT, Thorpe KJ, Fibuch EE, et al: A clinical evaluation of the accuracy of the Nellcor N-100 and Ohmeda 3700 pulse oximeters. *J Clin Monit* 1988; 4:31–36.

35. Nikerson BG, Sarkisian C, Tremper K: Bias and precision of pulse oximeters and arterial oximeters. *Chest* 1988; 93:515–517.

36. Thorson SH, Marini JJ, Pierson DJ, et al: Variability of arterial blood gas values in stable patients in the ICU. *Chest* 1983; 84:14–18.

37. Wagener JS, Hendricker C: Intrasubject variability of noninvasive oxygen measurements. *Chest* 1987; 92:1047–1049.

38. Sloan T: Finger injury by an oxygen saturation monitor probe. *Anesthesiol* 1988; 68:936–938.

39. Murphy KG, Secunda JA, Rockoff MA: Severe burns from a pulse oximeter *Anesthesiol* 1990; 73:350–352.

40. Shellock FG, Slimp G: Severe burn of the finger caused by using a pulse oximeter during MR imaging. *Am J Roentgenol* 1989; 153:1105.

41. Kanal E, Shellock FG: Burns associated with clinical MR examinations. *Radiology* 1990; 176:585.

42. Bashein G, Syrory G: Burns associated with pulse oximetry during magnetic resonance imaging (letter). *Anesthesiol* 1991; 75:382–383.

43. Finlay B, Couchie D, Boyer L: Electrosurgery burns resulting from use of miniature EKG electrodes. *Anesthesiol* 1974; 41:263–269.

44. Hall SV, Malhotra IV, Hedley-White J: Electrosurgery burns (correspondence). *Anesthesiol* 1975; 42:641.

45. Finlay B, Couchie D, Boyer L, et al: Electrosurgery burns (reply). *Anesthesiol* 1975; 421:641–642.

46. Shrake K, Blonshine S, Brown R, et al: AARC Clinical Practice Guidelines: Pulse oximetry. *Respir Care* 1991; 36:1406–1409.

47. King T, Simon RH. Pulse oximetry for tapering supplemental oxygern in hospitalized patients. *Chest* 1987; 92:713–716.

48. Smoker JM, Hess DR, Frey-Zeiler VL, et al: A protocol to assess oxygen therapy. *Respir Care* 1986; 21:35–39.

49. Carlin BW, Clausen JL, Ries AL: The use of cutaneous oximetry in the prescription of long-term oxygen therapy. *Chest* 1988; 94:239–241.

50. Golish JA, McCarthy K: Limitation of pulse oximetry in detecting hypoxemia. (abstract). *Chest* 1988; (suppl) 94:50S.

51. Loggan M, Kerby GR, Pingleton SK: Is routine assessment of arterial oxygen saturation in pulmonary outpatients indicated? *Chest* 1988; 94:242–244.

52. Escourru PJ, Delaparche MF, Visseaux A: Reliability of pulse oximetry during exercise in pulmonary patients. *Chest* 1990; 97:635–638.

53. American Society of Anesthesiologists. Standards for basic intraoperative monitoring. *ASA Newsletter* 1986; 50:12.

54. Cooper JB, Cullen DJ, et al: Effects of information feedback and pulse oximetry on the incidence of anesthesia complications. *Anesthesiol* 1987; 67:686–694.

55. Tyler IL, Tantisira B, Winter PM, et al: Continuous monitoring of arterial oxygen saturation with pulse oximetry during transfer to the recovery room. *Anesth Analg* 1984; 64:1108–1112.

56. Elling A, Hanning CD: Oxygenation during perioperative transportation, in Payne JP, Severinghaus JW (eds): *Pulse Oximetry.* Dorchester, Springer-Verlag, 1986, pp. 161–164.

57. Blair I, Holland R, Lau W, et al: Oxygen saturation during transfer from operating room to recovery after anesthesia. *Anesth Inten Care* 1987; 15:147–150.

58. Niehoff J, DelGuercio C, LaMorte W, et al: Efficacy of pulse oximetry and capnometry in postoperative ventilatory weaning. *Crit Care Med* 1988; 16:701–705.

59. Rasanen J, Downs JB, DeHaven B: Titration of continuous positive airway pressure by real-time dual oximetry. *Chest* 1987; 92:853–856.

60. Mok J, Pintar M, Benson L, et al: Evaluation of noninvasive measurements of oxygenation in stable newborns. *Crit Care Med* 1986; 14:960–963.

61. Bucher HU, Fanconi S, Baickert P, et al: Hyperoxemia in newborn infants: Detection by pulse oximetry. *Pediatrics* 1989; 84:226–230.

62. Baeckert P, Bucher HU, Fallenstein F, et al: Is pulse oximetry reliable in detecting hyperoxemia in the neonate? *Adv Exp Med Biol* 1987; 220:165–169.

63. Hodgson A, Horbar J, Sharp G, et al: The accuracy of the pulse oximeter in neonates. *Adv Med Exp Biol* 1987; 220:177–179.

64. Blanchette T, Dziodzio J, Harris K: Pulse oximetry and normoxemia in neonatal intensive care. *Resp Care* 1991; 36:25–32.

65. Russell RI, Helms PJ: Comparative accuracy of pulse oximetry and transcutaneous oxygen in assessing arterial saturation in pediatric intensive care. *Crit Care Med* 1990; 18:725–727.

66. Jones J, Heiselman D, Cannon L, et al: Continuous emergency department monitoring of arterial saturation in adult patients with respiratory distress. *Ann Emerg Med* 1988; 17:463–468.

67. Brouwers JW: Pulse oximeters, one lung disease and the rotabed (letter). *Anesth Analg* 1987; 66:1346–1347.

68. Cheng EY, Lauer KK, Stommel KA, et al: Evaluation of the palmar circulation by pulse oximetry. *J Clin Monit* 1989; 5:1–3.

69. Lawson D, Norley I, Korbon G, et al: Blood flow limits and pulse oximeter signal detection. *Anesthesiol* 1987; 67:599–603.

70. Graham B, Paulus DA, Caffee HH: Pulse oximetry for vascular monitoring in upper extremity replantation surgery. *J Hand Surg* 1986; 11A:687–692.

71. Narang VPS: Utility of the pulse oximeter during cardiopulmonary resuscitation. (letter). *Anesthesiol* 1986; 65:239–240.

72. Choi HJ, Little MS, Garber SZ, et al: Pulse oximetry for monitoring during ward analgesia: Epidural morphine versus parenteral narcotics. *J Clin Monit* 1989; 5:87–89.

73. Farney RJ, Walker LE, Jensen RL, et al: Ear oximetry to detect apnea and differentiate REM and NREM sleep, screening for sleep apnea syndrome. *Chest* 1986; 89:533–539.

74. Tiep BL, Burns M, Kao D, et al: Pursed lip breathing training using ear oximetry. *Chest* 1986; 90:218–221.
75. Bowton DL, Scuderi PE, Harris L, et al: Pulse oximetry monitoring oustide the intensive care unit: Progress or Problem? *Ann Intern Med* 1991; 115:450–454.
76. Komara JJ: Postoperative pulmonary care: Low flow oxygen therapy and pulse oximetry monitoring audit. (personal communication).

Chapter 11

Transcutaneous Oxygen and Carbon Dioxide Measurements

Patricia B. Koff, M.Ed. R.R.T.
Dean Hess, M.Ed., R.R.T.

"Although I had hoped it might work, I was really surprised when it did."

Leland Clark[1]

INTRODUCTION

The above words, spoken by Dr. Clark regarding the first blood gas electrode in 1954, were similar to the thoughts of many clinicians when the first transcutaneous electrodes were placed on infants in the 1970s. Although early skepticism surrounded their use, transcutaneous monitors have been used in the management of neonates, children, and adults. In addition to their use to track arterial blood gases, they also provide information related to perfusion; they have been used to evaluate tissue blood flow during shock, resuscitation, and peripheral vascular disease.

Transcutaneous monitors are trend monitors for the assessment of tissue oxygenation and carbon dioxide levels. The transcutaneous values approximate arterial values by hyperperfusing the area under the electrode. Hyperperfusion is created by heating the skin surface; transcutaneous electrodes function at ~42.5 to 45°C. Gases diffuse into the electrodes, which are similar to the Clark and Stowe-Severinghaus electrodes used in blood gas analyzers. The continuous display of oxygen and/or carbon dioxide allows noninvasive assessment of respiratory gases and perfusion.

HISTORY

Transcutaneous gas measurements were conducted as early as 1851 (Table 11–1) by Von Gerlach,[2, 3] who was an instructor at the Royal Veterinarian School of Berlin. His investigations focused on shellacking the shaved skin of horses, dogs, and men and measuring the content of the gas bubbles that formed underneath. He identified two of the key concepts in transcutaneous gas measurements that are used today: (1) gases diffuse through the skin and (2) gas diffusion varies with perfusion.

Oxygen

In 1951, oxygen was measured through the skin by Baumgardner and Goodfriend.[2, 3] Their experiment involved placing a human finger into a heated phosphate buffer solution. After 15 minutes, they found the Po_2 of the solution nearly equaled the Pao_2.

Clark, who began his work on an oxygen electrode in 1954, produced an electrode in 1956 that made routine Po_2 measurements practical.[1] His electrode was adapted for bloodless determination of oxygen tension by Rooth et al. in 1957. In 1969, Huch et al. reported the use of Po_2 electrodes on the skin of newborns.

Carbon Dioxide

Huch et al. also first reported transcutaneous Pco_2 measurements in 1973 using a Severinghaus electrode.[1] Severinghaus had developed a carbon dioxide electrode in 1958 that made blood gas analysis possible and laid the groundwork for transcutaneous measurements.[4] Some confusion surrounded early transcutaneous carbon dioxide values because they were found to be much higher than arterial values. This lead to the development of correction factors, which allowed transcutaneous values to be closer to arterial values.[5, 6]

TABLE 11–1.
History of Transcutaneous Gas Measurements

Date	Individual	Accomplishment
1851	Von Gerlach	Determined that gas diffuses through skin, and this varies with perfusion
1951	Baumgardner	Measured oxygen diffusion
1954	Clark	Developed oxygen electrode
1957	Rooth	Adapted Clark electrode for bloodless determinations
1969	Huch	Reported use of Po_2 electrodes
1973	Huch	Reported use of Pco_2 electrodes

PHYSIOLOGY

The skin (integument) is composed of several layers (Fig 11–1). The outermost layer is referred to as the *stratum corneum* or horny layer. It is composed of flattened epithelial cells from which most of the fluid has evaporated; it has been described as having "beeswax" characteristics.[7] Its composition includes keratin filaments in a matrix of lipid and nonfibrous protein.[3] The skin surface that is created by the stratum corneum provides an efficient, tough, protective mechanism for the body, as well as a barrier to diffusion of gases. Removal of the stratum corneum results in a dramatic increase in gas exchange across the skin.[8] Van Duzee[9] studied the effect of temperature on this layer and concluded that the lipid portion melted at approximately 41°C. The diffusion of gases through this melted layer appears to be enhanced. According to Tremper and Waxman, the diffusion ability may increase by 1000 times due to heating and may result in physiologic melting of a diffusion window to the living tissue beneath.[3]

The other layers of the epidermis are the lucidum, granulosum, and Malpighii. They are composed of living cells that consume oxygen and produce carbon dioxide. They do not provide a diffusion barrier to gases as does the stratum corneum layer, but they may be partially responsible for the underestimation of arterial oxygen levels and overestimation of

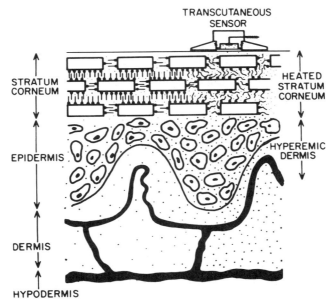

FIG 11–1.
Schematic cross section of the electrode and skin: stratum corneum, epidermis, dermis, and hypodermis. The irregular structure of the stratum corneum beneath the electrode represents the melted lipid. The dots represent oxygen. (*From Tremper KK, Waxman K, Shoemaker WC: Effects of hypoxia and shock on transcutaneous PO2 values in dogs.* Crit Care Med *1979; 7:526–531. © by Williams and Wilkins. Used by permission.*)

arterial carbon dioxide levels in adult patients evaluated by transcutaneous monitors. Patel et al.[10] have suggested that the use of a topical metabolic inhibitor, 4-allyl-2-methoxyphenol (Eugenol), may reduce the oxygen consumption in this layer and allow closer estimations of arterial values based on transcutaneous measurements.

The dermis portion of the skin is tough, flexible, and highly elastic. It is composed of connective tissue, blood vessels, lymphatics, and nerves. The presence of blood vessels allows for the regulation of body temperature by varying blood flow. Approximately one-third of all blood in the body circulates to the skin.[7]

Arterializing capillary blood with a transcutaneous monitor is accomplished by increasing the blood flow under the area of the monitor, thus hyperperfusing the dermis layer. The increased blood flow generated by the heat provides an increase in the oxygen delivery to the tissue or epidermis area, so that an approximation of arterial oxygen levels can be reached (Fig 11–2). In the case of carbon dioxide, however, heating results in a carbon dioxide level higher than that of the arterial level (Fig 11–3).

In addition to the arterializing effect, the usual countercurrent gas exchange that occurs between ascending and descending limbs of the capillaries is reduced due to heating. The velocity of the blood flow does not allow for carbon dioxide from the descending limb to be added to the ascending limb, or oxygen in the ascending limb to diffuse into the descending limb.[11] Thus the gas levels diffusing toward the electrode tend to be more similar to those in the arterial system.

Some transcutaneous units monitor the energy needed to maintain the temperature of the electrode. Because blood flow cools the skin under the electrode, an increase in energy required to maintain electrode temperature implies that blood flow under the electrode has increased. Although theoretically the energy required to maintain electrode temperature (the so-called "local perfusion reference") should provide an index of perfusion, this has not been found to be very useful clinically.

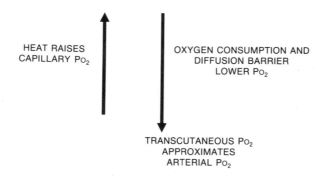

FIG 11–2.
Heating raises the Po_2 under the transcutaneous electrode, which nearly balances the effects of local oxygen consumption and the effects of the diffusion barrier. Under ideal conditions, this results in a transcutaneous Po_2 that nearly equals the arterial Po_2.

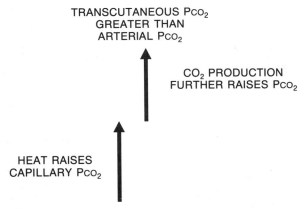

FIG 11–3.
Heating raises the P_{CO_2} under the transcutaneous electrode, and the P_{CO_2} further increases due to local CO_2 production. This results in a transcutaneous P_{CO_2} that is greater than the arterial P_{CO_2}; most manufacturers incorporate a correction factor into the transcutaneous CO_2 monitor so that the transcutaneous P_{CO_2} will approximate the arterial P_{CO_2} (under ideal conditions).

In summary, by applying a heated transcutaneous electrode to the skin, one is able to functionally melt the stratum corneum layer and increase the perfusion through the dermal layer. By doing this, skin electrodes can be used to approximate the oxygen and carbon dioxide levels in the arterial blood. However, for a variety of reasons described in this chapter, transcutaneous and arterial values are often not identical.

TECHNOLOGY

Figure 11–4 shows an example of a transcutaneous unit. All such units consist of a base monitor, a cable and electrode, calibration gases, and accessory items. Accessory items include adhesive disks, contact solution, and membrane kits. The transcutaneous electrode attaches to the skin via an adhesive ring. Gas diffuses across the skin surface, passes through a contact gel, crosses the membrane of the electrode, goes through the electrolyte solution, and reaches the measuring electrode. By listing these steps for passage, one can appreciate the potential technical (or technique) areas in which problems may occur (Fig 11–5). This section will address each of these areas.

Adhesion

The electrode must be attached to the skin so that it will not become disconnected or allow room air to be present between it and the skin surface. This is usually accomplished by use of a double-sided adhesive disk (Fig 11–6). Correct placement of this disk on the electrode can

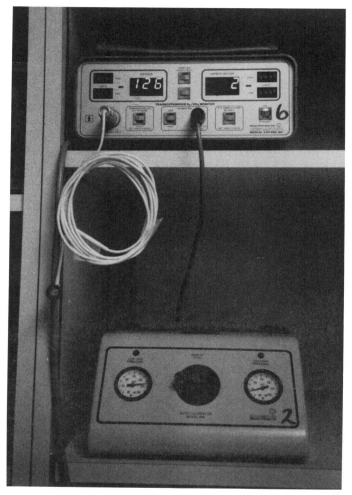

FIG 11–4.
Novametrix transcutaneous O$_2$/CO$_2$ monitor. Base unit is shown on top shelf, patient probe is attached to the left lower side of the unit. Center probe is connected to the gas calibrating unit, which is on the lower shelf.

be tedious; working with a disk that is sticky on both sides often causes adhesion to occur where it is not wanted (e.g., stuck to the operator's fingers, folded and stuck to itself, stuck to clothing or other equipment). Once it is in place, it is helpful to use a cotton ball to cover the remaining sticky surface so that intravenous lines and monitoring cables do not become attached to the adhesive disk. Care must also be exercised to assure that the cable is not in a precarious position (e.g., between bed rails, under other pieces of equipment).

PATH OF GAS TRANSFER DURING TRANSCUTANEOUS MONITORING

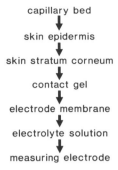

capillary bed

↓

skin epidermis

↓

skin stratum corneum

↓

contact gel

↓

electrode membrane

↓

electrolyte solution

↓

measuring electrode

FIG 11–5.
The steps for passage of gases from the blood to the transcutaneous electrode.

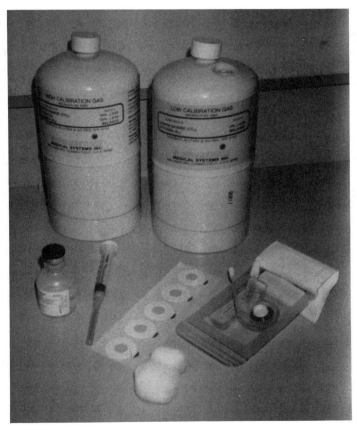

FIG 11–6.
Transcutaneous accessories include calibration tanks, electrode membrane kit, cotton balls, adhesive disks, and contact solution.

Contact

Prior to placing the electrode with the adhesive disk on the patient, a small drop of fluid must be placed on the center of the electrode to enhance gas diffusion (some practitioners place the drop of fluid directly on the skin surface and place the electrode over it). This fluid is either deionized water, or contact gel supplied by the manufacturer.[12] Patel et al.[10] have suggested the use of a metabolic inhibitor fluid as another alternative, but this is not commonly used. Carefully placing this fluid is a challenging aspect of the use of a transcutaneous monitor. It may get placed on the adhesive ring, which will reduce adhesion ability and allow room air to seep under the electrode. It may also be too large, hence reducing the adhesion ability of the ring by being moved out from under the electrode.

Membrane

The membranes used with transcutaneous electrodes are typically polymer films or Teflon.[3] They must be permeable to gases, but impermeable to the electrolyte solution. Anesthetic agents may affect the accuracy of transcutaneous monitors, and the type of membrane material used can also influence that accuracy.[3] Halothane is an anesthetic agent known to interfere with the reliability of transcutaneous measurements.[12]

The membrane covering the electrode should be routinely inspected. Tears in the membrane may allow the electrolyte to leak and cause analytical errors. Changing the membrane on the transcutaneous electrode has become easier with new units; most manufacturers now produce membrane kits that reduce technical problems. Even with these kits, membrane changes still require time to perform. Following a membrane and electrolyte change, a stabilization period is required before the system will function properly. Some systems require an equilibration period of as long as a 4-hours after a membrane change.

Electrolyte

Electrolyte solution is used as a conduction medium in blood gas analyzers and transcutaneous monitors. Different solutions may be needed for some oxygen electrodes and carbon dioxide electrodes, although some of the combined CO_2/O_2 units use only one type. One of the errors in transcutaneous monitoring is the use of oxygen electrolyte in carbon dioxide electrodes and vice versa. It is not uncommon for electrolyte solution to evaporate from the electrode, and a membrane change may be necessary if electrolyte is depleted.

Oxygen Electrode

The oxygen electrode used for transcutaneous measurements is a miniaturized Clark electrode, similar to those used in blood gas analyzers (Fig 11–7). The electrode consists of an anode and cathode in an electrolyte medium. Figure 11–8 demonstrates schematically the reaction that

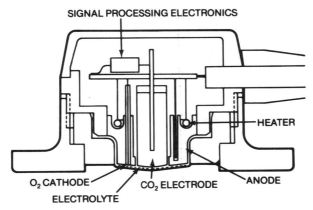

FIG 11–7.
Schematic diagram of the O_2/CO_2 sensor. (*From Mahutte CK et al: Evaluation of a singe transcutaneous PO2-PCO2 sensor in adult patients.* Crit Care Med *1984; 12:1063–1066. © by Williams and Wilkins. Used by permission.*)

takes place within the Clark electrode. Oxygen diffuses through the membrane, reacts at the platinum cathode with water, according to the following reaction:

$$O_2 + 2H_2O + 4e^- \rightleftarrows 4OH^-$$

The production of four electrons flowing through the circuit for each oxygen reduced produces a current, which is measured.

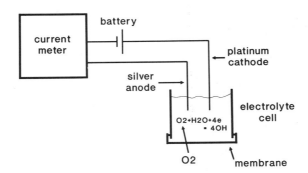

FIG 11–8.
Schematic of a Clark polarographic oxygen electrode. The circuit consists of a voltage source (battery) and a current meter connecting platinum and silver electrodes. The electrodes are immersed in an electrolyte cell. A membrane permeable to oxygen, but not to the electrolyte, covers one surface of the cell. Oxygen diffuses through the membrane and reacts at the platinum cathode with water to produce hydroxyl ions. The current meter measures the current produced by the electrons consumed in this reaction at the cathode.

Periodic cleaning of the transcutaneous oxygen electrode may be necessary because silver may deposit on the cathode and alter oxygen sensor current. Manufacturers vary on their recommendations for cleaning. Some provide special cloths or instruments with their membrane kits, while others recommend polishing with a soft cloth or gauze.[12-14] Polishing may be done during a membrane change, and in most cases an equilibration time will be necessary following this procedure.

Electrodes must be calibrated prior to their use. Some manufacturers use gases, while others may use solutions with known values. Two calibration points are used; a high value which is a room air or arterial value and a low value of zero. As electrode sites are changed (approximately every 2 to 4 hours), recalibration is recommended.

The temperature at which the electrode is maintained will influence the time required between site changes. Most units can regulate temperature between 42.5 to 45°C. On premature neonates who have thin skin, a temperature of 43°C may be tolerated for 2 to 3 hours,[15] and some suggest 44°C for neonates.[12] Given that skin thickness differs between patients, the susceptibility to blisters varies. Some babies seen 3 to 4 months after monitoring in the neonatal intensive care unit have small circular areas on their skin.[15] Eventually these areas do fade. Older pediatric patients and adults are often monitored at electrode temperatures of 44°C. For these patients, sites may only need to be changed every 4 to 6 hours.[12]

With the transcutaneous Po_2 electrode, the heating effect is nearly balanced by the effects of skin oxygen consumption and the diffusion barrier across the skin (Fig 11–2). However, this balancing effect is very variable, so that the transcutaneous Po_2 often differs from the arterial Po_2.

Carbon Dioxide Electrodes

The Stowe-Severinghaus electrode measures carbon dioxide via a reaction with water that produces hydrogen ions:

$$CO_2 + H_2O \rightleftarrows H_2CO_3 \rightleftarrows HCO_3^- + H^+$$

A glass hydrogen ion (pH) electrode is immersed in an electrolyte solution and referenced to a silver/silver-chloride electrode. As the level of hydrogen ions changes, the potential generated changes (Fig 11–9).

The carbon dioxide electrode must be calibrated with gases of known values. High and low levels in the range of 4 to 5% carbon dioxide for the low value and 10% for the high value are used.[12, 13]

The transcutaneous carbon dioxide electrode requires[16-19] a temperature of 42°C. Because the carbon dioxide electrode is often combined into one unit with the oxygen electrode, higher temperatures often must be used. Uncorrected transcutaneous carbon dioxide values are generally higher than arterial values. Although the reasons for this are varied, it is generally accepted that this is a result of skin metabolism and heating of the skin by the electrode. Thus the transcutaneous Pco_2 will be greater than the arterial Pco_2 (Fig 11–3). Fixed correction factors are incorporated into most monitors to allow the display of transcutaneous Pco_2 to be

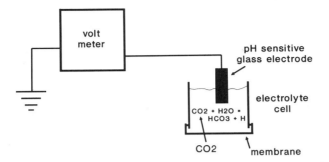

FIG 11–9.
A schematic of a Stowe-Severinghaus P_{CO_2} electrode. It consists of a pH-sensitive glass electrode, referenced to a silver/silver-chloride electrode. The glass electrode is immersed in an electrolyte cell with a CO_2 permeable membrane covering on the surface. The CO_2 diffuses into the cell, reacts with water in the cell, producing carbonic acid, and the pH electrode detects the pH change.

close to arterial P_{CO_2}. As with oxygen monitoring, the transcutaneous values should be used as trend indicators and not absolute values of arterial blood gases.

PROCEDURE

A procedure for using a transcutaneous monitor is outlined in Table 11–2. While the related technology and accessories have been discussed above, site selection requires some additional discussion. Regardless of the age of the patient being monitored, use of a transcutaneous monitor requires a site that is relatively well perfused and is flat so that the probe can lay

TABLE 11–2.
Procedure for Use of Transcutaneous Monitor

I. Obtain monitor	Place unit at bedside and allow warm-up time as recommended by the manufacturer.
II. Inspect membrane	Membrane should be free of air bubbles and scratches or tears. Change membrane according to manufacturer recommendations if indicated.
III. Select patient site	Evaluate perfusion, skin thickiness, and absence of bones.
IV. Prepare sensor	Attach double-sided adhesive ring and apply contact solution.
V. Set appropriate probe temperature	Consider patient's age and skin thickness.
VI. Prepare site	Rub site with alcohol swab and shave if necessary.
VII. Attach to patient	Assure probe is securely attached. Allow stabilization time of 10 to 20 min.
VIII. Set timer for site duration	Provide reminder of site change time.
IX. Set alarms	Monitor high and low alarms.
X. Monitor	Routinely monitor and record results according to institutional guidelines.
XI. Change site	Change site at appropriate intervals.

TABLE 11–3.
Transcutaneous Probe Placement Sites

NEONATAL	*FETAL*
General use	Scalp
Abdomen	
Thigh	*ADULT*
Lower back	General use
Chest	Chest
Ductal assessment	Abdomen
Upper right chest	Lower back
	Special assessments
PEDIATRIC	CPR—shoulder
Chest	Perfusion—limb
Abdomen	
Lower back	

evenly on the skin. Placing the probe over large bones or hair is not recommended. Table 11–3 lists potential placement sites. After placement of the electrode, an equilibration time of 10 to 20 minutes is required before valid transcutaneous readings are obtained.

Neonatal Placement

When using a transcutaneous monitor with neonatal patients, the abdomen, inner thigh, lower back, or chest can be used.[12-14] These areas are relatively well perfused, have minimal bone interference, and are large enough to allow the probe to lay evenly.

If the monitor is being used to assess the presence of a patent ductus arteriosus and potential right-to-left shunt, it is placed on the upper right quadrant (chest). Because the ductus adds blood flow to the descending aorta, placing the electrode on the upper right chest allows monitoring of preductal blood. To have a continuous trend assessment of ductal function, a patient may be monitored with two transcutaneous monitors; one electrode is placed on the upper right chest, and the other is placed on the abdomen or lower extremities.[20]

The use of continuous transcutaneous monitoring of the fetus during labor has been described.[21] For that use, Lofgren described the placement (via an amnioscope) on the fetal scalp.

Pediatric and Adult Placement

The chest, abdomen, and lower back are sites for transcutaneous monitoring in pediatric and adult patients.[12-14] Monitoring sites are chosen according to the specific clinical problem being monitored. For example, to evaluate the perfusion to an extremity, an electrode may be placed in that area. Hauser and Shoemaker[22] placed transcutaneous electrodes on the chest, the medial distal thigh, the medial mid-calf, and the dorsum of the foot. Mustapha et al.[23] also reported using electrodes below the knees in addition to the chest to assess ischemic lower limbs. Electrodes used in the emergency department to assess oxygen delivery during resuscitation are placed on the anterior shoulder of adult patients.[24]

CLINICAL USES OF TRANSCUTANEOUS MONITORS

Transcutaneous monitors are used in a variety of clinical settings with neonatal, pediatric, and adult patients. Clinical reports of that use have been found in the medical literature since the early 1970s. In 1978 two significant international meetings were held on the subject.[25, 26] This section will summarize the studies, which have provided clinical direction for the use of these monitors.

Neonatal

Transcutaneous monitors have been used extensively in neonatal intensive care units since the mid-1970s (Table 11–4).[27] This monitoring, in a noninvasive manner, provides real-time information on the oxygenation and ventilation status of infants. It was once thought that use

TABLE 11–4.
Transcutaneous Monitors: Selected Neonatal Studies

Reference	Date	O_2/CO_2	Contribution
Huch[27]	1973	O_2	Described the use of transcutaneous Po_2 in perinatal medicine.
Huch[29]	1976	O_2	Described routine use of transcutaneous Po_2 monitoring in infants and children.
Huch[30]	1981	O_2	Described simultaneous transcutaneous Po_2 monitoring of mothers and fetuses during labor.
Martin[31]	1982	O_2	Transcutaneous monitors are less accurate with hyperoxemia.
Heaf[35]	1983	O_2	Neonatal patients positioned with good lung up had better transcutaneous Po_2.
Gleason[36]	1983	O_2	Used transcutaneous $Po2$ to determine optimal position for spinal tap.
Kilbride[28]	1984	O_2	Frequency of blood gas determinations did not change with transcutaneous monitoring.
Bancalari[33]	1987	O_2	Retinopathy of prematurity may be reduced by use of transcutaneous monitors in infants >1000 g.
Mok[39]	1988	O_2	Raised awareness that monitors produce numbers that may not require treatment if overall clinical picture is considered.
Pearlman[20]	1989	O_2	Described use of transcutaneous monitors to assess ductal function.
Brustler[19]	1982	CO_2	Changes in hematocrit, scleredema, and tolazoline did not affect transcutaneous Pco_2.
Epstein[37]	1985	CO_2	Found that transcutaneous Pco_2 estimated arterial Pco_2 to within ±6 to 8 mm Hg; transcutaneous Pco_2 was a better indicator of arterial Pco_2 than end-tidal Pco_2.
Bucher[17]	1986	CO_2	Used transcutaneous Pco_2 monitors for 24 hours at 42°C.
Martin[16]	1988	CO_2	Found that higher $Paco_2$ levels affected the accuracy of transcutaneous Pco_2.
Hand[38]	1989	CO_2	pH <7.30 negatively affected correlation between transcutaneous and arterial Pco_2 values; transcutaneous Pco_2 better indicator of arterial Pco_2 than end-tidal Pco_2 monitoring.

of these monitors would reduce the number of arterial blood gases required, but this remains controversial. Kilbride and Merenstein[28] reported that transcutaneous monitoring did not decrease the frequency of arterial blood gas determinations. Although the introduction of pulse oximetry in the 1980s has reduced the use of transcutaneous monitors, they are still commonly used in neonatal intensive care units (ICUs).

Studies evaluating the correlation between arterial and transcutaneous oxygen have been reported[29-31] since 1976 (Fig 11–10). In 1978, Peabody[32] evaluated the effect of extreme hypotension and intravascular infusion of tolazoline (vasodilator) on the accuracy of transcutaneous Po_2 (Fig 11–11). While transcutaneous Po_2 showed close correlation to arterial Po_2 in most cases, two patients had low transcutaneous oxygen values relative to their arterial values. A blood pressure of more than 2.5 standard deviations below the predicted mean caused low transcutaneous PO_2 values due to reduced peripheral perfusion. The use of tolazoline presumably causes widespread vasodilation, so that preferential vasodilation through use of the heated electrode does not occur.

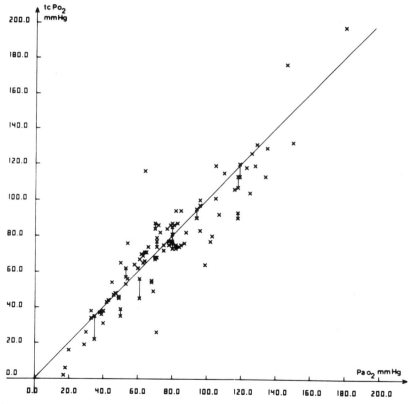

FIG 11–10.
Arterial Po_2 values and $Ptco_2$ and their relation to the line of identity. (*From Huch R et al:* Pediatrics, *1976; 57:681–690. Reproduced by permission of Pediatrics.*)

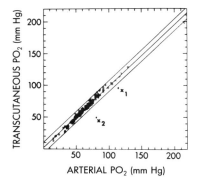

FIG 11–11.
Comparison of 159 simultaneous measurements of transcutaneous and arterial Po_2 in 30 sick infants made on 60 occasions. X1 represents measurements made in an infant receiving tolazoline; X2, measurements made in an infant with arterial blood pressure of 16/0 mm Hg. (*From Peabody et al: Transcutaneous oxygen tension in sick infants.* Am Rev Resp Dis *1978; 118:8387. Used by permission.*)

Transcutaneous monitors have also been used to document and correct episodes of hypoxemia in neonates. By continuously monitoring patients, steps can be taken to correct hypoxemic episodes and hopefully lessen morbidity associated with these. Kilbride and Merestein,[28] in a study of 20 neonatal patients, found that infants who were being monitored transcutaneously had fewer hypoxemic episodes.

During hyperoxemia, transcutaneous monitors are less accurate, and caution is advised[31] in using the monitors with neonates who are being maintained with an arterial Po_2 near 100 mm Hg. In the study by Kilbride and Merenstein[28] they found that hyperoxic time did not change by using transcutaneous monitors. These monitors also do not seem to reduce the incidence of retinopathy of prematurity (ROP). Bancalari et al.[33] reported that the incidence of ROP may be reduced in infants with birth weights of more than 1000 g who they monitored, but smaller infants (in whom ROP occurs more frequently and more severely) did not seem to be protected from ROP by the transcutaneous monitoring.

Transcutaneous monitors have been used to determine optimal positioning of infants. In 1979, Martin et al.[34] reported a 15 to 25% increase in the transcutaneous Po_2 values of infants in the prone position. Heaf et al.[35] evaluated infants with unilateral lung disease (diaphragmatic hernia patients, hypoplastic right lung patient, a patient with right-sided atelectasis) and showed that positioning the good lung uppermost produced the best oxygenation, which is in contrast to adult positioning. The optimal position for a spinal tap in preterm infants was also determined using transcutaneous monitors; the flexed position showed the greatest risk of morbidity. A modified flex with neck extension or upright positioning were recommended during spinal tap.[36]

Transcutaneous carbon dioxide electrodes were first used primarily in neonates.[6, 37, 38] These provide a means of continuous assessment of ventilatory status (Table 11–4). As mentioned in the electrode section of this chapter, electrode temperatures of 42°C are optimal,[18] and have been used for 24-hour monitoring when using an electrode that does not also measure transcutaneous oxygen.[17] Changes in hematocrit, the presence of scleredema, and treatment with tolazoline do not affect the accuracy of transcutaneous carbon dioxide.[19] Martin et al.[16] evaluated the effect of increasing arterial carbon dioxide levels on transcutaneous carbon dioxide accuracy and found that at higher carbon dioxide levels the reliability of transcutaneous values decreased (Fig 11–12). Hand[38] reported that acidosis (pH < 7.30) negatively affected correlation between transcutaneous and arterial carbon dioxide values. Transcutaneous carbon dioxide monitors should thus be used as *trend* monitors. Like transcutaneous Po_2, transcutaneous Pco_2 should be considered qualitative rather than quantitative.

One neonatal study has addressed the issue of appropriate indications for transcutaneous monitoring. Mok et al.[40] used transcutaneous monitors and pulse oximeters to assess the effect of age and wakefulness on oxygenation. As part of their study they found surprisingly low values of oxygenation in some babies who were clinically normal and free of cardiopulmonary disease. These patients exhibited no respiratory distress or cyanosis, so supplemental oxygen was not initiated. This illustrates the fact that use of these and other monitors may produce tendencies to treat the *numbers* instead of the patients, and prudent evaluation of the entire clinical picture is necessary.

Pediatric

The use of transcutaneous monitors in the pediatric population has had mixed reviews (Table 11–5). Some studies have documented the underestimation of arterial Po_2 values as infants become older and in infants who have bronchopulmonary dysplasia.[40, 41] Rome et al.[42] found an underestimation of arterial Po_2 and overestimation of arterial Pco_2 by transcutaneous monitors in premature infants with bronchopulmonary dysplasia when they were 8 to 12

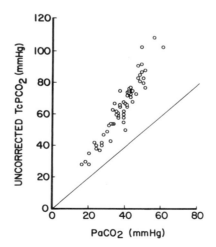

FIG 11–12.
Relationship between uncorrected transcutaneous Pco_2 and arterial Pco_2 in 60 infants. Line of identity is indicated. (*From Martin et al: Increasing arterial carbon dioxide tension: Influence on transcutaneous carbon dioxide tension measurements. Pediatrics 1988; 81:684–687. Reproduced by permission of Pediatrics.*)

TABLE 11–5.

Transcutaneous Monitors: Selected Pediatric Studies

Reference	Date	O_2/CO_2	Contribution
Monaco[39]	1982	O_2/CO_2	Found a $Pao_2/Ptco_2$ index of 0.84 and $Paco_2/Ptcco_2$ index of 1.6.
Rome[42]	1984	O_2/CO_2	Underestimation of Pao_2 and overestimation of $Paco_2$ by transcutaneous monitors in patients with bronchopulmonary dysplasia.
Hamilton[41]	1985	O_2	Suggested that the decreased $Ptco_2/Pao_2$ with increasing age was due to changes in the texture and thickness of the skin, changes in the capillary bed, and the effects of chronic lung disease.
Durand[43]	1986	O_2	Found that pulse oximetry could offer more accuracy than transcutaneous Po_2 in infants with chronic lung disease.
Fanconi[44]	1990	CO_2	Reported the use of transcutaneous Po_2 monitoring in predicting intubation needs of croup.
Russell[45]	1990	O_2	In hemodynamically stable infants and children, the accuracy limits of transcutaneous Po_2 and pulse oximetry were similar.

weeks postnatal age. Durand and Ramanathan[43] found that pulse oximetry was more accurate than transcutaneous Po_2 monitoring in infants with bronchopulmonary dysplasia.

A ratio or index is often used to compare transcutaneous oxygen values to arterial oxygen values ($Ptco_2/Pao_2$) (Table 11-6). As an infant grows and becomes older, this ratio decreases. The reasons for this are not clear; Hamilton et al.[41] suggested that this decrease may relate to changes in the texture and thickness of the skin, changes in the capillary bed with increasing age, and the effects of chronic lung disease.

Fanconi et al.[44] were able to determine when intubation was required in croup patients based on deteriorating transcutaneous Pco_2 values. Monitoring by this method proved more useful than monitoring clinical signs, and it also helped to track deterioration following epinephrine treatments. The use of transcutaneous oxygen monitoring has decreased since the introduction of pulse oximetry. In a group of infants and children, Russell and Helms[45] found

TABLE 11–6.

Transcutaneous Oxygen Ratio ($Ptco_2/Pao_2$)
Based on Age

Newborns:	≈ 1.0
Children:	≥ 0.85
Adults:	≥ 0.75

that transcutaneous P_{O_2} and pulse oximetry have similar accuracy limits; they suggested that both types of monitors have advantages and disadvantages such that neither is clearly superior to the other.

Adult

In 1976, Rooth et al.[46] reported the use of transcutaneous oxygen measurements in adults. These monitors may be useful in selected adults, even though their skin thickness is greater and the number of capillaries below the skin varies from site to site.[46-49] Many papers have described the use of transcutaneous monitors in a variety of adult settings (Table 11-7). The ratio of transcutaneous and arterial oxygen (Table 11-6) in healthy adults is ≥ 0.75.

Transcutaneous P_{CO_2} has a better correlation[64, 68] with arterial P_{CO_2} than the correlation of transcutaneous P_{O_2} with arterial P_{O_2}. Stokes et al.[50] evaluated a combination CO_2/O_2 transcutaneous monitor in 38 critically ill, mechanically ventilated patients and concluded that accurate estimates of arterial values can be obtained from transcutaneous measurements. They consistently found that transcutaneous P_{O_2} predicted changes in their patients' clinical status. Mahutte et al.[47] studied 47 critically ill patients, and found that a combined O_2/CO_2 transcutaneous monitor provided reliable trend information; in that study, changes of >5 mm Hg in transcutaneous P_{CO_2} nearly always indicated a similar change in Pa_{CO_2}. Following withdrawal of mechanical ventilation, Healey et al.[59] found that changes in transcutaneous P_{CO_2} were predictive of important arterial P_{CO_2} increases. Phan et al.[58] evaluated transcutaneous P_{CO_2} in anesthetized patients and concluded that transcutaneous P_{CO_2} could be used to estimate arterial P_{CO_2} with acceptable accuracy. Lanigan, Ponte, and Moxham,[61] however, concluded that dual O_2/CO_2 transcutaneous monitors have a limited role in anesthetic practice, and they suggested that these monitors should be used only as qualitative (*not* quantitative) indicators of changes in arterial blood gases.

TABLE 11-7.
Transcutaneous Monitors; Selected Adult Studies

Reference	Date	O_2/CO_2	Contribution
Matsen[51]	1980	O_2	Described use of transcutaneous P_{O_2} to evaluate peripheral perfusion.
Tremper[52]	1980	O_2	Transcutaneous P_{O_2} correlated well with arterial P_{O_2} with normal hemodynamic status; transcutaneous P_{O_2} decreased with a decrease in cardiac output.
Tremper[53]	1981	O_2	Found transcutaneous P_{O_2} reliable in adult surgical patients who were hemodynamically stable; with low flow shock, transcutaneous P_{O_2} decreased relative to arterial P_{O_2}.
Tremper[54]	1981	CO_2	Found transcutaneous P_{CO_2} reliable in patients with adequate cardiac function; during circulatory shock, the severity of the shock could be roughly determined by comparing the transcutaneous P_{CO_2} to arterial P_{CO_2}.

TABLE 11–7. (*Continued*)

Reference	Date	O_2/CO_2	Contribution
Waxman[24]	1983	O_2	Found that an initial transcutaneous Po_2 value of <60 mm Hg during resuscitation implied either the presence of hypoxia or poor tissue perfusion; also found transcutaneous monitors were helpful in evaluating fluid resuscitation.
Hauser[22]	1983	O_2	Used transcutaneous Po_2 to predict exercise-induced limb ischemia.
Mustapha[23]	1983	O_2	Found transcutaneous Po_2 reliable in assessing perfusion of the skin of healthy legs, ischemic legs, and prediction of healing potential following amputation.
Mahutte[47]	1984	O_2/CO_2	Found O_2/CO_2 dual monitor reliable with adult patients.
Abraham[55]	1984	O_2	During severe hypotension and cardiopulmonary resuscitation, transcutaneous Po_2 was a sensitive indicator of cardiac function and peripheral perfusion.
Abraham[56]	1984	O_2	During cardiopulmonary resuscitation, transcutaneous Po_2 provided useful information about the effectiveness of resuscitation and peripheral perfusion.
Abraham[57]	1984	O_2	Transcutaneous Po_2 provided useful information relative to peripheral perfusion during resuscitation.
Reed[48]	1985	O_2	Used transcutaneous Po_2 to predict changes in tissue perfusion.
Green[49]	1987	O_2	Found that transcutaneous Po_2 reliably reflected Pao_2 values at 50 to 100 mm Hg.
Phan[58]	1987	CO_2	Transcutaneous Pco_2 estimated arterial Pco_2 with a small bias, whereas end-tidal Pco_2 had a large negative bias.
Healey[59]	1987	CO_2	After withdrawal of mechanical ventilation, changes in both transcutaneous Pco_2 and end-tidal Pco_2 were predictive of important arterial Pco_2 increases.
Stokes[50]	1987	O_2/CO_2	Developed regression corrected values to more accurately predict arterial values from transcutaneous values.
Batay-Csorba[60]	1987	O_2	Used transcutaneous Po_2 to detect iliac and femoral artery disease.
Lanigan[61]	1988	O_2/CO_2	Transcutaneous monitoring provided qualitative, but not quantitative, estimates of blood gases during anesthesia.
Patel[10]	1989	O_2	Used Eugenol as the contact solution, and showed closer estimations of arterial oxygen levels from transcutaneous values.
Shoemaker[62]	1989	O_2	Studied the use of transcutaneous Po_2 values in 247 high-risk surgical patients; concluded these values were helpful in assessing circulatory changes.
Rooke[63]	1989	O_2	Demonstrated reproducibility of transcutaneous values in assessment of peripheral vascular disease.
Palmisano[64]	1990	O_2/CO_2	Transcutaneous Pco_2 was a relatively accurate predictor of arterial Pco_2, whereas transcutaneous Po_2 was a relatively inaccurate predictor of arterial Po_2.
Elborn[65]	1990	O_2	Found transcutaneous Po_2 useful in assessing perfusion to legs, and development of muscle hypoxia during exercise in patients with chronic cardiac failure.
Modesti[66]	1990	O_2	Used transcutaneous Po_2 during treadmill exercise to differentiate between normal subjects, patients with mild peripheral vascular disease, and patients with significant peripheral vascular disease.
Rooke[67]	1990	O_2	Found that diabetes in patients with arterial occlusive disease had a lower transcutaneous Po_2 than similar patient with only arterial occlusive disease.
Kesten[68]	1991	O_2/CO_2	Transcutaneous Pco_2 was a more accurate indicator of arterial blood gas values than transcutaneous Po_2.

Perhaps the most extensive study of the accuracy of transcutaneous Po_2 and Pco_2 in the prediction of arterial blood gases was conducted by Palmisano and Severinghaus.[64] This was a multicenter study conducted in 12 institutions that used 756 samples from 251 patients (neonatal, pediatric, and adult). They found that transcutaneous Po_2 was a poor predictor of arterial Po_2, particularly when Pao_2 was >80 mm Hg (Fig 11–13). Transcutaneous Po_2 was a better indicator of arterial Po_2 in neonates, particularly at a Pao_2 < 80 mm Hg. For carbon dioxide, however, they found that transcutaneous Pco_2 could be used to estimate arterial Pco_2 accurately in all age groups (Fig 11–14).

Transcutaneous oxygen monitoring has been used in adults to assess peripheral perfusion. Elborn et al.[65] used transcutaneous Po_2 to assess the legs of exercising patients with chronic heart failure. They found a significant decrease in transcutaneous Po_2 in these patients' legs and attributed this to abnormalities in perfusion and the development of muscle hypoxia. Modesti et al.[66] performed a similar evaluation in patients with early peripheral artery disease. Rooke and Osmundson[67] found a lower than expected lower limb transcutaneous Po_2 in patients with diabetes and peripheral vascular disease. Rooke and Osmundson[63] have also

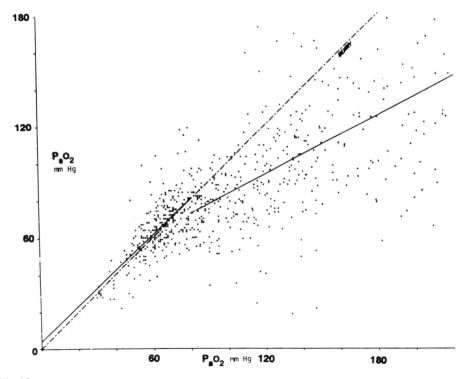

FIG 11–13.
The relationship of $Ptco_2$ to arterial Po_2; regression lines are shown for Pao_2 below and above 80 mm Hg; *n* = 723. (*From Palmisano BW, Severinghaus JW: Transcutaneous PCO2 and PO2: A multicenter study of accuracy. J Clin Monit 1990; 6:189–195. Used by permission.*)

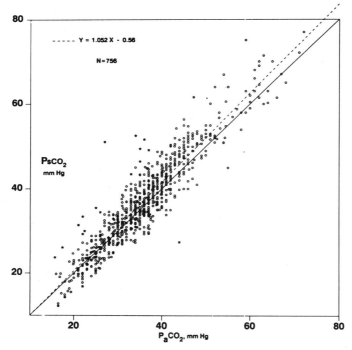

FIG 11–14.
The relationship of Ptcco₂ to Paco₂; the solid line is the line of identity. (*From Palmisano BW, Severinghaus JW: Transcutaneous PCO2 and PO2: A multicenter study of accuracy.* J Clin Monit *1990; 6:189–195. Used by permission.*)

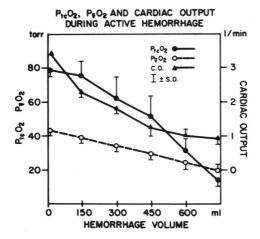

FIG 11–15.
Sequential values of mean transcutaneous Po₂ (Ptco₂), mixed venous Po₂ (Pv̄o₂), and cardiac output (C.O.) plotted against the volume of blood loss during active hemorrhage in dogs. (*From Tremper KK, Waxman K, Shoemaker WC: Effects of hypoxia and shock on transcutaneous PO2 values in dogs.* Crit Care Med *1979; 7:526–531. © by Williams and Wilkins. Used by permission.*)

TABLE 11–8.
Education Requirements for Personnel Using
Transcutaneous Monitors, as Recommended by
the American Academy of Pediatrics

- Technical aspects including:
    Quality control
    Application
    Maintenance
    Accuracy
    Response characteristics
    Limitations
- Interpretation including physiologic
  principles underlying the technique

reported the reproducibility of transcutaneous oxygen data in the assessment of peripheral vascular disease.

Canine[69–72] and human studies[52–56] have shown the relationship between cardiac output and transcutaneous Po_2. A decrease in cardiac output due to hemorrhage, shock, or cardiac arrest results in a decrease in transcutaneous Po_2 and an increase in transcutaneous Pco_2 (Fig 11–15). Transcutaneous Po_2 is a function of oxygen delivery to the tissue bed under the transcutaneous electrode. With a stable cardiac output, transcutaneous Po_2 reflects changes in arterial Po_2; with a stable arterial Po_2, transcutaneous Po_2 reflects changes in cardiac output. Several studies have also described the use of transcutaneous Po_2 during resuscitation to evaluate cardiac

TABLE 11–9.
Factors Affecting Transcutaneous and Arterial
Relationships

Electrode
    Calibration gases or substances
    Membrane condition
    Contact solution
    Probe placement and adhesion
    Temperature

Patient
    Oxygen:
        Skin thickness
        Perfusion
        Blood pressure
        Vasodilators
        Age
    Carbon Dioxide:
        Acidotic conditions
        perfusion

output.[54-56] Because the technical aspects of its use during resuscitation are not practical, transcutaneous Po_2 is uncommonly used in this application.

SUMMARY

Because use of transcutaneous monitors requires meticulous technical attention, they have become less popular in comparison to other monitors such as pulse oximeters. Despite their deceptive simplicity, specific education and training is required for the use of these monitors (Table 11–8).[73, 74] Clinicians using transcutaneous monitors must appreciate that transcutaneous Po_2 and Pco_2 are often different than arterial Po_2 and Pco_2, and that there are many factors that affect the relationship between transcutaneous and arterial values (Table 11–9). Even with the meticulous care that transcutaneous technology requires, these monitors still have clinical use as noninvasive trend monitors of oxygenation and ventilation status. Their accuracy, usefulness, and limitations in neonatal, pediatric, and adult patients have been documented. Yet their future use remains questionable in light of their technical requirements as compared to other noninvasive monitors. These monitors may be more useful in the future to evaluate peripheral vascular disease and other circulatory disturbances than to evaluate arterial blood gases.

REFERENCES

1. Clark LC: Measurement of oxygen tension: A historical perspective. *Crit Care Med* 1981; 9:690–692.
2. Lubbers DW: Theory and development of transcutaneous oxygen pressure measurement. *Int Anesthesiol Clin* 1987; 25:31–65.
3. Tremper KK, Waxman KS: Transcutaneous monitoring of respiratory gases, in Nochomovitz CN (ed): *Noninvasive Respiratory Monitoring.* 1986; 3:1–28.
4. Severinghaus JS, Bradley FA: Electrodes for blood PO2 and PCO2 determination. *J Appl Physiol* 1958; 13:515–520.
5. Severinghaus JS, Stafford M, Bradley AF: tcPCO2 electrode design, calibration and temperature gradient problems. *Acta Anaesthesiol Scand* 1978; 68(suppl):118–122.
6. Hansen TN, Tooley WH: Skin surface carbon dioxide tension in sick infants. *Pediatrics* 1979; 64:942–945.
7. Gray H. *Anatomy, Descriptive and Surgical*, ed 15. New York, Bounty Books, 1977.
8. Tolle CD, Beran AV, Johnston WD, et al: Transcutaneous gas monitoring through dermal window in adults (abstract). *Respir Care* 1982; 27:1240.
9. Van Duzee BF: Thermal analysis of human stratum corneum. *J Invest Dermatol* 1975; 65:404–408.
10. Patel BT, Delpy DT, Hillson PJ, et al: A topical metabolic inhibitor to improve transcutaneous estimation of arterial oxygen tension in adults. *J Biomed Eng* 1989; 11:381–383.
11. Lubbers DW: Theoretical basis of the transcutaneous blood gas measurements. *Crit Care Med* 1981; 9:721–733.
12. Novametrix 850B Auto-cal Operating Manual. Wallingford, CT, Novametrix Medical Systems.
13. Transend Cutaneous Gas System Operating Instructions. Anaheim, CA, Sensormedics Corporation.
14. Oxymonitor Operating Manual, Elk Grove, IL, Litton Company.

15. Martin R: Transcutaneous monitoring: Instrumentation and clinical applications. *Respir Care* 1990; 35:577–583.
16. Martin RJ, Beoglos A, Miller MJ, et al: Increasing arterial carbon dioxide tension: Influence on transcutaneous carbon dioxide tension measurements. *Pediatrics* 1988; 81:684–687.
17. Bucher HU, Fanconi S, Fallenstein F, et al: Transcutaneous carbon dioxide tension in newborn infants: Reliability and safety of continuous 24-hour measurement at 42 degrees C. *Pediatrics* 1986; 78:631–635.
18. Herrell N, Martin RJ, Pultusker M, et al: Optimal temperature for the measurement of transcutaneous carbon dioxide tension in the neonate. *J Pediatr* 1980; 97:114–117.
19. Brustler I, Enders A, Versmold HT: Skin surface PCO2 monitoring in newborn infants in shock. *J Pediatr* 1982; 100:454–457.
20. Pearlman SA, Maisels J: Preductal and postductal transcutaneous oxygen tension measurements in premature newborns with hyaline membrane disease. *Pediatrics* 1989; 83:98–100.
21. Lofgren O. Continuous transcutaneous oxygen monitoring in the fetus during labor. *Crit Care Med* 1981; 9:698–701.
22. Hauser CJ, Shoemaker WC: Use of a transcutaneous PO2 regional perfusion index to quantify tissue perfusion in peripheral vascular disease. *Ann Surg* 1983; 197:337–343.
23. Mustapha NM, Redhead RG, Jain SK, et al: Transcutaneous partial oxygen pressure assessment of the ischemic lower limb. *Surg Gynecol Obstet* 1983; 156:582–584.
24. Waxman K, Sadler R, Eisner ME, et al: Transcutaneous oxygen monitoring of emergency department patients. *Am J Surg* 1983; 146:35–38.
25. Severinghaus JW, Peabody J, Thurstrom A, Eberhard P, Zappia E (eds): Workshop on methodologic aspects of transcutaneous blood gas analysis. *Acta Anaesthesiol Scand* 1978, suppl. 68.
26. Huch A, Huch R, Lucey JF (eds): Continuous transcutaneous blood gas monitoring. *Birth Defects* 1979; Vol. 15, March
27. Huch R, Huch A, Lubbers DW: Transcutaneous measurement of blood PO2: Method and application in perinatal medicine. *J Perinat Med* 1973; 1:183–186.
28. Kilbride HW, Merenstein GB: Continuous transcutaneous oxygen monitoring in acutely ill preterm infants. *Crit Care Med* 1984; 12:121–124.
29. Huch R, Huch A, Albani M, et al: Transcutaneous PO2 monitoring in routine management of infants and children with cardiorespiratory problems. *Pediatrics* 1976; 57:681–690.
30. Huch R, Huch A. Fetal and maternal PtcO2 monitoring. *Crit Care Med* 1981; 9:694–697.
31. Martin RJ, Robertson SS, Hopple MM: Relationship between transcutaneous and arterial oxygen tension in sick neonates during mild hyperoxemia. *Crit Care Med* 1982; 10:670–672.
32. Peabody JL, Gregory GA, Willis MM, et al: Transcutaneous oxygen tension in sick infants. *Am Rev Resp Dis* 1978; 118:83–87.
33. Bancalari E, Flynn J, Goldberg RN, et al: Influence of transcutaneous oxygen monitoring on the incidence of retinopathy of prematurity. *Pediatrics* 1987; 79:663–669.
34. Martin RJ, Herrell N, Rubin D, et al: Effect of supine and prone positions on arterial oxygen tension in the preterm infant. *Pediatrics* 1979; 63:528–531.
35. Heaf DP, Helms P, Gordon I, et al: Postural effects on gas exchange in infants. *N Engl J Med* 1983; 308:1505–1508.
36. Gleason CA, Martin RJ, Anderson JV, et al: Optimal position for a spinal tap in preterm infants. *Pediatrics* 1983; 71:31–35.
37. Epstein MF, Cohen AR, Feldman HA, et al: Estimation of PaCO2 by two noninvasive methods in the critically ill newborn infant. *J Pediatrics* 1985; 106:282–286.
38. Hand IL, Shepard EK, Krauss AN, et al: Discrepancies between transcutaneous and end-tidal carbon dioxide monitoring in the critically ill neonate with respiratory distress syndrome. *Crit Care Med* 1989; 17:556–559.

39. Monaco F, Nickerson BG, McQuitty JC: Continuous transcutaneous oxygen and carbon dioxide monitoring in the pediatric ICU. *Crit Care Med* 1982; 10:765–766.

40. Mok JYQ, Hak H, McLaughlin FJ, et al: Effect of age and state of wakefulness on transcutaneous oxygen values in preterm infants: A longitudinal study. *J Pediatr* 1988; 113:706–709.

41. Hamilton PA, Whitehead MD, Reynolds ER: Underestimation of arterial oxygen tension by transcutaneous electrode with increasing age in infants. *Arch Dis Child* 1985; 60:1162–1165.

42. Rome ES, Stork EK, Carlo WA, et al: Limitations of transcutaneous PO2 and PCO2 monitoring in infants with bronchopulmonary dysplasia. *Pediatrics* 1984; 74:217–220.

43. Durand M, Ramanathan R: Pulse oximetry for continuous oxygen monitoring in sick newborn infants. *J Pediatr* 1986; 109:1052–1056.

44. Fanconi S, Burger R, Maurer H, et al: Transcutaneous carbon dioxide pressure for monitoring patients with severe croup. *J Pediatr* 1990; 117:701–705.

45. Russell RIR, Helms PJ: Comparative accuracy of pulse oximetry and transcutaneous oxygen in assessing arterial saturation in pediatric intensive care. *Crit Care Med* 1990; 18:725–727.

46. Rooth G, Hedstrand U, Tyden H, et al: The validity of the transcutaneous oxygen tension method in adults. *Crit Care Med* 1976; 4:162–165.

47. Mahutte CK, Michiels TM, Hassell KT, et al: Evaluation of a single transcutaneous PO2-PCO2 sensor in adult patients. *Crit Care Med* 1984; 12:1063–1066.

48. Reed LR, Maier RV, Landicho D, et al: Correlation of hemodynamic variables with transcutaneous PO2 measurements in critically ill adult patients. *J Trauma* 1985; 25:1045–1053.

49. Green GE, Hassell KT, Mahutte CK: Comparison of arterial blood gas with continuous intra-arterial and transcutaneous PO2 sensors in adult critically ill patients. *Crit Care Med* 1987; 15:491–494.

50. Stokes CD, Blevins S, Siegel JH, et al: Prediction of arterial blood gases by transcutaneous O2 and CO2 in critically ill hyperdynamic trauma patients. *J Trauma* 1987; 27:1240–1260.

51. Matsen III F, Wyss C, Pedegana L, et al: Transcutaneous oxygen tension measurement in peripheral vascular disease. *Surg Gynecol Obstet* 1980; 150:525–528.

52. Tremper K, Waxman K, Bowman R, et al: Continuous transcutaneous oxygen monitoring during respiratory failure, cardiac decompensation, cardiac arrest, and CPR. *Crit Care Med* 1980; 8:377–381.

53. Tremper KK, Shoemaker WC, Shippy CR, et al: Transcutaneous PCO2 monitoring on adult patients in the ICU and the operating room. *Crit Care Med* 1981; 9:752–755.

54. Tremper K, Shoemaker W: Transcutaneous oxygen monitoring of critically ill adults, with and without low flow shock. *Crit Care Med* 1981; 9:706–709.

55. Abraham E, Smith M, Silver L: Conjunctival and transcutaneous oxygen monitoring during cardiac arrest and cardiopulmonary resuscitation. *Crit Care Med* 1984; 12:419–421.

56. Abraham E, Smith M, Silver L: Continuous monitoring of critically ill patients with transcutaneous oxygen and carbon dioxide and conjunctival oxygen sensors. *Ann Emerg Med* 1984; 13:1021–1026.

57. Abraham E, Ehrlich H: Conjunctival and transcutaneous oxygen monitoring during resuscitation. *Ann Emerg Med* 1984; 13:287–289.

58. Phan CQ, Tremper KK, Lee SE, et al: Noninvasive monitoring of carbon dioxide: A comparison of the partial pressure of transcutaneous and end-tidal carbon dioxide with the partial pressure of arterial carbon dioxide. *J Clin Monit* 1987; 3:149–154.

59. Healey CJ, Fedullo AJ, Swinburne AJ, et al: Comparison of noninvasive measurements of carbon dioxide tension during withdrawal from mechanical ventilation. *Crit Care Med* 1987; 15:764–768.

60. Batay-Csorba P, Provan J, Ameli M: Transcutaneous oxygen tension measurements in the detection of iliac and femoral arterial disease. *Surg Gynecol Obstet* 1987; 164:102–104.

61. Lanigan C, Ponte J, Moxham J: Performance of transcutaneous PO2 and PCO2 dual electrodes in adults. *Br J Anaesth* 1988; 60:736–742.

62. Shoemaker WC, Appel PL, Kram HB: Incidence, physiologic description, compensatory mechanisms, and therapeutic implications of monitored events. *Crit Care Med* 1989; 17:1277–1285.

63. Rooke TW, Osmundson PJ: Variability and reproducibility of transcutaneous oxygen tension measurements in the assessment of peripheral vascular disease. *J Vasc Dis* 1989; 40:695–700.
64. Palmisano BW, Severinghaus JW: Transcutaneous PCO_2 and PO_2: A multicenter study of accuracy. *J Clin Monit* 1990; 6:189–195.
65. Elborn JS, Riley M, Stanford CF, et al: Transcutaneous oxygen tension in the leg during exercise in patients with chronic cardiac failure. *Int J Cardiol* 1990; 28:51–58.
66. Modesti PA, Boddi M, Gensini GF, et al: Transcutaneous oximetry monitoring during the early phase of exercise in patients with peripheral artery disease. *J Vasc Dis* 1990; 40:553–558.
67. Rooke TW, Osmundson PJ: The influence of age, sex, smoking and diabetes on lower limb transcutaneous oxygen tension in patients with arterial vascular occlusive disease. *Arch Intern Med* 1990; 150:129–132.
68. Kesten S, Chapman KR, Rebuck AS: Response characteristics of a dual transcutaneous oxygen/carbon dioxide monitoring system. *Chest* 1991; 99:1211–1215.
69. Tremper KK, Waxman K, Shoemaker WC: Effects of hypoxia and shock on transcutaneous PO_2 values in dogs. *Crit Care Med* 1979; 7:526–531.
70. Fink S, Ray CW, McCartney S, Ehrlich H, et al: Oxygen transport and utilization in hyperoxia and hypoxia: Relation of conjunctival and transcutaneous oxygen tensions to hemodynamic and oxygen transport variables. *Crit Care Med* 1984; 12:943–948.
71. Dronen SC, Manigas PA, Foutch R: Transcutaneous oxygen tension measurements during graded hemorrhage and reinfusion. *Ann Emerg Med* 1984; 14:534–539.
72. Gottrup R, Gellett S, Kirkegaard L, et al: Effect of hemorrhage and resuscitation on subcutaneous, conjunctival, and transcutaneous oxygen tension in relation to hemodynamic variables. *Crit Care Med* 1989; 17:904–907.
73. Avery GB, Bancalari EH, Engler A, et al: American Academy of Pediatrics Task Force on Transcutaneous Oxygen Monitors. Report of consensus meeting. *Pediatrics* 1989; 83:122–126.
74. Rennie JM: Transcutaneous carbon dioxide monitoring. *Arch Dis Child* 1990; 63:345–346.

Chapter 12

Capnography: Technical Aspects and Clinical Applications

Dean Hess, M.Ed., R.R.T.

INTRODUCTION

The ability to measure a patient's inhaled and exhaled CO_2 has existed for many years.[1] In recent years, this technology has evolved so that it is now available in virtually all operating rooms, in most critical care units, and in some emergency departments. In anesthesia, capnography has become a standard of care.[2-4] In spite of several comprehensive reviews of the topic,[5-9] the understanding of capnography by health care practitioners has not evolved as quickly as the technology. In fact, there are many misconceptions and unrealistic expectations of capnography. This chapter will discuss the technical and physiologic aspects of capnography.

TECHNICAL ASPECTS

Definitions

Capnometry is the measurement of CO_2 at the patient's airway during the ventilatory cycle.[5, 10] The *capnometer* provides a numeric display of inhaled and exhaled P_{CO_2}. *Capnography* is the graphic waveform display of CO_2 (either as percent or mm Hg) as a function of time (or volume). When the waveform is displayed, capnography includes *capnometry*. A device that measures CO_2 and displays a waveform is called a *capnograph*. The waveform displayed by a capnograph is called a *capnogram*. Although there is some controversy regarding the usefulness of a capnometer that does not display a CO_2 waveform,[11, 12] it is generally believed that capnography is superior to capnometry alone. Capnography allows the validity of the measured P_{CO_2} to be assessed. If the CO_2 waveform does not appear plausible, then the data provided should be questioned. Further, evaluation of the shape of the CO_2 waveform can be useful in the diagnosis of certain abnormal conditions, as discussed later in this chapter. Although capnography is technically different than capnometry, for simplicity the term *capnography* will be used throughout the remainder of this chapter.

Mainstream Versus Sidestream Capnographs

With the mainstream (nondiverting or in-line) capnograph, the measurement chamber (sometimes called the *cell* or *cuvette*) is placed directly at the airway (Fig 12–1). This results in a very crisp capnogram that is generated almost instantaneously. However, some problems are associated with this configuration. The mainstream sensor is subject to damage during handling (e.g., if it is dropped), it places additional weight on the airway (increasing the possibility of airway displacement), it increases mechanical dead-space, and it is difficult to use in spontaneously breathing patients. However, there are low-dead-space, low-weight, reasonably rugged mainstream sensors that are now commercially available (e.g., Novametrix).

With the sidestream (diverting or aspirating) capnograph, gas from the airway is aspirated through fine-bore tubing to the measurement chamber inside the device (Fig 12–2). This eliminates many of the problems associated with the mainstream sensor. However, it introduces other problems related to the aspiration of gas from the airway.[13–18] The sample tubing tends to become obstructed with secretions and water, and a delay in analysis occurs because of the time required for the sample to move from the airway to the measurement chamber. This delay depends on the length of the tubing, the diameter of the tubing, and the aspiration rate. Many commercially available sidestream capnographs use a sample flow of 150 mL/min. Use of a flow that is too slow has been shown to result in artifacts in the resultant capnogram.[3, 19] When a sidestream capnograph is used, care must be taken to position the sample port so that room air or fresh gas flow contamination does not occur. In anesthesia applications, the outlet of the capnograph must be fitted with a scavenger system or routed back to the patient circuit to avoid contamination of the environment with anesthetic gas.[20, 21]

With the sidestream capnograph, excess water and secretions must be removed from the

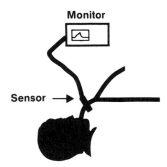

FIG 12–1.
Schematic illustration of mainstream capnograph, with the sensor placed directly at the airway. (*From Hess D: Capnometry and capnography: Technical aspects, physiologic aspects, and clinical applications. Respir Care 1990; 35:557–576. Used by permission.*)

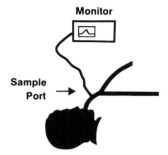

FIG 12–2.
Sidestream capnograph, with gas aspirated rrom the airway to the measurement chamber in the device. (*From Hess D: Capnometry and capnography: Technical aspects, physiologic aspects, and clinical applications.* Respir Care *1990; 35:557–576. Used by permission.*)

sample before it enters the measurement chamber. This is often accomplished by use of water traps and filters. Nafion tubing, which is water vapor permeable, also can be used. Some systems also use reverse flow, or a purge, to clear water and secretions from the sample tube. However, this technique is not recommended because of infection control reasons, and because it can compromise oxygenation if the purge gas is room air and the patient is being ventilated with high oxygen concentrations. If a purge is used, it should be manually controlled (rather than automatic), and it should use filtered gas to minimize patient contamination. For accurate detection of CO_2, it is also important that the sample tubing be impermeable to CO_2 and leak free.[22, 23]

A variation of the sidestream capnograph is the proximal-diverting system (used in the Nellcor N-1000). In this design, the measurement chamber is removed from the airway, but kept close to the patient. The intent of this configuration is to take advantage of the best features of the mainstream and sidestream designs, yet minimize the disadvantages of these designs.

There is no clear superiority between the mainstream and sidestream capnograph.[24] This is true for adults, and may be true for infants and children as well (see discussion later in this chapter). There are advantages and disadvantages of both (Table 12–1); the choice between these is one of personal preference.

The Infrared Capnograph

Most bedside capnographs used in respiratory care measure CO_2 by infrared absorption.[5] As seen in Figure 12–3, the absorption peak for CO_2 at 4.26 μm lies between those for H_2O. The peak for N_2O is close enough to that of CO_2 to produce a problem with interference. Another problem with infrared capnography is pressure (or collision) broadening,[5, 25–29] in which collisions between CO_2 and other gases (such as N_2O) affect the infrared absorption of CO_2. The magnitude of pressure broadening is dependent on the filter and detector of the capnograph.

TABLE 12–1.
Advantages and disadvantages of Mainstream and Sidestream Capnographs

• MAINSTREAM CAPNOGRAPH

Advantages:
  Sensor at patient airway
  Fast response (crisp waveform)
  Short lag time (real-time readings)
  No sample flow to reduce tidal volume

Disadvantages:
  Secretions and humidity blocks sensor window
  Sensor requires heating to prevent condensation
  Requires frequent calibration
  Bulky sensor at patient airway
  Does not measure N_2O
  Difficult to use with nonintubated patients
  Reusable adapters requires cleaning and sterilization

• SIDESTREAM CAPNOGRAPH

Advantages:
  No bulky sensors or heaters at airway
  Ability to measure N_2O
  Disposable sample line
  Ability to use with nonintubated patients

Disadvantages:
  Secretions block sample tubing
  Water trap required to remove water from the sample
  Frequent calibration required
  Slow response to CO_2 changes
  Lag time between CO_2 change and measurement
  Sample flow may decrease tidal volume

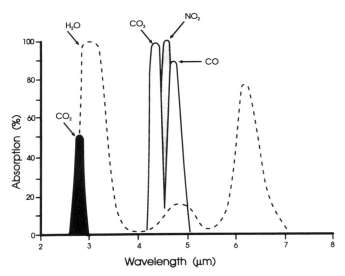

FIG 12–3.
Infrared absorption spectra for CO_2, H_2O, and N_2O; the CO_2 peak for capnography is at 4.26 μm.

The relative influence of any gas is such that if the influence of a specific gas is known, then the influence of other gases can be estimated. Pressure broadening is independent of the CO_2 concentration at $\leq 10\%$. The pressure-broadening influence[5] on CO_2 is in the following order: $He < O_2 < N_2 < N_2O$. Examples of pressure-broadening correction factors are found in Table 12–2. These factors can be used to correct for the presence of gases other than CO_2 in the mixture being analyzed.

A typical nondispersive double-beam positive-filter capnograph is illustrated[5] in Figure 12–4. The detector is filled with CO_2. Radiation that comes through the reference and sample cells affects the absorption by CO_2 in the detection chamber. CO_2 in the sample cell decreases the radiation transmitted to the detector. The increased radiation transmitted from the reference cell (relative to that from the sample cell) produces movement of a diaphragm, which is translated into a display of the amount of CO_2 present in the sample cell. Interference from N_2O is removed by a filter that absorbs the radiation from the N_2O absorption band. A chopper periodically permits measurement of the reference signal, the sample signal, and the dark signal (neither reference or sample signals).

A chopper is used in most capnographs and is important for several reasons. First, it allows a common source and detector to be used with the double-beam capnograph. Second, it provides an alternating signal from the reference and sample cells. Third, it produces a null signal (i.e., no signal from either sample or reference cell) that helps to eliminate drift and interference.

To provide accurate measurements, capnographs must be calibrated at regular intervals. This involves occasional use of a 5% CO_2 gas mixture and more frequent zero calibration with room air. The accuracy of a capnograph should be $\pm 12\%$ or ± 4 mm Hg, whichever is larger.[30] The performance of some commercially available capnographs has been reported.[31–37] When the capnograph is calibrated, it is important to consider the effects of water vapor pressure.[38]

TABLE 12–2.

Pressure Broadening Correction Factors for Various Gases*

Diluent Gas	Correction Factor
Helium	1.11
Oxygen	1.06
Nitrogen	1.00
Hydrogen	0.87

* Data from Gravenstein JS, Paulus DA, Hayes TJ: *Capnography in Clinical Practice.* Boston, butterwoths, 1989.
Multiplying the measurement in various diluent gases by the correction factor corrects to a calibration curve where the diluent gas is nitrogen (for the Beckman IR215 analyzer.)

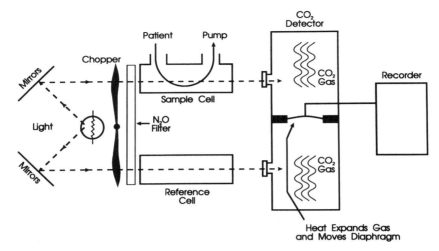

FIG 12–4.
Schematic representation of a nondispersive double-beam positive-filter capnograph.

Mass Spectrometry

The mass spectrometer can be used to measure inspired and expired CO_2, and also O_2, N_2, and anesthetic agents.[39–46] A typical mass spectrometer is illustrated in Figure 12–5. The sample is aspirated into a vacuum chamber. In the vacuum chamber, the gas is ionized by an electron beam. The charged fragments are accelerated into a dispersion chamber where they are separated according to mass and charge. Detectors (collectors) measure the component gases. Many mass spectrometers used in anesthesia and critical care are multiplex units, and

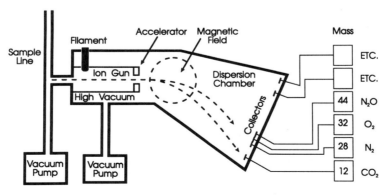

FIG 12–5.
Schematic representation of a mass spectrometer.

as such alternately sample gases from several patients. A problem associated with the use of mass spectrometry to measure CO_2 is that N_2O and CO_2 have nearly identical gram molecular weights. This problem is overcome by measuring N_2O as N_2O^+ and by measuring CO_2 as C^+. Because of their cost, mass spectrometers are used less often than infrared capnographs to measure inspired and expired CO_2.

PHYSIOLOGIC ASPECTS

The Normal Capnogram

The normal capnogram is illustrated in Figure 12–6. It is usually displayed with P_{CO_2} on the ordinate and time on the abscissa. However, the ordinate can be in units of percent CO_2. The abscissa can be displayed as exhaled volume, although this is unusual because most capnographs cannot measure a flow signal. The capnogram can be displayed in either fast speed or slow speed. The fast speed allows evaluation of the fine detail of each breath, whereas the slow speed allows the evaluation of trends in P_{ETCO_2}.

During inspiration, P_{CO_2} is zero (Fig 12–6). At the beginning of exhalation, P_{CO_2} remains zero as gas from the anatomic dead-space leaves the airway (*A*, phase I). The capnogram then rises sharply as alveolar gas mixes with dead-space gas (*A–B*, phase II). The curve then levels and forms a plateau during most of exhalation (*B–C*, phase III), which represents gas flow from alveoli and is thus called the *alveolar plateau*. The P_{CO_2} at the end of the alveolar plateau is called the end-tidal P_{CO_2} (P_{ETCO_2}). The end-tidal P_{CO_2} may not occur at end-exhalation (i.e., immediately before inhalation). This is particularly true with sidestream capnographs, where fresh gas will be aspirated when expiratory flow ceases. For this reason, some clinicians refer to P_{ETCO_2} and "peak-exhaled P_{CO_2}" or "maximal exhaled P_{CO_2}." It is also important not to confuse changes in exhaled P_{CO_2} with changes in flow. If the capnogram records P_{CO_2} as a

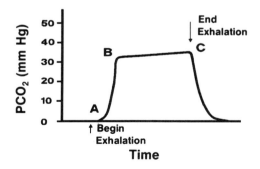

FIG 12–6.
The normal capnogram. Point *A* represents anatomic dead-space, *B* represents the beginning of the alveolar plateau, and *C* represents the end of the alveolar plateau. The P_{CO_2} at *C* is the end-tidal P_{CO_2}. (*From Hess D: Capnometry and capnography: Technical aspects, physiologic aspects, and clinical applications. Respir Care 1990; 35:557–576. Used by permission.*)

function of time (which is usually the case), then flow is only a factor if it affects this relationship.

The $Petco_2$ presumably represents alveolar Pco_2 ($Paco_2$). $Paco_2$ is determined by the rate at which CO_2 is added to the alveolus and the rate at which CO_2 is cleared from the alveolus. The rate at which CO_2 is added to the alveolus is determined by tissue CO_2 production and venous blood flow (perfusion). The rate at which CO_2 is cleared from the alveolus is determined by alveolar ventilation. Thus, $Paco_2$ is the result of the relationship between ventilation and perfusion, the V/Q ratio. With a normal V/Q, the $Paco_2$ will approximate the $Paco_2$ (Fig 12–7). If ventilation is decreased compared to perfusion, there will be more time for equilibration between $P\overline{v}co_2$ and $Paco_2$, and thus the $Paco_2$ will rise toward $P\overline{v}co_2$. With a high V/Q (i.e., dead-space), $Paco_2$ will approach the inspired Pco_2 ($Pico_2$), which is usually zero. $Petco_2$ is a mixture of gas flowing simultaneously from millions of alveoli and represents the mixture of many different $Paco_2$'s. Theoretically, $Petco_2$ could be as low as the $Pico_2$ (zero) or as high as the $P\overline{v}co_2$ (but not higher than this).

An increase or decrease in $Petco_2$ can be the result of changes in CO_2 production and delivery to the lungs,[47–49] changes in alveolar ventilation, or an equipment malfunction (Tables 12–3 and 12–4). However, because of homeostasis, compensatory changes may occur so that $Petco_2$ does not change. For example, if CO_2 production increases (such as with fever) and alveolar ventilation increases proportionately (the normal homeostatic response), then $Petco_2$ may not change. In clinical practice, $Petco_2$ is a nonspecific indicator of cardiopulmonary homeostasis and usually does not indicate a specific problem or abnormality.

Capnography has been suggested as a useful backup disconnect alarm in mechnically ventilated patients.[50, 51] The rationale for this is that the capnograph will detect no CO_2 if the ventilator is disconnected from the airway. However, no data exist to suggest that addition of capnography to properly functioning ventilator disconnect alarms improves the detection of a ventilator disconnect in the critical care unit. This may actually contribute to alarm-noise-pollution secondary to false-positive alarms, thus decreasing the sensitivity of staff to real alarm conditions. Failure of capnography to detect disconnection has been reported.[52]

If the $Paco_2$ is measured, then the gradient between the $Paco_2$ and $Petco_2$ (the $Paco_2$–$Petco_2$

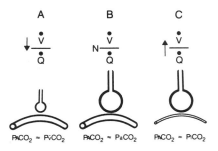

FIG 12–7.
$Paco_2$ with **A,** low V/Q, **B,** normal V/Q, and **C,** high V/Q. (*From Hess D: Capnometry and capnography: Technical aspects, physiologic aspects, and clinical applications. Respir Care 1990; 35:557–576. Used by permission.*)

TABLE 12–3.
Causes of Increased Petco$_2$

Increased CO$_2$ Production and Delivery to the Lungs
- Fever
- Sepsis
- Bicarbonate administration
- Increased metabolic rate
- Seizures

Decreased Alveolar Ventilation
- Respiratory center depression
- Muscular paralysis
- Hypoventilation
- COPD

Equipment Malfunction
- Rebreathing
- Exhausted CO$_2$ absorber
- Leak in ventilator circuit

TABLE 12–4.
Causes of Decreased Petco$_2$

Decreased CO$_2$ Production and Delivery to the Lungs
- Hypothermia
- Pulmonary hypoperfusion
- Cardiac arrest
- Pulmonary embolism
- Hemorrhage
- Hypotension

Increased Alveolar Ventilation
- Hyperventilation

Equipment Malfunction
- Ventilator disconnect
- Esophageal intubation
- Complete airway obstruction
- Poor sampling
- Leak around endotracheal tube cuff

gradient) can be calculated. This gradient is normally small, being less that 5 mm Hg. However, with dead-space-producing disease (high V/Q), the P_{ETCO_2} may be considerably less than the $Paco_2$ (Table 12–5). In patients with airway obstruction, Tulou and Walsh[53] found that the $Paco_2$–P_{ETCO_2} gradient decreased significantly if P_{ETCO_2} was measured at maximal exhalation. Although shunting may result in a large gradient between Pao_2 and Pao_2, it will only have a small effect on the $Paco_2$–P_{ETCO_2} gradient.

On occasion, the P_{ETCO_2} may be greater than the $Paco_2$.[54, 55] The physiologic reasons for a P_{ETCO_2} greater than $Paco_2$ are not well understood,[56] and may relate to low (but finite) V/Q regions within the lung. Fletcher and Jonson[57] have reported that P_{ETCO_2} is more often greater than $Paco_2$ when the tidal volume is high. With a larger tidal volume, there is a greater expiratory time that may allow lung units with a low V/Q (and thus a longer time constant) to empty. Jones et al.[58, 59] found P_{ETCO_2} greater than $Paco_2$ during exercise, and attributed this to an increase in $Paco_2$ because of increased CO_2 that is emitted into a lung volume becoming smaller during exhalation.

One technical point is important when $Paco_2$ is compared with P_{ETCO_2}. That is, the $Paco_2$ must be adjusted to the patient's body temperature if it is not 37°C.[60–62] Failure to adjust the $Paco_2$ for temperature will result in an incorrect $Paco_2$–P_{ETCO_2}.

Much of the reported research on the relationship between P_{ETCO_2} and $Paco_2$ has been done in anesthesia. In a frequently cited paper, Nunn and Hill[63] reported a mean $Paco_2$–P_{ETCO_2} of 4.7 ± 2.5 mm Hg, which was determined from 12 "fit" patients during anesthesia. Phan et al.[61] reported a $Paco_2$–P_{ETCO_2} of 5.8 ± 5.9 mm Hg from 211 measurements in 23 anesthesized patients.

There has been little reported on the relationship between P_{ETCO_2} and $Paco_2$ in stable critically ill patients. Donati et al.[60] found a $Paco_2$–P_{ETCO_2} gradient of 3.2 ± 2.8 in 20 patients following coronary artery bypass surgery, and Russell, Graybeal, and Strout[64] found a gradient of 5.5 ± 5.2 mm Hg in a similar patient population. Hoffman et al.[65] found that P_{ETCO_2} was misleading when used to estimate $Paco_2$ at various levels of mechanical ventilation in critically ill patients, primarily because of a large variability in the $Paco_2$–P_{ETCO_2} gradient. In a series of 200 measurements from 26 stable but critically ill trauma patients, Hess and Agarwal[66] found a mean $Paco_2$–P_{ETCO_2} of 0.9 ± 3.6 mm Hg; it was not unusual for the P_{ETCO_2} to be slightly greater than the $Paco_2$. The "normal" relationship between $Paco_2$ and P_{ETCO_2} in stable critically ill patients has not been clearly established.

Several investigators have evaluated the stability of the $Paco_2$–P_{ETCO_2}. In a canine model, Das, Joshi, and Philippart[67] found good correlation between P_{ETCO_2} and $Paco_2$ over a wide range of $Paco_2$'s (14 to 104 mm Hg). Takki, Aromaa, and Kauste[68] evaluated $Paco_2$–P_{ETCO_2}

TABLE 12–5.
Causes of Increased $Paco_2$–P_{ETCO_2}

- Pulmonary hypoperfusion
- Pulmonary embolism
- Cardiac arrest
- Positive pressure ventilation (especially PEEP)
- High-rate low-tidal volume ventilation

---

during five types of ventilation and found that the gradient was stable. Perrin et al.[69] varied the ventilation in a series of patients and found that changes in P_{ACO_2} could be used to predict changes in $Paco_2$. Whitesell et al.[62] found that the $Paco_2$–$Petco_2$ was stable during anesthesia and suggested that $Petco_2$ could be used to predict $Paco_2$ for an individual patient once the gradient was determined for that patient. However, Raemer et al.[70] found that the $Paco_2$–$Petco_2$ was too variable during anesthesia to allow precise prediction of $Paco_2$ from $Petco_2$. In a series of 26 critically ill but stable mechanically ventilated trauma patients, Hess and Agarwal[66] found that the short-term (1-hour) variability in $Petco_2$ was similar to the short-term variability in $Paco_2$.

Hoffman et al.[65] evaluated $Petco_2$ in 20 critically ill patients during changes in mechanical ventilation. The relationship between $Petco_2$ and $Paco_2$ was evaluated after changes in the rate and/or tidal volume settings of the ventilator. They found that changes in $Petco_2$ did not correlate well with changes in $Paco_2$, and that the trends in $Petco_2$ were opposite the trends in $Paco_2$ in four patients. These investigators concluded that $Petco_2$ may be a misleading indicator of changes in $Paco_2$. In a group of 59 patients following cardiac surgery, Russell, Graybeal, and Strout[64] found that the relationship between $Paco_2$ and $Petco_2$ was not significant in many individual patients. They concluded that the individual variations demonstrated in $Paco_2$–$Petco_2$ in postoperative cardiac patients make periodic assessments of ventilatory adequacy by arterial blood gas measurements necessary.

Capnographic Waveforms

Capnography involves not only the measurement of inspired and expired CO_2 concentration, but evaluation of the capnogram as well. The shape of the capnogram can be characteristic for many clinical conditions.[71–74]

The capnogram with airflow obstruction is characterized by the lack of a true alveolar plateau, or the slope of the alveolar plateau is increased. With severe airflow obstruction, there also may be an increase in $Petco_2$ (Fig 12–8). The lack of an alveolar plateau is because of alveoli with long time constants that contribute CO_2-rich gas to the expired gas flow. With reversible airflow obstruction, the shape of the capnogram may normalize with bronchodilator therapy.

With bradypnea, cardiac oscillations may be seen on the capnogram (Fig 12–9).[75] These

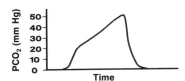

FIG 12–8.
Capnogram produced with airflow obstruction. (*From Hess D: Capnometry and capnography: Technical aspects, physiologic aspects, and clinical applications.* Respir Care 1990; 35:557–576. Used by permission.)

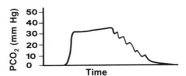

FIG 12–9.
Capnogram with cardiac oscillations. (*From Hess D: Capnometry and capnography: Technical aspects, physiologic aspects, and clinical applications.* Respir Care *1990; 35:557–576. Used by permission.*)

oscillations are thought to be the result of the heart beating against the lungs. The presence of cardiac oscillations on the capnogram is a normal finding.

Rebreathing is characterized by an increase in both inspired and expired CO_2 (Fig 12–10).[76] This is the result of a malfunction in the respiratory equipment, such as a malfunctioning exhalation valve or excessive mechanical dead-space. This might also be the result of depletion of the CO_2 absorbent in an anesthesia circuit.

A downward spike may be seen in the expiratory capnogram of patients recovering from neuromuscular blockade (Fig 12–11), which is commonly called a *curare cleft*. However, this is more commonly seen in patients who are not breathing in synchrony with the ventilator or in patients with uneven expiratory flow. Thus, note that curare cleft is not necessarily associated with nueromuscular blockade.

CLINICAL APPLICATIONS

Capnography to Detect Esophageal Intubation

Esophageal intubation is a serious problem.[77] It can occur at the time of intubation, during manipulation of the endotracheal tube, or during movement of the head.[78] Esophageal intubation can be difficult to recognize, particularly in obese patients, or in patients in whom the vocal cords cannot be easily visualized. Of the methods available to detect esophageal intubation, measurement of Petco$_2$ is regarded as the most reliable, and it has been suggested that Petco$_2$ should be used routinely to determine proper endotracheal tube position.[77]

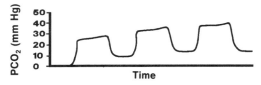

FIG 12–10.
Capnogram produced with rebreathing. (*From Hess D: Capnometry and capnography: Technical aspects, physiologic aspects, and clinical applications.* Respir Care *1990; 35:557–576. Used by permission.*)

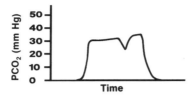

FIG 12–11.
Capnogram with curare cleft. (*From Hess D: Capnometry and capnography: Technical aspects, physiologic aspects, and clinical applications.* Respir Care 1990; 35:557–576. Used by permission.)

Using a dog model, Murray and Modell[79] found $Petco_2$ useful in the recognition of esophageal intubation. Monitoring of esophageal Pco_2 produced very low levels of $Petco_2$ (Fig 12–12). Total obstruction of the endotracheal tube also resulted in a drop in $Petco_2$, and evaluation of the capnographic waveform was useful in the detection of partial obstruction of the endotracheal tube. In this study, it was also shown that movement of the endotracheal tube from the trachea into the pharynx resulted in changes in the capnogram (Fig 12–13).

In a study of 20 patients, Linko, Paloheimo, and Tammisto[80] found $Petco_2$ useful in the detection of esophageal intubation. They did find that esophageal Pco_2 could be quite high (4.4 to 4.9%) following exhaled gas ventilation with associated inadvertent gastric distention. However, the esophageal Pco_2 dropped to 1 to 1.6% following six ventilations of the stomach. Guggenberger, Lenz, and Federle[81] reported rapid detection by capnography of accidental esophageal intubation in 21 patients during anesthesia.

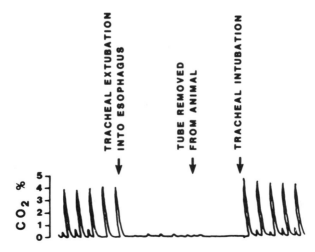

FIG 12–12.
Capnogram using an animal (canine) model, illustrating the difference between tracheal and esophageal intubation. (*From Murray IP, Modell JH: Early detection of endotracheal tube accidents by monitoring carbon dioxide concentration in respiratory care.* Anesthesiol 1983; 59:344–346. Used by permission.)

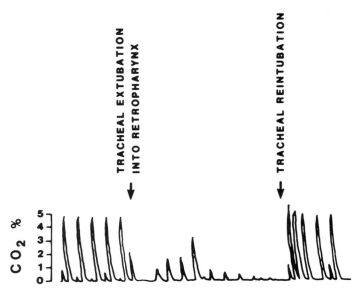

FIG 12–13.
Capnogram using an animal (canine) model, illustrating the effect of movement of the endotracheal tube from the trachea into the pharynx. (*From Murray IP, Modell JH: Early detection of endotracheal tube accidents by monitoring carbon dioxide concentration in respiratory care. Anesthesiol 1983; 59:344–346. Used by permission.*)

Zbinden and Schupfer[82] reported a case in which the capnogram revealed a pattern compatible with tracheal intubation following esophageal intubation for a few breaths in a child who had ingested carbonated beverage before intubation. Garnett, Gervin, and Gervin[83] evaluated the effects of ingested carbonated beverages on esophageal Pco_2. They instilled beer into the stomachs of dogs and compared esophageal Pco_2 to tracheal Pco_2. Ingestion of the carbonated beverage resulted in an increased esophageal Pco_2, but there was a rapid decrease in this following 10 to 15 seconds of gastric ventilation. Thus, high gastric Pco_2's were quickly washed out, allowing $Petco_2$ to be useful in detection of esophageal intubation following ingestion of carbonated beverages.

Owen and Cheney[84] have reported the usefulness of a CO_2 apnea monitor to detect esophageal intubation. This method is qualitative rather than quantitative, in that only the presence or absence of CO_2 is detected. This device offers the advantage of lower cost than capnography, but suffers a significant limitation in that it does not provide either a capnographic waveform or a display of $Petco_2$. Other portable battery-operated CO_2 monitors (e.g., MSA MiniCAP) are also available to confirm endotracheal intubation; these devices are convenient to use outside of the operating room because they are simple to use, they do not require calibration, and they have no warm-up time. Such devices may be particularly useful to prehospital providers in the field.

Simple colorimetric techniques to evaluate the presence of CO_2 in exhaled gas have been available for more than 50 years. In 1919, Marriott[85] described the use of phenolsulphonephthalein, which produced a color change in the presence of CO_2. By collection of alveolar gas, subjecting that gas to the indicator, and comparison with color standards, Marriott was able to determine the concentration of alveolar P_{CO_2}. In 1959, Smith and Volpitto[86] described a barium hydroxide precipitation reaction that could be used to evaluate alveolar CO_2 concentration. In 1984, Berman, Furgiuele, and Marx[87] described the "Einstein carbon dioxide detector," which uses cresol red and phenothalein to produce a color change from red to yellow in the presence of exhaled CO_2. They suggested that this device might be useful to confirm tracheal intubation or to detect esophageal intubation.

A portable nonelectronic disposable device (Fig 12–14) has recently become commercially available to detect esophageal intubation (Easy Cap, Nellcor, Hayward, California, formerly Fenem).[89–99] This device is designed to produce a color change (colorimetric end-tidal CO_2 detection) in the presence of exhaled CO_2, and bench evaluation has indicated that it produces appropriate color changes over a wide range of P_{CO_2}s and ventilatory patterns.[94] In a study of 62 intubations in anesthetized patients, Goldberg et al.[95] found that colorimetric end-tidal CO_2 monitoring using the Easy Cap was a safe, reliable, rapid, simple, and portable method for determining endotracheal tube position. In that study, the Easy Cap confirmed tracheal intubation and detected esophageal intubation 100% of the time. Anton et al.[96] evaluated the Easy Cap in 60 hospitalized adult patients undergoing intubation. They found that the sensitivity for detection of tracheal placement was nearly 100% for patients in respiratory failure, but was not as good for patients in cardiac arrest. MacLeod et al.[97] evaluated the use of the Easy Cap during 250 emergency intubations. In that study, it was found that the sensitivity was greater for tracheal intubation in nonarrested patients (100%) than arrested patients (72%), but that the specificity was greater in arrested patients (100%) than nonarrested patients (86%). Others have found that the Easy Cap is less reliable in the detection of esophageal intubation in cardiac arrested patients.[100–102] The Easy Cap may be useful to confirm tracheal intubation; however, its use is less reliable in cardiac arrest. Use of the Easy Cap during intrahospital transport of mechanically ventilated patients has also been described and may be useful to detect ventilator disconnect and airway misplacement in such patients during transport.[103] The Easy Cap can only be used short term; it becomes ineffective in the presence of humidity (in the patient's exhaled gas), as well as pulmonary edema fluid and endotracheal-administered epinephrine and other drugs (if they contaminate the device).

Several limitations of the use of P_{ETCO_2} to detect esophageal intubation must be recognized. First, significant levels of CO_2 can be present in the stomach following exhaled gas ventilation or ingestion of carbonated beverage. However, this CO_2 is quickly cleared with esophageal ventilation.[83] Second, exhaled CO_2 from the lung can be very low in the presence of low pulmonary perfusion. Thus, monitoring of P_{ETCO_2} to detect esophageal intubation may be of limited usefulness in the presence of cardiac arrest. However, it has been shown in dogs that P_{ETCO_2} is useful in the detection of esophageal intubation even in the presence of cardiac arrest.[104] Finally, capnography cannot be used to confirm endotracheal tube placement if exhaled gas ventilation is being performed.

Generally, capnography does not guarantee that the endotracheal tube is not in a mainstem

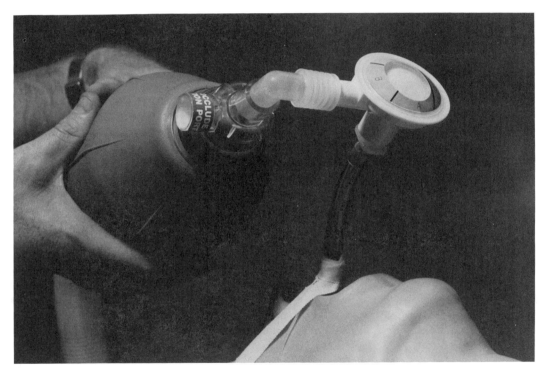

FIG 12–14.
Disposable device (Fenem) to detect esophageal intubation. (*From Hess D: Capnometry and capnography: Tecnnical aspects, physiologic aspects, and clinical applications.* Respir Care *1990; 35:557–576. Used by permission.*)

bronchus. However, Gandhi et al.[105] reported a case in which $Petco_2$ decreased from 28 to 22 mm Hg following movement of the endotracheal tube from the trachea into the right mainstem bronchus in an anesthetized patient. This effect was then duplicated in a canine model. These authors attributed this effect to an increase in V/Q of the ventilated lung, resulting in a decrease in $Petco_2$. Further work is needed to determine the usefulness of capnography to detect mainstem intubation in critically ill patients.

Capnography During Cardiac Arrest

It has been known for many years that decreased pulmonary blood flow (i.e., cardiac output) results in decreased $Petco_2$.[106, 107] Many animal and clinical studies have evaluated the ability of $Petco_2$ to monitor pulmonary blood flow during resuscitation. Because $Petco_2$ is determined by V/Q, if V is held constant, then changes in Q will be reflected by changes in $Petco_2$.

Porcine,[108–110] canine,[111, 112] and sheep[113] models of cardiac arrest have suggested that $Petco_2$ is useful in the evaluation of the effectiveness of cardiopulmonary resuscitation. Typically, the onset of cardiac arrest results in a drop of $Petco_2$ to zero. With the initiation of CPR, there is an increase in $Petco_2$. $Petco_2$ correlates with cardiac output (i.e., pulmonary blood flow) during CPR,[108] as well as coronary perfusion pressure (aortic pressure minus right atrial pressure).[109]

One of the exciting results of animal studies on the use of $Petco_2$ during CPR is the reported usefulness of $Petco_2$ as a prognosticator of resuscitability.[110] Animals who are successfully resuscitated typically have a higher $Petco_2$ during resuscitation. Thus, a very low $Petco_2$ during CPR is unlikely to be associated with a positive outcome.

There have also been reports of the usefulness of $Petco_2$ during resuscitation of humans.[114–124] Kalenda[114] observed that $Petco_2$ decreased when a resuscitator became fatigued, and that $Petco_2$ increased when resuscitation was continued with another resuscitator. Garnett et al.[115] evaluated $Petco_2$ in 23 patients following cardiac arrest, and found that $Petco_2$ increased immediately in patients who had a return of spontaneous circulation. Similar results were reported by Falk, Rackow, and Weil[116] in an evaluation of 13 episodes of cardiac arrest in 10 patients. Sanders et al.[117] found that $Petco_2$ during CPR was useful in the identification of patients likely to be resuscitated. In that study, patients who were resuscitated had a $Petco_2$ of 15 ± 4 mm Hg during resuscitation, but patients who were not resuscitated had a $Petco_2$ of only 7 ± 5 mm Hg. Similar findings have been reported by Callaham and Barton.[122, 123] They found that an initial $Petco_2$ of 15 mm Hg during resuscitation correctly identified 71% of the patients who were successfully resuscitated, with a specificity of 98%. Colorimetric end-tidal CO_2 monitoring may also be useful to evaluate pulmonary blood flow during resuscitation,[96, 100, 102] but more work is needed in this area.

If bicarbonate is adminstered during CPR, this may affect the usefulness of $Petco_2$ as an indicator of pulmonary blood flow, because it will result in an increase in $Petco_2$ independent of pulmonary blood flow. Although it is premature to recommend the routine use of capnography during resuscitation, the use of $Petco_2$ as a real-time objective indicator of the effectiveness of resuscitation is promising.

Capnography in Head-Injured Patients

Iatrogenic hyperventilation is commonly used to induce cerebral vasoconstriction in patients with severe head injury. MacKersie and Karagianes[125] evaluated the use of Petco$_2$ monitoring in 36 head-injured patients. They found very good correlation between Petco$_2$ and Paco$_2$ ($r = 0.95$). Because many head-injured patients are young and free of lung disease (at least early in their hospital courses), Petco$_2$ may be useful to monitor Paco$_2$. However, Petco$_2$ may not be a very good predictor of Paco$_2$ in these patients if previous lung disease is present, if the patient has acute lung injury or adult respiratory distress syndrome (ARDS), or if pulmonary blood flow if reduced secondary to hypotension or pulmonary embolism.

Capnography with Increased Dead-Space Ventilation

Several studies have evaluated the relationship between the Paco$_2$–Petco$_2$ gradient and Vd/Vt.[49, 52, 126–130] Fletcher et al.[127] have found that patients with increased alveolar dead-space ventilation has an increased slope of the alveolar plateau on the capnogram. Yamanaka and Sue[128] have shown that the Paco$_2$–Petco$_2$ gradient correlated closely with Vd/Vt ($r = 0.80$). This is similar to data reported by Poppius, Korhonen, and Kreus,[129] who also found that the Paco$_2$–Petco$_2$ gradient correlated well with Vd/Vt ($r = 0.74$). Bermudez and Lichtiger[130] found an increased Paco$_2$–Petco$_2$ following cardiopulmonary bypass; they attributed this to an increase in dead-space ventilation.

Several studies have found that occlusion of branches of the pulmonary circulation resulted in a decrease in Petco$_2$ compared to Paco$_2$. This has been reported in experimental studies in dogs,[131] in children during heart surgery,[132] and in children during the repair of congenital cardiac defects.[133]

Since the late 1950s, there has been interest in the use of capnography to detect acute pulmonary embolism.[134–139] Unfortunately, this use for capnography seems to be more sensitive than specific. In a comparison of capnography to angiography in the diagnosis of pulmonary embolism in 44 adult patients with COPD, Chopin et al.[138] reported a sensitivity of 100%, but a specificity of only 65% (i.e., a false-positive rate of 35%); although the negative predictive value was 100%, the positive predictive value was only 74%. The Paco$_2$–Petco$_2$ gradient is usually increased when pulmonary embolism is present, but the gradient is also increased for a variety of other causes when pulmonary embolism is not present (i.e., any dead-space-producing disease). Although capnography, with other diagnostic criteria, may be useful in the diagnosis of pulmonary embolism, the Petco$_2$ by itself is of limited usefulness in the diagnosis of pulmonary embolism. A normal Paco$_2$–Petco$_2$, however, is unlikely if significant pulmonary embolism is present. Hatle and Rokseth[136] found that the Paco$_2$–Petco$_2$ gradient measured at forced exhalation was more useful in the evaluation of acute pulmonary embolism. Eriksson et al.[137] extrapolated phase III of the capnogram to determine the Pco$_2$ at 15% of the predicted total lung capacity, and found that this was useful in the diagnosis of pulmonary embolism. With maximal exhalation, the gradient approached zero in patients with obstructive lung disease, but remained high in patients with pulmonary embolism. In a canine model, Byrick, Kay, and Mullen[139] found that monitoring of pulmonary artery pressure was more sensitive than capnography in the detection of fat and marrow embolism.

Capnography in Infants and Children

Due to their smaller tidal volumes and more rapid respiratory rates, monitoring of Petco$_2$ is more difficult in infants and children than adults. This causes difficulty in producing a valid capnogram and in the identification of the Petco$_2$. There has also been less interest in capnography in infants and children because transcutaneous Pco$_2$ is commonly monitored in this patient population.

Epstein et al[140] evaluated peak-expired CO$_2$ in 24 mechanically ventilated neonates, and found that expired CO$_2$ consistently underestimated Paco$_2$ (mean 7.5 mm Hg). Further, they found that the airway adaptor used to measure CO$_2$ led to CO$_2$ retention in half of the patients. Watkins and Weindling[141] evaluated end-tidal Pco$_2$ in 19 infants with respiratory disease, and found poor correlation between Paco$_2$ and Petco$_2$ ($r = 0.388$). They concluded that capnography might only be useful in infants with normal lung function. Hand et al.[142] evaluated Petco$_2$ in 12 infants and concluded that this monitor was not useful because it severely underestimated Paco$_2$ in the most severely ill infants. McEvedy et al.[143] found that Petco$_2$ measured from the distal endotracheal tube was significantly greater than proximal Petco$_2$ in 27 intubated neonates, and they found distal Petco$_2$ useful in neonates with mild to moderate lung disease, but not in those with severe lung disease.

Others have found capnography useful in infants and children. Using a rabbit model, Evans, Hogg, and Rosen[144] concluded that Petco$_2$ is a good estimate of Paco$_2$ at respiratory rates of 10 to 100/min. Lindahl, Yates, and Hatch[145] reported a high correlation between Petco$_2$ and Paco$_2$ in normal children ($r = 0.94$) and children with acyanotic congenital heart disease ($r = 0.98$). Meny, Bhat, and Aranas[146] reported moderate correlation between Paco$_2$ and Petco$_2$ ($r = 0.69$), and found that the Paco$_2$–Petco$_2$ gradient was greater for patients with severe disease than those with moderate disease. Nelson et al[147] found a mean Paco$_2$–Petco$_2$ gradient of 1.7 mm Hg in infants, and Valentin, Lomholt, and Thorup[148] reported a median Paco$_2$–Petco$_2$ gradient of 5 mm Hg (range -4 to 13 mm Hg) in children during halothane anesthesia. Fletcher[149] found that monitoring of Petco$_2$ was useful during anesthesia in children with cardiac disease if significant right to left shunting was not present. Burrows[150] found that Vd/Vt was a primary determinant of Paco$_2$–Petco$_2$ in infants and children undergoing cardiac surgery. Cote et al.[151] found CO$_2$ monitoring to be useful in the diagnosis of intraoperative events such as malignant hyperthermia, circuit disconnection or leak, equipment failure, accidental extubation, endobronchial intubation, or kinked entotracheal tube. Dumbit and Brady[152] used a nostril catheter to measure Petco$_2$ in spontaneously breathing infants, and found a mean Paco$_2$–Petco$_2$ gradient of 2.4 mm Hg in normal term infants, 3.5 mm Hg in preterm infants who had recovered from respiratory distress syndrome, and 9 mm Hg in infants with bronchopulmonary dysplasia; they concluded that measurements of Petco$_2$ in infants was useful.

There is some controversy regarding the use of sidestream versus mainstream capnography with infants and the appropriate flow to be used if a sidestream monitor is used.[153–161] Using a mainstream monitor, Meredith and Monoco[158] found Petco$_2$ monitoring useful in preterm and term infants. Pascucci, Schena, and Thompson[153] compared the use of sidestream and mainstream monitors in infants and concluded that the mainstream device produced a more accurate representation of the expired CO$_2$ waveform. However, they used a flow of 50 mL/min with the sidestream monitor. Others have shown that this flow may be too slow.[154–156] As shown by Gravenstein,[156] at a flow of 50 mL/min, the $Petco_2$ is artifactually low, the waveform is rounded, and inspired CO_2 is artifactually displayed. These artifacts can be eliminated by increasing the flow to 150 mL/min or greater. Using a rabbit model, Evans, Hogg, and Rosen[144] suggested that a flow of 300 mL/min be used during capnography in neonates. Badgwell et al.[157] found that $Petco_2$ measurements were more accurate in children weighing less than 12 kg if gas was sampled from the distal endotracheal tube rather than the proximal endotracheal tube. However, they found no difference in the accuracy of $Petco_2$ measures between the proximal and distal ends of the endotracheal tube in children weighing more that 12 kg. This may be the result of the continuous flow past the endotracheal tube that occurs in neonatal ventilator circuits, and differences between proximal and distal $Petco_2$ may be minimized if care is taken to prevent contamination of the sample with fresh gas flow.[162–164]

The usefulness of capnography in infants and children has not been clearly established. Much work remains to be done to establish the appropriate role of capnography in neonatal and pediatric respiratory care, as well as appropriate systems for this monitoring (mainstream versus sidestream, proximal versus distal).

Capnography During Spontaneous Ventilation

Capnography is most often used with intubation and mechanical ventilation. However, techniques to measure $Petco_2$ during spontaneous breathing have been described.[165–177] Bowe et al.[164] described the construction of a modified nasal cannula for capnography (Fig 12–15) and evaluated its use in 21 patients. They found $Paco_2$–$Petco_2$ gradients using the modified cannula that were similar to those following intubation. McNulty et al.[176] sampled $Petco_2$ from a 16-gauge intravenous catheter pierced through one of the prongs of a nasal cannula. They found that $Petco_2$ most closely approximated $Paco_2$ when optimal waveforms were selected for analysis; although the bias between $Paco_2$ and $Petco_2$ was nearly zero, there were relatively wide limits of agreement ($\pm$ 6 to 8 mm Hg). Capnography using a mouthpiece has also been described,[165] but this method is virtually impossible to use for continuous monitoring. When a capnograph is used with a nasal cannula, it is important that the sample is not contaminated with room air or oxygen flow. Such contamination will result in significant underestimation of $Petco_2$. Capnography is technically difficult in nonintubated patients, and further work is needed to determine which patient populations might benefit from this monitoring.

The use of capnography during exercise has also been described.[58, 59, 178] Jones et al.[59] developed a regression equation to predict $Paco_2$ from $Petco_2$ during exercise. Chambers et al.[178] found that measurement of $Petco_2$ during ECG stress testing provided objective data to support a clinical suspicion of chest pain induced by hyperventilation; they found a greater incidence of hypocapnia during exercise testing in patients with nonischemic chest pain than in patients with ischemia and control subjects.

Capnography During Weaning from Mechanical Ventilation

It can be difficult to predict which patients can be successfully weaned from mechanical ventilation. The success of weaning is often judged by clinical findings (e.g., respiratory rate and effort, cardiac status, neurologic status) and the patient's ability to maintain adequate

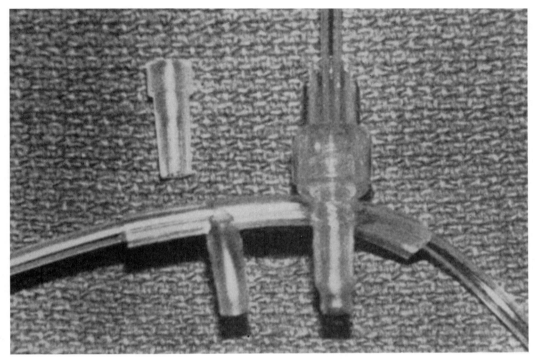

FIG 12–15.
Modified nasal cannula for capnography during spontaneous breathing. Syringe cap with tip removed (*left*); cannula is modified by insertion of syringe cap, and attachment of sampling line. (*From Bowe EA, Boysen PG, Broome JA, et al: Accurate determination of end-tidal carbon dioxide during administration of oxygen by nasal cannula. J Clin Monit 1989; 5:105–110. Used by permission.*)

arterial blood gases. Because capnography is noninvasive and continuous, its use to evaluate the adequacy of ventilation during weaning is attractive. It is also interesting that one study suggested that a $Paco_2$–$Petco_2$ of less than 8 mm Hg may be useful to predict patients who may be successfully weaned from the ventilator.[179]

Healey et al.[180] evaluated the usefulness of $Petco_2$ monitoring during the weaning of 10 postoperative patients, and found that changes in $Petco_2$ correlated well with changes in $Paco_2$ ($r = 0.82$). However, the change in $Petco_2$ incorrectly predicted the change in $Paco_2$ in 25% of the cases in that study. Niehoff et al.[181] found that patients monitored with capnography and pulse oximetry required fewer blood gases during weaning. They also found that capnography was insensitive to hypercarbia ($Paco_2 > 45$ mm Hg), and the $Paco_2$ was >60 mm Hg when the $Petco_2$ was <40 mm Hg in some patients in that study. Withington et al.[182] found that $Petco_2$ predicted $Paco_2$ to within ±2 mm Hg in 89% of readings, and it had a sensitivity of 78.6% for the detection of hypercarbia ($Paco_2 > 45$ mm Hg). Thrush, Wayne, and Downs[183] found that continuous monitoring of $Petco_2$ was useful during weaning of patients from ventilatory support after cardiac surgery. Hess et al.[184] also evaluated the use of capnography during weaning of postcardiac surgery patients. They reported a moderate correlation between

Petco$_2$ and Paco$_2$ during weaning ($r = 0.82$). Although Hess et al. found no statistically significant difference between the changes in Petco$_2$ and Paco$_2$ ($P = 0.63$), the change in Petco$_2$ incorrectly predicted the direction of change in Paco$_2$ in 43% of cases.

Weinger and Brimm[185] found considerable variation in Petco$_2$ during the weaning of postcardiotomy patients. During weaning with intermittent mandatory ventilation (IMV), they found that the Petco$_2$ following spontaneous breaths was often greater than that following ventilator breaths. After comparing several ways to deal with this variability, they concluded that the maximal Petco$_2$ independent of breathing pattern, provides a clinically useful indicator of Paco$_2$ during weaning with IMV. Smith, Novak, and Venus[186] found that Petco$_2$ was breathing-pattern dependent, but remained consistent for mechanical and for spontaneous breaths during weaning from mechanical ventilation using SIMV. They recommended that the breath-specific or maximum Petco$_2$ be used to calculate the Paco$_2$–Petco$_2$ gradient at the start of weaning, and then be used as the reference for estimating Paco$_2$.

Capnography to Determine PEEP Levels

Positive end-expiratory pressure (PEEP) is commonly used in the care of patients with acute respiratory failure. "Best" or "optimal" PEEP may be difficult to determine clinically, and requires the use of a pulmonary artery catheter to measure cardiac output and Qs/Qt. Murray et al.[187] used a canine model to evaluate use of the Paco$_2$–Petco$_2$ gradient to determine appropriate PEEP levels. They found that the Paco$_2$–Petco$_2$ gradient was a sensitive indicator of the appropriate amount of PEEP. Generally, they found that the Paco$_2$–Petco$_2$ was the lowest at the appropriate level of PEEP; in other words, the lowest Paco$_2$–Petco$_2$ corresponded to the best V/Q.

Unfortunately, others have not been able to replicate the work of Murray et al. in patients. Jardin et al.[188] studied 11 patients in acute respiratory failure and found no difference between the Paco$_2$–Petco$_2$ gradients in patients on zero PEEP, "best" PEEP, or excessive PEEP. Blanch et al.[189] found the Paco$_2$–Petco$_2$ gradient useful in patients with acute respiratory failure, but only if an initial inflection point was present on the pressure-volume curve. Clinically, this is of limited usefulness because most critical care units are not equipped to measure pressure-volume curves. At present, the use of the Paco$_2$–Petco$_2$ gradient to determine appropriate PEEP levels in critically ill patients has not been clearly established.

SUMMARY

In patients who have a stable hemodynamic status, Petco$_2$ may be useful to track changes in Paco$_2$. This might be useful, for example, in patients with head injury whose intracranial pressure is sensitive to changes in Paco$_2$. In patients with unstable hemodynamics, capnography may be useful to monitor changes in pulmonary blood flow. Following a difficult intubation, capnography may be useful to determine endotracheal tube placement. However, there are many areas related to capnography in which further work is necessary. These include areas such as neonatal and pediatric respiratory care, cardiac arrest, and determination of "best"

PEEP. More work is also needed to determine appropriate means to measure $Petco_2$ in nonintubated patients.

Perhaps the most important thing to recognize about $Petco_2$ is that it is *NOT* $Paco_2$. When capnography is used, it is most important that those responsible for its use appreciate the physiologic as well as technologic basis for capnography, and recognize that capnography is *not* a noninvasive monitor of $Paco_2$ *per se*. Assuming that $Petco_2$ is similar to $Paco_2$ will deceive those caring for the patient and could result in mismanagement of the patient's care. Capnography is not indicated for every intubated or mechanically ventilated patient. The challenge to clinicians is to determine objectively when this monitor is indicated in the care of patients.

REFERENCES

1. Hess D: An overview of noninvasive monitoring in respiratory care: Present, past, and future. *Respir Care* 1990; 35:482–499.
2. Eichorn JH, Cooper JB, Cullen DJ, et al: Standards for patient monitoring during anesthesia at Harvard Medical School. *JAMA* 1986; 256:1017–1020.
3. Choi HJ: End-tidal PCO2: Should it be a standard of care in obstetric anesthesia? (letter). *Anesthesiol* 1986; 64:829–830.
4. Swedlow DB: Capnometry and capnography: The anesthesia disaster early warning system. *Seminars in Anesthesia* 1986; 5:194–205.
5. Gravenstein JS, Paulus DA, Hayes TJ: *Capnography in Clinical Practice*. Boston, Butterworths, 1989.
6. Hess D: Capnometry and capnography: Technical aspects, physiologic aspects, and clinical applications. *Respir Care* 1990; 35:557–576.
7. Paulus DA: Capnography. *Intern Anesthesiol Clin* 1989; 27:167–175.
8. Stock MC: Noninvasive carbon dioxide monitoring. *Crit Care Clin* 1988; 4:511–526.
9. Weingarten M: Respiratory monitoring of carbon dioxide and oxygen: A ten year perspective. *J Clin Monit* 1990; 6:217–225.
10. Mogue LR, Rantala B: Capnometers. *J Clin Monit* 1988; 4:115–121.
11. Paloheimo MPJ: A carbon dioxide monitor that does not show the waveform has value. *J Clin Monit* 1988; 4:210–212.
12. Block FE: A carbon dioxide monitor that does not show the waveform is worthless. *J Clin Monit* 1988; 4:213–214.
13. Schena J, Thompson J, Crone RK: Mechanical influences on the capnogram. *Crit Care Med* 1984; 12:672–674.
14. Gravenstein N, Lampotang S, Beneken JEW: Factors influencing capnography in the Bain circuit. *J Clin Monit* 1985; 1:6–10.
15. Epstein RA, Reznik AM, Epstein MAF: Determinants of distortions in CO2 catheter sampling systems: A mathematical model. *Respir Physiol* 1980; 41:127–136.
16. From RP, Scamman FL: Ventilatory frequency influences accuracy of end-tidal CO2 measurements. Analysis of seven capnometers. *Anesth Analg* 1988; 67:884–886.
17. van Genderingen HR, Gravenstein N: Capnogram artifact during high airway pressures caused by a water trap. *Anesth Analg* 1987; 66:185–187.
18. Lerou JGC, van Egmond J, Kolmer HHB: The influence of tube geometry on the performance of long sampling tubes in respiratory mass spectrometry. *Clin Phys Physiol Meas* 1986; 7:125–137.

19. Doyle DJ: Time constant related distortion in side-stream capnography (abstract). *Can J Aenesth* 1990; 37:S70.

20. Lawson D, Jelenich S: Capnographs: A new operating room pollution hazard? (letter) *Anesth Analg* 1985; 64:377–382.

21. Cozanitis DA, Paloheimo MPJ: Operating room pollution from "capnographs" (letter). *Anesth Analg* 1986; 65:990–991.

22. Zupan J, Martin M, Benumof JL: End-tidal CO2 excretion waveform and error with gas sampling line leak. *Anesth Analg* 1988; 67:579–581.

23. Koebert RF, Munster R: One-way leak in mass spectrometer sampling system (letter). *Anesthesiol* 1987; 67:606–607.

24. Nelson LD, Safesak K: Sidestream vs. in-line sensing for capnography in adult surgical patients (abstract). *Chest* 1990; 98:114S.

25. Collier CR, Affeldt JE, Farr AF: Continuous rapid infrared CO2 analysis. *J Lab Clin Med* 1955; 45:526–539.

26. Severinghaus JW, Larson CP, Eger EI: Correction factors for infrared carbon dioxide pressure broadening by nitrogen, nitrous oxide and cyclopropane. *Anesthesiol* 1961; 22:429–432.

27. Ammann ECB, Galvin RD: Problems associated with the determination of carbon dioxide by infared absorption. *J Appl Physiol* 1968; 25:333–335.

28. Cormack RS, Powell JN: Improving the performance of the infra-red carbon dioxide meter. *Brit J Anaesth* 1972; 44:131–141.

29. Kennell EM, Andrews RW, Wollman H: Correction factors for nitrous oxide in the infrared analysis of carbon dioxide. *Anesthesiol* 1973; 39:441–443.

30. Capnometers. ASTM Standard F-20.03.11 (draft). Philadelphia, ASTM, 1989.

31. Olsson SG, Fletcher R, Jonson B, et al: Clinical studies of gas exchange during ventilatory support—A method using the Siemens-Elema CO2 analyzer. *Br J Anaesth* 1980; 52:491–499.

32. Fletcher R, Werner O, Nordstrom L, et al: Sources of error and their correction in the measurement of carbon dioxide elimination using the Siemens-Elema CO2 analyzer. *Br J Anaesth* 1983; 55:177–185.

33. Carbon dioxide monitors. *Health Dev* 1986; 15:255–284.

34. End-tidal carbon dioxide measurement in emergency medicine and patient transport. *Health Dev* 1991; 20:35–54.

35. Hicks GH, Haynes G, Boyd T, et al: The comparative accuracy of four infrared PetCO2 analyzers (abstract). *Respir Care* 1988; 33:951–952.

36. Seaman FL, from RP: High frequency response of six capnometers (abstract). *Anesthesiol* 1989; 71:A360.

37. Selby DG, Ilsey AH, Runciman WB: An evaluation of five carbon dioxide analyzers for use in the operating theatre and intensive care unit. *Anesth Intens Care* 1987; 15:212–216.

38. Severinghaus JW: Water vapor calibration errors in some capnometers: Respiratory conversions misunderstood by manufacturers? *Anesthesiol* 1989; 70:996–998.

39. Fowler KT, Hugh-Jones P: Mass spectrometry applied to clinical practice and research. *Br Med J* 1957; 1;1205–1211.

40. McAslan TC: Automated respiratory gas monitoring of critically injured patients. *Crit Care Med* 1976; 4:255–260.

41. Ayres SM: Use of mass spectrometry for evaluation of respiratory function in the critically ill patient. *Crit Care Med* 1976; 4:219–222.

42. Riker JB, Haberman B: Expired gas monitoring by mass spectrometry in a respiratory intensive care unit. *Crit Care Med* 1976; 4:223–229.

43. Yakulis R, Snyder JV, Powner D, et al: Mass spectrometry monitoring of respiratory variables in an intensive care unit. *Respir Care* 1978; 23:671–679.

44. Ozanne GM, Young WG, Mazzei WJ, et al: Multipatient anesthetic mass spectrometry: Rapid analysis of data stored in long catheters. *Anesthesiol* 1981; 55:62–70.
45. Grevisse P, Delcambre Y, Picart P, et al: Turning the mass-spectrometer into an easy to handle clinical instrument for routine multipatient surveillance of respiratory and anesthetic gases during anesthesia. *Acta Anaesth Belg* 1987; 38:37–44.
46. Blank ST, King P, Smith BE: Anesthesia gas monitoring: Central system or stand-alone? *Med Instrum* 1988; 22:155–160.
47. Patel AJ, Choi C, Giuffrida JG: Changes in end tidal CO2 and arterial blood gas levels after release of tourniquet. *S Med J* 1987; 80:214–216.
48. Baudendistel L, Goudsouzian N, Cote C, et al: End-tidal CO2 monitoring. Its use in the diagnosis and management of malignant hyperthermia. *Anesthesia* 1984; 39:1000–1003.
49. Stockwell MA, Bruce W, Soni N: The influence of CO2 production and physiological deadspace on end-tidal CO2 during controlled ventilation: A study using a mechanical model. *Anaesth Intens Care* 1989; 17:482–486.
50. Food and Drug Administration. Recommendations for increasing early detection of accidental disconnections. Proposal under review by the U.S. Food and Drug Administration.
51. Cooper JB, Couvillown LA: *Accidental Breathing Disconnections.* HHS Publications, FDA 86-4205 (1985).
52. Levins FA, Francis RI, Burnley SR: Failure to detect disconnection by capnography (letter). *Anaesthesia* 1989; 44:79.
53. Tulou PP, Walsh PM: Measurement of alveolar carbon dioxide tension at maximal expiration as an estimate of arterial carbon dioxide tension in patients with airway obstruction. *Am Rev Respir Dis* 1970; 102:921–926.
54. Moorthy SS, Losasso AM, Wilcox J: End-tidal PCO2 greater than PaCO2. *Crit Care Med* 1984; 12:534–535.
55. Shankar KB, Moseley H, Kumar Y: Arterial to end tidal carbon dioxide tension differences during caesarean section anesthesia. *Anesthesia* 1986; 41:678–702.
56. Piiper J: Blood-gas equilibrium of carbon dioxide in lungs: A continuing controversy. *J Appl Physiol* 1986; 60:1–8.
57. Fletcher R, Jonson B: Deadspace and the single breath test for carbon dioxide during anesthesia and artificial ventilation. Effects of tidal volume and frequency of respiration. *Br J Anaesth* 1984; 56:109–119.
58. Jones NL, McHardy JR, Naimark A, et al: Physiological dead space and alveolar-arterial gas pressure differences during exercise. *Clin Sci* 1966; 31:19–29.
59. Jones NL, Robertson DG, Kane JW: Difference between end-tidal and arterial PCO2 in exercise. *J Appl Physiol* 1979; 47:954–960.
60. Donati F, Maille J, Blain R, et al: End-tidal carbon dioxide tension and temperature changes after coronary artery bypass surgery. *Can Anaesth Soc J* 1985; 32:272–277.
61. Phan CQ, Tremper KK, Lee SE, et al: Noninvasive monitoring of carbon dioxide: A comparison of the partial pressure of transcutaneous and end-tidal carbon dioxide with the partial pressure of arterial carbon dioxide. *J Clin Monit* 1987; 3:149–154.
62. Whitesell R, Asiddao C, Gollman D, et al: Relationship between arterial and peak expired carbon dioxide pressure during anaesthesia and factors influencing the difference. *Anesth Analg* 1981; 60:508–512.
63. Nunn JF, Hill DW: Respiratory dead space and arterial to end-tidal CO2 tension difference in anesthetized man. *J Appl Physiol* 1960; 15:383–389.
64. Russell GB, Graybeal JM, Strout JC: Stability of arterial to end-tidal carbon dioxide gradients during postoperative cardiorespiratory support. *Can J Anaesth* 1990; 37:560–566.

65. Hoffman R, Kreiger BP, Kramer MR, et al: End-tidal carbon dioxide in critically ill patients during changes in mechanical ventilation. *Am Rev Respir Dis* 1989; 140:1265–1268.

66. Hess D, Agarwal NN: Variability of blood gases, pulse oximetry saturation, and end-tidal carbon dioxide pressure in stable, mechanically ventilated patients. *J Clin Monit* 1992; 8:111–115.

67. Das JB, Joshi ID, Philippart Al: End-tidal CO_2 and tissue pH in the monitoring of acid-base changes: A composite technique for continuous, minimally invasive monitoring. *J Ped Surg* 1984; 19:758–763.

68. Takki S, Aromaa U, Kauste A: The validity and usefulness of the end-tidal PCO_2 during anesthesia. *Ann Clin Res* 1972; 4:278–284.

69. Perrin F, Perrot D, Holzapfel L, et al: Simultaneous variations of $PaCO_2$ and $PACO_2$ in assisted ventilation. *Br J Anaesth* 1983; 55:525–530.

70. Raemer DB, Francis D, Philip JH, et al: Variation in PCO_2 between arterial blood and peak expired gas during anesthesia. *Anesth Analg* 1983; 62:1065–1069.

71. Kalenda Z: Capnography during anesthesia and intensive care. *Acta Anaesth Belg* 1978; 29:201–228.

72. Carlon GC, Ray C, Miodownik S, et al: Capnography in mechanically ventilated patients. *Crit Care Med* 1988; 16:550–556.

73. Smalhout B, Kalenda Z: *Atlas of Capnography.* The Netherlands, Kerckebosch-Zeist, 1975, Vol 1.

74. Watson R, Benumof J, Clausen J, et al: Expiratory CO_2 plateau slope predicts airway resistance (abstract). *Anesthesiol* 1989; 71:A1072.

75. Fowler KT, Read J: Cardiac oscillations in expired gas tensions, and regional pulmonary blood flow. *J Appl Physiol* 1961; 16:863–868.

76. Miller DM: Early detection of "rebreathing" in afferent and efferent reservoir breathing systems using capnography. *Br J Anaesth* 1990; 64:251–255.

77. Birmingham PK, Cheney FW, Ward RJ: Esophageal intubation: A review of detection of techniques. *Anesth Analg* 1986; 65:886–891.

78. Conrardy PA, Goodman LR, Lainge F, et al: Alteration of endotracheal tube position. Flexation and extension of the neck. *Crit Care Med* 1976; 4:7–12.

79. Murray IP, Modell JH: Early detection of endotracheal tube accidents by monitoring carbon dioxide concentration in respiratory care. *Anesthesiol* 1983; 59:344–346.

80. Linko K, Paloheimo M, Tammisto T: Capnography for detection of accidental oesophageal intubation. *Acta Anaesthiol Scand* 1983; 27:199–202.

81. Guggenberger H, Lenz G, Federle R: Early detection of inadvertent oesophageal intubation: pulse oximetry vs. capnography. *Acta Anaesthesiol Scand* 1989; 33:112–115.

82. Zbinden S, Schupfer G: Detection of oesophageal intubation: The cola complication (letter). *Anesthesia* 1989; 44:81.

83. Garnett AR, Gervin CA, Gervin AS: Capnographic waveforms in esophageal intubation: Effect of carbonated beverages. *Ann Emerg Med* 1989; 18:387–390.

84. Owen RL, Cheney FW: Use of an apnea monitor to verify endotracheal intubation. *Respir Care* 1985; 30:974–976.

85. Marriott WM: The determination of alveolar carbon dioxide tension by a simple method. *JAMA* 1916; 66:1594–1596.

86. Smith RH, Volpitto PP: Simple method of determining CO_2 content of alveolar air (letter). *Anesthesiol* 1959; 20:702–703.

87. Berman JA, Furgiuele JJ, Marx GF: The Einstein carbon dioxide detector (letter). *Anesthesiol* 1984; 60:613–614.

88. Jones BR, Dorsey MJ: Disposable end-tidal CO_2 detector: Minimal CO_2 requirements (abstract). *Anesthesiol* 1989; 71:A359.

89. Feinstein R, White PF, Westerfield SZ: Intraoperative evaluation of a disposable end-tidal CO_2 detector (abstract). *Anesthesiol* 1989; 71:A461.

90. Strunin L, Williams T: The FEF end-tidal carbon dioxide detector (letter). *Anesthesiol* 1989; 71:621–622.

91. King H, Wooten DJ: Blind nasal intubation by monitoring end-tidal CO2 (letter). *Anesth Analg* 1989; 69:412–413.

92. Gerald J, MacLeod BA, Heller MB, et al: Verification of endotracheal intubation using a disposable end-tidal CO2 detector (abstract). *Prehospital Disaster Med* 1989; 4:74.

93. O'Callaghan JP, Williams RT: Confirmation of tracheal intubation using a chemical device (abstract). *Can J Anaesth* 1988; 35:S59.

94. Hess D, Ruppert T, McClure S: A bench evaluation of the FEF end-tidal CO detector (abstract). *Respir Care* 1989; 34:1047–1048.

95. Goldberg JS, Rawle PR, Zehnder JL, et al: Colorimetric end-tidal carbon dioxide monitoring for tracheal intubation. *Anesth Analg* 1990; 70:191–194.

96. Anton WR, Gordon RW, Jordan TM, et al: A disposable end-tidal CO2 detector to verify endotracheal intubation. *Ann Emerg Med* 1991; 20:271–275.

97. MacLeod BA, Heller M, Gerard J, et al: Verification of endotracheal tube placement with colorimetric end-tidal CO2 detection. *Ann Emerg Med* 1991; 20:267–270.

98. O'Flaherty D, Adams AP: The end-tidal carbon dioxide detector. *Anaesthesia* 1990; 45:653–655.

99. Denman WT, Hayes M, Higgins D, et al: The Fenem CO2 detector device. An apparatus to prevent unnoticed oesophageal intubation. *Anaesthesia* 1990; 45:465–467.

100. Varon AJ, Morrina J, Civetta JM: Use of colorimetric end-tidal carbon dioxide monitoring to prognosticate immediate resuscitation from cardiac arrest (abstract). *Anesthesiol* 1990; 73:A412.

101. Varon AJ, Morrina J, Civetta JM: Clinical utility of a colorimetric end-tidal carbon dioxide detector in emergency intubation (abstract). *Anesthesiol* 1990; 73:A413.

102. Higgins D, Hayes M, Denman W, et al: Effectiveness of using end tidal carbon dioxide concentration to monitor cardiopulmonary resuscitation. *Br Med J* 1990; 300:581.

103. Daugherty A, Hess D, Simmons M: Evaluation of the Fenem end-tidal CO2 detector during in-hospital patient transport (abstract). *Respir Care* 1991; 35:1116–1117.

104. Sayah AJ, Peacock WF, Overton DT: End-tidal CO2 measurement in the detection of esophageal intubation during cardiac arrest. *Ann Emerg Med* 1990; 19:857–860.

105. Gandi SK, Munshi CA, Coon R, et al: Capnography for detection of endobronchial migration of an endotracheal tube. *J Clin Monit* 1991; 7:35–38.

106. Sealy WC, Ogino S, Lesage AM, et al: Functional and structural changes in the lung in hemorrhagic shock. *Surg Gynecol Obstst* 1966; 122:754–760.

107. Ayres SM, Mueller H, Giannelii S, et al: The lung in shock. Alveolar-capillary gas exchange in the shock syndrome. *Am J Cardiol* 1970; 26:588–594.

108. Weil MH, Bisera J, Trevino RP, et al: Cardiac output and end-tidal carbon dioxide. *Crit Care Med* 1985; 13:907–909.

109. Trevino RP, Bisera J, Weil MH, et al: End-tidal CO2 as a guide to successful cardiopulmonary resuscitation: A preliminary report. *Crit Care Med* 1985; 13:910–911.

110. Gudipati C, Weil MH, Bisera J, et al: Expired carbon dioxide: A noninvasive monitor of cardiopulmonary resuscitation. *Circulation* 1988; 77:234–239.

111. Sanders AB, Atlas M, Ewy GA, et al: Expired PCO2 as an index of coronary perfusion pressure. *Am J Emerg Med* 1985; 3:147–149.

112. Sanders AB, Ewy GA, Bragg S, et al: Expired PCO2 as a prognostic indicator of successful resuscitation from cardiac arrest. *Ann Emerg Med* 1985; 14:948–952.

113. Ornado JP, Garnett AR, Glauser FL: Relationship between cardiac output and the end-tidal carbon dioxide tension. *Ann Emerg Med* 1990; 19:1104–1106.

114. Kalenda Z: The capnogram as a guide to the efficacy of cardiac massage. *Resuscitation* 1978; 6:259–263.

115. Garnett AR, Ornato JP, Gonzalez ER, et al: End-tidal carbon dioxide monitoring during cardiopulmonary resuscitation. *JAMA* 1987; 257:512–515.

116. Falk JL, Rackow EC, Weil MH: End-tidal carbon dioxide concentration during cardiopulmonary resuscitation. *N Engl J Med* 1988; 318:607–611.

117. Sanders AB, Kern KB, Otto CW, et al: End-tidal carbon dioxide monitoring during cardiopulmonary resuscitation. A prognostic indicator for survival. *JAMA* 1989; 262:1347–1351.

118. Ornato JP, Gonzalez ER, Garnett R, et al: Effect of cardiopulmonary resuscitation compression rate on end-tidal carbon dioxide concentration and arterial pressure in man. *Crit Care Med* 1988; 16:241–245.

119. Ornato JP, Levine RL, Young DS, et al: The effect of applied chest compression force of systemic arterial pressure and end-tidal carbon dioxide concentration during CPR in human beings. *Ann Emerg Med* 1989; 18:732–737.

120. Lepilin MG, Vasilyev AV, Bildinov OA, et al: End-tidal carbon dioxide as a noninvasive monitor of circulatory status during cardiopulmonary resuscitation. *Crit Care Med* 1987; 15:958–959.

121. Ward KR, Sullivan RJ, Zelenck RR, et al: A comparison of interposed abdominal compression CPR and standard CPR by monitoring end-tidal PCO2. *Ann Emerg Med* 1989; 18:831–837.

122. Callaham M, Barton C: Prediction of cardiopulmonary resuscitation from end-tidal carbon dioxide concentration. *Crit Care Med* 1990; 18:358–362.

123. Barton C, Callaham M: Lack of correlation between end-tidal carbon dioxide concentrations and PaCO2 in cardiac arrest. *Crit Care Med* 1991; 19:108–110.

124. Steedman DJ, Roberson CE: Measurement of end-tidal carbon dioxide concentration during cardiopulmonary resuscitation. *Arch Emerg Med* 1990; 7:129–134.

125. MacKersie RL, Karagianes TG: Use of end-tidal carbon dioxide tension for monitoring induced hypocapnia in head-injured patients. *Crit Care Med* 1990; 18:764–765.

126. Severinghaus JW, Stupfel MA, Bradley AF: Alveolar dead space and arterial to end-tidal carbon dioxide differences during hypothermia in dog and man. *J Appl Physiol* 1957; 10:349–355.

127. Fletcher R, Jonson B, Cumming G: The concept of deadspace with special reference to the single breath test for carbon dioxide. *Br J Anaesth* 1981; 53:77–88.

128. Yamanaka MK, Sue DY: Comparison of arterial-end-tidal PCO2 difference and dead space/tidal volume ratio in respiratory failure. *Chest* 1987; 92:832–835.

129. Poppius H, Korhonen O, Kreus KE: Arterial to end-tidal CO2 difference in respiratory disease. *Scand J Resp Dis* 1975; 56:254–262.

130. Bermudez J, Lichtiger M. Increases in arterial to end-tidal CO2 tension differences after cardiopulmonary bypass. *Anesth Analg* 1987; 66:690–692.

131. Julian DG, Travis DM, Robin ED, et al: Effect of pulmonary artery occlusion upon end-tidal CO2 tension. *J Appl Physiol* 1960; 15:87–91.

132. Schuller JL, Bovill JG, Nijveld A: End-tidal carbon dioxide concentration as an indicator of pulmonary blood flow during closed heart surgery in children. *Br J Anaesth* 1985; 57:1257–1259.

133. Heneghan CPH, Scallan MJH, Branthwaite MA: End-tidal carbon dioxide during thoracotomy. Its relation to blood level in adults and children. *Anaesthesia* 1981; 36:1017–1021.

134. Robin ED, Julian DG, Travis DM, et al: A physiologic approach to the diagnosis of acute pulmonary embolism. *N Engl J Med* 1959; 260:586–591.

135. Nutter DO, Massumi RA: The arterial-alveolar carbon dioxide tension gradient in diagnosis of pulmonary embolus. *Dis Chest* 1966; 50:380–387.

136. Hatle L, Rokseth R: The arterial to end-expiratory carbon dioxide tension gradient in acute pulmonary embolism and other cardiopulmonary diseases. *Chest* 1974; 66:352–357.

137. Eriksson L, Wollmer P, Olsson C, et al: Diagnosis of pulmonary embolism based upon alveolar dead space analysis. *Chest* 1989; 96:357–362.

138. Chopin C, Fesard P, Mangalaboyi J, et al: Use of caponography in diagnosis of pulmonary embolism during acute respiratory failure of chronic obstructive pulmonary disease. *Crit Care Med* 1990; 18:353–357.

139. Byrick RJ, Kay JC, Mullen JB: Capnography is not as sensitive as pulmonary artery pressure monitoring in detecting marrow microembolism. *Anesth Analg* 1989; 68:94–100.

140. Epstein MF, Cohen AR, Feldman HA, et al: Estimation of PaCO2 by two noninvasive methods in the critically ill newborn infant. *J Pediatr* 1985; 106:282–286.

141. Watkins AMC, Weindling AM: Monitoring of end tidal CO2 in neonatal intensive care. *Arch Dis Child* 1987; 62:837–839.

142. Hand IL, Shepard EK, Krauss AN, et al: discrepancies between transcutaneous and end-tidal carbon dioxide monitoring in the critically ill neonate with respiratory distress syndrome. *Crit Care Med* 1989; 17:556–559.

143. McEvedy BAB, McLeod ME, Mulera M, et al: End-tidal, transcutaneous, and arterial PCO2 measurements in critically ill neonates: A comparison study. *Anesthesiol* 1988; 69:112–116.

144. Evans JM, Hogg IJ, Rosen M: Correlation of alveolar PCO2 estimated by infra-red analysis and arterial PCO2 in the human neonate and the rabbit. *Br J Anaesth* 1977; 49:761–764.

145. Lindahl SGE, Yates AP, Hatch DJ: Relationship between invasive and noninvasive measurements of gas exchange in anesthetized infants and children. *Anesthesiol* 1987; 66:168–175.

146. Meny RG, Bhat AM, Aranas E: Mass spectrometer monitoring of expired carbon dioxide in critically ill neonates. *Crit Care Med* 1985; 13:1064–1068.

147. Nelson NM, Prod'hom LS, Cherry RB, et al: Pulmonary function in the newborn infant. I. Methods: Ventilation and gaseous metabolism. *Pediatrics* 1962; 30:963–974.

148. Valtin N, Lomholt B, Thorup M: Arterial to end-tidal carbon dioxide tension difference in children under halothane anesthesia. *Can Anaesth Soc J* 1982; 29:12–15.

149. Fletcher R: Invasive and noninvasive measurement of the respiratory deadspace in anesthetized children with cardiac disease. *Anesth Analg* 1988; 67:442–447.

150. Burrows FA: Physiologic dead space, venous admixture, and the arterial to end-tidal carbon dioxide difference in infants and children undergoing cardiac surgery. *Anesthesiol* 1989; 70:219–225.

151. Cote CJ, Szyfelbein SK, Goudsouzian NG, et al: Intraoperative events diagnosed by expired carbon dioxide monitoring in children. *Can Anaesth Soc J* 1986; 33:315–320.

152. Dumpit FM, Brady JP: A simple technique for measuring alveolar CO2 in infants. *J Appl Physiol* 1978; 45:548–650.

153. Pascucci RC, Schena JA, Thompson JE: Comparison of a sidestream and mainstream capnometer in infants. *Crit Care Med* 1989; 17:560–562.

154. Sasse FJ: Can we trust end-tidal carbon dioxide measurements in infants? (editorial) *J Clin Monit* 1985; 1:147–148.

155. Schieber RA, Namnoum A, Sugden A, et al: Accuracy of expiratory carbon dioxide measurements using the coaxial and circle breathing circuits in small subjects. *J Clin Monit* 1985; 1:149–155.

156. Grevenstein N: Capnometry in infants should not be done at lower sampling flow rates (letter). *J Clin Monit* 1989; 5:63.

157. Badgwell JM, McLeod ME, Lerman J, et al: End-tidal PCO2 measurements sampled at the distal and proximal ends of the endotracheal tube in infants and children. *Anesth Analg* 1987; 66:959–964.

158. Meredith KS, Monaco F: End tidal carbon dioxide (PetCO2) monitoring in the intensive care nursery (abstract). *Crit Care Med* 1989; 17:S106.

159. Hillier SC, Lerman J: Mainstream vs. sidestream capnography in anesthetized infants and children (abstract). *Anesthesiol* 1989; 71:A357.

160. Badgwell JM, Heavner JE, May WS, et al: End-tidal PCO2 monitoring in infants and children ventilated with either a partial rebreathing or a nonrebreathing circuit. *Anesthesiol* 1987; 66:405–410.

161. Hillier SC, Badgwell JM, McLeod ME, et al: Accuracy of end-tidal PCO2 measurements using a sidestream capnometer in infants and children ventilated with the Sechrist infant ventilator. *Can J Anaesth* 1990; 37:318–321.

162. Rich GF, Sconzo JM: Continuous end-tidal CO2 sampling within the proximal endotracheal tube estimates arterial CO2 tension in infants. *Can J Anaesth* 1991; 38:201–203.

163. Rich GF, Sullivan MP, Adams JM: Is distal sampling of end tidal CO2 necessary in small subjects? (abstract) *Anesthesiol* 1989; 71:A1005.

164. Bowe EA, Boysen PG, Broome JA, et al: Accurate determination of end-tidal carbon dioxide during administration of oxygen by nasal cannula. *J Clin Monit* 1989; 5:105–110.

165. Hess D, Golden W, Hinderer J, et al: Capnometry in nonintubated patients (abstract). *Respir Care* 1989; 34:1040–1042.

166. Ibarra Eduardo, Lees DE: Mass spectrometer monitoring of patients with regional anesthesia (letter). *Anesthesiol* 1985; 63:572–573.

167. Machin JR, MacNeil A: Gas sampling from a facemask for capnography. *Anesthesia* 1986; 41:971–972.

168. Turner KE, Sandler AN, Vosu HA, et al: Noninvasive monitoring of carbon dioxide in non-intubate postoperative patients: Comparison of PaCO2 versus etCO2 versus tcPCO2 (abstract). *Anesth Analg* 1989; 68:S295.

169. Norman EA, Zieg NJ, Ahmad I: Better design for mass spectrometer monitoring of the awake patient (letter). *Anesthesiol* 1986; 64:664.

170. Huntington CT, King H: A simpler design for mass spectrometer monitoring of the awake patient (letter). *Anesthesiol* 1986; 65:565–566.

171. Goldman JM: A simple, easy, and inexpensive method for monitoring etCO2 through nasal cannulae (letter). *Anesthesiol* 1987; 67:806.

172. Urmey WF: Accuracy of expired carbon dioxide partial pressure sampled from a nasal cannula. I (letter). *Anesthesiol* 1988; 68:959–960.

173. Bonsu AK, Tamilarasan A, Bromage PR: A nasal catheter for monitoring tidal carbon dioxide in spontaneously breathing patients (letter). *Anesthesiol* 1989; 71:318.

174. Dunphy JA: Accuracy of expired carbon dioxide partial pressure sampled from a nasal cannula. II (letter). *Anesthesiol* 1988; 68:960–961.

175. Goldman JA: Accuracy of expired carbon dioxide partial pressure sampled from a nasal cannula. Reply (letter). *Anesthesiol* 1988; 68:961–962.

176. McNulty SE, Roy J, Torjman M, et al: Relationship between arterial carbon dioxide and end-tidal carbon dioxide when a nasal sampling port is used. *J Clin Monit* 1990; 6:93–98.

177. Ackerman WE, Juneja MM, Reaume D: Measurement of etCO2 and respiratory rate from a nasal cannula during cesarean section (abstract). *Anesthesiol* 1989; 71:A976.

178. Chambers JB, Kiff PJ, Gardner WN, et al: Value of measuring end tidal partial pressure of carbon dioxide as an adjunct to treadmill exercise testing. *Br Med J* 1988; 296:1281–1285.

179. McNabb L, Globerson T, St. Clair R, et al: The arterial-end tidal PCO2 difference in patients on ventilators (abstract). *Chest* 1981; 80:381.

180. Healey CJ, Fedullo AJ, Swinburne AJ, et al: Comparison of noninvasive measurements of carbon dioxide tension during withdrawal from mechanical ventilation. *Crit Care Med* 1987; 15:764–767.

181. Niehoff J, DelGuercio C, LaMorte W, et al: Efficiency of pulse oximetry and capnography in postoperative ventilatory weaning. *Crit Care Med* 1988; 16:701–705.

182. Withington DE, Ramsay JG, Saoud T, et al: Weaning from ventilation after cardiopulmonary bypass: evaluation of a noninvasive technique. *Can J Anaesth* 1991; 38:15–19.

183. Thrush DN, Wayne S, Downs JB: Weaning without blood gases: A possibility (abstract). *Anesthesiol* 1989; 71:A208.

184. Hess D, Schlottag A, Levin B, et al: An evaluation of the usefulness of end-tidal PCO_2 to aid weaning from mechanical ventilation following cardiac surgery. *Respir Care* 1991; 36:837–843.
185. Weinger MB, Brimm JE: End-tidal carbon dioxide as a measure of arterial carbon dioxide during intermittent mandatory ventilation. *J Clin Monit* 1987; 3:73–79.
186. Smith RA, Novak RA, Venus B: End-tidal CO2 monitoring utility during weaning from mechanical ventilation. *Respir Care* 1989; 34:972–975.
187. Murray IP, Modell JH, Gallagher TJ, et al: Titration of PEEP by the arterial minus end-tidal carbon dioxide gradient. *Chest* 1984; 85:100–104.
188. Jardin F, Genevray B, Pazin M, et al: Inability to titrate PEEP in patients with acute respiratory failure using end-tidal carbon dioxide measurements. *Anesthesiol* 1985; 62:530–533.
189. Blanch L, Fernandez R, Benito S, et al: Effect of PEEP on the arterial minus end-tidal carbon dioxide gradient. *Chest* 1987; 92:451–454.

Chapter 13

Indirect Calorimetry

Ray Ritz, R.R.T.

John Cunningham, Ph.D.

INTRODUCTION

Calorimetry is defined as the measurement of *heat production*. As we will see, this is not done at the bedside *per se*. Rather, the energy expended for what Kleiber[1] eloquently described as the "fire of life" is measured by a quantification of the reduction-oxidation (redox) chemistry required to fuel the fire at the cellular level. Thus, clinical medicine employs the variant of calorimetry termed *indirect calorimetry* to assess the energy requirements of individual patients. These energy needs are most easily expressed either in Calories (kcal) or in joules (J) as units of energy. Both the delivery of one obligate substrate and the removal of one obligate product of this redox chemistry occur through *respiratory gas exchange* so that this provides a convenient sampling site from which the corresponding *energy expenditure* can be calculated, in conjunction with several assumptions. These assumptions mathematically describe the principles of cellular chemistry and interorgan physiology. The derived energy needs of an ill patient are often expressed in relation to the expected normal needs available from tables or prediction equations.

The term "caloric" has its origin in the works of Antoine Lavoisier who coined it in the 1780s with reference to the "matter of fire." Lavoisier considered air to contain two components, the "vital air," which he later termed *oxygen*, and the "azote" (nitrogen) that did not support life.[2] He measured calories as the heat energy needed to melt ice water in an "ice calorimeter." Lavoisier established that calories were liberated from "vital air" in association with the release of "charbonneuse" (fixed carbon) into the air. Other contemporaries contributed enormously to the advancement of our present knowledge concerning animal metabolism, including Cavendish, who discovered hydrogen, and Crawford, who proposed that water was produced during metabolism. Fifty years later, Leibig demonstrated that carbohydrate, fat, and protein served as the oxidant substrates for this redox chemistry (and also proposed that urinary nitrogen quantitatively reflected protein catabolism). Simultaneously, Joule defined a more general unit of mechanical energy.[3] Thus, by 1850 one could confidently write the general equation for human energy expenditure as follows:

$$\text{Carbohydrate, fat or protein} + \text{oxygen} \rightarrow \text{fixed carbon} + \text{water} + \text{kcal/joule}$$

Two centuries after Lavoisier, a lively debate centered on the expression of metabolic energy as either *calories* or *joules*.[4, 5] Both are metric units. The calorie emphasizes that, ultimately, energy exits the body as heat (despite its seldom direct measurement), while the joule emphasizes the accomplishment of work during this transition from food to heat. That is, food energy is converted to useful kinetic energy, such as for muscular contraction, or stored as potential energy during anabolism (e.g., protein synthesis, fat deposition, etc.) prior to its requisite exit as heat during life. At present the literature from the United States remains largely calorie based (i.e., in kilocalories) while most other publications express energy expenditure in joules (i.e., in magajoules). While this is of some importance for the comparison of data derived by calorimetry, a call for a renaming of the clinical procedures as "joulemetry" has, fortunately, not yet occurred. The *Calorie* values assigned to foods are kilocalories in the metric system. The conversion to kilojoules is kcal $\times$ 4.184 = kJ, with expression as magajoules in human energetics (1 MJ = 1000 kJ).

Respiration should be appreciated as a term that has a dual meaning in animal energetics. At the organ system level, respiration describes the muscular work associated with ventilation during breathing. It connotes the inhalation and exhalation of air through the tracheobronchal passages servicing the alveolar clusters driven by muscular contraction/relaxation sequences. A uniform replacement of this term with the term "ventilation" would be appropriate. At the cellular level, respiration defines the process of stepwise energy transfer from the covalent chemical bonds of the calorigenic substrates, such as glucose or fatty acids, to the phosphate bonds in adenosine triphosphate (ATP). The basis of clinical calorimetry is the estimation of "metabolizable energy," that is, the sum of that transferred to cellular work via ATP plus that directly "wasted" as heat. Truly then, life is sustained by the combined actions of external respiration (ventilation) and internal respiration (cellular energetics) acting in concert.

Calorimetry may be either *direct* or *indirect*, depending on the procedure for measuring heat production. Mammals are only 60 to 70% efficient at converting the energy from foods into ATP or other cellular energy stores (such as creatine phosphate in muscle), so there is an appreciable escape of energy as heat during cellular respiration. This inefficiency is not deleterious for a homeotherm such as man whose core temperature at 37°C exceeds that of comfortable environments. Calorimetric procedures that measure heat production during cellular respiration are classified as direct. These require specialized chambers surrounded by thermal insulation to prevent unmeasured heat losses. Variants of direct calorimeters were constructed in the late 1800s and early 1900s, such as the *Armsby calorimeter*.[6] Later, the application of a gradient-layer principle enabled rapid response times to changes in heat emission. *Bomb calorimeters*, which completely combust food samples and liberate maximal calories, were a prior application of direct calorimetry with profound importance to the modern equations employed in clinical nutrition as discussed later. Unfortunately, a presentation of the details of direct calorimetry is beyond the present scope.

INDIRECT CALORIMETRY

The parallel development of indirect calorimetry is well described elsewhere in great detail[2] and, in fact, the Atwater-Rosa-Benedict calorimeter evolved to include both direct and indirect systems operating simultaneously.[7] All indirect calorimetry procedures substitute measurements of either the substrates consumed or the excretion products produced during cellular chemistry for the measurement of heat production *per se*. The close agreement between simultaneous measurements of energy expenditure by direct and indirect methods has been documented to the extent that errors are expected to occur only from mechanical or operational failures. Although the details of the procedure employed by Lavoisier and his assistant Armand Sequin remain unknown, (and were lost to the guillotine in Paris on May 8, 1794), they involved the analysis of exhaled air traversing through a long tube exiting a copper face mask.[8] Drawings of the apparatus in use[2] suggest that carbon dioxide was trapped with alkali and that oxygen was measured by a eudiometric method (the absorption by phosphorous). This was the earliest of many methods that analyzed respiratory gas exchange. The analysis of *expired air* during indirect calorimetry quantifies the whole body uptake of the oxidant for metabolism (oxygen disappearance) and may also measure the excretion of metabolic waste from energy metabolism (carbon dioxide appearance). The earliest details of specific techniques, likely descendant from Lavoisier, were reported[2] in 1817. A valve was used to separate inspired air from the expired air, which was collected in an impermeable bladder. Alkali extraction of carbon dioxide was followed by the eudiometric (gravimetric) measurement of oxygen from its absorption on a known weight of phosphorous.

One novel approach to indirect calorimetry in the past two decades has been the implementation of a "nonrespiratory" procedure. This is advantageous because it frees the individual under study from the restraints of physical attachment to some collection apparatus, but is limited because the duration of study must be at least several days. In this *doubly labeled water technique* a measurement of the rate of disappearance of isotopes of hydrogen and oxygen from the body following their introduction into the body water pool permits estimation of total carbon dioxide production without collection or analysis of expired air.[9, 10] Refinements to this procedure include the analysis of these isotopes in urine or saliva. The presentation of the details of doubly labeled water calorimetry, however, is beyond the present scope.

RESPIRATORY GAS EXCHANGE

Man and most other mammals may be viewed as "terrestrial water tanks" whose bodies consist of more than 60% water. Water balance is, thus, a major driving force for lifestyle adaptations. This, however, can be satisfied by episodic intakes, as can the need for acquisition of calorigenic substrates and other nutrients. Standing in singular contrast to these classically recognized nutrient needs is the need for oxygen as the obligate co-oxidant in cellular energy metabolism. In our opinion, *oxygen is a nutrient* for which: (1) the requirement is huge and continuous; (2) a deficiency is devastating and swiftly manifested; (3) a specialized organ, the lung, is present; and (4) storage is minimal and *the requirement is continuous*. It is this direct link between oxygen need and energy production that permits the use of methods of indirect calorimetry employing respiratory gas analysis.

The analysis of oxygen consumption has become the cornerstone of clinical indirect calorimetry. Several approaches are available, and each may be done over a defined time interval for subsequent extrapolation to the complete day; however, significant daily variations are common. The lineage from Lavoisier is obvious among modern technologies. Some early clinical systems were constructed to be *closed circuits*.[11] All air inspired by the subject originated from a cylinder of 100% oxygen and the expired air was completely captured, "scrubbed" of carbon dioxide, and recirculated. Thus, the disappearance of oxygen from the cyclinder replaced exactly the volume of oxygen consumed by the subject and could be recorded. The development of mass spectrometry for the measurement of both oxygen and carbon dioxide concentrations in air samples vastly simplified the alternate *open-circuit system* of indirect calorimetry at the bedside. In open-circuit systems, subjects breathe room air through a one-way valve that also permits the complete capture of all expired air into an impermeable "Douglas bag."[12] Both the total expired air volume and the gas composition of the expired air are measured. Since the inspired air is not rebreathed and its volume is not recorded, the breathing circuit is considered to be open. The oxygen and carbon dioxide contents of the inspired air are assumed to be those of fresh ambient air in the circulations. This is clinically useful as long as the room is not confining or subject to low air circulation or crowded with numerous personnel during the measurement. Modern *metabolic carts* are the descendants of these two "Douglas lineages," either as closed circuits employing the scrubbing of carbon dioxide and sophisticated oxygen analyzers in place of volume replacement or as open circuits combining flow measurement (in place of expired air volume measurement) with gas analysis of oxygen and carbon dioxide in the expired air or both inspired and expired air. The analysis of inspired air adds the advantage of monitoring energy expenditure during ventilator-assisted breathing at oxygen concentrations above ambient.

We now turn to a discussion of with indirect calorimetry through the analysis of respiratory gas exchange. One final noteworthy point is the potentially unfortunate connotation that could be associated with the procedure—that is, direct calorimetry might be interpreted as being more useful, by virtue of its adjective, although it merely measures the total "thermogenic" output and requires a prolonged measurement period. Conversely, indirect calorimetry could, by virtue of its adjective, seem perhaps less valuable, even though it can provide both a rapid assessment of energy output and the *respiratory quotient* (RQ), which has value in inputting the fuel mixture being utilized (see the section on partitioning of fuels later in this chapter). In this last respect the open and closed indirect systems may be considered equivalent only when the closed loop includes a measurement of carbon dioxide production prior to scrubbing. Otherwise, the omission of a carbon dioxide measurement introduces a difference in utility (namely the loss of the RQ data) to be reckoned with by the clinician.

INDIRECT CALORIMETRY AND ENERGY METABOLISM

Man is subject to the laws of thermodynamics. The tandem operations of respiration at the organ system level, oxygen delivery to cells by the cardiovascular system, and respiration at the cellular level are coordinated to postpone transiently the second law of thermodynamics (entropy). As a multicellular organism organized into organ systems, the energetics within individual cells vary at any point in time, as do the energetics among the tissues and organs they compose. For example, cells of the brain are able to metabolize only glucose (or ketones during severe fuel deficits) even at times when the body as a whole is deriving more than 60% of its energy from fat. This phenomenon occurs nightly in sound sleepers and, obviously, is not aberrant. The partitioning of calorigenic substrates among major organs is depicted in Table 13–1 for two extreme metabolic states.[13, 14] It is useful to recall the episodic nature of the acquisition of these energy substrates from foods in contrast to the continuous nature of cellular energy needs. In the hospital setting, this normal counterplay is sometimes overidden by continuous enteral or parenteral feeding modalities.

Indirect calorimetry by the analysis of respiratory gas exchange provides an acceptable approximation of the whole body energy metabolism *under the conditions that exist during the study*. Often these data are extrapolated to a 24-hour day; however, this practice carries over the limitations of interpretation. If the subject has fasted for 12 hours and has been lying comfortably in a thermoneutral environment for an equilibration period of approximately 15 to 30 minutes, then the measured metabolic rate is termed "basal" or BMR in the older literature. Since the meaning of "basal" is imprecise, given that metabolic rate decreases from basal during sleep by approximately 5 to 8% modern authors refer to this condition as the *resting energy expenditure* (REE) or resting metabolic rate (RMR). These equivalent measures, BMR and REE (or RMR) are standardized and permit comparisons with expectations on a per hour or per day basis. However, this measurement does not estimate the energy costs associated with physical activity, anxiety, or other disturbances during patient care, the reduction in

TABLE 13–1.
Energy Requirements of Organs and Substrate Partitioning in Metabolic States*

Organ	Size % wt	Energy Need % total	Fed RQ	Fasted RQ
Brain	2.0	15–20	1.0	1.0–0.90
Heart	0.5	9–11	0.9	0.8–0.75
Liver	2.5	25–33	0.9	0.75–0.70
Kidney	0.5	4–8	1.0	0.75–0.70
SUBTOTAL	5.0	50–75	0.94–1.0	0.80–0.75
Muscles	30–40	15–30	1.0	0.75–0.70
Fat and skeletal	30–35	3–5	1.0	
TOTAL		100	0.96–1.0	0.79–0.73

* % values rounded from data cited in Refs. 13 and 14, fed state RQ data presumes glucose as fuel coupled with minor fatty acid oxidation by heart and muscle; fasting state RQ presumes gluconeogenesis (conversion of amino acids to glucose) plus fatty acid oxidation.

expenditure that occurs during sleep, or the heat losses that occur with food ingestion. Thus, REE measurements are of limited value when extrapolated to a 24-hour day in patient care settings unless adjustments for nonbasal or nonresting components of metabolism are applied. Obviously, significant assumptions are required for the correction from BMR or REE to *total energy expenditure* (TEE). Finally, when energy expenditure is measured at the bedside in settings characterized by effects from medications, continuous or recent feedings, significant nursing interventions, etc., the resulting metabolic rate is better termed the *metabolic energy expenditure* (MEE) to denote potential deviations from the conditions for REE.

Sufficient clinical precision can be achieved with the measurement of either CO_2 production (the volume of CO_2, abbreviated as Vco_2 and usually displayed in milliliters per minute) or O_2 consumption (volume at Vo_2, also in ml/min) plus a knowledge of the metabolic state. The ratio of Vco_2/Vo_2 is defined as the *respiratory quotient* (RQ). The RQ reflects, in a general way, the metabolic state. When only one respiratory gas is measured (i.e., only Vco_2 or Vo_2), an RQ consistent with the clinical conditions must be assumed. A energy value for the total Vo_2 is then assigned from a table of standard values based on the RQ. Table 13–2 (from Lusk[15]) is the classic presentation of this procedure. Note that the units are kilocalories per liter of oxygen consumed for the period of time measured and must be correctly applied to Vo_2 recoreded in ml/min.

The energy value for use in calculations when only Vco_2 is measured can also be found in other versions of the above-mentioned table. However, measurement of Vco_2 alone is so rare as to be obsolete in clinical calorimetry (with the exception of the doubly labeled water method).[16] When both Vco_2 and Vo_2 are measured, the estimation of energy expenditure using the derived RQ is improved by 0 to 10%. The magnitude of improvement depends on: (1) the difference between the true RQ and the otherwise assumed RQ and (2) the single gas measured. That is, up to a 6% improvement in MEE can occur versus that derived from Vo_2 data if the metabolic state were completely misclassified or up to 10% improvement in MEE derived from Vco_2 data in the same situation.

The substrates that are aerobically metabolized to yield energy can be mathematically partitioned into two categories, *glucose* and *fat*, when both Vco_2 and Vo_2 are measured during indirect calorimetry. Again, several assumptions are necessary as detailed later, and the interpretation of the fuel partition must be made with caution given that the limitations are greater than for estimation of MEE.

Following sufficient collection of data, generally 10 minutes or longer, MEE can be derived from standard equations. Most often, the *Weir equation*[17] is used, either with the correction term for protein oxidation as calculated from urinary nitrogen (UN) or without a correction for protein oxidation. Weir showed that this latter correction introduces only a minor error when ignored. This is, in part, attributable to the low absolute amount of protein used as a substrate for energy production and in part to the similarity of calorigenesis from amino acid oxidation relative to glucose and fat. Very rarely is the UN excretion measured simultaneously with MEE in clinical practice. Some workers substitute an average UN from an equivalent metabolic period of interest (such as the 24-hour UN from the prior day). This would be acceptable when the conditions of feeding and illness are stable. Alternatively, both mathematical procedures and confirmatory measurements show that the error resulting from the omission of the protein oxidation factor estimated by UN is less than 5% for individuals and averages

TABLE 13–2.
Analysis of the Oxidation of Mixtures of Carbohydrate and Fat*

| R.Q. | Percentage of Total Oxygen Consumed by | | Calories per liter O₂ | RQ | Percentage of Total Oxygen Consumed by | | Calories per liter O₂ |
	Carbohydrate %	Fat %	kcal		Carbohydrate %	Fat %	kcal
0.707	0	100.0	4.686	0.86	52.2	47.8	4.875
0.71	1.02	99.0	4.690	0.87	55.6	44.4	4.887
0.72	4.44	95.6	4.702	0.88	59.0	41.0	4.899
0.73	7.85	92.2	4.714	0.89	62.5	37.5	4.911
0.74	11.3	88.7	4.727	0.90	65.9	34.1	4.924
0.75	14.7	85.3	4.739				
0.76	18.1	81.9	4.751	0.91	69.3	30.7	4.936
0.77	21.5	78.5	4.764	0.92	72.7	27.3	4.948
0.78	24.9	75.1	4.776	0.93	76.1	23.9	4.961
0.79	28.3	71.7	4.788	0.94	79.5	20.5	4.973
0.80	31.7	68.3	4.801	0.95	82.9	17.1	4.985
0.81	35.2	64.8	4.813	0.96	86.3	13.7	4.998
0.82	38.6	61.4	4.825	0.97	89.8	10.2	5.010
0.83	42.0	58.0	4.838	0.98	93.2	6.83	5.022
0.84	45.4	54.6	4.850	0.99	96.6	3.41	5.035
0.85	48.8	51.2	4.862	1.00	100.0	0	5.047

A hypothetical patient produces 220 ml/min of CO_2 (Vco_2) and consumes 235 ml/min of O_2 (Vo_2). The RQ is thus 220/235 = 0.94. The MEE is 1683 kcal/d by Table 13–2 or 1684 kcal/d by the Weir equation.

Substrate partitioning is 80% glucose and 20% fatty acids by Table 13.2. An error in calibration is found, such that the Vco_2 is truly 213 ml/min. This 3% error results in the following data. The RQ is now 0.91 and the MEE is now 1670 kcal/d by Table 13–2 or 1672 kcal/d by the Weir equation (a 1% error versus that above).

However, the substrate partitioning is now 70% glucose and 30% fatty acids (a 10% error for each of these versus that above).

* Modified from Lusk G: *J Biol Chem* 1924; 59:41–42.

below 2%. The calculated MEE from the following equation is the total kcal or (kJ) for the period of time measured and is usually converted into a daily total. This equation has stood the test of time (Table 13–3) and provides a clinically meaningful estimate.[18] The Weir equation:

$$\text{MEE} = 3.94 \times Vo_2 + 1.106 \times Vco_2 - 2.17 \times UN$$

where MEE is the total kcal/time (and can be per day when multiplied by 1440/minutes of analysis), Vo_2 and Vco_2 are expressed in liters, and UN is the correction for protein oxidation.

More recently, Ferrannini derived the same "nonprotein" equation [see Equation (9) in Ref. 19] independently, starting with the principles of "free energy" (enthalpy minus entropy). His and several other equations present alternate coefficients for the protein correction from UUN

TABLE 13–3.
Equations for Calculating MEE from Indirect Calorimetry Data*

Author	Equation Coefficients			RQ/kcal: Assumptions		
	___ × VO$_2$ +	___ × VCO$_2$ –	___ × UN	P	C	F
Weir	3.94	1.06	2.17	0.80/4.463	1.00/5.047	0.718/4.735
Consolazio et al.	3.78	1.16	2.98	0.81/4.244	1.00/4.945	0.707/4.606
Peters & Van Slyke	3.82	1.22	2.01	0.80/4.468	1.00/5.049	0.711/4.685
Ben-Porat et al.	3.913	1.093	3.341	0.81/4.244	1.00/5.007	0.705/4.684
Brouwer	3.87	1.20	1.43†	0.81/4.594	1.00/5.066‡	0.711/4.719
Livesey & Elia§	3.80	1.25	1.09	0.835/4.656	1.00/5.047	0.710/4.685

* Intended for fasting state.
† Includes a subtraction for methane productions: –0.518 × CH$_4$.
‡ See text for starch versus glucose (5.013kcal/L) as substrate.
§ Calculated using the Weir method and values in Table 6 of the paper.
From Ref. 18. P = protein; C = carbohydrate; F = Fot; RQ/kcal = respiratory quotient for pure substrate oxidation of kcal relased per liter of oxygen consumed.

or from urine total N. As noted, the correction itself does not seem necessary for clinical practice.

It is didactically illustrative to solve the Weir equation to the appropriate coefficients as multipliers for Vo_2 alone when the RQ is assumed to vary from its physiologic extremes of 1.0 to 0.7, reflecting different metabolic states. This is, in fact, a reversal of the steps used by Weir to derive the two-variable equation above. The coefficient is $5.0 \times Vo_2$ at RQ = 1.0 and $4.7 \times Vo_2$ at RQ = 0.70. That these coefficients are quite comparable to the extremes of values listed by Lusk for use when only Vo_2 is measured (Table 13–2) is not coincidental. This synchrony arises, rather, from the use by Weir of substantially the same data for his derivation. Namely, both Lusk and Weir used carbohydrate oxidation data published by Zuntz in 1897, while their data for fat oxidation were from Zuntz or from Cathcart and Cuthbertson,[20] respectively.

PARTITIONING FUEL OXIDATION

In 1842 Leibig first reported[3] that carbohydrate, fat, and protein were the substrates for MEE. Workers including Rubner and Zuntz determined the heats of combustion for these substrates from "bomb calorimetry". These heats were manipulated by Lusk, and later by Weir with minor modification to derive their equations for MEE. Combustion data assumed by various workers are reproduced in Table 13–3. The accuracy of the original data is remarkable. Also in Table 13–3 are the RQ values for the oxidation of starch (or glucose) and triglyceride assumed by each author. The RQ values are derived from the *molar stoichiometry* of cellular respiration. They are identical for starch or glucose since all starch is converted to glucose for metabolism, but the RQs do differ slightly for triglyceride oxidation, depending on the presumed content of depot fat energy stores. The values for energy produced are those measured by bomb calorimetry of known weights of each substrate. For starch or glucose:

$$\text{1 mole } C_6H_{12}O_6 + 6 \text{ moles } O_2 \rightarrow 6 \text{ moles } CO_2 + 6 \text{ moles } H_2O + \text{energy}$$

$$RQ = 6 \, CO_2/6 \, O_2 = 1.0$$

producing 670 kcal from 1 mole of substrate consumed (665 to 675, depending on the reference author chosen).

For lipid oxidation (including oxidation of the glycerol moiety released with fatty acid mobilization), the RQs are very similar but the energy produced varies with the fatty acid chain lengths presumed to be oxidized. For *tripalmitate* (glycerol with 3 palmitic acids, each C_{16} saturated):

$$\text{1 mole } C_{51}H_{98}O_6 + 72.5 \text{ moles } O_2 \rightarrow 51 \text{ moles } CO_2 + 49 \text{ moles } H_2O$$

$$RQ = 51 \, CO_2/72.5 \, O_2 = 0.703$$

producing 7660 kcal from 1 mole of substrate (806 grams) or 9.63 kcal/gram.

For *tristearin* (glycerol with 3 stearic acids, each C_{18} saturated):

$$1 \text{ mole } C_{57}H_{110}O_6 + 81.5 \text{ moles } O_2 \rightarrow 57 \text{ moles } CO_2 + 55 \text{ } H_2O + \text{energy}$$
$$RQ = 57 \text{ } CO_2/81.5 \text{ } O_2 = 0.699$$

producing 8490 kcal from 1 mole of substrate (890 grams) or 9.54 kcal/gram. For a *typical adipose triglyceride* [glycerol with fatty acids from the distribution of 50% saturated fat (2/3 C_{16}, 1/3 C_{18}), 40% monounsaturated C_{18} and 10% polyunsaturated C_{18}]:

$$1 \text{ mole } C_{54}H_{104}O_6 + 77 \text{ moles } O_2 \rightarrow 54 \text{ moles } CO_2 + 52 \text{ moles } H_2O$$
$$RQ = 54 \text{ } CO_2/77 \text{ } O_2 = 0.701$$

producing 8040 kcal from 1 mole of substrate (848 grams) or 9.48 kcal/gram. Livesay and Elia[21] report that direct measurements of adult human fat have an RQ = 0.710 to 0.715 and yield 9.45 to 9.5 kcal/gram. This would appear to result from production of 8090 kcal/mole.

Readers desiring to write other substrate stoichiometries and calculate caloric equivalents need only the following constants: all gases are 22.4 liters per mole; the conversion of moles to grams uses C = 12 g × #/mole, H = 1 g × #/mole and O = 16 g × #/mole.

One important piece of notation is needed for the calculation of the energy delivered by nutritional support to patients. One mole of glucose is of variable weight in foods. That is, when the substrate is glucose (powder), the weight of one mole is 180 grams and the energy value is 670 kcal/180 gram = 3.72 kcal/gram. With 97% absorbed, approximately 3.6 kcal/gram is available when fed. *The "general" value of 4 kcal/gram often (mis)used is derived from calculations based on starch as a food.* Although all starch is converted into glucose, starch is a polymer of glucose formed by dehydration synthesis, resulting in the loss of one HO molecule for each bond. Thus, one mole of starch weighs less when fed (162 grams/mole rather than 180) but becomes "rehydrated" by hydrolysis during digestion. The calorie value for starch is 670 kcal/162 gram per mole = 4.1 kcal/gram with a 97% absorption, or 4 kcal/gram fed. Alas, much of metabolism carries over similar remnants of the presumption that starch (glycogen) rather than glucose is the substrate for cellular energy. Consider the terms *glycolysis* for glucose oxidation, *hypoglycemia* for low blood glucose, and *glycosuria* for glucose loss in urine. When the energy substrate is *intravenous dextrose*, the value becomes 670 kcal/198 gram/mole = 3.4 kcal/gram as a result of the hygroscopic nature of anhydrous glucose. However, 100% is "absorbed" (intravenous gut bypass), to that 3.4 kcal/gram infused is close to the 3.6 kcal/gram when fed as powder.

In healthy persons, the MEE at any time can range from below the REE (during sleep) to a level reflecting muscular work during active periods. A few minutes' "window" of REE may reflect in a general sense the habitual daily total MEE (as related to lean body mass), but says little about EE on a specific day. In ill patients, the range of MEEs around the REE is usually narrowed by minimal muscular work and sedative medications. There may be a degree of hypermetabolism from fever or as associated with a specific disease. All of these factors are reasonably constant throughout the day so that a short duration measurement of MEE is appropriate for extrapolation to the total daily EE in patients.

At the same time, clinicians are tempted to assign percentages for glucose oxidation and fatty acid oxidation from the RQ value when it is available from measurements of both V_{CO_2} and V_{O_2} (Table 13–2). This approach is subject to a greater error than is generally appreciated. An error of only 0.03 in the RQ produces a 10% error in the partitioning of glucose versus fat as detailed in the example that accompanies Table 13–2. An RQ error can result from a combination of errors in the measurement of V_{O_2} and V_{CO_2}. Secondly, an erroneous RQ may be "carried over" to the table for substrate partitioning by using the assumption that amino acid (protein) oxidation is negligible as shown earlier for the Weir equation. If UN is unmeasured during substantial protein oxidation, the error in MEE is of the order of 5%, while the error carried over for substrate partitioning from the overall RQ ranges from 10 to 30%.[22] This is because the RQ for amino acid oxidation, which averages 0.8, simulates 50% glucose and 50% fat as substrates when the V_{O_2} and V_{CO_2} from amino acid oxidation are not factored out (subtracted) prior to calculating the nonprotein RQ to partition the substrates as glucose and fat. If 4% of the total V_{O_2} were due to amino acid oxidation, then this would mimic the oxidation of 2% glucose plus 2% fatty acid, but would most likely occur in a setting of a true total glucose oxidation of less than 10% (e.g., starvation). The error thus becomes 12.5% "apparent" versus 10% "true" glucose oxidation.

Other errors in substrate partitioning can result during ketosis and when *medium chain triglycerides* (MCTs) are included in the fat regimen. These errors are generally small and are presented for completeness. The stoichiometric equations for these processes shown below are written with the assumptions detailed elsewhere by other authors.[19, 23]

A loss of ketones in the urine and breath (as acetone) during *ketosis* eliminates approximately 10% of the total substrate produced from fatty acids. Since their formation (RQ = 0.57, Ref. 19) is not counterbalanced by their oxidation as carbohydrate equivalents (RQ = 0.90 for hydroxbutyrate or RQ = 1.0 for acetoacetate or acetone), the whole body RQ is skewed downward. An estimate of the glucose/fat substrate partition from the whole body RQ will be likewise skewed.

Ketone formation and oxidation involves a complex set of reactions. Ketone formation from fatty acids is illustrated by palmitic acid:

$$1 \text{ mole } C_{16}H_{32}O_2 + 7 \text{ moles } O_2 \rightarrow 4 \text{ moles AcAc} + 4 \text{ moles } H^+ + 4 \text{ moles } H_2O$$

$$RQ = 4\ CO_2/7\ O_2 = 0.57$$

The AcAc thus formed can be converted to hydroxbutyrate (OH-b) or acetone and these reactions confound the RQ data:

$$1 \text{ mole AcAc} + 1 \text{ mole NADH} \rightarrow 1 \text{ mole OH-b} + 0.5 \text{ mole } O_2$$

$$RQ = 0\ CO_2/0.5\ O_2 = 0\ !!$$

or

$$1 \text{ mole AcAc} \rightarrow 1 \text{ mole Acetone} + 1 \text{ mole } CO_2$$

$$RQ = 1\ CO_2/0\ O_2 = \text{undefined } !!$$

The oxidation of ketones proceeds essentially as for glucose:

$$1 \text{ mole AcAc} + 4 \text{ moles } O_2 + H^+ \rightarrow 4 \text{ moles } CO_2 + 3 \text{ moles } H_2O$$

$$RQ = 4 \, CO_2/4 \, O_2 = 1.0$$

or

$$1 \text{ mole OH-b} + 4.5 \text{ moles } O_2 + H^+ \rightarrow 4 \text{ moles } CO_2 + 4 \text{ moles } H_2O$$

$$RQ = 4 \, CO_2/4.5 \, O_2 = 0.89$$

or

$$1 \text{ mole acetone} + 3 \text{ moles } O_2 \rightarrow 3 \text{ moles } CO_2 + 3 \text{ moles } H_2O$$

$$RQ = 3 \, CO_2/3 \, O_2 = 1.0$$

The oxidation of ketones produces approximately 3500 kcal from 1 mole (100 grams) = 3.5 kcal/gram. If all ketones formed from fatty acids are oxidized, the RQ is unaffected (since their formation at 0.57 and oxidation at 0.9 to 1.0 average out to fatty acid oxidation at 0.75). Only the condition of severe ketosis with urinary and breath losses of unoxidized substrates results in errors. Ketones formed with an RQ of 0.57, but not oxidized, reduce the overall body RQ measured by indirect calorimetry; this occurs in a metabolic state where the overall RQ itself is close to 0.7. Thus, it is possible to measure a true RQ of 0.69 to 0.67 in uncontrolled ketoacidosis.

The oxidation of MCTs may be a major source of energy for patients fed commercial liquid tube feeding products. Enteral MCTs leave intestinal cells via the portal vein (unlike long chain triglycerides), appear to trigger insulin release (unlike long chain triglycerides), and are preferentially oxidized by the liver.[24] This hepatic oxidation occurs even when abundant glucose is available (unlike long chain triglycerides) and is thermogenic (unlike long chain triglycerides). When intravenously infused, MCTs are subject to lipoprotein lipase action and the resulting fatty acids (MCFAs) are presumably extracted by the liver, muscle, and other organs for oxidation. Overall, the oxidation of MCTs appears to have an RQ of 0.74 (see equation below and Ref. 23), mimicking a 10% glucose plus 90% fat pattern (Table 13–2) despite the actual oxidation of 100% fat. Thus, for each 10% of calories fed as MCTs, a misclassification of 1% glucose oxidation will occur from the overall body RQ using Table 13–2. MCT oxidation:

$$1 \text{ mole } C_{28}H_{52}O_6 + 38 \text{ moles } O_2 \rightarrow 28 \text{ moles } CO_2 + 26 \text{ moles } H_2O$$

$$RQ = 28 \, CO_2/38 \, O_2 = 0.736$$

producing 3990 kcal from 1 mole of substrate (484 grams) or 8.2 kcal/gram.

The reader is cautioned to suspect RQ determinations that, in practice, exceed the limits of 1.0 to 0.7. As shown previously, neither substantial protein catabolism nor moderate ketosis should result in an RQ below 0.7 overall. An RQ higher than 1.0 is possible and may be real, but only if the subject is being substantially overfed with glucose when studied. Here the upper limit will approach 1.2 as a result of the conversion of excess glucose to triglyceride by adipose and liver cells:

$$13.5 \text{ mole } C_6H_{12}O_6 + 3 \text{ moles } O_2 + ATP \rightarrow 1 \text{ mole } C_{54}H_{104}O_6 + 26 \text{ moles } CO_2 + 29 \text{ moles } H_2O$$

$$RQ = 26 \text{ } CO_2/3 \text{ } O_2 = 8.7$$

If only 2% of the whole body oxygen consumption were used for NET lipogenesis, then the whole body RQ would be $(0.98 \times 1.0) + (0.02 \times 8.7) = 1.15$. This represents 98% for whole body MEE entirely from glucose (since it is in excess) and 2% of V_{O_2} for lipogenesis from the excess glucose substrate.

TECHNICAL ASPECTS OF INDIRECT CALORIMETRY

As previously described, assessment of energy expenditure can be performed by three basic methods or calculated by the Fick equation. The direct calorimetry technique utilizes a chamber into which a subject is placed and their heat loss is directly measured. This technique, although accurate, is not practical for most hospitalized patients. The second (nonrespiratory) method involves the administration of doubly labeled water. Last, there is the measurement of energy expenditure using indirect calorimetry. By measuring the volume of oxygen consumed and the volume of carbon dioxide produced per unit of time, an accurate assessment of energy expenditure can be made. This last method is utilized in numerous patient care applications today.

Designing indirect calorimetry systems that provide precise and reliable measurements of oxygen consumption and carbon dioxide production requires the use of highly sophisticated devices. Additionally, to utilize this technology practically, these systems must be portable and capable of interfacing with patients who may be mechanically ventilated or who are spontaneously breathing either room air or some amount of supplemental oxygen with or without positive end expiratory pressure (PEEP). Even with the current microprocessor-controlled systems this is not an easy task. A well-trained clinician is required who has a reasonable understanding of the technical limitations of the calorimeter being used. The clinician must also have the skill to assess and control the clinical setting for a variety of factors that can adversely affect the accuracy of a study.

The following sections review the fundamental principles that apply to the operation of various indirect calorimeters and the methods that can be employed to assure optimal performance. Various clinical considerations will be discussed which can impact the accuracy of a study. Last, the key issues required to develop essential protocols for an indirect calorimetry program will be reviewed.

CALCULATIONS

The basis of all bedside indirect calorimetry systems is the determination of the volume of oxygen consumed (V_{O_2}) and the volume of carbon dioxide produced (V_{CO_2}) per unit of time by the patient. The relationship between these two components yields the respiratory quotient (RQ). These values are calculated from the following formulas:

Respiratory quotient:

$$RQ = V_{CO_2}/V_{O_2}$$

Carbon dioxide production:

$$V_{CO_2} = V_E(F_{ECO_2}) - V_I(F_{ICO_2})$$

Since the ambient concentration of CO_2 is negligible, this formula can then be simplified to:

$$V_{CO_2} = V_E(F_{ECO_2})$$

Oxygen consumption:

$$V_{O_2} = V_I(F_{IO_2}) - V_E(F_{EO_2})$$

This calculation imposes the greatest degree of complexity. Inspiratory minute ventilation measurements are not done by most calorimeters. If V_I is not measured, it must then be calculated using the Haldane transformation. Assuming that there is no uptake or release of nitrogen (N_2) during ventilation, V_I can be calculated by:

$$V_I = \frac{F_{EN_2}}{F_{IN_2}} V_E$$

Assuming no other gases are present other than O_2, CO_2, and N_2, F_{EN_2} and F_{IN_2} are obtained by:

$$F_{EN_2} = 1.0 - F_{EO_2} - F_{ECO_2}$$

and

$$F_{IN_2} = 1.0 - F_{IO_2} - F_{ICO_2}$$

Substituting the right-hand portions of the above two formulas into the original V_I calculations results in:

$$V_I = \frac{1.0 - F_{EO_2} - F_{ECO_2}}{1.0 - F_{IO_2} - F_{ICO_2}} V_E$$

By further substituting the formula for V_I into the formula for V_{O_2}, the final formula employed by most open-circuit calorimeters is:

$$V_{O_2} = \frac{(1 - F_{E_{O_2}} - F_{E_{CO_2}})}{1 - F_{I_{O_2}}} (F_{I_{O_2}} - F_{E_{O_2}}) \, V_E$$

When attempting to measure and compare the inspiratory and expiratory minute ventilation, one quickly realizes that the difference between the two is often small but critical. Failure to correct for the difference between V_I and V_E will result in significant errors in the V_{O_2} calculation.[25]

TYPES OF INDIRECT CALORIMETERS

The two basic design classifications of indirect calorimeters are the open-circuit system and the closed-circuit type. Each offers certain advantages and each is also limited by various factors associated with its design. The best calorimeter for a situation will be determined by the clinical setting in which it must be used and the operating characteristics of the instrument.

Open-Circuit Systems

Open-circuit calorimeters are so named because they sample the patient's inspiratory gas for O_2 and CO_2 content and then re-analyze the expiratory gas and measure its volume before discharging it into the ambient atmosphere. Most operate well with mechanically ventilated patients as long as the $F_{I_{O_2}}$ is less than 0.60,[35] but newer designs may allow measurements when the $F_{I_{O_2}}$ approaches 0.80.[37, 39] Open-circuit calorimeters employ three basics techniques of operation as discussed in the following.

Conventional Mixing Chamber Technique
This technique permits measurements of patients spontaneously breathing either room air or supplemental oxygen by using a mask, mouthpiece, or canopy and also allows the study of patients being mechanically ventilated. After analysis of the inspiratory gas is completed, expired gas is directed into a mixing chamber (Fig 13–1). The mixing chamber is sized to accommodate several of the patient's breaths and contains a set of baffles. These baffles facilitate the equilibration of the early and late portions of the tidal volumes and create a stable mean $F_{E_{O_2}}$ and $F_{E_{CO_2}}$. A gas sample is taken after this mixing is complete and compared against the concentrations obtained from the inspiratory gas. A simultaneous measurement of the exhaled V_E allows the calculation of V_{O_2} and V_{CO_2}.

Prior to entering the mixing chamber, the temperature of the expired gas is measured as well as the pressure so the appropriate temperature and pressure corrections can be applied.

During studies of patients who are breathing spontaneously but receiving supplemental oxygen at ambient pressure or in conjunction with PEEP/CPAP and during studies of patients being mechanically ventilated, the expired gas is passively exhaled into the mixing chamber.

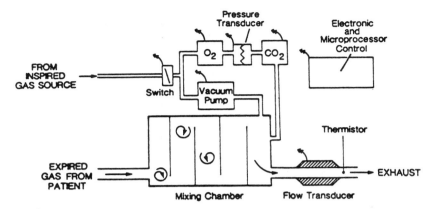

FIG 13–1.
A schematic of a generic conventional mixing chamber technique calorimeter. (*From Branson RD: The measurement of energy expenditure: instrumentation, practical considerations and clinical application. Respir Care 1990; 35:640–659. Used by permission.*)

When a canopy (a loose fitting shell covering the patient's head) is used to study patients spontaneously breathing room air, the calorimeter must be configured to draw ambient gas actively from the room through the canopy and into the mixing chamber. In this mode the mixing chamber calorimeter adopts the dilution (or flow-by) technique. The generated flow is high enough to ensure adequate washout of the canopy and a complete extraction of the patient's minute ventilation. The titration of this flow (which is done automatically by the calorimeter's flow generator) is important in order to avoid overdilution of the expired gas or an inadvertent buildup of CO_2 in the canopy. Again, the canopy technique is useful only if the patient is breathing room air.

Dilution Technique

This technique is used in some monitor designs and is a modification of the conventional mixing chamber method (Fig 13–2). The basic operation is consistent with that described in the previous section on canopy studies although the device is not limited to that technique alone. The unique component of this design is the lack of a direct volume measuring device. Instead, a flow generator ensures that a consistent flow of gas passes through the mixing chamber at all times. This flow is a combination of the patient's minute ventilation and the additional flow provided by the flow generator. By knowing the output of the flow generator that is needed to meet the desired total ouput, the patient's minute ventilation can be calculated.

Because the expired gases are diluted in this process, the accuracy and stability of the gas analyzers is critical. Oxygen analyzers must be accurate to the fourth decimal place and free of any drift through the course of the study.

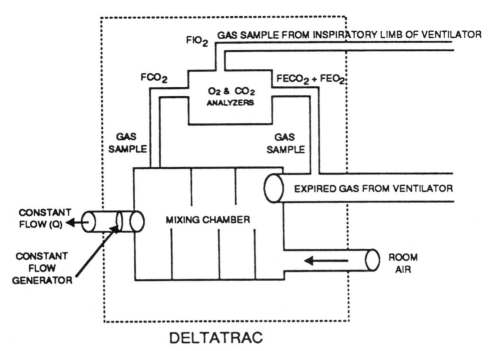

FIG 13–2.
A schematic of a dilution technique calorimeter (DeltaTrac). When a study is performed gathering exhaled gas from a canopy instead of a ventilator, no gas is drawn from the room. Instead, the entire volume of gas required is drawn through the canopy. (*From Weissman CW, Sadar A, Kemper MA: In vitro evaluation of a compact metabolic measurement instrument. JPEN 1990; 14:216–221. Used by permission.*)

Breath-by-Breath Technique

As indicated by its descriptive classification, this technique analyzes F_{IO_2}, F_{EO_2}, F_{ECO_2}, and tidal volume measurements on each breath. This obviates the need for a mixing chamber and provides immediate data on changes in V_{O_2} and V_{CO_2} (Fig 13–3). This allows the operator to see responses to therapy as well as detect system leaks or other malfunctions quickly. Tidal volume values are averaged over a period of time to calculate minute ventilation.

Breath-to-breath systems can be used on spontaneously ventilating patients who are breathing room air, supplemental oxygen, or receiving CPAP as well as on patients who are being mechanically ventilated. They employ the same types of gas analysis and volume measuring devices as mixing chamber systems.

Closed-Circuit Systems

Closed systems require the patient to inspire each tidal volume from a closed chamber and then return it on exhalation to that same chamber. A standard infrared analyzer determines

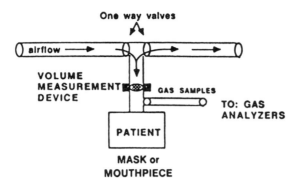

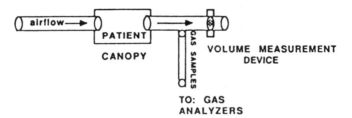

FIG 13–3.
The breath-by-breath calorimeter's gas flow patterns and sampling sites for both mechanically ventilated patients or patients breathing supplemental oxygen (*top*) and for canopy studies (*bottom*). (*From Kemper MA: Indirect calorimetry equipment and practical considerations of measurement, in: Weissman C (ed): Problems in Respiratory Care: Nutrition and respiratory disease. Philadelphia, JB Lippincott Co, 1989; 2:479–490. Used by permission.*)

the CO_2 content of the exhaled gas so that Vco_2 may be calculated. The carbon dioxide is then removed by passing the expired gas through a soda lime CO_2 absorber before it returns to the spirometer. This type of design is somewhat simpler since it does not utilize an oxygen analyzer but instead determines Vo_2 by measuring the volume lost from the closed system as metabolism occurs. This technique also offers the advantage of being able to perform studies on Fio_2's of 1.0.

Oxygen Replenishment Technique

The closed system illustrated in Figure 13–4 allows the patient to breath to-and-fro from a filled bellows. As oxygen is consumed, a like amount is added to the system by a precisely controlled oxygen flow source. The replenishment is controlled by monitoring changes in the bellows position with an ultrasonic sensor. This method of Vo_2 measurement has been

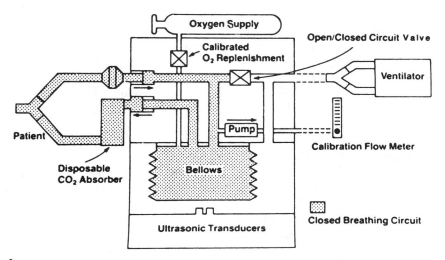

FIG 13–4.
A schematic of the closed-circuit oxygen replenishment technique calorimeter. Changes in the bellows position between the beginning of an inspiration and the end of the following expiration are detected by the ultrasonic transducer below the bellows. The V_{O_2} is determined from this position change. (*Courtesy Vital Signs, Totawa, New Jersey.*)

demonstrated to be very accurate compared to other methods.[26–28] Carbon dioxide production is determined with a standard infrared CO_2 analyzer supplying F_{ECO_2} and the ultrasonic sensor providing V_E data. Calculation of V_{CO_2} is the product of the two.

One of the limitations of closed systems is encountered when interfacing them with mechanical ventilators. This requires that the ventilator be connected not to the patient but to the chamber surrounding the bellows. Tidal volumes delivered by the ventilator enter the chamber, compressing the bellows, which then drives a like volume from the bellows into the patient. This increases the compressible volume of the breathing circuit significantly. To deliver a specific tidal volume to the patient, the ventilator must deliver the desired V_T plus an additional amount equal to the volume compressed in the calorimeter. The higher the ventilating pressures, the greater the compressed volume and the ventilator must therefore deliver an even greater total volume. Unless inspiratory flow rates are increased, inspiratory times can be unacceptably extended. Also, spontaneous triggering of the ventilator is impaired creating an increase in the work of breathing for the patient. The only way to compensate for this last problem is to adjust the ventilator frequency,[28] which then alters the work of breathing (and hence the metabolic rate) of the patient. By increasing the set ventilator rate to match or exceed the patient's spontaneous rate, triggering work may be reduced. Also, by increasing the set ventilator rate the set V_T may not need to be significantly increased. Therefore, the patient's minute ventilation may be maintained while avoiding the need to force the ventilator to deliver unacceptably large (and slow) tidal volumes. This alteration in patient work and breathing pattern may invalidate the study.

Another problem associated with the all-closed-circuit techniques is that changes in FRC will effect the V_{O_2} measurements. Since it is a closed circuit, a rise in Functional Residual Capacity (FRC) will transfer a volume of gas from the spirometer into the patient's lungs. This decrease of gas volume in the spirometer will be interpreted as a volume of oxygen consumed. Conversely, a decrease of FRC will add volume to the spirometer and be erroneously reported as a decrease in V_{O_2}.

Last, canopy measurements are not possible. Studies on spontaneously breathing patients must be performed using either a face mask or with a mouthpiece and nose clip.

Oxygen Depletion Technique

Using a design similar to the oxygen replenishment technique, this system differs by not adding oxygen to the circuit as it is consumed (Fig 13–5). Oxygen consumption is measured by a loss of volume as recorded by a spirometer.

In addition to the problems described above that are associated with closed-circuit calorimeters, this design also poses the potential threat of allowing the F_{IO_2} of the gas in the closed circuit to fall below therapeutic (or even ambient) levels if the study is performed at some F_{IO_2} below 1.0. If the study was performed with the spirometer filled with room air ($F_{IO_2} = 0.21$), the patient during the course of the test would consume oxygen, thus lowering the F_{IO_2} to subambient levels. This is avoided by filling the spirometer with 100% oxygen prior to starting the study.

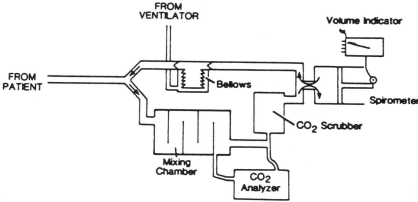

FIG 13–5.
A schematic of the closed-circuit oxygen depletion technique calorimeter. Decreases in the volume contained in the spirometer between the start and the end of the test determine the oxygen consumed. Failure to fill the spirometer with 100% oxygen at the start of the test can result in the patient breathing a hypoxic gas mixture. (*From Branson RD: The measurement of energy expenditure: Instrumentation, practical considerations and clinical application.* Respir Care *1990; 35:640–659. Used by permission.*)

MAINTENANCE OF AN INDIRECT CALORIMETER

Maintaining precise calibration of an indirect calorimetry system is essential in order to obtain accurate physiologic data. The three basic components whose accuracy and function must be verified daily are the oxygen analyzing cell, the infrared carbon dioxide analyzer, and the volume measuring device.

The heart and soul of an indirect calorimeter are its gas analyzers and volume measuring device. Carbon dioxide analysis is almost exclusively performed using the infrared light absorption technique. By placing a sampling cell between an infrared source and a photometer, the amount of CO_2 of a gas sample being aspirated through the cell can be determined. Contamination of the cell by water or debris will result in an overestimation in the level of CO_2. Also, the aspirating pump must function within certain specified parameters to ensure accurate operation.

Perhaps the most difficult sensor to develop was the oxygen sensor. Oxygen sensors require an accuracy of four decimal places since the difference between the F_{IO_2} and the F_{EO_2} can be extremely small. They also require a reliability factor which allows that accuracy to be maintained while the calorimeter is transported to numerous study locations.

Open-circuit calorimeters generally employ oxygen sensors that are either a paramagnetic analyzer or a zirconia cell. The paramagnetic device depends on the magnetic properties of oxygen to apply torque to a quartz crystal. This in turn produces a specific electrical potential related to the oxygen concentration. These sensors are fragile and frequent jarring and vibrations can have deleterious effects on their accuracy.

Zirconia cells use the migration of oxygen ions across the cell wall to create an electrical potential. The unique feature of this technique is that the zirconia cell must be maintained at a temperature of 700 to 800°C to function.[29] Frequent temperature changes can shorten the cell's life so there may be some advantage to leaving calorimeters with this type of sensor turned on at all times. It is also important to protect them from contamination with excess water vapor. While the heated zirconia sensors may fare better if left on continuously, the pumps that draw gas samples through the system will receive less wear and tear if they are turned off when not in use. Since the calorimeter must be unplugged for transport, it should be allowed a warm-up period similar to the time spent in transit.

Sensor Calibration

Both gas analyzers are generally exposed to two calibration gases. The first is a low point calibration conveniently using ambient atmosphere for the control. Room air will provide a stable F_{IO_2} of 0.209 and a F_{ICO_2} of 0.0003 (or essentially 0.0). The only potential error in this part of the calibration process occurs if the calibration is performed in an area where the environment is contaminated with a constant flow of above-ambient oxygen. This could happen if calibration was done, for example, at an intensive care unit (ICU) bedside where an oxygen administration device was inadvertently positioned near the gas entrainment port of the calorimeter. A calibration performed away from this type of potential interference will eliminate this source of error.

A second high point calibration is then done using a precisely analyzed gas usually containing a mixture of 95% oxygen and 5% carbon dioxide. The exact composition of the mixture may vary, and one may choose to use a combination that more closely matches the clinical range in which the study will be done (for example, $O_2 = 0.400$ and $CO_2 = 0.035$). This gas is usually provided by the manufacturer and is often continuously attached to the monitor to allow periodic, automatic recalibrations. The specific methods of calibration may vary depending on the manufacturer, but failure to meet the high and low controls in either O_2 or CO_2 analyzers renders the monitor inoperative.

Most open-circuit calorimeters use a pneumotachograph, a turbine spirometer, or heated wire to measure gas volumes and these must be accurate within a range of 0.01 to 2.0 L. Calibration of these devices is generally accomplished by providing specific amounts of room air through the monitor with a pulmonary function calibration syringe. These 1- to 3-L syringes provide precise volumes and allow the operator to establish quickly an accurate gas volume measurement. By entering into the calorimeter the expected calibration volume, internal gain and span controls will be automatically adjusted until the volume monitoring device agrees with the delivered volume. Again, with the fully automated calorimeters currently manufactured, little interaction is required by the operator other than correct delivery of the specific volume of gas at a flow rate that does not violate the linear threshold of the device. High delivered flow, during calibration may render the monitor insensitive to small tidal volumes or the low flows that can occur at the end of a breath. A failure to achieve proper volume calibration will generally require service by a qualified individual.

Closed-circuit calorimeters measure V_{O_2} without the use of an oxygen analyzer but still require the standard calibration of their CO_2 analyzer. Although they measure volumes by analyzing spirometer (or bellows) displacement, the volume calibration procedure is similar.

Total System Validation

Once the individual accuracy of the gas analyzers and volume monitoring device is verified, it may be prudent periodically to ascertain that the interaction between them is appropriate. One goal of a calorimeter is to produce an RQ that requires input from all three along with the cooperation of other essential calorimeter components such as gas drying mechanisms, blowers, and miscellaneous electrical systems, and software algorithms. Testing the entire system operation can be useful. This has been described using several techniques, some specific to individual devices. One method[30] is to use a methanol flame chamber as a substitute for a patient (Fig 13–6). The predicted RQ produced during the combustion of this alcohol is 0.67. This system has been shown to be reliable and is offered as a calibration aid designed for use with the dilution technique calorimeter (DeltaTrac, SensorMedics Corp, Yorba Linda, CA) though it may be adaptable for calibrating other systems.

Another method[31, 32] described utilizes a butane flame (giving an RQ of 0.615) controlled by a soap film bubble flowmeter and a rather complicated test circuit (Fig 13–7). This system appears compatible with most calorimeters and permits normal operation of the monitor during mechanical ventilation and, in place of the patient, provides a "metabolically active" control. The complexity of the circuity of Figure 13–7 and its use of uncommon components make it

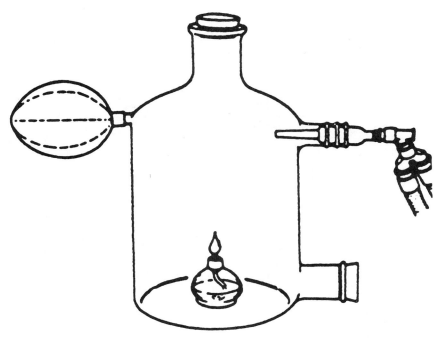

FIG 13–6.
A calorimeter validation device that uses a methanol flame in a closed system to produce an RQ of 0.67. (*From Damask MC, Weissman C, Askanazi J, et al: A systematic method for validation of gas exchange measurements. Anesthesiol 1982; 57:213–218. Used by permission.*)

somewhat difficult to construct. Also both of the above techniques' dependency on an open flame require the operator to exercise a degree of caution when they are in use.

The method depicted in Figure 13–8 avoids the use of an open flame and may offer (arguably) a simpler and more readily available apparatus. This system utilizes a two-chambered test lung (Model 1600 TTL, Michigan Instruments Inc, Grand Rapids, MI), which is configured such that one lung is a "master lung," which receives a VT of room air gas from a ventilator. The master lung is connected by a metal latch to a "slave lung." As the master lung is inflated, it causes the slave lung to be raised (or to "inspire") at the same time. Both lungs are separated by a series of one-way valves. The slave lung inspires from a Douglas bag filled with a precisely analyzed mixture of 17.5% oxygen, 4% carbon dioxide, and the balance of nitrogen. During expiration, the master lung's volume is directed out of the test circuit by a second exhalation valve, which operates synchronously with the ventilator's. The "metabolized" gas (gas that is consistent with normal exhaled concentrations) drawn from the Douglas bag by the slave lung is directed through the expiratory limb of the ventilator circuit. A one-way valve between the Douglas bag and the slave lung prevents any gas from reentering the Douglas bag. To the calorimeter that is connected appropriately to the standard ventilator circuit, it appears that the "patient" has inspired fresh gas and exhaled metabolized gas.

BF Bacterial filter

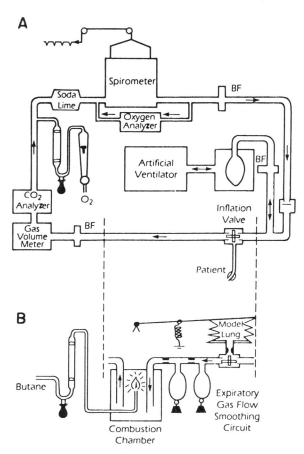

FIG 13–7.
The schematic illustrates, **A,** a closed-circuit O_2 replenishment calorimeter, although an open system could be substituted, interfaced with a validation apparatus that uses a butane flame to consume O_2 and produce CO_2. **B,** the validation circuit employs a series of capacitance bags and resistors to smooth the flow of gas through the apparatus. (*From Nunn JF, Makita K, Royston B: Validation of oxygen consumption measurements during artificial ventilation. J Appl Physiol 1989; 67:2129–2134. Used by permission.*)

The calibration gas must be accurately analyzed to the fourth decimal place (for example, for oxygen a F_{IO_2} of 0.1753) to allow for adequate resolution of the gas analyzer. Given this gas mixture, an RQ of 0.70 would be obtained. The circuitry of this system can be modified to test a calorimeter for proper function during mechanical ventilation, hood or canopy studies, or mouthpiece or face mask studies. Once the function of the calorimeter is confirmed, it may be taken to the bedside where the real challenge awaits.

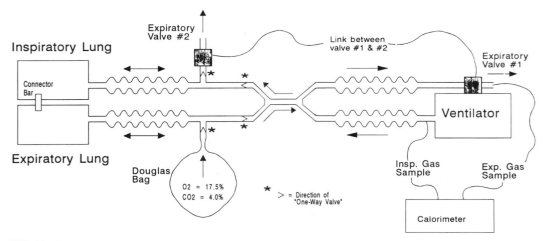

FIG 13–8.
The validation appratus shown uses a two-chambered test lung with appropriate valving to separate the gas delivered on inspiration to one chamber from the gas exhausted from the other. A Douglas bag filled with gas consistent with normal exhaled gas mimics a patients Vo_2 and Vco_2 without an open flame.

THE PATIENT INTERFACE

Metabolic studies are performed on patients under three distinct conditions: (1) patients spontaneously breathing room air studied with a canopy, (2) patients breathing unassisted but receiving supplemental oxygen (with or without PEEP being applied), which requires the patient to use a mouthpiece or face mask, or (3) patients being mechanically ventilated. Each circumstance requires some adjustment in study technique.

Canopy Studies

Studying the spontaneously breathing patient who is not receiving supplemental oxygen is perhaps the simplest procedure to perform. Most open-circuit calorimeters come with a canopy system (Fig 13–9), which allows the patient to be studied comfortably in the supine position. The canopy is placed over the patient's head and connected to the calorimeter.

The calorimeter, when configured for this type of study, will draw a specific flow of gas from the room through the canopy. Large gaps between the patient and the canopy should be avoided, but there is no need to enclose the patient tightly since the system requires room air to enter the hood in an unrestricted fashion. It is important that the patient remain quiet. Upper body or arm movement can create a "bellows" effect and cause some exhaled gas to escape from the canopy and not be drawn through the monitor. This will cause the Vo_2 and Vco_2 to be reduced and result in inaccurate estimations of energy expenditures. The canopy

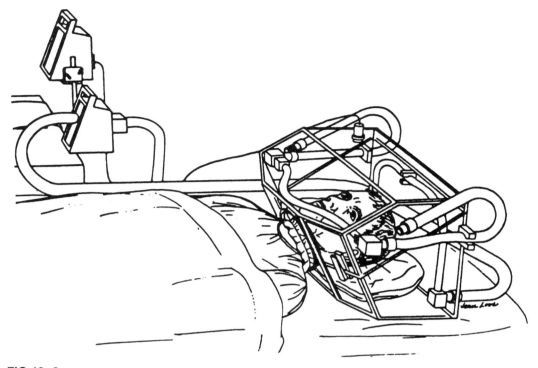

FIG 13–9.
An example of a canopy device that covers the patient's head during spontaneous ventilation with room air. It is impossible to employ this technique if the patient requires supplemental oxygen since the F_{IO_2} sample is obtained from the ambient atmosphere. (*From Branson RD: The measurement of energy expenditure: Instrumentation, practical considerations and clinical application.* Respir Care 1990; 35:640–659. *Used by permission.*)

method is not applicable to closed-circuit calorimeters since those systems require the patient to inhale and exhale their entire minute ventilation through the monitor during the test.

Mouthpiece/Mask Studies

Spontaneously breathing patients receiving supplemental oxygen may be the most difficult group on which to perform a metabolic study. The canopy technique is not applicable since the patient's entire minute ventilation must be inspired from a controlled oxygen source and exhaled into the calorimeter. The canopy would allow contamination of the supplemental oxygen with room air, causing an instability of the F_{IO_2}. Therefore, an oxygen administration circuit must be used that provides an adequate flow rate and a inspiratory gas reservoir that ensures the patient's inspiratory flow demands are met during the test. The gas delivery system must provide a stable F_{IO_2}, which makes a venturi-based O_2 therapy device inappropriate for these studies. During the course of the study, a simple option is to use an air/O_2 blender to provide a stable high flow of precisely controlled supplemental oxygen. Since excess water can adversely effect the calorimeter's sensors, continuous aerosol generators should be replaced with nonaerosol generating humidifiers if humidification is required during the test.

The patient must breathe through a mouthpiece or mask that is connected to a nonrebreathing valve. The nonrebreathing valve forces the patient to inspire from the oxygen source and exhale into the calorimeter. During exhalation, excess flow from the oxygen supply must be vented to the room to avoid any inadvertent increase in system pressure. This overpressure vent must be configured with a one-way valve, which prevents contamination of the inspiratory gas with room air. If PEEP (CPAP) is being applied to the patient, then a matching PEEP valve must be placed on the inspiratory limb overpressure vent to equalize pressures on both sides of the nonbreathing valve. Figure 13–10 illustrates a system that meets all of these criteria.

Once the circuity is properly assembled, the next challenge is to prevent any leaks during the study. The most common site of leaks is at the patient interface. If a mouthpiece is used, it should be the type with a built-in lip seal such as those commonly used for pulmonary function tests. The seal is placed between the lip and the gum and will help prevent ambient

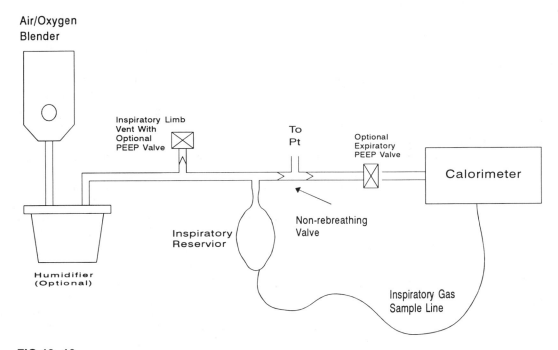

FIG 13–10.
A system for providing a stable F_{IO_2} with or without PEEP during a metabolic study. The humidifier may be included for patients with artificial airways in place. The nonrebreathing valve at the patient connection serves two purposes: (1) preventing rebreathing and (2) preventing the mixing of inspiratory and expiratory gases.

gas contamination during inspiration or an accidental loss of the patient's minute ventilation. Also a nose clip must be used to prevent nose breathing. Although the mouthpiece and nose clip may be tolerated well by a cooperative patient, others may find it uncomfortable, the nose clip may slip off, or the patient may simply fatigue and permit circuit leaks.

Replacing the nose clip and mouthpiece with a face mask may reduce the incidence of accidental leaks associated with patient cooperation. Unfortunately, maintaining a competent seal with a mask may not be much easier. With either system, any leak of exhaled gas out into the room will result in lower Vo_2 and Vco_2 measurements. On the other hand, if room air is entrained during inspiration, the Vo_2 will appear to climb dramatically on that breath.

Mask or mouthpiece studies require diligent and continuous observation by the clinician. The patient should be evaluated for changes in work of breathing caused by the circuit. Sudden alterations in Vo_2 or Vco_2 merit an assessment of the circuit and patient interface for leaks.

Mechanical Ventilation Studies

A well-calibrated and -maintained indirect calorimeter can provide a simple and accurate assessment of the energy expenditure of many mechanically ventilated patients. There are some limitations, depending on the type of monitor used.

The closed-circuit calorimeter, as previously discussed, separates the patient from the ventilator. Volumes delivered by the ventilator are used to drive similar volumes out of the calorimeter and into the patient. This design makes the delivery of any constant flow from the ventilator to the patient impossible. The discontinuance of this constant flow during the study can cause a change in breathing pattern or alter the work of breathing for the patient. Also the interference with the patient's ability to trigger the ventilator and any alterations in set rates and delivered volumes, and changes in inspiratory times must be considered before proceeding with a measurement of energy expenditure. Under some conditions, studies may be impossible or inappropriate to perform.

The function of open-circuit calorimeters is complicated by the presence of a constant flow in the breathing circuit. If the open-circuit system is to correctly measure V_E, the inspiratory and expiratory gases must be separated. This is accomplished with the placement of a second synchronously operating exhalation valve at the patient's airway, which directs exhaled gas into the monitor without contaminating it with the constant flow gas[33, 34] (Fig 13–11).

These valves may interfere with the patient's ability to trigger the ventilator since they include a one-way valve between the patient and the constant flow in the breathing circuit. When they are used, patients should be assessed for any alterations in breathing patterns caused by the valve's inclusion in the breathing circuit. Ventilators that provide flow from a demand valve in response to spontaneous efforts by the patient do not need this adaptation and expired gas can be collected from the exhaust port of the ventilator.

The volume of gas compressed in the ventilator circuit will not affect the measurement of Vo_2 and Vco_2 although V_E will be mildly overestimated.[35]

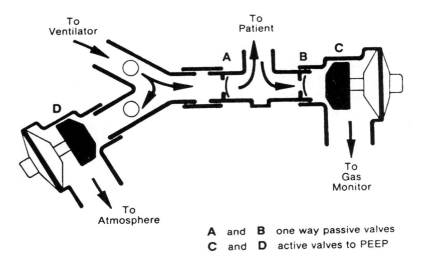

A and B one way passive valves
C and D active valves to PEEP

FIG 13–11.
The valve system shown prevents the exhaled gas from the patient from being contaminated by any constant flow gas in the ventilator circuit. The two pneumatically powered exhalation valves (C and D) are controlled by the ventilator and operate synchronously, applying equal levels of PEEP and opening and closing simultaneously. (*From Nelson LD, Anderson HB, Garcia H: Clinical validation of a new metabolic monitor suitable for use in critical care patients.* Crit Care Med *1987; 15:951–957. Used by permission.*)

TECHNICAL CONSIDERATIONS

Numerous technical requirements must be met in order to ensure an accurate and reproducible assessment of energy expenditure. Careful setup of the testing apparatus and frequent assessment of its operation is necessary.

F_{IO_2} Stability

Open-circuit calorimeters generally only make periodic measurements of the inspired oxygen concentrations. Because of this, fluctuations in the delivered oxygen concentration will result in serious errors in measuring REE.[36] Some ventilators may utilize gas blending mechanisms, which include internal reservoirs that dampen any minor fluctuations, thus providing stable inspiratory oxygen concentrations. Other ventilators with proportional solenoid gas delivery valves may have very small internal volumes. Consequently, they may not provide adequate F_{IO_2} stability to perform a metabolic study. These normal fluctuations are clinically insignificant but when performing a metabolic study it is necessary to modify the gas supply to the ventilator by attaching both high-pressure air and oxygen inlet hoses to the single high-pressure outlet of an air/O_2 blender and preblend the air and oxygen to the desired concentration before it enters the ventilator. The ventilator is then operated with its F_{IO_2} control set to 1.0. This should be done any time the clinician suspects fluctuations in the delivered oxygen concentration of any ventilator.

Those calorimeters that measure F_{IO_2} and F_{ECO_2} on a breath-to-breath basis minimize the effect of fluctuating F_{IO_2}. Closed-circuit systems also avoid this complication because the patient takes and returns his or her entire minute ventilation from the calorimeter. As previously described, one closed-circuit system, the MRM-6000 (Waters Instrument Inc, Rochester, MN), measures V_{O_2} by the volume depletion of the closed system, and the F_{IO_2} can fall as the test progresses if the spirometer is not filled with 100% oxygen. This could lead to inadvertent administration of inadequate (or even subambient) levels of oxygen.[28] Another closed-circuit system, the VVR-Q (Vital Signs, Totowa, NJ) avoids this potential problem by adding oxygen at the rate at which it is consumed.

Limitations of High F_{IO_2}

Performing studies with open-circuit calorimeters at high F_{IO_2}'s will result in grossly magnified errors in V_{O_2} calculations of the F_{IO_2} is not stable.[37–40.] Newer open-circuit calorimeters are generally limited to measurements where the F_{IO_2} does not exceed 0.60 to 0.80 depending on the instrument, although some may be limited to maximum F_{IO_2}'s as low as 0.40. The reason for this F_{IO_2} limitation is the open-circuit system's dependence on the Haldane transformation equation to calculate V_{O_2}:

$$V_{O_2} = \frac{(1 - F_{EO_2} - F_{ECO_2})}{1 - F_{IO_2}} (F_{IO_2} - F_{EO_2}) \, V_E$$

As the F_{IO_2} increases, the denominator of the above formula becomes smaller (this results in the mathematical dilemma of the denominator equaling 0 when the F_{IO_2} is 1.0). It has been demonstrated that an F_{IO_2} analysis error of 0.01 at 0.40 will result in a 15% error in V_{O_2}, and a similar error at an F_{IO_2} of 0.80 will result in an error of greater than 90% in the calculation of the V_{O_2}.

Closed-circuit systems are not affected by high F_{IO_2}'s and can even produce an accurate V_{O_2} in the presence of 100% oxygen.

Effects of Other Gases

Aside from oxygen, carbon dioxide, and nitrogen the next most commonly encountered gas during a metabolic study is water vapor. Unfortunately, this gas will impair the function of both O_2 and CO_2 analyzers, pneumotachographs, and turbine spriometers.[41] Effectively removing excess water vapor from the analyzed gases is accomplished by various methods dependent on the design of the monitor. These methods include heating or cooling the sample gas,[42, 43] placing water traps or specially constructed tubing which allows the water vapor in the gas sampling line to equilibrate with that in the room,[44] or by drawing the sample gas through a chamber filled with a desiccant.[45]

Perhaps the most problematic of the above drying systems is the use of desiccants. This technique can slow the gas sampling time and the desiccant columns need to be changed frequently. They also create the potential for leaks that would contaminate the gas samples leading to errors. Each of the systems could fail, hence, the need for the periodically employing one of the methods described to validate the accurate performance of the calorimeter.

The other unusual gas (or gases) that may be encountered is an anesthetic agent. The presence of these agents creates errors in the Haldane transformation equaiton, which makes accurate tests impossible.

System Leaks

Both open- and closed-circuit systems are intolerant of any leak of expired gas out of the circuit or inadvertent entrainment of room air into the inspiratory sample. Circuits must be checked prior to beginning a study and periodically during its course.

Entrainment of room air into an inspiratory circuit that is intended to supply an F_{IO_2} greater than 0.209 will result in an unstable F_{IO_2} and the appearance of an increase in V_{O_2}. Leaks on the expiratory side will lower the measured V_E, V_{O_2}, and V_{CO_2}. These leaks, although commonly found in the breathing circuit, can also occur around the airway cuff or through chest tubes. Actively leaking chest tubes are a form of expiratory leak and will reduce the measured V_E and V_{CO_2} even though the F_{ECO_2} obtained from the airway may remain unchanged.[46] This would result in an accurate RQ but a grossly altered REE. Also, the nonventilatory extraction of CO_2 or the addition of oxygen to the blood, which occurs during extracorporeal membrane oxygenation (ECMO), makes the meaursrement of REE impossible.

In closed-circuit systems a volume leak out of the circuit is represented by a falsely elevated V_{O_2}. The accidental entrainment of room air into the system results in the opposite effect.

Maintaining a Portable System

When a monitor is turned off for transport to another location for a study, it should be allowed to warm up for the same period of time it was shut off.[35] Frequent transportation throughout a hospital invariably exposes the instrument to numerous jars and vibrations. For this reason, calibration should be done daily and periodic total system validation as described earlier should be performed at least monthly based on our clinical experience.

PROTOCOL DECISIONS

The presence of an indirect calorimeter is not in and of itself the hallmark of a quality nutritional assessment program. This is to a great extent dependent on having a systematic approach to who is tested, how they are tested, how often they are tested, and what is done with the data. One survey of nutritional support teams found that only 101 of 420 respondents owned indirect calorimeters and, of those, only 60 actually used them.[47] Of the 60 users, only 20 did more than 10 tests per month and 39 had no standard protocol for preforming studies. Studies have shown that attempting to predict appropriate nutritional support is difficult in many patients,[48-50] so providing a precise reproducible method of REE assessment would seem valuable. Given the cost of indirect calorimeters (approximately \$15,000 to \$40,000) an organized approach to utilizing them would seem to be a priority.

Patients who are candidates for periodic or serial testing are described in Table 13–4. It has been suggested that after the initial study, patients should be studied weekly or more frequently if their clinical picture is altered.[51] It is advocated that clinically unstable patients be studied two to three times per week.[52] The study should be performed after preparing the patient according to the guidelines described in Table 13–5 if possible. The goal of the guidelines is to achieve a resting metabolic state. Perhaps one of the greatest challenges is to prevent any interruptions or disturbances of the patient during the study period.

The length of measurement time will vary depending on the clinical conditions. Resting steady state should be achieved prior to beginning data collection. Monitoring the V_{O_2} for periods of its smallest variability (5 to 10%) may be an acceptable way of determining steady state. Once steady state is achieved, data collection should be done in most cases for 15 to 30 minutes. Some calorimeters will provide data that excludes variations in energy expenditure that exceed certain defined limits. This may be helpful in defining for that patient what is a resting state, but one could easily argue that measuring all expenditure levels gives a more accurate picture of the patient. Of course, Figure 13–12 clearly demonstrates that energy expenditure varies greatly during the course of 24 hours but the goal of data collection during steady state is to ensure that subsequent tests are performed in similar conditions.

Interaction between physicians, nutritionists, respiratory therapists, and nurses utilizing a well-calibrated and -maintained calorimeter and operated within the guidelines of a well-organized protocol can be of great clinical value. Without this collaboration and organization, an indirect calorimeter becomes an expensive and useless toy.

TABLE 13–4.
Target Patients for Metabolic Studies*

- Recipients of parental or enteral support
- Burn injuries
- Major surgery
- Multiple trauma
- Obesity/eating disorders
- Neuromuscular disease
- Organ failure
- Failure to wean from mechanical ventilation

* From Ref. 47.

TABLE 13–5.
Patient Preparation for a Metabolic Study*

• Supine position for more than 30 minutes prior to test
• Nothing by mouth for more than 2 hours prior to test
  or
  receiving continuous nutrient infusion
• Measurement performed in quiet thermoneutral surroundings
• No voluntary movement during testing
• Measurements should be made after a state of equilibrium has been reached.

* From Ref. 47.

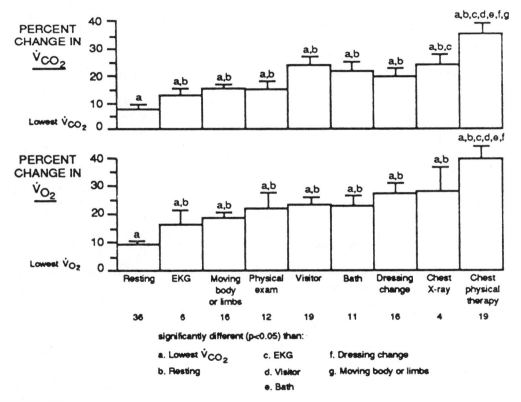

FIG 13–12.
Variations in the patient's V_{O_2} and V_{CO_2} from that of the resting state can be dramatic and accompany virtually every bedside activity. This serves to highlight the need for doing serial studies in the resting state so that like data may be compared. (*From Weissman C, Kemper M, Hyman AI: Variation in the resting metabolic rate of the mechanically ventilated critically ill patients.* Anesth Analg *1989; 68:457–461. Used by permission.*)

REFERENCES

1. Kleiber M: *The Fire of Life. An Introduction to Animal Energetics.* Huntington, NY, 1975. Robert E Kreiger Publishing Co, 1975.
2. Holmes FL: *Lavoisier and the Chemistry of Life. An Exploration of Scientific Creativity.* Madison, The University of Wisconsin Press, 1985.
3. Lusk G: *The Elements of the Science of Nutrition*, ed 4. Philadelphia, WB Saunders Co, 1928, pp. 18–20.
4. Ames SR: The joule—unit of energy. *J Am Dietet Assoc* 1970; 57:415–416.
5. Kleiber M: Joules versus calories in nutrition. *J Nutr* 1972; 102:309–312.
6. Brown NM: Armsby's calorimeter. *Nutr Today* 1990; July/Aug:7–12.
7. Atwater WO, Snell JF: Description of a bomb calorimeter and a method of its use. *J Am Chem Soc* 1903; 25:659–699.
8. Lusk G: Mementoes of Lavoisier: Trip to Chateau de la Caniere. *JAMA* 1925; 85:1246.
9. Lifson N, Gordon GB, McClintock R: Measurement of total carbon dioxide production by means of D_2O^{18}. *J Appl Physiol* 1955; 7:704–710.
10. Schoeller DA, Ravusin E, Schutz Y, et al: Energy expenditure by doubly labeled water: Validation in humans and proposed calculation. *Am J Physiol* 1986; 250:R823–R830.
11. Benedict FG: A portable respiration apparatus for clinical use. *Bost Med Surg J* 1918; 178:667–668.
12. Douglas F: A method for determining the total respiratory exchange in man. *J Physiol (Lond)* 1911; 42:xvii–xviii.
13. Grande F: Energy expenditure of organs and tissues, in: *Assessment of Energy Metabolism in Health and Disease. First Ross Conference on Medical Research.* Columbus, OH, Ross Laboratories, 1980, pp 88–92.
14. Holliday MA: Metabolic rate and organ size during growth from infancy to maturity and during late gestation and early infancy. *Pediatrics* 1971; 47:169–179.
15. Lusk G: Analysis of the oxidation of mixtures of carbohydrate and fat. A correction. *J. Biol Chem* 1924; 59:41–42.
16. Brown AC: CH-4 Energy metabolism. In Ruch TC, Patton HD (eds.) Howell's Textbook of Physiology and Biophysics ed 20, Vol III. Philadelphia, WB Saunders Co, 1973, p. 94.
17. Weir JB deV: New methods for calculating metabolic rate with special reference to protein metabolism. *J Physiol* 1949; 109:1–9.
18. Cunningham JJ: Calculation of energy expenditure from indirect calorimetry: assessment of the Weir equation. *Nutrition* 1990; 6:222–223.
19. Ferrannini E: The theoretical bases of indirect calorimetry: A review. *Metabolism* 1988; 37:287–301.
20. Cathcart EP, Cuthbertson DP: The composition and distribution of the fatty substances of the human subject. *J Physiol* 1931; 72:349–360.
21. Livesay G, Elia M: Estimation of energy expenditure, net carbohydrate utilization, and net fat oxidation and synthesis by indirect calorimetry: Evaluation of errors with special reference to the detailed composition of fuels. *Am J Clin Nutr* 1988; 47:608–628.
22. Elia M, Livesay G: Theory and validation of indirect calorimetry during net lipid synthesis. *Am J Clin Nutr* 1988; 47:591–607.
23. Bursztein S, Saphar S, Singer S, et al: A methematical analysis of indirect calorimetry measurements on acutely ill patients. *Am J Clin Nutr* 1989; 50:277–230.
24. Bach AC, Frey A, Lutz O: Clinical and experimental effects of medium-chain triglyceride-based fat emulsions: A review. *Clin Nutr* 1989; 8:223–225.
25. Weissman C: Measuring oxygen uptake in the clinical setting, in Bryan-Brown CW, Ayres SM (eds): *Oxygen Transport and Utilization.* Fullerton, CA, Society of Critical Care Medicine, 1987; pp 25–64.
26. Ravrich JM, Ibanez J, Marse P: Validation of a new closed circuit indirect calorimetry method compared with the open Douglas bag method. *Inten Care Med* 1989; 15:274–278.

27. Branson RD, Hurst JM, Davis K, et al: A laboratory evaluation of the Biergy VVR calorimeter. *Respir Care* 1988; 33:341–347.
28. Keppler T, Dechert RE, Arnoldi DK, et al: Evaluation of the Waters MRM-6000 and Biergy VVR closed circuit indirect calorimeters. *Respir Care* 1989; 34:28–35.
29. Kocache RMA, Swan J, Holman DF: A minature rugged and accurate solid electrolyte oxygen sensor. *J Physics Environ Sci Instrum* 1984; 17:447–482.
30. Damask MC, Weissman C, Askanazi J, et al: A systematic method for validation of gas exchange measurements. *Anesthesiol* 1982; 57:213–218.
31. Nunn JF, Makita K, Royston B: Validation of oxygen consumption measurements during artificial ventilation. *J Appl Physiol* 1989; 67:2129–2134.
32. Makita K, Nunn JF, Royston B: Evaluation of metabolic measuring instruments for use in critically ill patients. *Crit Care Med* 1990; 18:638–644.
33. Nelson LD, Anderson HB, Garcia H: Clinical validation of a new metabolic monitor suitable for use in critical care patients. *Crit Care Med* 1987; 15:951–957.
34. Head CA, Grossman GD, Jordan JC, et al: A valve system for the accurate measurement of energy expenditure in mechanically ventilated patients. *Respir Care* 1985; 30:969–973.
35. Kemper MA: Indirect calorimetry equipment and practical considerations of measurement, in Weissman C (ed): *Problems in Respiratory Care: Nutrition and Respiratory Disease.* Philadelphia, JB Lippincott CO, 1989; 2:479–490.
36. Browning JA, Lindberg SE, Turney SF, et al: The effects of fluctuating FIO2 on metabolic measurements in mechanically ventilated patients. *Crit Care Med* 1982; 10:82–85.
37. Ultman JS, Bursztein S: Analysis of error in the determination of respiratory gas exchange at varying FIO2. *J Appl Physiol* 1981; 50:210–216.
38. Weissman CW, Sadar A, Kemper MA: In vitro evaluation of a compact metabolic measurement instrument. *JPEN* 1990; 14:216–221.
39. Takala J, Keinanen O, Vaisanen P, et al: Measurement of gas exchange in intensive care: Laboratory and clinical evaluation of a new device. *Crit Care Med* 1989; 17:1041–1047.
40. Halmagyi DFJ, Kinney JM: Metabolic rate in active respiratory failure complicating sepsis. *Surgery* 1975; 77:492–499.
41. Norton AC: Accuracy in pulmonary measurement. *Respir Care* 1979; 24:131–137.
42. Bohrn S, Hogman B, Olsson S, et al: A new device for continuous measurement of gas exchange during mechanical ventilation. *Crit Care Med* 1980; 8:705–709
43. Metabolic gas monitor operator's manual. Midvale, UT, Utah Medical Products, 1988.
44. DeltaTrac metabolic monitor operator's manual. Yorba Linda, CA, SensorMedics Corp.
45. Metascope operator's manual. Louisville, CO, Cybermedic, 1990.
46. Bishop MJ, Benson MS, Pierson DJ: Carbon dioxide excretion via bronchopleural fistulas in adult respiratory distress syndrome. *Chest* 1989; 91:400–404.
47. Campbell SM, Kudsk KA: "High tech" metabolic measurements: Useful in daily clinical practice? *JPEN* 1988; 12:610–612.
48. Daly JM, Heymsfield SB, Head CA, et al: Human energy requirements: Overestimation by widely used prediction equation. *Am J Clin Nutr* 1985; 42:1170–1174.
49. Schane J, Goede M, Silverstein P: Comparison of energy expenditure measurement techniques in severly burned patients. *J Burn Care Rehab* 1987; 8:366–370.
50. Hunter DC, Jaksic T, Lewis D, et al: Resting energy expenditure in the critically ill: Estimation versus measurement. *Br J Surg* 1988; 75:875–878.
51. Mullen J, Feurer ID: Protocol: Indirect calorimetric measurement of resting energy expenditure. Philadelphia, Hospital of the University of Pennsylvania 1986.
52. Weissman C, Kamper M, Hyman AI: Variation in the resting metabolic rate of the mechanically ventilated critically ill patients. *Anesth Analg* 1989; 68:457–461.

Chapter 14

Cardiovascular Function

David P. Meeker, M.D.

Herbert P. Wiedemann, M.D.

INTRODUCTION

The introduction of the balloon-tipped pulmonary artery catheter in the early 1970s ushered in a new era of clinical medicine. Enamored, and perhaps overly emboldened by the new technology, physicians applied it widely. Invasive monitoring of cardiovascular function became, and still remains, an integral and virtually routine aspect of intensive care.[1]

Despite its widespread application and apparent value in the management of critically ill patients, invasive monitoring has certain major drawbacks. The most important disadvantage of invasive monitoring is the inherent physical risk to the patient. The application of invasive monitoring techniques also tends to be time-consuming and labor intensive. Coincident with the growing appreciation of the disadvantages of invasive monitoring, new technological developments are raising the prospects that reliable and practical methods of noninvasive cardiovascular monitoring may become available in the foreseeable future.[2]

This chapter reviews the emerging, and still evolving, methods by which blood pressure and cardiac output can be measured noninvasively.

NONINVASIVE MONITORING OF ARTERIAL BLOOD PRESSURE

Normal Arterial Pressures and Traditional Invasive Monitoring

The current standard practice in seriously ill patients is to measure systemic blood pressure by invasive arterial cannulation and direct transduction of the pressure waveform.[1] The method is reliable and accurate when utilized correctly and therefore is considered the "gold standard" for measuring arterial pressure. For this reason, and in view of its relative safety, peripheral artery cannulation is commonly performed in intensive care units (ICUs) and operating rooms.

The radial artery usually is chosen due to its accessibility and generally good collateral circulation supplied by the ulnar artery. However, pheripheral artery cannulation can be performed at other sites, including the brachial, femoral, dorsalis pedis, and axillary arteries.

It is important to recognize that the arterial pressure and waveform changes as the pressure wave travels from the proximal aorta toward the periphery. As the arterial pressure wave moves distally from the aorta, there is a gradual increase in systolic pressure and a gradual decrease in diastolic pressure, whereas mean pressure remains relatively constant.[3] Thus, for example, femoral artery pressure more closely approximates aortic pressure than does radial artery pressure. The systolic pressure can increase as much as 15 to 20 mm Hg from the central aorta to the brachial artery, but in normal adults, much less change occurs between the brachial and radial arteries.

It is helpful to remember the "site-specific" nature of arterial pressure when evaluating investigations reporting the accuracy (or inaccuracy) of noninvasive pressure monitoring techniques. For example, the systolic and diastolic pressures recorded from the new noninvasive finger cuff devices should not be expected to correspond precisely to simultaneous intra-arterial pressures measured from a brachial artery catheter. Furthermore, it is worthwhile pointing out that under certain pathophysiologic conditions, normal assumptions regarding the relative blood pressure relationships at different anatomic sites may not hold. Stern et al.[4] found reversal of the usual relationship between aortic and radial artery pressure in patients following cardiopulmonary bypass. Relative to aortic pressure, radial artery systolic (and often radial mean) pressures were lower immediately after cardiopulmonary bypass than before bypass. In many patients, the pressure difference was large enough to be clinically significant (12 to 32 mm Hg). The change persisted for 10 to 60 minutes, gradually returning toward normal, and seemed to be associated with rewarming at the end of bypass and lowered forearm vascular resistance. These findings suggest that pressure relationships could potentially be altered in a variety of other circumstances (e.g., vasopressor use, sepsis, peripheral vascular disease) that have yet to be studied extensively. Thus, although radial artery pressure is frequently utilized as a "gold standard," it may not always consistently reflect central arterial pressure.

Although peripheral artery cannulation can be performed reasonably safely in clinical settings, there is some risk of local infection or arterial occlusion and embolization. In addition, cannulation must be performed by trained personnel. These considerations are stimulating the development of automated noninvasive monitoring devices.

Methods for Automated Noninvasive Blood Pressure Measurement

Although blood pressure can be measured noninvasively via the manually operated sphygmomanometer, this technique is not ideal or practical in settings where continuous or very frequent monitoring is necessary. Development of automated noninvasive monitors has generally proceeded along one of two lines: (1) the oscillometric method or (2) the Penaz method.[5]

Oscillometric Technique

The majority of automated noninvasive monitors utilizes some variant of the oscillometric method.[6] The first commercially viable device became available in 1976 under the trade name

Dinamap (an acronym for "device for indirect noninvasive mean arterial pressure"). The first Dinamap model measured only mean arterial pressure, since with the oscillometric technique this is a more reliable and accurate measurement than either systolic or diastolic pressures. This is true because mean arterial pressure is measured when oscillations of cuff pressure reach the greatest magnitude. Later models of the Dinamap measured and displayed the systolic and diastolic pressures also, in a concession to the clinical tradition of recording these values.

The principles that govern the oscillometric method have been reviewed recently in detail.[6] Briefly, the process depends on the detection of oscillations—and quantification of their amplitude—during automated stepwise decrements (usually 5 mm Hg intervals) of cuff pressure. Various algorithms have been utilized to translate these data into arterial pressures, and further refinements continue to be tested and recommended. Simply put, the systolic blood pressure is the cuff pressure where the amplitude of oscillations increases rapidly, and the diastolic pressure is where such amplitude decreases rapidly. The mean arterial pressure is generally the lowest cuff pressure with the greatest oscillation amplitude.

The oscillometric technique has certain inherent limitations and problems. Low pulse pressure and significant hypotension may reduce the amount of oscillation to the degree that only mean arterial pressure is measurable and, in extreme situations, even mean pressure may be unmeasurable. Another problem is the presence of motion artifact, especially when the motion is rhythmic, as may occur during patient shivering (or seizures) or during transport in ambulances and helicopters. During such circumstances, the algorithm-based measurements are confounded and machine performance degrades. Often, stabilization of the limb around which the cuff is placed will allow for accurate results.

Penaz Method

The method of Penaz[5] is utilized by the Finapress device, a new noninvasive automatic blood pressure monitor that provides continuous blood pressure and arterial waveform display by means of a finger cuff.[7] The Penaz method relies on the volume-clamp principle. Circumferential pressure applied by a finger cuff can be varied in order to maintain constant digital arterial size (as assessed by a photoplethysmograph); under such circumstances, the cuff pressure equals arterial pressure. A rapidly responding servomechanism continuously adjusts finger cuff pressure to maintain zero transmural arterial pressure; the stored cuff pressure trace is used to derive arterial pressures (systolic, mean, diastolic) and heart rate.[7, 8]

Clinical Evaluation of Noninvasive Blood Pressure Monitors

The accuracy of both the Dinamap and Finapress devices has been studied rather extensively in various clinical settings, although head-to-head comparisons of the two devices are few. Experience with the Dinamap is far greater, since this device was introduced much earlier. Furthermore, the Finapress is currently in a more dynamic phase of its development, with comparatively more rapid and significant improvements in the finger cuff and calculation algorithms occurring recently. Thus, current studies may not be directly comparable with previous investigations.

According to standards recommended by the Association for the Advancement of Medical

Instrumentation (AAMI), blood pressure devices should have an accuracy of less than 5 mm Hg mean error with a standard deviation of less than 8 mm Hg when compared with an arterial catheter.[6] In most studies, the Dinamap device fulfills these criteria, but with some important exceptions in individual patients.[6] Some factors that cause problems with Dinamap measurements include patient shivering or seizures, external vibrations (e.g., ambulance or helicopter transport), shock (with low pulse pressure and vasoconstriction), and large cyclic or beat-to-beat variations of blood pressure (10 to 50 mm Hg within 4 to 15 seconds) or pulse rate (beat-to-beat variation greater than 15%), which may occur during mechanical ventilation, hypovolemia, and dysrhythmias.[6]

Venus et al.[9] evaluated the Dinamap in 43 critically ill patients requiring extensive hemodynamic monitoring in ICUs. The Dinamap underestimated systolic blood pressure by a mean of 9.2 ± 16.4 mm Hg and overestimated diastolic blood pressure by a mean of 8.7 ± 10.6 mm Hg. Although mean arterial pressure was measured more accurately than systolic or diastolic pressures, significant individual variation was still observed. Gravlee and Brockschmidt[10] studied 38 adults undergoing cardiac surgery; all patients had a pulmonary artery catheter in place to monitor circulatory hemodynamics. They found that the relationship between Dinamap and directly measured blood pressure varied substantially over time, sometimes with systemic hemodynamic conditions. The accuracy guidelines proposed by AAMI (intrapatient mean error less than 5 mm Hg; SD less than 8 mm Hg) were not reliably fulfilled.

The accuracy of the Finapress device may be affected by hypothermia, low cardiac output, hypotension, vasoconstrictor drugs, one-lung anesthesia, and poor physical condition.[11, 12] However, the presence of peripheral vascular disease did not seem to affect performance of the device in one study.[13] Very recently published studies have evaluated the performance of the Finapress during the induction of anesthesia and during open heart or other major surgery.[8, 12, 14, 15] Each of these studies concluded that currently available Finapress devices are insufficiently accurate for routine clinical use. Although accurate readings were obtained in many patients most of the time, significant deviations occurred. Of further concern, many of these deviations appeared to be random and not clearly associated with clinical events known or suspected to affect Finapress accuracy. It is likely that the performance would even be worse than that observed in these four studies[8, 12, 14, 15] if the Finapress was evaluated in patients with hypotension, cardiac arrest, or major dysrhythmia.

Few studies have directly compared the Finapress and Dinamap in individual patients. Gorback, Quill, and Levine[16] concluded that the two devices were equally accurate for diastolic and mean arterial pressures in 32 patients undergoing general anesthesia. Epstein, Huffnagle, and Bartkowski[17] evaluated 10 patients undergoing general anesthesia, and found that the Dinamap was more reliable, chiefly due to the fact the Finapress was markedly inaccurate in 20% of the study population (the same percentage of Finapress "outliers" these investigators had found in an earlier study[8]). In those cases where the Dinamap and Finapress measurements exhibited discrepancies, the Dinamap correlated much more closely with directly measured intra-arterial pressure.

In summary, present techniques for automated noninvasive measurement do not meet standards for ideal clinical performance, especially when circulatory instability exists. However, future technological advances may allow for reliable indirect blood pressure measurements.

NONINVASIVE MEASUREMENT OF CARDIAC OUTPUT

Development of the Swan-Ganz catheter has made invasive monitoring of cardiac output (CO) routine in the intensive care and intraoperative setting.[1] In addition to the inherent disadvantages of invasive monitoring in the inpatient settting, invasive measurement of cardiac ouput is rarely appropriate in the outpatient setting. Doppler ultrasound and transthoracic electrical bioimpedance (TEB) are two promising noninvasive technologies for measurement of CO.

Doppler Ultrasound

Doppler Principle

The Doppler effect was originally described by Johann Christian Doppler[18, 19] in 1842. A century later, this principle was extended to the noninvasive measurement of cardiac output.[20, 21]

The Doppler principle states that an apparent shift in the transmitted frequency of sound occurs as a result of motion of either the source or the target.[19] Ultrasound waves directed through flowing blood are backscattered with a shifted frequency by the moving erythrocytes—a phenomenon known as the Doppler shift.[22, 23] The frequency change or Doppler shift is proportional to the velocity of the erythrocytes moving along the axis of the ultrasound beam. The blood velocity may be determined from the formula:

$$V = \frac{F \times C}{2f \times \cos\theta}$$

where V = velocity of blood, F = the measured Doppler frequency shift, f = the known frequency of the emitted ultrasound signal, C = the speed of sound in the tissue (1540 m/s), and θ = the angle between the direction of blood flow and the direction of the ultrasound signal.[22]

The ultrasound beam is reflected when it strikes an interface between two different materials. The marked difference between tissue and blood results in a strong intensity signal recognized by standard imaging echocardiography, whereas the acoustical impedance difference between plasma and red blood cells produces a low-amplitude signal. The red blood cell is the primary target of the Doppler ultrasound, which is able to process the low-amplitude signals. Unlike two-dimensional echocardiography, where the best images are obtained when the ultrasound beam is perpendicular to the heart, the best Doppler signals are obtained when the ultrasound beam is parallel to flow.[19]

The Doppler ultrasound transducer consists of one or more piezoelectric crystals that function as transmitter and receiver. An electrical signal causes the crystal to oscillate, which, when placed against tissue, creates a pressure wave front that passes through the tissue with a given frequency. Reflected wave fronts are picked up by the nonoscillating crystal and converted back into an electrical signal. For the purpose of measuring cardiac output, Doppler ultrasound instruments have been designed that record from the transesophageal, transtracheal, or transcutaneous (e.g., suprasternal notch or intracostal) positions.

Three conventional Doppler ultrasound modes are pulsed, continuous wave, and high pulse repetition frequency Doppler. In pulse wave Doppler, a single crystal functions as both transmitter and receiver. Following an initial oscillation, the crystal stops transmitting and waits for the reflected signal. The major advantage of pulse Doppler is that it permits sampling of a volume at a known distance from the crystal.[19, 24] Since the speed of ultrasound through tissue is fixed, it is possible to determine the time required for the reflected signal from a given depth to return to the crystal. The instrument can then be set to interpret only signals from that depth—a characteristic known as *range-gating*. However, maximum measurable velocity is limited since only a single pulse can be in the examining range at any time, and the maximum recordable velocity is dependent on pulse repetition frequency. The maximum discernible velocity is reduced for deeper measurements since more time must be allowed for the reflected signal to reach the crystal.[24] Conversely, a shorter distance results in a higher transmitted frequency and greater measurable velocity.

Continuous wave Doppler consists of two crystals with one continuously sending signals and the other continuously recording. Maximal recordable velocity is unlimited since the pulse frequency is high. However, with continuous transmission and reception, information from the full length of the beam is recorded, making it impossible to determine the exact depth of the flow signal.

High pulse repetition frequency represents an intermediate form between pulse and continuous wave Doppler.[19] The higher frequency signal allows for measurement of greater blood velocities while sacrificing depth specificity since more than one signal is in the body at a time sampling blood flow at more than one depth.

The use of Doppler ultrasound to calculate blood velocity requires quantification of the frequency shift (i.e., the received frequency must be compared to the transmitted frequency). Early units employed a zero crossing detector, which simply determined the time interval between zero crossings of the transmitted sinewave. Most current, commercially available instruments incorporate a linear detector, which allows simultaneous analysis of numerous sine waves within the sample volume. Two available methods are fast Fourier transformation (FFT), which is a digital method permitting simultaneous analysis of the various frequency components within the sample volume, and CHIRP Z analysis, which provides similar information using analog electronics.[19] As shown in Figure 14–1, peak flow velocity, ejection time, flow velocity integral, and acceleration time may be determined from the Doppler waveform. On-line visual display of the spectral analysis, available on some instruments, allows for easy focusing of the ultrasound beam and rapid recognition of misalignment of the beam to the desired level of flow (Fig 14–2). Visual inspection of the velocity waveform may provide additional hemodynamic information as will be discussed.[25]

The majority of available studies have used transcutaneous Doppler ultrasound to determine blood velocity. Velocity measurements from the aortic root are obtained by placing the transducer in the suprasternal notch and angling the transducer so that the signal is parallel to blood flow in the ascending aorta (Figure 14–3). Care must be taken to differentiate confounding signals from the innominate artery and the pulmonary artery.[26] As a rule, detected velocities in the pulmonary artery will be less than in the aorta. Although blood velocity in the innominate

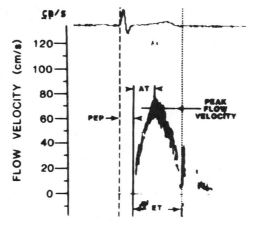

FIG 14–1.
Doppler flow velocity tracing. The vertical axis displays flow velocity and the horizontal axis represents time. AT = acceleration time; ET = ejection time; PEP = preejection period. (*From Dabestani A et al:* Am J Cardiol *1987; 59:662–668. Used by permission.*)

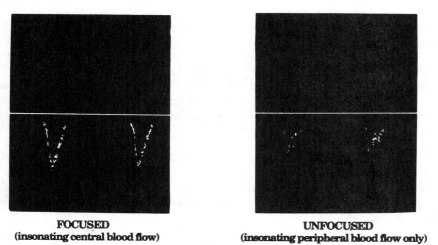

FOCUSED
(insonating central blood flow) UNFOCUSED
(insonating peripheral blood flow only)

FIG 14–2.
Recognition of midstream aortic flow. (*From Singer M et al:* Crit Care Med *1989; 17:447–452. Used by permission.*)

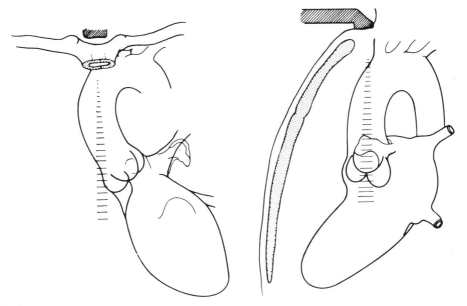

FIG 14–3.
Representative anterior and left lateral views of the left ventricular cavity and aortic root. Doppler transducer is positioned in the suprasternal notch. (*From Huntsmal LL, et al:* Circulation *1983; 67:593–602. Used by permission.*)

artery may exceed blood velocity in the aorta, the duration of systolic flow is longer and the acceleration of flow is less rapid, allowing the observer to discriminate between signals.

Cardiac Output Calculation

Cardiac output may be calculated from blood velocity using the following formula: stroke volume (SV) × heart rate (HR), where stroke volume is equal to the systolic velocity integral (SVI) × the cross-sectional area (CSA) of the aorta. Therefore, a reliable CO measurement depends not only on an accurate Doppler measurement of blood velocity, but on a separate accurate measurement of aortic diameter. The current technique and subsequent calculation of CO is founded on three basic assumptions[27]:

1. That the aorta is a circle whose area, defined by the equation $A = \pi R^2$, can be accurately measured
2. That there are uniform conditions of laminar flow with blunt velocity profiles such that measuring the velocity of flow at one point is representative of flow across the aortic channel
3. That the angle between the ultrasound beam and blood flow is <20 degrees, since cosine 20 degree = 0.94 and approaches unity as the angle narrows; larger angles require accurate measurement of the angle or the calculated CO may be significantly underestimated.

Measurement of the aortic cross-sectional area introduces the largest potential error into Doppler ultrasound CO calculations. A small change in measured diameter may significantly alter the area measurement since this result is squared. The aorta is not perfectly circular but is rather oval shaped and no true area calculation exists for ovals. Furthermore, aortic diameter may vary from systole to diastole with a 14% increase in diameter of the proximal aortic root noted in one study.[28] The diameter of the outflow tract, the aortic orifice, and distal aortic root did not change significantly. Aortic compliance decreases with age, minimizing the importance of systolic to diastolic changes in diameter in older patients.[29]

Conflicting data exist regarding the optimal level at which to calculate the aortic area. Ideally, the aortic diameter and blood velocity should be measured at the same level. Ihlen et al.[28] reported Doppler ultrasound derived COs of 49 to 102% higher than simultaneously obtained invasive measurements when the cross-sectional area of the aortic root was used in the calculation. The best correlation was obtained using the aortic orifice area.[28, 30] Ihlen et al.[28] proposed that a plug of formed flow leaves the left ventricle, emptying into the larger proximal aortic root; therefore, the effective area over which blood flow occurs in the aortic root is smaller than the anatomical aortic root area. However, other studies have reported good correlation with invasive measurements of CO using cross-sectional area measurements from the proximal aorta, leaving this issue undecided.[22, 26] Interestingly, Ihlen et al.[28] obtained identical maximum velocities at three different levels, suggesting the level of velocity measurement is a less important variable.

Echocardiographic aortic area measurements may be more difficult in surgical patients due to a shift of mediastinal structures or the presence of mediastinal and subcutaneous air.[22] Direct intraoperative measurement of aortic diameter has variably correlated with indirect echocardiographic measurements, further confirming that aortic area measurements contribute significantly to the inherent variability of this technique.[22, 31]

In addition to accurate measurement of the aortic area, the Doppler measurement of cardiac output assumes uniform conditions of laminar flow and flat velocity profiles. Evidence that the velocity profile in the ascending aorta is relatively flat is supported by several animal studies.[32–34] In an open chest dog model where CO was controlled, the mean Doppler ultrasound calculated COs correlated[32] with an *r* of 0.98 to 0.99 with the artificially set level of CO. The correlation was equally tight when comparing four different sampling sites in the ascending and four sites in the descending aorta, suggesting the presence of uniform flow. Lucas et al.,[33] in a similar model, calculated intraluminal aortic velocity from sample volumes obtained by moving an intraluminal Doppler crystal in 2-mm intervals from the anterior to the posterior wall. Systolic velocity profiles were skewed with slightly higher velocities near the posterior wall. However, the impact of a skewed profile was minimized when measurements were taken over the entire cardiac cycle with the result that the mean velocity profile was relatively flat. The most reliable point for estimating vessel mean velocity from point mean velocity was along an axis 5 mm from the anterior wall. Misalignment of the axis of the left ventricular outflow tract and the axis of the ascending aorta may account for the observed skewing of the velocity profile.[23, 35]

A skewed velocity profile in the proximal aorta has also been documented in human studies.[36, 37] Segadal and Matre[36] used an intraluminal Doppler ulstrasound to measure blood velocity in 2-mm increments across the ascending aorta from the point of maximum convexity to the point of maximum concavity. In five patients with normal aortic values, the velocity profile was flat and symmetric in early systole; skewed, but flattened during late systole, with the highest velocities along the left posterior wall; and bidirectional in late systole and early diastole with retrograde velocities along the left posterior wall. Unlike the dog model, the mean velocity profile was also skewed, with higher mean velocities calculated from samples taken close to the convex wall. The most representative sampling site was one-third the diameter away from the convex wall. Sampling from other sites produced as much as an 85% underestimate to a 135% overestimate. One patient did have a flat mean velocity profile in the setting of a marked tachycardia, which preferentially shortens diastole, minimizing the impact of the negative velocity profile in diastole.

The above recommendations for determining mean velocity from point velocity assume a state of laminar flow. Turbulent flow may develop at higher flow rates in animals.[34] Turbulent flow has also been documented in the ascending aorta of normal patients with high cardiac outputs and occurs consistently in patients with abnormal aortic valves.[38] Aortic valve disease produces irregular velocity profiles and appears to preclude reliable calculation of cardiac output.[36] The optimal site for determining mean velocity in patients with valvular disease or prosthetic valves is unknown, and both skewed mean velocity profiles and turbulent flow introduce a potential source of error, which may be magnified depending on the intraluminal sampling site. Skewed mean velocity profiles and turbulent flow are more likely to be a factor in the high catecholamine state characteristic of the ICU patient.[27]

Finally, most Doppler ultrasound blood velocity determinations are made with the ultrasound beam paralleling the direction of blood flow. An angle of interrogation <20 degrees introduces an error of <6% into the calculation since cosine 20 = 0.94 and approaches unity as the angle narrows. However, failure to measure accurately an angle of interrogation >20 degrees introduces a significant source of error into the calculation, resulting in an underestimation of the actual cardiac output.[8]

Clinical Applications

Published reports comparing CO measured by noninvasive Doppler ultrasound with various invasive modalities [i.e., thermodilution (TD), the Fick principle, or dye dilution] suggest good correlation between the two techniques in the majority of cases.[22, 26, 30, 39–41] Reported correlation coefficients range from 0.83 to 0.98 in patients where an adequate study is performed. Unfortunately, the gold standard, which, in this case, is the invasive measurement of CO, has its own inherent variability (e.g., CO measured by a thermodilution catheter may vary by 12 to 15%).[42] Some authors suggest Doppler ultrasound measurement of CO may actually be superior to that of TD in certain situations.[43]

Interobserver variability ranges from 9 to 11% as determined by experienced observers.[30] Reported intraobserver variability ranges from 1.9 ± 1.8% to 3.2 ± 2.9% for peak flow velocity, ejection time, and flow velocity integral with higher variability (7.9 ± 6.6%) for acceleration time.[44] The authors[44] conclude that a >13% change on serial recordings by the same observer reflects a true hemodynamic change.

Wong et al.[45] examined the time required for a novice to learn the technique. The volunteer group included an internist, nurses, a medical student, and an anesthesiologist. The novice observers required an average of 12.9 ± 3.5 attempts to obtain reproducible readings within

10% of the reference value. The authors acknowledge that a longer training period would be required to obtain reproducible values from a critically ill patient.

While most studies suggest the technique is accurate, reproducible, and relatively easily mastered, this has not been a universal experience.[46] Adequate transcutaneous studies are not obtained in all patients. Patients who pose particular problems include those with neck deformities, subcutaneous emphysema, and pulmonary emphysema, where measurements from the suprasternal notch may not be possible. Patients with aortic stenosis and aortic prosthetic valves will have altered hemodynamics in the aortic root such that the effective flow channel is less than the measured aortic diameter.[26] In aortic insufficiency, Doppler ultrasound measures the total left ventricular CO, whereas thermodilution measures net forward output.[39] Patients with a CO <1.5 L/min may not generate an adequate signal for accurate determination of blood velocity. Finally, cardiac arrhythmias may alter calculated CO even though most systems average velocity readings over a number of beats.

Most studies have excluded these technically difficult patients from the study group. However, even with careful patient selection, adequate studies may still be difficult to obtain. Nishimura et al.[22] obtained an adequate measurement of aortic area in 45 of 54 (83%) patients and an adequate Doppler signal permitting velocity measurement in 38 of 45 (84%). Thus, an adequate study was obtained in only 70% of patients in which it was attempted. However, in this 70% of patients, the correlation between thermodilution and Doppler CO was good, with a correlation coefficient of 0.94 in the medical patients and 0.85 in the surgical patients.

Conversely, Donovan et al.[47] reported a less favorable experience. They obtained 145 CO determinations in 38 critically ill patients using a Doppler ultrasound in the suprasternal notch angled so as to parallel blood flow in the ascending aorta and 2-D and M-mode echocardiography to measure the internal diameter of the ascending aortic root just above the aortic valve. The patients included 16 postoperative cardiothoracic surgery patients, 10 patients with a recent myocardial infarction, and 12 critically ill medical ICU patients. The mean ± standard deviation difference between thermodilution and Doppler CO was 0.51 ± 1.6 L/min, (range −0.49 to 5.6 L/min) yielding an overall correlation coefficient of 0.58. The correlation was equally poor when each group was analyzed separately.

The reasons for such disparate results may simply reflect more careful patient selection in those studies reporting favorable correlations. The study by Donovan et al.[47] was performed in critically ill patients; they required up to 1 hour in some patients to obtain a satisfactory pulsed Doppler tracing. However, in addition to patient selection, variability in other factors, such as aortic area measurement and Doppler angle measurement, integral to the calculation of CO by Doppler may explain the conflicting results.[27]

Concentric Beam Doppler

Concentric beam or dual-beam Doppler ultrasound is a recently developed, stand-alone Doppler technology capable of determining both the total cross-sectional area of the ascending aorta and the blood flow velocity.[48-51] The ultrasound transducer emits a narrow cylindrical beam and a wider diverging exterior beam (Fig 14–4)[50]; the combination provides for a velocity measurement and a cross-sectional area measurement from the same instrument, thereby

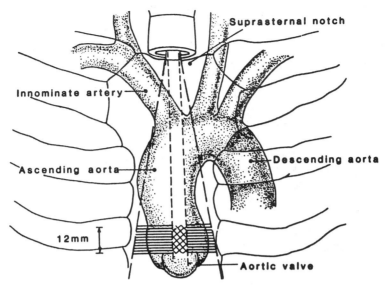

FIG 14–4.
Doppler probe aiming. The Doppler probe is placed in the suprasternal notch and aimed at the ascending aorta. The narrow beam sample volume should be entirely within the aorta; the wide beam sample volume should include the entire aortic cross section. (*From Wong DH, et al:* Crit Care Med *1990; 18:443–437. Used by permission.*)

theoretically overcoming some of the limitations of traditional Doppler instrumentation. The 2-D or M-mode echocardiographic measurement of aortic diameter is no longer necessary, and the calculated CO is independent of the angle of insonation.

The intensity of each Doppler shift frequency is proportional to the number of erythrocytes moving at a specific velocity. The sum of all these intensities equals the power return.[49] The cross-sectional area is determined from the ratio of the power return of the narrow and wide beam as defined by the equation

$$\text{CSA} = kP_n/P_w$$

where k equals a constant, P_n equals the power reture from the narrow beam, and P_w equals the power return from the wide beam.[48] The mean velocity is measured by the wide beam over the width of the ascending aorta, negating the impact of a skewed velocity profile. Furthermore, the measurement is independent of the angle of insonation since a change in the angle from acute to oblique will have an equal and opposite effect on the measurement of blood velocity and cross-sectional area; these changes effectively cancel each other, leaving the CO measurement unaffected.

In theory, concentric beam Doppler eliminates significant potential sources of error associated with traditional Doppler ultrasound. Looyenga et al.,[49] in a group of carefully selected patients, reported a significant correlation between concentric beam Doppler and thermodilution derived CO ($r = 0.96$, SEE $= 0.55$ L/min). Measurements were taken from the suprasternal notch; patients with anatomic variants of the chest wall, trachea, or ascending aorta and aortic valve were excluded. The time required to perform the study ranged from 3 to 5 minutes in those patients easily insonated to 30 to 40 minutes in the technically difficult patient. Adequate measurements were obtained in 27/40 ventilator patients. In 3 patients, the endotracheal tube appeared to obstruct the Doppler signal. Adequate studies were not obtained in 2 patients with severe respiratory distress since movement of the chest cage prevented consistent focusing of the beam. Niclou, Teague, and Lee[48] reported a similarly tight correlation in a series of high-quality studies ($r = 0.86$). However, 17 technically difficult studies in patients with obesity, emphysema, and uncooperative patients on ventilators correlated poorly with thermodilution CO ($r = 0.45$, SEE $= 2.62$ L/min).

At present, CO measurements reported with concentric beam Doppler at best approach the accuracy of traditional Doppler methods. Furthermore, individual patient measurements may vary[48, 50] by more than 1.5 L/min. Multiple factors may account for the observed individual patient variability. Accurate measurement of CO by dual-beam Doppler ultrasound requires that the narrow beam sample volume be within the aorta, that the wide beam encompass the full cross section of the aorta, and that the axis of the insonating beam be close to the axis of blood flow.[50] Nevertheless, the inherent advantage of measuring aortic cross-sectional area and velocity with the same instrument warrants further development of this technique.

Continuous Monitoring

Unlike transcutaneous Doppler techniques, which must be held in place, transesophageal[25, 32, 52] and transtracheal[53] ultrasound devices offer the potential for continuous monitoring. The initial transesophageal instrument consisted of a modified esophageal stethoscope[31, 52]; a simple esophageal transducer fixed in a larger rigid tube has also been described.[25]

The transducer is positioned in the esophagus at the level of the fifth and sixth vertebrae, approximately 35 cm from the mouth where the esophagus runs parallel to the descending aorta. The probe is directed posteriorly so as to insonate midstream descending aortic blood flow. A higher ultrasound frequency (5.1 mHz) is used to reduce beam depth and minimize the risk of insonating blood flow from other thoracic blood vessels. As shown in Figure 14–2, on-line visual monitoring of the spectral display allows rapid readjustment of the probe. Changes in the pitch of an auditory signal may also facilitate focusing of the beam.

The esophageal transducer is easily placed with adequate signals obtained in 2 to 10 minutes.[25, 31] The transducer has been left in place for up to four days without significant complications.[25] Movement of the patient in the ICU or manipulation of the mediastinum during cardiac surgery may necessitate refocusing the beam. The larger, more rigid esophageal tube[25] appears to require less repositioning than the esophageal stethoscope.[31, 52]

The transducer insonates blood moving away from it in the descending aorta, generating a negatively deflected velocity waveform. Information available from the waveform includes peak velocity, stroke distance (which equals the velocity time integral and correlates with stroke volume), the flow time, and the cycle time (Fig 14–5). However, actual measurement of CO is not possible with this technique since the transesophageal ultrasound insonates descending aortic bood flow, which carries only a portion of the total CO.

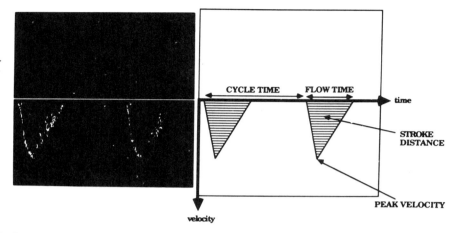

FIG 14–5.
Esophageal Doppler recordings. (*From Singer M, et al:* Crit Care Med *1989; 17:447–452. Used by permission.*)

Freund[52] derived a proportionality factor for measurement of CO using transesophageal echo. A one-time measurement of CO was obtained by means of transcutaneous Doppler ultrasound positioned in the suprasternal notch and a separate 2-D echocardiographic aortic diameter measurement from the left fourth or fifth parasternal space. The average correlation coefficient was 0.67 ± 0.31, compared to TD CO in 23 surgical patients. The correlation improved to 0.85 ± 0.15 for the last 13 patients, suggesting a learning effect. As shown in Figure 14–6, esophageal CO accurately tracked TD CO although absolute CO measurements differed significantly.[31] The authors postulated that transcutaneous Doppler measurement of CO to determine a proportionality factor introduces a large calibration error. The error appears to be random, both overestimating and underestimating thermodilution CO (Fig 14–6). Furthermore, the calibration error changed post bypass grafting, suggesting a redistribution of aortic blood flow. Recalibration with transcutaneous echocardiographic measurements is not possible during thoracic surgery, underscoring a further limitation of this technique.

The experience with transtracheal Doppler ultrasound has been similar to that with the transesophageal probe. Abrams, Weber, and Holmen[53] fixed a transducer to the end of an endotracheal tube so as to ensure atraumatic contact between the probe and the tracheal wall. In 18 surgical patients comparing TD and Doppler CO, a linear regression line could be fit over a range of COs from 2.69 to 8.62 L/min with a correlation coefficient squared of 0.84. However, the slope of the line equaled 0.75, with Doppler ultrasound both under- and overestimating TD COs.

While limited in their ability to measure CO accurately, transesophageal and transtracheal technologies offer the ability to track changes in CO accurately.[25, 31, 53] Both single measurements via transcutaneous Doppler and continuous monitoring of blood velocity via transtracheal or transesophageal probes afford a noninvasive means of assessing the hemodynamic response to physiologic maneuvers such as exercise[54] or therapeutic interventions such as

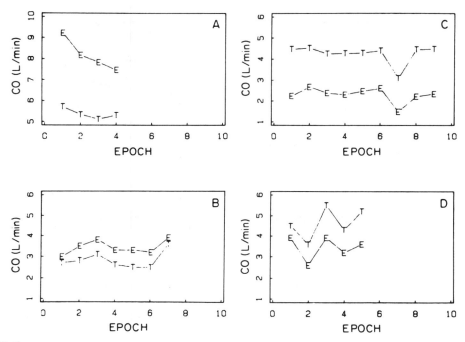

FIG 14–6.
Thermodilution cardiac output (*T*) and esophageal Doppler cardiac output (*E*) values for each epoch recorded in four different patients. Note that in **A** and **B**, *E* overestimates *T*, whereas in **C** and **D**, *E* underestimates *T*. (*From Mark JB, et al:* Anesth Analg *1986; 65:1013–1020. Used by permission.*)

volume replacement,[25] inotrope administration,[9, 25, 32, 40, 55] afterload reduction,[9, 25, 55] and pacing.[55] Lange et al.[56] reported using continuous wave Doppler measurements of aortic blood flow velocity before and after antiarrhythmic drug testing to determine which patients were susceptible to the negative inotropic effect of the drug and might be prone to develop congestive heart failure. Five of nine patients receiving a drug with negative inotropic properties showed a decline in the rate correlated stroke distance or flow velocity integral exceeding the 95% confidence limit of day-to-day variability, which was 13%. Two of these five patients subsequently developed clinical signs of congestive heart failure, suggesting that this strategy may provide early evidence of myocardial depression.

In each of the above examples, actual measurement of CO is not required. Errors introduced in the measurement of the cross-sectional aortic area or the calculation of a proportionality factor if flow is being measured in the descending aorta are avoided. Clinically important information may be gleaned from comparison of stroke distance, minute distance (equal to stroke distance × heart rate), and peak aortic velocity before and after a physiologic or therapeutic maneuver. Furthermore, analysis of the shape of the waveform provided both diagnostic information and assessment of therapeutic response.[25] As shown in Figure 14–7, hypovolemia presents as a narrow-based waveform that widens with volume replacement. Afterload reduc-

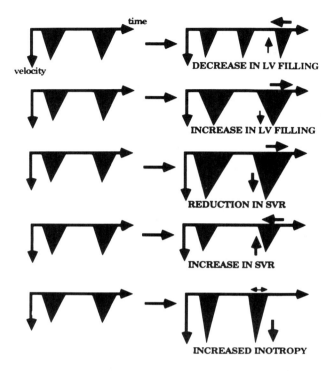

STYLIZED CHANGES OCCURING WITH HEMODYNAMIC CHANGES

FIG 14-7.
Alterations in waveform shape with hemodynamic changes. (*From Singer M, et al:* Crit Care Med *1989; 17:442–452. Used by permission.*)

tion increases stroke distance through an increase in peak velocity and flow time, whereas dobutamine increases peak velocity without significantly affecting other variables. In the acute care setting, such qualitative information allows rapid assessment of a response to therapy.

Pulmonary Artery Occlusion Pressure

Several studies have attempted to correlate pulmonary artery occlusion pressure (PAOP, or "wedge" pressure) with information derived from Doppler echocardiography.[25, 56–58] Singer, Clarke, and Bennett,[25] as discussed previously, suggested that the velocity waveform provided information regarding the volume status of the patient. In addition to a narrow-based waveform, both the stroke distance to peak velocity ratio and the flow time (FT) to cycle time (CT) ratio were decreased in the hypovolemic patient. They concluded that significant hypovolemia could be ruled out if the product of stroke distance/peak velocity and flow time/cycle time was >0.05. Unfortunately, these variables are not useful in the diagnosis of volume overload.

Transmitral pulsed Doppler echocardiography has provided a more accurate estimate of PAOP.[57, 58] Measurements are obtained[57] with 2-D Doppler echocardiography and a pulsed

Doppler flowmeter with an ultrasonic frequency of 2.5 mHz. Mitral pulsed Doppler spectra may be obtained from the apical forechamber view with the Doppler beam aligned perpendicular to the mitral valve annulus. As shown schematically in Figure 14–8, left ventricular diastolic function is characterized by passive early diastolic filling, represented by the E wave. Late diastolic active filling associated with atrial contraction is represented by the A wave. Time velocity integrals are averaged over five cardiac cycles. In a study of 104 critically ill patients, 91 with coronary artery disease (CAD), the ratio of A/E time velocity integrals showed a significant linear correlation with simultaneous PAOP readings ($r = 0.98$, SEE = 0.10)(Fig 14–9). The interobserver correlation coefficient[57] for two experienced observers was 0.95. Channer et al.[58] reported a similarly high linear correlation with PAOP in 22 patients with CAD ($r = 0.84$).

The above technique requires validation in a broader patient population that includes mechanically ventilated patients both with and without positive end-expiratory pressure. Although the A/E ratio of integrals continued to correlate[57, 58] with PAOP at values >30 mm Hg, the numbers of patients were small, and these results will require verification. Finally, the reported tight correlation between invasive and noninvasive measures of PAOP were obtained by experienced observers. The transferability of this technique to the intensivist or allied health professional remains to be tested.

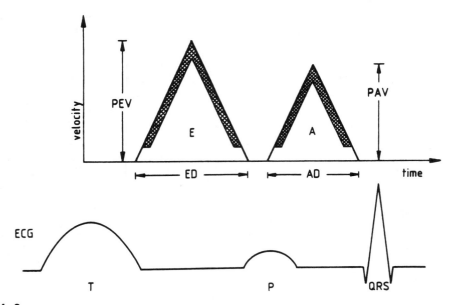

FIG 14–8.
Diagram of Doppler mitral flow velocity profile demonstrating the various characteristics of the profile that was measured. *A,A* wave = (atrial contraction; *E,E* wave = early filling; *AD,* = A-wave velocity; ED = E-wave duration; PAV = peak A-wave velocity; and PEV = peak E-wave velocity. (*From Stork STV, et al:* Crit Care Med *1990; 18:1158–1160. Used by permission.*)

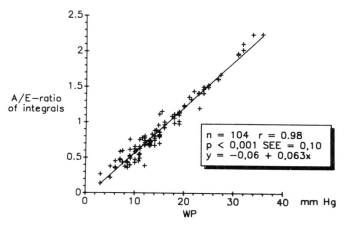

FIG 14–9.
Regression of *A/E* ratio of integrals to invasively measured WP (wedge pressure or PAOP). (*From Stork TV et al:* Crit Care Med *1990; 18:1158–1160. Used by permission.*)

Pulmonary Artery Pressure

Doppler ultrasound also provides reasonable estimates of pulmonary artery pressure (PAP)[59–63] Three commonly employed methods to calculate PAP include measurement of (1) the interval between pulmonic valve closure (Pc) and tricuspid valve opening (To)(2), the acceleration time (AcT) determined from pulmonary flow analysis, and (3) the systolic transtricuspid gradient, which is calculated from Doppler-detected tricuspid regurgitation.

The Pc-To interval increases proportionately with increasing PAP. The actual PAP is estimated from a previously derived nomogram. Accurate measurement of the Pc-To interval is critical since a 10-ms difference results in a 10 mm Hg difference in estimated PAP. In 48 patients with pulmonary hypertension (PHTN),[64] estimated PAP correlated with the invasive measurement of PAP with an $r = 0.89$. However, measurement of the Pc-To interval may not be accurate in patients with significantly elevated right atrial pressures or tricuspid regurgitation, which often accompanies PHTN. These patients were excluded from the above study.

AcT or time to peak velocity (TPV), defined as the time from onset of ejection to peak velocity (Figure 14–10), correlates negatively[60, 65, 66] with mean PAP ($r = -0.82$ to -0.72). The acceleration time index defined as AcT/right ventricular ejection period (RVEP) also correlates negatively[59–61, 66] with invasive measurements of PAP with an r ranging from -0.85 to -0.78. In one study, the regression line was not perfectly linear at higher values and more closely resembled a logarithmic function. AcT/RVEP versus log 10 PAP improved the correlation coefficient to -0.90. However, Dabestani et al.[59] did not find that use of a logarithmic function improved the correlation over that determined by simple linear regression, therefore leaving this issue undecided.

The AcT may not provide reliable estimates[67] of PAP in the patient with a heart rate greater than 100 bpm or the patient with atrial fibrillation where the value may change from beat to beat. Averaging a sufficient number of beats may minimize the impact of beat-to-beat variability.[62] Patients with an atrial septal defect may have a prolonged AcT due to increased pulmo-

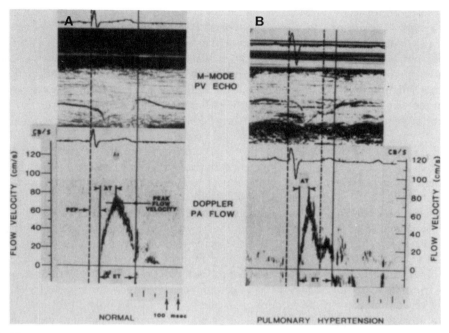

FIG 14–10.
A, M-mode pulmonary valve echogram (*top*) and Doppler pulmonary artery (PA) flow velocity tracing (*bottom*) in a normal subject. On the Doppler tracing, the vertical axis displays flow velocity and the horizontal axis represents time. Doppler peak flow velocity occurs in midsystole. **B,** Pulmonary valve (PV) echogram (*top*) and PA flow velocity (*bottom*) in a patient with pulmonary hypertension (mean presure 52 mm Hg). The Doppler recording shows a rapid acceleration to peak flow velocity in early systole, with a rapid deceleration to a nadir in midsystole, followed by a brief secondary increase in flow velocity in late systole. Note the temporal relation of midsystolic notching on the M-mode pulmonic valve echogram and PA flow velocity tracing. AT = acceleration time; ET = ejection time; and PEP = preejection period. (*From Dabestani A, et al: Am J Cardiol 1987; 59:662–668. Used by permission.*)

nary blood volume with values falling in the normal range despite the presence of an elevated PAP.[62] Similarly, patients with severe RV dysfunction may have an abnormally prolonged AcT in the setting of a normal or slightly elevated PAP. Finally, the AcT may be shortened in patients with tricuspid regurgitation.

Chan et al.,[67] in 50 consecutive patients undergoing cardiac catheterization, compared the above two methods with the systolic transtricuspid gradient method for determining PAP. The gradient is determined from Doppler-detected tricuspid regurgitation and added to a clinical measurement of jugular venous distention or a fixed value of 14 mm Hg. Calculation of the transtricuspid gradient was possible in 36/50 (72%) of patients and yielded a correlation coefficient of 0.87. The Pc-To interval correlated well with invasive measurements of PAP ($r = 0.87$), but adequate studies were obtained in only 11/50 (22%) patients. The high incidence of atrial and or ventricular arrhythmias precluded reliable measurement of the interval. The AcT method yielded an r of -0.65, which improved to -0.85 if only patients with a heart rate of 60 to 100 bpm were analyzed. In summary, the transtricuspid gradient technique was the most reliably consistent method for analyzing PAP in this study.

The transtricuspid gradient technique proved less effective in 41 patients with COPD.[68] PAP could not be estimated in 14/41 (34%) patients due to poor signal quality, absence of Doppler-detected tricuspid regurgitation, and inadequate tricuspid regurgitation, Estimated PAP in the remaining studies yielded an *r* value of 0.65 (SEE = 9 mm Hg), suggesting that the technique may be less reliable in the COPD population. Furthermore, the relative accuracy of continuous wave Doppler used in this study compared to pulse Doppler remains to be defined.

As in the aorta, analysis of the Doppler waveform provides qualitative information on PAP. As shown in Figure 14–10, a dome-shaped waveform characterizes the normal pulmonary artery tracing, whereas a triangular configuration with a sharper upstroke characterizes the patient with PHTN.[59–61] A smaller percentage of patients with PHTN exhibit a spike and dome configuration with midsystolic notching of the waveform.

The optimal site from which to determine PAP remains to be defined. Recent studies have estimated PAP from Doppler blood flow velocity measurements in the right ventricular (RV) outflow tract, pulmonary orifice, or main pulmonary artery. Graettenger, Greene, and Voyles[69] obtained adequate tracings in 100% of patients from the RV outflow tract as opposed to only 75% from the main pulmonary artery. Okamoto et al.[61] noted similar technical difficulties insonating the pulmonary trunk, obtaining an adequate signal in only 14/23 (60%) patients. Systolic fluttering of the pulmonic cusp and/or eddy currents in patients with pulmonary hypertension may account for the inability to consistently obtain adequate signals from the pulmonary trunk.[66] When adequate studies were obtained, velocity measurements were comparable between the two sites,[60, 62] although the quality of the recording was better from the RV outflow tract.

The optimal transducer site from which to assess blood flow velocity may vary from patient to patient. The short axis parasternal view has been used with reasonable success in the majority of cases, with the ultrasound beam angled so as to insonate central blood flow.[59, 60, 67] In patients with COPD, the short axis parasternal view may not be an option secondary to lung hyperinflation. Ferrazza et al.[70] reported adequate studies in 52/59 (88%) COPD patients using the left oblique subcostal view and 38/59 (64%) using the right oblique subcostal view, compared to only 12/59 (20%) using the short axis parasternal view. Peak flow velocity measurements were consistently higher using the left oblique view.

The use of multiple views may be required in routine studies of pulmonary artery blood flow. Lighty et al.[71] reported view-dependent differences in measured flow velocity ranging from 7 to 48% in 20/32 (62%) adult patients studied. They attributed the difference to variations in the angle between the Doppler beam and insonated blood flow. Multiple views should be attempted, with the highest recorded velocity used to approximate PAP.

Thoracic Electrical Bioimpedance

Observations that body impedance varied with the cardiac cycle when exposed to a high-frequency electrical current date back to the early 1900s. Nyboer et al.[72, 73] in 1940 passed a high-frequency current across the human thorax and recorded the associated impedance changes with each heart beat; they called the recording a *radiogram*. Kubicek et al.[74] in 1966 susequently developed a more sophisticated method of determining aortic velocity from observed impedance changes. Recent studies have extended the use of thoracic electrical bioimpedance (TEB) to the clinical arena.

Physiologic Principle

Electricity moves through tissue via ions as opposed to the free flow of electrons mediating metallic conduction. Tissue conduction depends on the concentration, type, charge, and mobility of the available ions. The relationship between current (I), voltage (V), and impedance (Z) is defined by Ohm's law $(V = I \times Z)$. Voltage is defined as the potential difference across a circuit measured in joules per coulomb. Current is defined as the number of coulombs of charge flowing per unit time or amperes. The resistance or impedance is measured in volts per ampere or ohms and reflects the ease with which charges move through the system.[72] TEB measures the impedance change between two electrodes related to the cyclical change in thoracic blood volume. An increase in blood volume within a segment of conducting tissue results in a fall in the impedance.[72]

The use of TEB to measure SV and CO consists of passing a constant high-frequency, low-amplitude, sinusoidal alternating current longitudinally through the thorax between two electrodes. A tetrapolar electrode system is superior to the bipolar system since it minimizes the interface artifact and allows for a uniform current density distribution in the segment of interest.[72] As shown in Figure 14–11, conductive strip electrodes or pairs of spot electrodes are placed around the neck—one as low as possible with the higher electrodes (#1) spaced at least 3 cm away from the lower electrodes. Electrodes #3 are placed at the level of the xiphoid with electrodes #4 at least 3 cm below. Use of constant landmarks ensures consistent placement of the electrodes. The voltage drop between electrodes #2 and #3 is determined by a high-input impedance linear amplifier.[75, 76] Since a constant current is used, Ohm's law dictates[72] that a change in the detected voltage between electrodes #2 and #3 reflects a change in impedance $(\triangle Z)$.

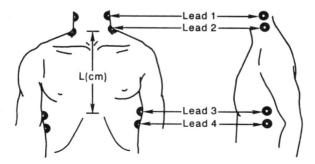

FIG 14–11.
Placement of impedance electrodes. (*From Gotshall RW, et al:* Crit Care Med *1989; 17:806–810. Used by permission.*)

Stroke Volume and Cardiac Output

Kubicek's original equation to calculate stroke volume from impedance changes made the following assumptions[77]:

1. The thorax is a cylinder with base circumference equal to the circumference of the thorax at the xiphoid level. The cylinder has electrical length L (cm), which is the measured distance between the voltage sensing electrodes #2 and #3.
2. The cylindrical conductor has a steady-state mean base impedance (Z_0). The resistance of the conductor is directly proportional to its length and inversely proportional to its cross-sectional area as summarized in the equation:

$$R = \rho b \cdot L/A$$

where L is the length of the conductor, A is the cross-sectional area occupied by the blood, and ρb equals the specific resistivity of the blood, which varies with hematocrit.[72] At the frequencies employed (20 to 100 kHz), impedance (Z) may be substituted for the resistance (R). Since the cross-sectional area of blood changes as the volume of blood within the defined electrical cylinder changes, the following equation may be algebraically derived:

$$SV = \rho b \cdot L^2/Z_0^2 \cdot (\triangle Z)$$

Kubicek et al.[74] in 1966 proposed using the first derivative of the cardiac component of $\triangle Z$ (dZ/dt) to calculate stroke volume, which is less affected by movement and respiratory artifact. Peak ascending aortic blood flow (PF) was calculated from the following equation:

$$PF = \rho b \cdot L^2/Z_0^2 \cdot (dZ/dt)_{max}$$

Multiplying PF by left ventricular ejection time (LVET) in seconds yields the SV. LVET may be measured from the dZ/dt tracing. However, as shown in Figure 14–12, a clearly defined point signaling the end of ventricular ejection is not always present. A phonocardiogram or carotid pulse tracing has been used in some studies to determine LVET more accurately. A final summary of the equation used to calculate stroke volume can be expressed[77] as follows:

$$SV = \rho b \cdot L^2/Z_0^2 \cdot LVET \cdot (dZ/dt)_{max}$$

Cardiac output is then determined by multiplying SV × heart rate (HR).

Bernstein[77] critically evaluated Kubicek's original equation and a subsequent modification proposed by Sramek.[77–79] Criticisms of the initial Kubicek equation were that it consistently overestimated cardiac output in normal populations and generated variable results in critically ill populations.[77] Bernstein argues for elimination of ρb based on evidence that ρb does not vary significantly with hematocrit[80] and therefore contributes little to the variability of the equation.

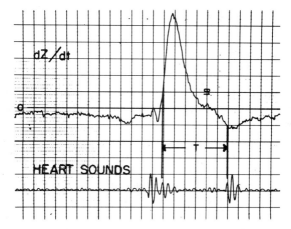

FIG 14–12.
A *dZ/dt* waveform where the end of ventricular ejection is not clearly defined. (*From Kubicek WG, et al:* Ann NY Acad Sci *1970; 170:724–732. Used by permission.*)

Sramek[77–79] made the observation that the thorax is not a true cylinder, but as shown in Figure 14–13, more closely approximates a truncated cone whose volume equals one-third the volume of a larger thoracic encompassing cylinder. The volume of electrically participating tissue (VET) was estimated from the height and circumference of the thorax. Based on anthropometric observations that the circumference of the rib cage at the level of the xiphoid was three times the height of the thoracic cone, and the height of the thoracic cone was 70%

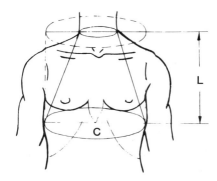

FIG 14–13.
Schematic representation of an adult thorax showing Kubicek's thoracic encompassing cylinder of length L (*dashed lines*). Sramek's smaller volume conductor, the frustum (*truncated cone*), of equal base circumference and L are noted to extend from the common base to the root of the neck (*solid lines*). (*From Bernstein DP:* Crit Care Med *1986; 14:908–909. Used by permission.*)

of body height, the equation was modified to estimate VET from body height raised to the third power as shown:

$$SV = (0.17H)^3/4.2 \cdot LVET \cdot (dZ/dt)_{max}/Z_0$$

Use of the constant relationship, 17% of total body height, minimizes the impact of errors in measurement of L. A 2- to 3-cm error in measurement introduces a 20 to 30% error in the calculation of SV since L is raised to the third power.[77]

Bernstein[77] subsequently proposed a weight correction factor to account for alterations in weight or body surface area that are not considered in the Sramek equation. He notes that the relationship $L = 17\%$ toal body height is correct only for patients of ideal body weight and that systematic underestimation of SV occurs in patients 15 to 20% heavier than ideal body weight.[77] Basal impedance (Z_0) decreases as lower thoracic circumference increases, confirming the inverse relationship between Z_0 and its cross-sectional area as summarized in the equation $Z_0 = \rho b \cdot L/A$. Bernstein defined the correction factor as follows:

$$\sigma = B \text{ weight observed/weight ideal}$$

where B represents the relative blood volume index as determined by the ratio of the average basal steady-state blood volume at any given deviation from ideal body weight to the average basal steady state blood volume in milliliters per kilogram at ideal body weight.

In summary, Bernstein's modification of Sramek's equation is as follows:

$$SV = \sigma \cdot [(0.17H)^3/4.2] \cdot LVET \cdot (dZ/dt)_{max}/Z_0$$

Some commercially available noninvasive continuous cardiac output monitors (NCCOM-3) are designed to accept only a single value for L. Figure 14–14 is a nomogram that incorporates σ into the entered value of L.

Clinical Application

Thoracic electrical bioimpedance, as a noninvasive modality for measuring SV and CO, has tremendous potential applicability in both inpatient and outpatient settings. TEB has been studied in animal models,[81–83] healthy human subjects,[84–87] and critically ill patients.[81, 86, 88–90] CO as measured by TD or the Fick method was used as the gold standard in most studies. As noted previously, comparison of a new technique with a gold standard that has its own inherent variability precludes making a definitive assessment regarding the accuracy of the new technique. However, the variability of the technique, the ability to track changes in CO, and the bias as measured by the difference between TEB and the reference standard can be assessed.

Interpretation of the available TEB literature is complicated by the use of different instruments and formulas to calculate SV. Two commonly employed instruments are the Minnesota impedance cardiograph (MIC), which uses the original Kubicek equation, and a computerized system (NCCOM-3), which employs the Sramek or modified Bernstein-Sramek equation to calculate CO. The Kubicek equation requires entering a measured value of L and a value for

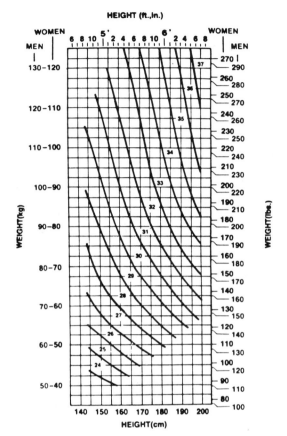

FIG 14–14.
Nomogram for determining the proper *L* entry into calculation for the modified Sramek SY equation. (*From Bernstein DP:* Crit Care Med *1986; 14:904–909. Used by permission.*)

ρb. The first derivative of basal impedance (*dZ/dt*) is manually calculated from the tracing. While clearly a more cumbersome method, it offers the advantage of visual inspection of the *dZ/dt* waveform and elimination of poor-quality tracings. NCCOM-3 offers the advantage of real-time measurement of CO, while sacrificing the ability to monitor the waveform visually. Interpretation of the available literature is further complicated by the failure of more recent studies using the NCCOM-3 to specify which generation of software was employed[91]; later generations have solved some of the problems associated with the earlier models. Studies examining the accuracy of instruments employing the original Kubicek equation in both normal individuals and critically ill patients and of instruments employing the Sramek or modified Bernstein-Sramek equations will be reviewed separately.

Reasonable correlation between TEB-derived CO using the Kubicek equation and other noninasive means of calculating CO has been reported in healthy individuals at rest and with exercise. Edmunds, Godfrey and Tooley[87] compared CO measured by TEB and the indirect Fick CO_2 rebreathing method in 23 normal individuals. Despite a close correlation ($r = 0.92$), TEB CO consistently overestimated CO as determined by the indirect Fick method at rest and with exercise. A correction factor based on packed cell volume yielded a relationship approaching the line of identity. The mean coefficient of variation measurement was 13% at rest and 5% with steady-state treadmill walking. Accurate results could not be obtained at higher levels of exercise on a bicycle ergometer. Teo et al.[92] reported a better correlation between TEB CO and a direct Fick measurement of CO in 20 patients undergoing routine catheterization ($r = 0.93$). Measurements were taken at rest and at levels of exercise up to 130 W. CO ranged from 3.5 to 18.0 L/min. No systematic error was observed and the random error was less than 5%. No correlation factors were employed in this study.

More variable results comparing TEB- and thermodilution-derived CO have been reported in the critically ill population (Table 14–1). Paired readings of TD and TEB CO produced[93] an acceptable correlation in 9 of 10 clinically stable preoperative patients ($r = 0.86$ to 0.99). The coefficient of variation for TEB was 4.8% compared to 9.9% for TD. TEB accurately tracked[93] small changes in SV (6.4%) induced by Dextran infusions with a correlation coefficient for the measurement of change of 0.88.

A much weaker correlation was reported by Donovan et al.[89] in 27 critically ill ICU patients comparing TD and TEB. A variety of values for the resistivity of blood ρb as well as three different values for L were employed. The minimum distance measured anteriorly or posteriorly between electrodes #2 and #3 or the mean distance of the two was substituted for L. LVET was determined from simultaneous carotid waveform tracings. Patients with intracardiac shunts, pleural effusions, pulmonary atelectasis, incompetent valves, or an intra-aortic balloon pump were excluded. CO ranged from 2.4 to 12.0 L/min. Correlation coefficients ranged from 0.48 to 0.64 in the 14 patients who survived and 0.46 to 0.79 in those who died over range of values for ρb and L. A constant value of 150 Ω/cm for ρb and utilization of the mean distance between inner electrodes yielded the best agreement between techniques (mean difference 0.17 ± 2.4 L/min). In summary, the inherent variability of the Kubicek equation is largely a function of the variability of ρb and L. The available literature precludes making a specific recommendation regarding determination of these values.

Most recent studies have employed the NCCOM-3. The earliest models utilized the Sramek equation to calculate SV with later models released since 1986–87 (NCCOM-3 revision 6) incorporating an adjustment for body weight as suggested by Bernstein.[77] Variable results

TABLE 14–1.
TD Versus TEB*

Author		Setting	(Pt. #)	r Value	Mean Difference
Eckman et al.	(93)	Preop	(10)	0.85	4.8%
Gotshall et al.	(86)	ICU	(10)	NA	-0.22 ± 1.0 L/min (SD)
Donovan et al.	(89)	ICU	(27)	0.63	0.17 ± 2.4 L/min (SD)
Muzi et al.	(108)	ICU	(14)	0.87	NA

* Kubicek equation. r = correlation coefficient; NA = not available.

have been reported in relatively healthy populations. Smith et al.[85] reported a relatively weak correlation ($r = 0.53$) comparing CO measured by an indirect Fick method using a CO_2 rebreathing technique and TEB CO. Results were widely scattered with 73% of the values lying outside limits defined by the line of identity $\pm 20\%$. TEB consistently underestimated the indirect Fick results at all levels of exercise up to 130 W. However, significantly better correlations have been reported comparing TD and TEB CO in clinically stable patients undergoing routine cardiac catheterization[94] ($r = 0.83$) or preoperative assessment.

Comparison of TD and TEB CO in the ICU and intraoperative setting has yielded r values ranging from 0.61[75] to 0.93[95] (Table 14–2). TEB CO correlated least closely with simultaneous TD-derived CO in the study by Wong et al.[90] ($r = 0.61$). They obtained satisfactory readings in 56/68 (84%) postoperative ICU patients. The best correlation was observed in those patients who had not undergone aortic or cardiac surgery and who were mechanically ventilated. Problems with electrode placement in patients with bandages covering internal jugular lines or thoracic wounds at the level of the xiphoid may have contributed to the poorer correlation in their study. Better results were reported by Appel et al.[96] in 16 critically ill patients ($r = 0.83$ with a mean difference between TEB and TD CO values of 16.2 ± 11.8 SD%), and Bernstein[88] in 17 ICU patients ($r = 0.88$). The greatest variability was observed in patients with a CO of less than 2 L/min where TEB overestimated TD CO by 50 to 100%.

The optimal choice of technology or equation to calculate CO from TEB measurements is unclear. Head to head comparisons have not clarified the issue. Huang et al.[97] compared the Sramek, the modified Sramek, and the Bernstein-Sramek equation using Doppler-derived CO as the gold standard. The original Sramek equation most closely approximated the Doppler-estimated CO. Unfortunately, as noted previously in this chapter, Doppler CO has its own variability. Gotshall, Wood, and Miles[86] compared the MIC utilizing the Kubicek method and the NCCOM-3 utilizing the modified Sramek equation in 7 normal individuals and 10 ICU patients. The MIC, NCCOM-3, and TD COs were comparable in the 10 ICU patients (6.3 ± 0.7, 6.4 ± 0.8, and 6.6 ± 0.6 L/min, respectively). However, NCCOM-3 yielded significantly higher values for CO in the normal individuals (9.2 ± 0.6 versus 6.2 ± 0.4 L/min) for reasons that were unclear to the authors.

TABLE 14–2.
TD versus TEB*

Author (ref)		Setting	(Pt.#)	r value	Mean Difference
Bernstein	(88)	ICU	(17)	0.88	NA
Spinola et al.	(81)	ICU	(10)	0.77	NA
Wong et al.	(90)	ICU	(68)	0.61	-0.67 ± 1.72 L/min
Appel et al.	(94)	Intraop	(16)	0.83	6.2 ± 11.8 %
Castor et al.	(95)	Intraop	(6)	0.93	$-0.78 \pm 12.11\%$

* Sramek, modified Sramek, or Sramek-Bernstein equation.
NA = Not available; r = Correlation coefficient.

Pediatric Population

Several studies have examined TEB CO in the neonatal and older pediatric populations. Gotshall and Miles,[98] using the MIC in seven canine pups, obtained a correlation coefficient of 0.96 as compared to TD over a range of COs produced by hemorrhage and blood reinfusion. The same authors[99] used the MIC to study 37 patients, aged 2 to 171 months, with a variety of congenital heart defects. Correlation coefficients ranged from 0.69 to 0.89 for patients with no shunts ($N = 11$), intracardiac left to right shunts via an atrial septal defect (ASD) ($N = 7$), or ventricular septal defect (VSD) ($N = 12$), and an extracardiac left to right shunt via a patent ductus arteriosus (PDA) ($N = 7$). The highest correlation ($r = 0.89$) was observed in the ASD group and the lowest ($r = 0.69$) in the VSD group.

Comparable results have been reported in studies using the NCCOM-3. A significant correlation between TD and TEB was obtained[100] in seven preterm and term lambs during volume contraction and expansion ($r = 0.82$). Braden et al.[101] in 26 children undergoing cardiac catheterization, reported a correlation coefficient of 0.84 between TD and TEB COs in the pediatric population for those without shunts and 0.70 in those patients with a left to right shunt.

In the ICU population, the NCCOM-3–derived CO correlated well with Doppler CO[102] ($r = 0.94$) and TD CO[103] ($r = 0.94$). However, thoracic length L in the latter study was determined by choosing a value that produced a TEB CO measurement within 10% of a simultaneous TD CO measurement. Although TEB accurately tracks changes in CO[104] a reliable measurement of the actual cardiac output awaits development of a nomogram for children that accounts for the different thoracic length-to-height ratio in this population.[103]

Technological Limitations

A variety of physiologic states and mechanical limitations compromises the accuracy of TEB. Tracheostomy dressings over surgical wounds and internal jugular line placements may prevent accurate electrode placement.[89, 98] Tracheostomies may also hinder electrode placement.[89, 98] A 2-cm error in the distance between neck and thoracic electrode placement may result in a 20% error in the calculated stroke volume, underscoring the importance of electrode placement. Additional mechanical problems include the use of electrocautery, which may temporarily disable the NCCOM-3,[88] the presence of metal within the chest, and extremely oily skin.[90] The problem of oily skin may be solved by thorough cleansing of the skin and use of special exercise electrodes (Vermont Med, Inc, Bellows Falls, VT).[98]

The impact of atelectasis, pleural effusions, and air on TEB CO is unclear. Patients with these conditions have been excluded from most studies. A normal first derivative waveform (dZ/dt) was observed in a patient with a thickened pericardium and pericardial effusion.[105] A subsequent pneumopericardium resulted in dampening of the curve and a significant underestimation of CO compared to the TD values. Air is a poor conductor, limiting the utility of TEB in such states. Pneumopericardium and possibly a pneumothorax can adversely affect TEB CO measurements.

Physiologic states that can compromise the accuracy of TEB include septic shock,[88] aortic insufficiency,[94] mitral regurgitation,[106] tachycardias,[82] dysrhythmias, and a pacemaker. Both animal[82, 83] and human studies have reported inaccuracies in TEB at low CO.[88, 95, 107, 108] As noted, TEB may overestimate[81, 88] CO by 50 to 100% in patients with TD CO measurements of less than 2.5 L/min. However, Muzi et al.[108] suggests this is not a consistent relationship. Despite a good correlation ($r = 0.87$), TEB CO actually underestimated TD CO at low levels (less than 5.0 L/min) in 14 ICU patients using the original Kubicek equation.

NCCOM-3–derived cardiac outputs may be inaccurate at heart rates greater than 150[96] to 180.[81] Newer generations of the NCCOM-3 have reportedly solved this problem with improved accuracy up to heart rates of 199.[91] Dysrhythmias and pacemakers may compromise computer measurement of CO due to the poor electrocardiogram *R*-wave recognition necessary[81] for computing *dZ/dt*. Finally, valvular abnormalities may compromise the accuracy of TEB CO. TEB may overestimate CO in patients with AI and these patients were excluded from most studies of TEB. As shown in Figure 14–15, mitral regurgitation (MR) changes the shape of the *dZ/dt* waveform and compromises the accuracy of the technique.[108] The presence of MR increases the size of the O-wave, which decreases in size following surgical correction.

Several studies have examined the impact of respiration on TEB. Early studies employed an end-expiratory breath hold to minimize respiratory variation in the *dZ/dt* signal. Several more recent studies using either the NCCOM-3 system[81] or an ensemble averaging technique[93] report reliable measurement of CO during spontaneous respirations. Edmunds, Godfrey, and Tooley,[106] using the Kubicek formula in 23 healthy volunteers, noted no significant difference

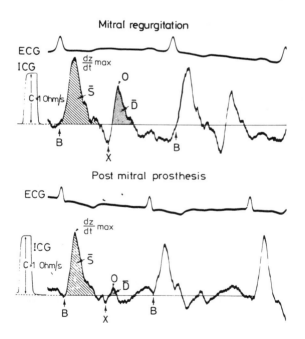

FIG 14–15.
Impedance cardiogram recordings in mitral regurgitation and postmitral prosthesis in the same patient. *B*-marks the beginning of isovolumetric contraction. The *X* point signals the end of ventricular ejection and occurs simultaneously with the aortic heart sound. The O-wave coincides with rapid early diastolic filling of the left ventricle and decreases in size following mitral valve replacement. (*From Schieken RM, et al: Br Heart J 1981; 45:166–72. Used by permission.*)

in measured CO at varying lung volumes or with spontaneous breathing. However, this assumption may not hold true for exercise where Du Quesnay, Stoule, and Hughson[109] did note significant differences in CO between normal breathing and an inspiratory or expiratory breath hold at exercise levels exceeding 100 W. These differences may reflect true changes in CO or simply an increased impact of respiratory variation at higher respiratory rates and tidal volumes. Mechanical ventilation with or without positive end-expiratory pressure does not appear to affect TB CO significantly.[95]

Reproducibility

TEB in most reported studies is a reproducible technique with a coefficient of variation ranging from 13% at rest[87] to less than 5% with exercise.[87, 92] The reproducibility of TEB approaches or exceeds that reported for TD. Eckman et al.[93] reported a coefficient of variation of 4.8% with TEB compared to 9.9% for TD in 10 preoperative patients. Nine untrained health professionals required an average of 8.4 ± 4.5 trials to obtain reproducible results within 10% of the reference value in a population of healthy volunteers.[45] Electrode misplacement accounted for the greatest source of error. In summary, TEB, like Doppler echocardiography, appears to be a reproducible and relatively easily mastered technique, although a similar study has not been performed in a critically ill ICU population.

SUMMARY

At present, the optimal technology and choice of equation to calculate stroke volume remains unknown. Both the original Kubicek equation and the computerized incorporation of the Sramek equation or its modification have proven reproducible and accurate in some studies.

TEB, like Doppler cardiac output, has its greatest potential as a noninvasive means of tracking changes in caridac output. Its ability to measure CO accurately in the inpatient and outpatient setting awaits further technological advancement and perhaps further refinement of currently employed equations to calculate SV.

REFERENCES

1. Wiedemann HP, Matthay MA, Matthay RA: Cardiovascular pulmonary monitoring in the intensive care unit. *Chest* 1984; 85:537–549, 656–668.
2. Shoemaker WC, Appel PL, Kram HB, et al: Multicomponent noninvasive physiologic monitoring of circulatory function. *Crit Care Med* 1988; 16:482–490.
3. O'Rourke MF, Yaginuma T: Wave reflections and the arterial pulse. *Arch Intern Med* 1984; 144:366–371.
4. Stern DH, Gerson JI, Allen FB, et al: Can we trust the direct radial artery pressure immediately following cardiopulmonary bypass? *Anesthesiol* 1985; 62:557–561.
5. Penaz J: Photoelectric measurement of blood pressure, volume and flow in the finger. *Digest 10th Int Conf Med Biol Eng* 1973; p. 104.
6. Ramsey M: Blood pressure monitoring: Automated oscillometric devices. *J Clin Monit* 1991; 7:56–67.

7. Boehmer RD: Continuous, real-time, noninvasive monitoring of blood pressure: Penaz methodology applied to the finger. *J Clin Monit* 1987; 3:282–287.

8. Epstein RH, Kaplan S, Leighton BL, et al: Evaluation of a continuous noninvasive blood pressure monitor in obstetric patients undergoing spinal anesthesia. *J Clin Monit* 1989; 5:157–163.

9. Venus B, Mathru M, Smith RA, et al: Direct versus indirect blood pressure measurements in critically ill patients. *Heart Lung* 1985; 14:228–231.

10. Gravlee GP, Brockschmidt JK: Accuracy of four indirect methods of blood pressure measurement, with hemodynamic correlations. *J Clin Monit* 1990; 5:284–298.

11. Kurki TS, Smith NT, Head N, et al: Noninvasive continuous blood pressure measurement from the finger; optimal measurement conditions and factors affecting reliability. *J Clin Monit* 1987; 3:6–13.

12. Kurki TS, Smith NT, Sanford TJ, et al: Pulse oximetry and finger blood pressure measurement during open-heart surgery. *J Clin Monit* 1989; 5:221–228.

13. East TD, Pace NL, Sorenson RM, et al: Effect of peripheral vascular disease on accuracy of noninvasive, continuous, blood pressure measurement from the finger (Finapress). *Anesthesiol* 1987; 67:A186.

14. Kermode JL, Davis NJ, Thompson WR: Comparison of the Finapress blood pressure monitor with intra-arterial manometry during induction of anaesthesia. *Anaesth Intens Care* 1989; 17:470–486.

15. Gibbs NM, Larach DR, Derr JA: The accuracy of Finapress noninvasive mean arterial pressure measurements in anesthetized patients. *Anesthesiol* 1991; 74:647–652.

16. Gorback MS, Quill TJ, Lavine ML: The relative accuracies of two automated noninvasive arterial pressure measurement devices. *J Clin Monit* 1991; 7:13–22.

17. Epstein RH, Huffnagle S, Bartkowski RR: Comparative accuracies of a finger blood pressure monitor and an oscillometric blood pressure monitor. *J Clin Monit* 1991; 7:161–167.

18. Doppler CJ: Uber das farbige Licht der Doppelsterne. *Abhandlungen der Koniglishen Bohmischen Gesellschaften der Wissenchaften* 1842; 11:465.

19. Goldberg S: *Doppler Echocardiography*. Philadelphia, Lea & Febiger, Pub, 1988, pp 1–69.

20. Sequeira RF, Light LH, Cross G, et al: Transcutaneous aortovelography: A quantitative evaluation. *Br Heart J* 1976; 38:443–450.

21. Light H: Transcutaneous aortovelography: A new window on the circulation? *Br Heart J* 1976; 38:433–442.

22. Nishimura RA, Callahan MJ, Schaff HV, et al: Noninvasive measurement of cardiac output by continuous-wave Doppler echocardiography: Initial experience and review of the literature. *Mayo Clin Proc* 1984; 59:484–489.

23. Side CD, Gosling RG: Nonsurgical assessment of cardiac function. *Nature* 1971; 232:335–336.

24. Come PC: The optimal Doppler examination: Pulsed, continuous wave or both? *J Am Coll Cardiol* 1986; 7:886–888.

25. Singer M, Clarke J, Bennett ED: Continuous hemodynamic monitoring by esophageal Doppler. *Crit Care Med* 1989; 17:447–452.

26. Huntsman LL, Stewart DK, Barnes SR, et al: Noninvasive Doppler determination of cardiac output in man: Clinical validation. *Circulation* 1983; 67:593–602.

27. Bernstein DP: Noninvasive cardiac output, Doppler flowmetry, and gold-plated assumptions. *Crit Care Med* 1987; 15:886–887.

28. Ihlen H, Amlie JP, Dale J, et al: Determination of cardiac output by Doppler echocardiography. *Br Heart J* 1984; 51:54–60.

29. Towfig BA, Weir J, Rawles JM: Effect of age and blood pressure on aortic size and stroke distance. *Br Heart J* 1986; 55:560–568.

30. Bouchard A, Blumlein S, Schiller NB, et al: Measurement of left ventricular stroke volume using

continuous wave doppler echocardiography of the ascending aorta and m-mode echocardiography of the aortic valve. *J Am Coll Cardiol* 1987; 9:75–83.

31. Mark JB, Steinbrook RA, Gugino LD, et al: Continuous noninvasive monitoring of cardiac output with esophageal Doppler ultrasound during cardiac surgery. *Anesth Analg* 1986; 65:1013–1020.

32. Fisher DC, Sahn DJ, Friedman MJ, et al: The effect of variations on pulsed Doppler sampling site on calculation of cardiac output: An experimental study in open-chest dogs. *Circulation* 1983; 67:370–376.

33. Lucas CL, Keagy BA, Hsiao HS, et al: The velocity profile in the canine ascending aorta and its effect on the accuracy of pulsed Doppler determinations of mean blood velocity. *Cardiovasc Res* 1984; 18:282–293.

34. Falsetti HL, Carroll RJ, Swope RD, et al: Turbulent blood flow in the ascending aorta of dogs. *Cardiovasc Res* 1983; 17:427–436.

35. Seed WA, Wood NB: Velocity patterns in the aorta. *Cardiovasc Res* 1971; 5:319–330.

36. Segadal L, Matre K: Blood velocity distribution in the human ascending aorta. *Circulation* 1987; 76:90–100.

37. Jenni R, Vieli A, Ruffmann K, et al: A comparison between single gate and multigate ultrasonic Doppler measurements for the assessment of the velocity pattern in the human ascending aorta. *European Heart J* 1984; 5:948–953.

38. Stein PD, Sabbah HN: Turbulent blood flow in the ascending aorta of humans with normal and diseased aortic valves. *Circ Res* 1976; 39:58–65.

39. Chandraratna PA, Nanna M, McKay C, et al: Determination of cardiac output by transcutaneous continuous-wave ultrasonic Doppler computer. *Am J Cardiol* 1984; 53:234–237.

40. Ihlen H, Myhre E, Amlie JP, et al: Changes in left ventricular stroke volume measured by Doppler echocardiography. *Br Heart J* 1985; 54:378–383.

41. Ihlen H, Endresen K, Myreng Y, et al: Reproducibility of cardiac stroke volume estimated by Doppler echocardiography. *Am J Cardiol* 1987; 59:975–978.

42. Stetz CW, Miller RG, Kelly GE, et al: Reliability of the thermodilution method in the determination of cardiac output in clinical practice. *Am Rev Respir Dis* 1982; 126:1001–1004.

43. Singer M, Bennett D: Pitfalls of pulmonary artery catheterization highlighted by Doppler ultrasound. *Crit Care Med* 1989; 17:1060–1061.

44. Gardin JM, Dabestani A, Matin K, et al: Reproducibility of Doppler aortic blood flow measurements: Studies on intraobserver, interobserver and day-to-day variability in normal subjects. *Am J Cardiol* 1984; 54:1092–1098.

45. Wong DH, Onishi R, Tremper KK, et al: Thoracic bioimpedance and Doppler cardiac output measurement: Learning curve and interobserver reproducibility. *Crit Care Med* 1989 17:1194–1198.

46. Waters J, Kwan OL, Kerns G, et al: Limitations of Doppler echocardiography in the calculation of cardiac output. *Circulation* 1982; 66:122.

47. Donovan KD, Dobb GJ, Newman MA, et al: Comparison of pulsed Doppler and thermodilution methods for measuring cardiac output in critically ill patients. *Crit Care Med* 1987; 15:853–857.

48. Niclou R, Teague SM, Lee R: Clinical evaluation of a diameter sensing Doppler cardiac output meter. *Crit Care Med* 1990; 18:428–432.

49. Looyenga DS, Liebson PR, Bone RC, et al: Determination of cardiac output in critically ill patients by dual beam Doppler echocardiography. *J Am Coll Cardiol* 1989; 13:340–347.

50. Wong DH, Mahutte CK: Two-beam pulsed Doppler cardiac output measurement: Reproducibility and agreement with thermodilution. *Crit Care Med* 1990; 18:433–437.

51. Perrino Jr AC, Barash PG: Concentric beam Doppler: Should we be going in circles? *Crit Care Med* 1990; 18:456–457.

52. Freund PR: Transesophageal Doppler scanning versus thermodilution during general anesthesia: An initial comparison of cardiac output techniques. *Am J Surg* 1987; 153:490–494.

53. Abrams JH, Weber RE, Holmen KD: Continuous cardiac output determination using transtracheal Doppler: Initial results in humans. *Anesthesiol* 1989; 71:11–15.

54. Maeda M, Yokota M, Iwase M, et al: Accuracy of cardiac output measured by continuous wave Doppler echocardiography during dynamic exercise testing in the supine position in patients with coronary artery disease. *J Am Coll Cardiol* 1989; 13:76–83.

55. Bojanowski LMR, Timmis AD, Najm YC, et al: Pulsed Doppler ultrasound compared with thermodilution for monitoring cardiac output responses to changing left ventricular function. *Cardiovasc Res* 1987; 21:260–268.

56. Lange H, Lampert S, St. John M, et al: Changes in cardiac output determined by continuous-wave Doppler echocardiography during propafenone or mexiletine drug testing. *Am J Cardiol* 1990; 65:458–462.

57. Stork TV, Muller RM, Piske GJ, et al: Noninvasive determination of pulmonary artery wedge pressure: Comparative analysis of pulsed Doppler electro-cardiography and right heart catheterization. *Crit Care Med* 1990; 18:1158–1163.

58. Channer KS, Wilde P, Culling W, et al: Estimation of left ventricular end-diastolic pressure by pulsed Doppler ultrasound. *Lancet* 1986; 1005–1007.

59. Dabestani A, Mahan G, Gardin JM, et al: Evaluation of pulmonary artery pressure and resistance by pulsed Doppler echocardiography. *Am J Cardiol* 1987; 59:662–668.

60. Martin-Duran R, Larman M, Trugeda A, et al: Comparison of Doppler-determined elevated pulmonary artery pressure with pressure measured at cardiac catheterization. *Am J Cardiol* 1986; 57:859–863.

61. Okamoto M, Miyatake K, Kinoshita N, et al: Analysis of blood flow in pulmonary hypertension with the pulsed Doppler flowmeter combined with cross sectional echocardiography. *Br Heart J* 1984; 51:407–415.

62. Matsuda M, Sekiguchi T, Sugishita Y, et al: Reliability of non-invasive estimates of pulmonary hypertension by pulsed Doppler echocardiography. *Br Heart J* 1986; 56:158–164.

63. Laaban JP, Diebold B, Zelinski R, et al: Noninvasive estimation of systolic pulmonary artery pressure using Doppler echocardiography in patients with chronic obstructive pulmonary disease. *Chest* 1989; 96:1258–1262.

64. Hatle L, Angelsen BAJ, Tromsdal A: Non-invasive estimation of pulmonary artery systolic pressure with Doppler ultrasound. *Br Heart J* 1981; 45:157–165.

65. Migueres M, Escamilla R, Coca F, et al: Pulsed Doppler echocardiography in the diagnosis of pulmonary hypertension in COPD. *Chest* 1990; 98:280–285.

66. Kitabatake A, Inoue M, Asao M, et al: Noninvasive evaluation of pulmonary hypertension by a pulsed Doppler technique. *Circulation* 1983; 68:302–309.

67. Chan KL, Currie PJ, Seward JB, et al: Comparison of three Doppler ultrasound methods in the prediction of pulmonary artery pressure. *J Am Coll Cardiol* 1987; 91:549–554.

68. Marchandise B, De Bruyne B, Delaunois L, et al: Noninvasive prediction of pulmonary hypertension in chronic obstructive pulmonary disease by Doppler echocardiography. *Chest* 1987; 91:361–365.

69. Graettinger WF, Greene ER, Voyles WF: Doppler predictions of pulmonary artery pressure, flow, and resistance in adults. *Am Heart J* 1987; 113:1426–1437.

70. Ferrazza A, Marino B, Giusti V, et al: Usefulness of left and right oblique subcostal view in the echo-Doppler investigation of pulmonary arterial blood flow in patients with chronic obstructive pulmonary disease: The subxiphoid view in the echo-Doppler evaluation of pulmonary blood flow. *Chest* 1990; 98:286–289.

71. Lightly GW, Gargiulo A, Kronzon I, et al: Comparison of multiple views for the evaluation of pulmonary artery blood flow by Doppler echocardiography. *Circulation* 1986; 74:1002–1006.

72. Nyboer J, Bango S, Barnett S, et al: Radiocardiograms. *J Clin Invest* 1940; 19:773.

73. Mohapatra SN: *Non-invasive Cardiovascular Monitoring by Electrical Impedance Technique.* London, Pitman Medical Pub, 1981, pp 1–30.

74. Kubicek WG, Karnegis JR, Patterson RP, et al: Development and evaluation of an impedance cardiac output system. *Aerosp Med* 1966; 37:1208–1212.

75. Kubicek WG, Kottke FJ, Ramos MU, et al: The Minnesota impedance cardiograph—theory and applications. *Biomedical Eng* 1974; 9:410–416.

76. Kubicek WG, Kottke FJ, Ramos MU, et al: Impedance cardiography as a noninvasive method of monitoring cardiac function and other parameters of the cardiovascular system. *Ann NY Acad Sci* 1970; 170:724–732.

77. Bernstein DP. A new stroke volume equation for thoracic electrical bioimpedance: Theory and rationale. *Crit Care Med* 1986; 14:904–909.

78. Sramek BB, Rose DM, Miyamoto A: Stroke volume equation with a linear base impedance model and its accuracy, as compared to thermodilution and magnetic flowmeter techniques in humans and animals. Proceedings of the Sixth International Conference on Electrical Bioimpedance, Zadar, Yugoslavia, 1983, p 38.

79. Sramek BB: Noninvasive technique for measurement of cardiac output by means of electrical impedance. Proceedings of the Fifth International Conference on Electrical Bioimpedance. Business Cent. for Academia Soc. Japan, Tokyo, Japan. Tokyo, Japan, 1981, p 39.

80. Quail AW, Traugott FM, Porges WL, et al: Thoracic resistivity for stroke volume calculation in impedance cardiography. *J Appl Physiol* 1981; 50:191–195.

81. Spinale FG, Reines HD, Crawford, Jr, FA: Comparison of bioimpedance and thermodilution methods for determining cardiac output: Experimental and clinical studies. *Ann Thorac Surg* 1988; 45:421–425.

82. Spinale FG, Smith AC, Crawford FA: Relationship of bioimpedance to thermodilution and echocardiographic measurements of cardiac function.

83. Tremper KK, Hufstedler SM, Barker SJ, et al: Continuous noninvasive estimation of cardiac output by electrical bioimpedance: An experimental study in dogs. *Crit Care Med* 1986; 14:231–233.

84. Eisenberg BM, Linb G, Vollmar R: Estimation of central haemodynamics during dynamic stress by impedance and radiocardiography. *Acta Cardiol* 1988; XLIII:253–258.

85. Smith SA, Russell AE, West MJ, et al: Automated noninvasive measurement of cardiac output: Comparison of electrical bioimpedance and carbon dioxide rebreathing techniques. *Br Heart J* 1988; 59:292–298.

86. Gotshall RW, Wood VC, Miles DS: Comparison of two impedance cardiographic techniques for measuring cardiac output in critically ill patients. *Crit Care Med* 1989; 17:806–811.

87. Edmunds AT, Godfrey S, Tooley M: Cardiac output measured by transthoracic impedance cardiography at rest, during exercise and at various lung volumes. *Clin Sci* 1982; 63:107–113.

88. Bernstein DP: Continuous noninvasive real-time monitoring of stroke volume and cardiac output by thoracic electrical bioimpedance. *Crit Care Med* 1986; 14:898–901.

89. Donovan KD, Dobb GJ, Woods PD, et al: Comparison of transthoracic electrical impedance and thermodilution methods for measuring cardiac output. *Crit Care Med* 1986; 14:1038–1044.

90. Wong DH, Tremper KK, Stemmer EA, et al: Noninvasive cardiac output: Simultaneous comparison of two different methods with thermodilution. *Anesthesiol* 1990; 72:784–792.

91. Masaki DI, Greenspoon JS, Ouzounian JG: Noninvasive determination of cardiac output by thoracic electrical bioimpedance. *Crit Care Med* 1990; 121–122.

92. Teo KK, Hetherington MD, Haennel RG, et al: Cardiac output measured by impedance cardiography during maximal exercise tests. *Cardiovasc Res* 1985; 19:737–743.

93. Ekman LG, Milsom I, Arvidsson S, et al: Clinical evaluation of an ensemble-averaging impedance cardiography for monitoring stroke volume during spontaneous breathing. *Acta Anaesthesiol Scand* 1990; 34:190–196.

94. Salandin V, Zussa C, Risica G, et al: Comparison of cardiac output estimation by thoracic electrical bioimpedance, thermodilution, and Fick methods. *Crit Care Med* 1988; 16:1157–1158.

95. Castor G, Molter G, Helms J, et al: Determination of cardiac output during positive end-expiratory pressure—noninvasive electrical bioimpedance compared with standard thermodilution. *Crit Care Med* 1990; 18:544–546.

96. Appel PL, Kram HB, Mackabee J, et al: Comparison of measurements of cardiac output by bioimpedance and thermodilution in severely ill surgical patients. *Crit Care Med* 1986; 14:933–935.

97. Huang KC, Stoddard M, Tsueda K, et al: Stroke volume measurements by electrical bioimpedance and echocardiography in healthy volunteers. *Crit Care Med* 1990; 18:1274–1278.

98. Gotshall RW, Miles DS: Noninvasive assessment of cardiac output by impedance cardiography in the newborn canine. *Crit Care Med* 1989; 17:63–65.

99. Miles DS, Gotshall RW, Golden JC, et al: Accuracy of electrical impedance cardiography for measuring cardiac output in children with congenital heart defects. *Am J Cardiol* 1988; 61:612–616.

100. Belik J, Pelech A: Thoracic electric bioimpedance measurement of cardiac output in the newborn infant. *J Pediatr* 1988; 113:890–895.

101. Braden DS, Leatherbury L, Treiber FA, et al: Noninvasive assessment of cardiac output in children using impedance cardiography. *Am Heart J* 1990; 120:1166–1172.

102. Tibballs J: A comparative study of cardiac output in neonates supported by mechanical ventilation: Measurement with thoracic electrical bioimpedance and pulsed Doppler ultrasound. *J Pediatr* 1989; 114:632–635.

103. Introna RPS, Pruett JK, Crumrine RC, et al: Use of transthoracic bioimpedance to determine cardiac output in pediatric patients. *Crit Care Med* 1988; 16:1101–1105.

104. Mickel JJ, Lucking SE, Chaten FC, et al: Trending of impedance-monitored cardiac variables: Method and statistical power analysis of 100 controll studies in a pediatric intensive care unit. *Crit Care Med* 1990; 18:645–650.

105. Lage SG, Bellotti G, Ramires JAF, et al: Pneumopericardium: A novel limitation for thoracic electrical bioimpedance? *Crit Care Med* 1987; 15:891–892.

106. Schieken RM, Patel MR, Falsetti HL, et al: Effect of mitral valvular regurgitation on transthoracic impedance cardiogram. *Br Heart J* 1981; 45:166–172.

107. Ebert TJ, Eckberg DL, Vetrovec GM, et al: Impedance cardiograms reliably estimate beat-by-beat changes of left ventricular stroke volume in humans. *Cardiovasc Res* 1984; 18:354–360.

108. Muzi M, Ebert TJ, Tristani FE, et al: Determination of cardiac output using ensemble-averaged impedance cardiograms. *J Appl Physiol* 1985; 58:200–205.

109. Du Quesnay MC, Stoute GJ, Hughson RL: Cardiac output in exercise by impedance cardiography during breath holding and normal breathing. *J Appl Physiol* 1987; 62:101–107.

Chapter 15 _____

Impedance Pneumography, Apnea Monitoring, and Respiratory Inductive Plethysmography

Richard D. Branson, R.R.T.

Robert S. Campbell, R.R.T.

INTRODUCTION

The techniques of respiratory inductive plethysmography (RIP) and impedance pneumography (IP) are unique among noninvasive respiratory monitoring methods due to the patient/monitor interface. Typical respiratory monitoring requires a flow and/or pressure sensor in the gas stream to determine ventilatory volumes. These two techniques utilize sensors on or around the chest wall and abdomen to monitor not only volumes, but breathing frequency and ventilatory pattern. This chapter will review the principles of operation and clinical uses of RIP and IP. Some consideration will also be given to apnea monitoring with techniques other than IP.

IMPEDANCE PNEUMOGRAPHY

Impedance pneumography is commonly used in the intensive care unit (ICU) to monitor respiratory frequency and breathing pattern, and it is the most frequent technique used in home apnea monitors.[1, 2] The use of IP to monitor respiratory volumes has been described, but is not routinely performed.[3, 4]

Principles of Operation

Impedance pneumography measures changes in electrical impedance (ΔZ) between two electrodes placed on the chest wall. The electrodes used are commonly the same electrodes used for monitoring the electrocardiogram (ECG). Changes in chest wall impedance are a result of changes in the blood/bone/tissue ratio between the electrodes. The technique of IP uses a constant, low-amplitude, high-frequency current of 100 KHz passed between electrodes on the chest wall, and the return voltage is measured to calculate impedance.

The most frequent cause of chest wall impedance change is respiration. During inspiration, as the lungs fill and the chest wall moves outward, chest wall impedance increases. During expiration, the chest wall moves inward as the lungs deflate, causing a fall in chest wall impedance (Fig 15–1). Note that the relative contribution of gas in the lungs is insignificant because air offers little change in impedance. Chest wall movement due to lung inflation is the measured variable. The resulting change in the amplitude of the high-frequency signal is processed by the monitor and a representative respiration waveform is produced as output to a monitor display or printer (Fig 15–2). Further software processing allows the respiratory rate to be calculated, and alarms for apnea may be set.

A diagram of a typical impedance pneumography system is shown in Figure 15–3. A reference generator creates the high-frequency current that is passed between the two electrodes. The relatively low voltage returned is amplified to produce the reference signal as shown in Figure 15–2. A demodulator processes the signal to a useful waveform for display. Further amplification allows software processing for calculation of respiratory frequency and apnea alarm settings.

Typically, an impedance pneumography system provides a constant display of the respiration waveform and calculates respiratory rate based on a 4 to 6 breath average. These monitors usually offer the clinician adjustable high and low respiratory rate alarms and an adjustable apnea alarm time. Some IP systems used for apnea monitoring and for critical care monitoring provide a sensitivity adjustment, which helps differentiate between impedance changes due to respiration and those due to motion artifact or cardiac activity.

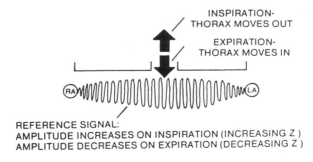

INSPIRATION-
THORAX MOVES OUT

EXPIRATION-
THORAX MOVES IN

REFERENCE SIGNAL:
AMPLITUDE INCREASES ON INSPIRATION (INCREASING Z)
AMPLITUDE DECREASES ON EXPIRATION (DECREASING Z)

FIG 15–1.
A constant high-frequency reference signal is passed between the left and right electrodes creating a baseline reference. As the chest wall expands during inspiration, impedance increases while expiration causes impedance to decrease.

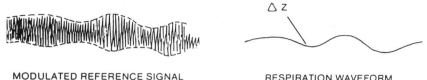

MODULATED REFERENCE SIGNAL   RESPIRATION WAVEFORM

FIG 15–2.
The raw reference signal created by respiration-related changes in chest wall impedance (*left*) and the processed waveform (*right*) displayed on the monitor.

Clinical Use of Impedance Pneumography

The most common use of IP is for home apnea monitoring of infants. This technique is widely accepted because of the monitor's ease of use and simplicity. Home apnea monitoring of infants is frequently employed and has been recommended for preterm infants and infants at risk for sudden infant death syndrome (SIDS).[5–8] Apnea has been demonstrated to occur in 25 to 84% of preterm infants, and the early identification of apnea in infants at risk for SIDS may be useful in preventing death.[7–9] This not only makes home apnea monitoring with IP an important technique, it also makes this a very lucrative business.[9] The appropriateness of home apnea monitoring, its effects on the family, and the efficacy of apnea monitoring are not considered here, but have been discussed elsewhere.[10–12]

Despite its relative ease of use, IP is not without problems. Several authors have described alarm failures with IP monitors during apneic episodes.[13–15] These failures are most often caused by upper airway obstruction and bradycardia coinciding with apnea. In the case of obstructive apnea, the patient continues breathing efforts despite the inability to draw gas into the lungs. These efforts create a change in chest wall impedance, despite the absence of lung

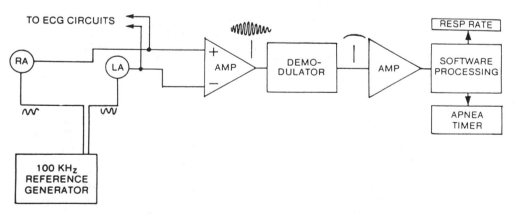

FIG 15–3.
Schematic diagram of impedance pneumograph.

inflation, and the monitor fails to alarm. The inability of IP to differentiate between obstructive and central apnea is a serious limitation of this monitoring technique.

If apnea and bradycardia occur simultaneously, a resultant rise in the amplitude of cardiac oscillations can cause the monitor to mistake cardiac activity for respiratory activity. Typically, cardiac and respiratory activity can be differentiated by signal amplitude, but bradycardia causes cardiac-related impedance changes to increase. When this occurs, apnea is not detected and no alarm is sounded. In this instance an alarm may not sound until the heart rate is less than the set low respiratory rate (usually <10/min), at which time resuscitation may not be successful. Figure 15–4 demonstrates a case of apnea followed by bradycardia (prior to the set apnea alarm time) that is not detected by IP. The newest generation of impedance pneumographs also continuously monitors ECG so that this life-threatening situation does not occur.

Weese-Mayer et al.[16] found that during apnea monitoring of infants, 69% of alarms were the result of patient movement and that 23% of all other alarms were false alarms. The use of IP monitors for detecting apnea in the hospital and home continues on a regular basis. The use of ECG monitoring with IP has significantly improved the safety and efficacy of the technique. However, IP cannot differentiate obstructive from central apnea.

Impedance pneumography is a common component of intensive care unit monitoring sys-

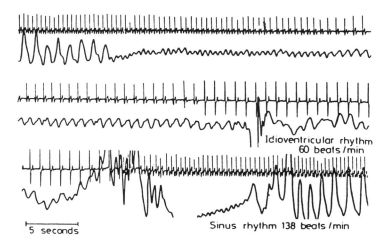

FIG 15–4.
A 24-hour ECG and respiration recording showing the ECG trace above a simultaneous respiration signal. The initial heart rate is 136/min. At 8 seconds after the onset of the recording, an apneic episode occurs that lasts 47 seconds. Twenty seconds after the onset of the apnoea sinus bradycardia with a junctional escape rhythm begins. Twenty seconds later there is an idioventricular escape rhythm of 60/min, which lasts for 7 seconds before a large breath occurs. A further apnoeic episode of 18 seconds follows this breath and an idioventricular rhythm continues during this apnoea until artificial ventilation with a bag and face mask is started. Almost immediately the heart rate increases and the ECG reverts to sinus rhythm. When the heart rate falls, the cardiac impression on the respiration trace becomes larger in amplitude. By the time of established junctional rhythm the cardiac impression resembles a shallow respiration signal. *(From Southall DP et al: An explanation for failure of impedance apnoea alarm systems.* Arch Dis Child *1980; 55:63–65. Used by permission.)*

tems. Using the ECG electrodes, a continuous waveform of respiratory effort is displayed (Fig 15–5) and respiratory frequency is calculated on a gliding average. During mechanical ventilation, more sophisticated ventilator alarms are used to detect apnea, and the IP display is rarely used for monitoring. In the nonintubated patient, IP measurement of respiratory frequency may be useful to detect apnea and abnormal breathing patterns. However, the clinician should never neglect the time-honored monitoring of respiratory rate by visual inspection for 60 seconds.

Other Apnea Monitoring Techniques

Although impedance pneumography is a popular apnea monitoring technique, other systems are available. Capnography can be utilized to detect apnea in intubated patients, and in nonintubated patients a modified nasal cannula is used (see Chapter 12). Briefly, capnography

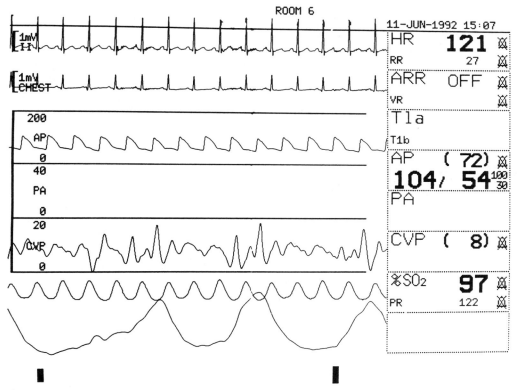

FIG 15–5.
Typical ICU monitoring screen. The top two tracings are ECG; the third, arterial blood pressure; the fourth, central venous pressure; the fifth is a plethysmographic display of the pulse waveform from a pulse oximeter; and the last is the respiration waveform as measured by impedance pneumography. The calculated respiratory frequency is displayed below the numeric HR (heart rate) display.

detects apnea when no exhaled carbon dioxide (CO_2) is measured by the sensor. Chief among the problems associated with capnography are untoward effects of humidity and secretions, and malposition of the sensor. In each case a false apnea alarm would result.

Airflow can also be measured at the airway using thermometry. In these cases a thermistor is placed in the expired gas path, again using a modified nasal cannula or nasal catheter in nonintubated patients. As inspired and expired gases travel over the thermistor, the cooling effect causes a change in resistance, reflected as a temperature change. Like IP, the resulting qualitative signal can be processed and displayed or printed. Using a thermistor to detect apnea is hindered by malposition of the sensor and depends on the sensitivity of the device or its inability to detect shallow breathing.

The use of either capnography or thermometry alone is not recommended. However, combining either of these with IP may allow detection of apnea and differentiation between central and obstructive apnea. Commercial systems are available for this combined monitoring.

RESPIRATORY INDUCTIVE PLETHYSMOGRAPHY

Respiratory inductive plethysmography is a noninvasive monitor of ventilatory frequency and pattern that uses transducer bands placed on the torso and abdomen.[17-19] RIP also has the ability to monitor changes in lung volumes from a known baseline, but it cannot make absolute volume measurements.

The RIP System

The basic principle by which RIP measures respiration was first described in 1967 by Konno and Mead.[20] This principle relies on the assumption that the respiratory system moves with two degrees of freedom, the rib cage (RC) and the abdomen (AB). During normal inspiration, the diaphragm descends and displaces the AB while the RC expands outward.

A commercially available RIP system (Respigraph) is manufactured by Noninvasive Monitoring Systems (NIMS, Miami, FL)(Fig 15–6). The system consists of two elastic cloth bands, each having two coils of insulated Teflon wire sewn sinusoidally to the cloth.[21] One band encircles the rib cage at the nipple level, or above the breasts in female patients, and the other encircles the abdomen at the level of the umbilicus (Fig 15–7). An oscillator produces a sine wave amplitude of approximately 20 mV at a frequency of 30 kHz to each of the transducer bands. Cross-sectional area changes in the bands cause the orientation of the Teflon wire to be altered, resulting in a change in oscillatory frequencies due to changes in self-inductance.

A microprocessor conditions the raw signals from the transducer bands by demodulating and amplifying the frequency changes and converting them to analog signals for display. Waveforms from both RC and AB bands can be displayed or printed in real time or digitized for later data processing.

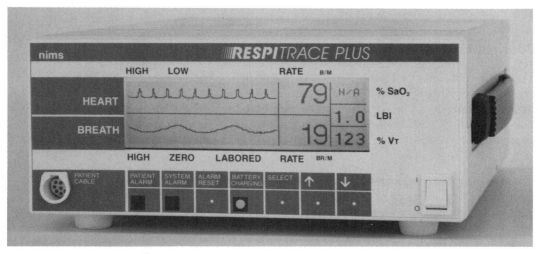

FIG 15–6.
RIP system (Respigraph). (*Courtesy of NIMS, Inc, Miami Beach, FL.*)

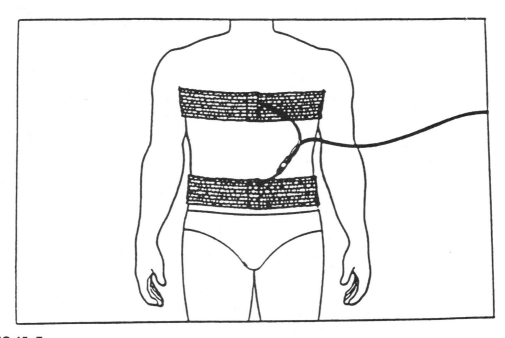

FIG 15–7.
Proper placement of RIP transducer bands, which are connected by snaps to the oscillator module. The RC band is placed on the upper chest above the breasts in female subjects or at the nipple level in male subjects; the AB band is placed at the level of the umbilicus. (*From Krieger BP: Ventilatory pattern monitoring. Respir Care 1990; 35:697–708. Used by permission.*)

Calibration and Accuracy

Many different calibration procedures have been described and assessed for the RIP.[21-25] These various procedures affect not only the accuracy and validity of RIP measurements, but also the measurements displayed. The level of understanding by both the practitioner and patient, ease of operation, and patient cooperation also play an important role in the clinical usefulness and success of RIP.

Isovolume Maneuver Calibration Procedure (IMC)

IMC is the standard method of calibrating any noninvasive respiratory monitor that measures both the RC and AB compartments contribution to tidal volume (V_T). Using this method, the sum change in volume of the RC and AB should equal the total volume change at the airway opening. With the airway occluded, the change in volume between the RC and AB should be equal but opposite to yield a sum volume of zero. The two-step procedure is performed in one body position and requires patient understanding and cooperation. First, the patient is instructed to shift volume gently between the RC and the AB compartments with the airway occluded. Pressure in the airway should remain less than 10 cm H_2O to minimize compression of thoracic gas volume. The RC and AB electrical signals are displayed graphically during the procedure, and each gain is adjusted to create a 45-degree angle (42 to 48 degrees is acceptable) on an oscilloscope. This determines the proportional factor K for the RIP, which plots RC and AB excursion for each individual patient. In addition to the 45-degree angle, the calibration may be verified if the RC and AB excursion waveforms are equal and opposite and yield a sum volume of zero.

The second step of the procedure involves the connection of a spirometer or pneumotachograph to the patient's airway opening to measure actual V_T. The gains of the RC and AB signals are adjusted equally such that V_T measured by RIP equals V_T measured by a spirometer. RIP may be useful to track trends in V_T even if the second step of the calibration is not done. In other words, spirometric measurement need only be done if absolute measurement of V_T is desired on a continuous basis. This method is required if V_T measurement on a continuous basis is desired. This calibration method is considered the standard for proportioning RC and AB contribution to V_T and for enabling RIP to detect obstructive apnea reliably. Measurement of V_T is accurate (within 10%) during tidal breathing if body position is constant. However, accuracy declines (within 20%) if body position changes or the V_T range changes from the calibration period. An additional clinical limitation of this method is that few patients can be trained to perform the isovolume maneuver correctly.

Qualitative Diagnostic Calibration (QDC)

This method was devised to overcome the fact that most patients cannot properly perform the isovolume maneuver. If the contribution of the RC and AB excursions to V_T is known, then the proportional factor K can be solved by the following equation:

$$K = -\text{SD (VAB)}/\text{SD (VRC)}$$

where SD is standard deviation. A constant V_T may be approximated by allowing the patient to breath normally for 5 minutes in a single body position and omitting any breath with ± 1.0 SD of the mean of the uncalibrated sum (VRC + VAB). Once the appropriate K factor is solved for the patient, a baseline is designated from which a trend of V_T may begin. This calibration may be updated by the computer as often as every 5 minutes. Automatic recalibration is important to assure proper assignment of the correct K, which is necessary for detection and distinction of obstructive apnea and hypopnea. However, when a trend of V_T is clinically important, automatic recalibration may increase the measurement error if changes in either body position or transducer band placement has occurred.

Two-Posture Simultaneous Equation Method (SEM)

This calibration method is also based on the principles of the IMC calibration and on the fact that the contribution of the RC and AB to V_T varies between each compartment as body position changes. With the patient in the supine position, a change in V_T is caused predominantly by AB excursion while RC excursion predominates in the standing position. Volume signals from RC and AB transducers are recorded with V_T measured by spirometry with the patient in both the supine and standing (upright) position. The gain factors for the RC (X) and AB (Y) signals are solved using the following formulas:

$$X = [(AB)(V_T') - (AB')(V_T)]/[(RC')(AB) - (RC)(AB')]$$

$$Y = [(RC)(V_T') - (RC')(V_T)]/[(RC)(AB') - (RC')(AB')]$$

where V_T = spirometer volume measurement of tidal breathing while supine, V_T' = spirometer volume measurement of tidal breathing while standing, RC = RC signal of the RIP with patient supine, RC′ = RC signal of the RIP with patient standing, AB = AB signal of the RIP with patient supine, and AB′ = AB signal of the RIP with patient standing. RIP volume measurement is made equal to that of the spirometer by multiplying the RC excursion signal by X and the AB excursion signal by Y. This calibration procedure improves the volume measuring accuracy of RIP when used on patients that undergo changes in body position or range of V_T. Obstructive apnea and hypopnea cannot be detected by RIP when the SEM calibration has been performed.

Variables Measured by RIP and Display Techniques

Waveforms produced by RIP can be separated into measurements of volume, flow, timing, and thoracoabdominal motion. These components are depicted in Figure 15–8. Processing of the data allows numerical means, variability, and trends to be displayed.

Volume Components

Tidal volume is determined from the trough-to-peak sum signal (Fig 15–8) and minute ventilation from the sum of inspiratory V_T signals over a 1-minute period. It should be noted that

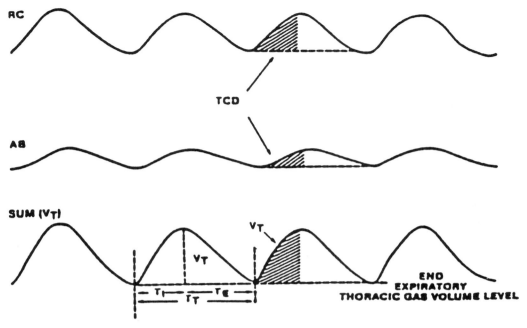

FIG 15–8.
RIP tracings showing RC and AB waveforms; the electrical sum of the RC + AB = VT. Total compartmental displacement (TCD) is the absolute sum of the area during inspiration (TI) of the RC + AB (*shaded areas*), irrespective of sign. When the RC and AB compartments are in synchrony (as depicted here), the TCD will equal the sum (VT), and the TCD/VT ratio will equal unity (1.00). The end-expiratory thoracic gas volume (or FRC level) is shown, as well as timing components (TE = expiratory time; TT = total respiratory cycle time).

RIP monitors inspiratory minute ventilation (VI), whereas most critical care measurements are expired minute ventilation (VE).

Volume components are used in the detection of apnea and are defined as a flat RC, AB, and sum signal for greater than 10 seconds. In clinical use, the sum signal is rarely absolutely zero due to changes in patient position, gas compression, and drift. As such, if the sum signal is less than 25% of the mean VT during the 5-minute calibration period, an apnea alarm will sound.

During critical care monitoring, RIP does not continuously monitor volumes. Instead a mean VT and VI are recorded from the QDC calibration. All subsequent measurements are recorded as a percent change from the QDC mean. For example, if during the QDC VT was 500 mL and over the following 2 hours VT fell to 375 mL, the RIP would display that VT was reduced from 100 to 75%. Changes in VI would likewise be displayed. If during QDC, the VI was 6 L/min and VI rose to 10 L/min, the RIP display would reflect an increase in minute ventilation from 100 to 160%.

Time Components

RIP is capable of displaying inspiratory time (T_I), expiratory time (T_E), and total cycle time (T_T). Respiratory frequency f is calculated on a breath-to-breath basis by dividing T_T by 60. This breath-by-breath updating of f can lead to confusion because the displayed value will not equal the f counted over 1 minute. A computed summary printout provides the f based on a 1-minute average. This value is more useful for calculating trends and making clinical decisions. The T_I/T_T ratio or duty cycle can also be calculated by RIP and is a reflection of ventilatory timing.[26]

Flow Components

Inspiratory flow can be calculated from V_T/V_I and used as a rough estimate of ventilatory drive.[26]

Thoracoabdominal Synchrony

By analyzing coordination between the RC and AB contribution to V_T, RIP can detect asynchrony of the ventilatory muscles. Asynchronous breathing can occur in patients with COPD, diaphragmatic paralysis, and respiratory muscle fatigue.[27-29] When asynchronous breathing is present, weaning from mechanical ventilation may not be possible.

RIP can perform sophisticated analyses of thoracoabdominal coordination using an index known as the *total compartmental displacement/tidal volume ratio* (TCD/V_T). TCD is the sum of the areas under the RC and AB tracings during an inspiration (Fig 15–8). If perfect synchrony is achieved, the TCD/V_T is 1.00. If dysynchrony or asynchrony occur, the TCD/V_T is greater than 1.00.

Rib Cage Contributions to Tidal Volume

The contribution of rib cage displacement to the V_T is calculated as the percent RC/V_T. The abdominal contributions can also be calculated (100 − %RC/V_T). Normal %RC/V_T is less than 50% in the supine position and greater than 50% in the upright position. A %RC/V_T greater than 100% suggests minute abdominal excursions, compared to RC or paradoxical respiration. If %RC/V_T is 0%, upper airway obstruction should be suspected.[30, 31]

Compressed Plots

While the continuous displays of RC, AB, and sum waveforms are useful, long-term monitoring requires some form of data reduction to allow interpretation of clinical trends. The microprocessor of the RIP system allows compressed plots or envelope data to be displayed or printed (Fig 15–9). The height of each vertical line is proportional to the V_T of a single breath. Additionally, the %RC/V_T is displayed from 0 to 100%, the end-expiratory thoracic gas volume (TGV) is shown as a solid line at the base of each V_T and the TCD as a dotted line above the V_T (Fig 15–10). Compressed plots may also include numerical data including respiratory frequency and oxygen saturation (Spo_2).

The clinical interpretation of these compressed plots is not readily accomplished by the novice, but the plots may be the most useful data supplied by RIP. The normal values for RIP components are shown in Table 15–1.

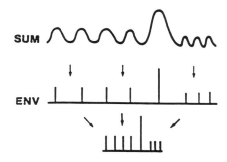

FIG 15–9.
Illustration showing how the Respigraph system reduces analog breath waveforms to a compound plot envelope (ENV) for convenient record collection. The height of each vertical bar is proportional to the size of the V_T as represented by the sum signal.

Usefulness of Monitoring RIP Components

Respiratory Frequency (f)

Although easy to measure, the value of monitoring f is underappreciated.[32–35] An abnormal f is a nonspecific, but very sensitive, sign of respiratory and/or central nervous system (CNS) dysfunction. Tobin et al.[34] have shown that a rise in f precedes the development of respiratory failure, and that bradypnea is a common sign of CNS depression (injury or drug overdose).

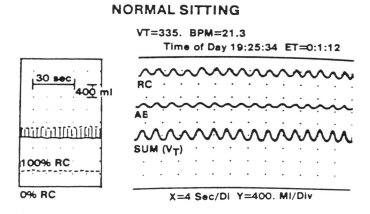

NORMAL SITTING

VT=335. BPM=21.3
Time of Day 19:25:34 ET=0:1:12

FIG 15–10.
Videodisplay of breath waveforms in a normal adult using Respigraph. The corresponding compressed plot is illustrated in the left panel. The envelope plot depicts VT as vertical lines; at the upper tip of these vertical lines is a hatched line representing TCD. The hatched horizontal line at the lower portion of the plot is the breath-by-breath plot of % RC/VT denoted as %RC. (*From Baker LE, Hill DW: The use of electrical impedance techniques for the monitoring of respiratory pattern during anaesthesia. Brit J Anaesth 1969; 41:2–17. Used by permission.*)

TABLE 15–1.
Breathing Pattern Components in Adults

	Mean	Range	Coefficient of Variation*
Respiratory frequency (breaths/min)			
Normal, at rest	17	12–22	21–29
Successfully extubated	24	15–35	28
Tidal volume (mL)			
Normal, at rest	383	200–500	22–28
Successfully extubated	435	155–700	34
Minute ventilation (L)			
Normal, at rest	6.0	N/A	23
Successfully extubated	9.7	3.4–16.0	N/A
TCD/VT			
Normal (at rest)	1.05	<1.10	4–14
Successfully extubated	1.17	1.03–1.47	N/A

* Coefficient of variation equals SD divided by the mean times 100; N/A, not available. MCA/VT is similar to TCD/VT.

Perhaps more important than the absolute f is its trend over time. While f may be variable, a sustained change is associated with significant clinical events.[32–35] Tobin et al.[35] have suggested that an increase in $f > 11$/min in critically ill patients indicates the need for ventilatory support. However, it should be noted that if a patient with tachypnea fails to increase f further, it may be a sign that the respiratory muscles are unable to meet the current demands.

In addition to f, the breathing pattern is also useful in detecting dysfunction. The compressed plots used by RIP can demonstrate the classic abnormal breathing patterns associated with CNS injury including Biot's breathing, Cheyne-Stokes breathing, neurogenic hyperventilation, and apneic episodes.

Tidal Volume and Minute Ventilation

Tidal volume is subject to even greater variability in normal persons than is respiratory f, and it is more difficult to assess.[36] Changes in VT occur normally with alterations in breathing pattern and sighing, or may result from airway obstruction and metabolic disturbances.

TCD/VT

As previously described, the TCD/VT is a measure of thoracoabdominal coordination. Krieger et al.[37] have shown that a normal TCD/VT is 1.17 ± 0.12, and this value remains relatively constant for a given patient. Temporary changes in TCD/VT are of little usefulness, while prolonged increases may be a sensitive indicator of respiratory failure.[38]

Clinical Uses of RIP

To date, RIP has been used far more often as a research tool than a clinical monitor. Yet there is some promise of potential clinical usefulness of RIP in the ICU, the step-down unit, the sleep laboratory, and the home. These applications will be considered individually below.

Use of RIP in the ICU

The role of RIP in the ICU is not necessarily as a monitor of acute events, but rather a system to forewarn of impending adverse events. RIP has the advantage of being continuous, whereas many respiratory measurements are performed intermittently. If it is to be effective, then RIP must provide clinically relevant information that allows the clinician to undertake therapy to prevent catastrophe.

Several authors have shown that respiratory frequency and breathing pattern changes during weaning from ventilatory support may be sensitive indicators of weaning success or failure.[35, 37] Krieger and Ershowsky[38] have also shown that respiratory muscle fatigue is characterized by rapid, shallow breathing and respiratory alternans. The use of RIP to monitor respiratory muscle coordination as evidenced by an increase in TCD/V_T or increasing variability of $\%RC/V_T$ may assist in identifying these problems early. Several authors have shown the usefulness of these variables in predicting weaning success of ICU patients,[35–39] although some of these data were retrospective.[39]

Kreiger et al. have also reported a reduction in time until extubation using a group of RIP monitors. They found that patients remained intubated for an average of 15 hours less, compared to a retrospective group from the preceding year.[40] Krieger et al. also stated that continuous monitoring with RIP was useful in determining the success of lung expansion techniques (i.e., incentive spirometry).

RIP may allow an estimation of auto-PEEP. If TGV is measured at end-expiration, it is essentially equivalent to functional residual capacity. Auto-PEEP then can be measured by adding external PEEP until end-expiratory TGV increases.[41] The amount of PEEP required to cause this change in TGV is equal to auto-PEEP. This is only effective if auto-PEEP is due to dynamic airway collapse.[42–44]

None of these papers addresses the problems associated with RIP. Chief of these problems is patient movement. The spontaneously breathing ICU patient tends to have frequent position changes. This, along with diaphoresis and patient activity, can cause the bands to slide out of position, rendering the entire system useless. This experience with RIP has typically precluded its use in the ICU for anything but short-term research projects.

Use in the Step-Down Unit

The establishment of step-down units for patients with primarily respiratory problems has been slow to develop when compared to cardiac step-down units.[45, 46] These new "pulmonary care" or "noninvasive monitoring" units are becoming more popular, however, due to the cost savings compared to intensive care.[45]

Krieger et al. have described a noninvasive monitoring unit (NIMU) that utilizes a multiplex RIP system for four beds. They found that through reductions in staff they were able to reduce costs by an average of $3500 per admission.[39, 47] Even with reduced staffing, their rate of successful weaning from mechanical ventilation and discharge rate remained unchanged. These results are quite promising and it has been suggested that NIMUs may save $500 million annually in the United States.[47] While this may be true, the role of RIP is, at best, suspect. The cost savings is in development of the NIMU. The value of using RIP or a combination of other noninvasive monitors (capnography, oximetry, etc.) in the NIMU has yet to be proven.

Use in Sleep Labs and Home Monitoring

As described earlier, impedance pneumography is the most common method of home apnea monitoring and, when combined with either capnography or a method of airflow detection, is frequently used in the sleep lab. It has been suggested that the ability of RIP to distinguish central and obstructive apnea may make it useful in the sleep lab. However, even the RIP can fail to differentiate between central and obstructive apnea if respiratory efforts are weak. In this instance, use of esophageal manometry may be indicated.[48] A modification of RIP that includes neck plethysmography (NIP) appears to be capable of detecting these minute respiratory efforts, even when RC and AB signals are flat.

The use of RIP in the home has the advantage of continuous recording of reams of data for later analysis. However, no method of respiratory monitoring has proven to be a reliable diagnostic tool in the home. It is hoped that further refinement of RIP for infants may lead to better apnea monitors, particularly for infants at risk for SIDS.

SUMMARY

Impedance pneumography and respiratory inductive plethysmography are monitoring techniques that are unique due to their site of patient attachment. Their clinical usefulness, however, appears questionable. While IP is used frequently for apnea monitoring, it has considerable limitations when used alone. Although common, the use of IP in the ICU appears to be of little value or interest.

RIP is a sophisticated research tool that continues to help us better understand clinical pulmonary physiology. However, as a clinical tool, it appears to be useful only in the hands of a few investigators involved in its development. The suggestion that RIP saves money is, we believe, unsubstantiated. The development of NIMUs saves money, regardless of which type of monitoring system is used.

REFERENCES

1. ECRI: Infant home apnea monitors. *Health Dev* 1987; March–April:79–91.
2. Pacela AF: Impedance pneumography—a survey of instrumentation techniques. *Med Biol Eng* 1966; 4:1–15.
3. Grenvik A, Ballou S, McGinley H, et al: Impedance pneumography. *Chest* 1972; 62:439–443.
4. Baker LE, Hill DW: The use of electrical impedance techniques for the monitoring of respiratory pattern during anaesthesia. *Brit J Anaesth* 1969; 41:2–17.
5. Daily WJR, Klaus M, Meyer HBP: Apnea in premature infants: Monitoring, incidence, heart rate changes, and an effect of environmental temperature. *Pediatrics* 1969; 43:510–518.
6. Alden ER, Mandelkorn T, Woodrum DE, et al: Morbidity and mortality of infants weighing less than 1000 grams in an intensive care nursery. *Pediatrics* 1972; 50:40–49.
7. Kelly DH, Shannon DC, O'Connell K: Care of infants with near miss sudden infant death syndrome. *Pediatrics* 1978; 61:511–514.
8. Steinschneider A: A re-examination of "the apnea monitor business." *Pediatrics* 1976; 58:1–5.
9. Stein IM, Shannon DC: The pediatric pneumogram: A new method for detecting and quantitating apnea in infants. *Pediatrics* 1975; 55:599–603.

10. Neuman MR: Apnea monitoring: Technical aspects, in Little GA (ed): *Report of a Consensus Development Conference*. Bethesda, MD, National Institutes of Health, 1987 (NIH 87-2905).
11. Thach BT: Sleep apnea in infancy and childhood. *Med Clin North Am* 1985; 69:1289–1315.
12. Black L, Hersher L, Steinschneider A: Impact of the apnea monitor on family life. *Pediatrics* 1978; 62:681–685.
13. Southall DP, Richards JM, Lau KC, et al: An explanation for failure of impedance apnoea alarm systems. *Arch Dis Child* 1980; 55:63–65.
14. Southall DP, Levitt GA, Richards JM, et al: Undetected episodes of prolonged apnea and severe bradycardia in preterm infants. *Pediatrics* 1983; 72:541.
15. Warburton D, Stark AR, Taeusch HW: Apnea monitor failure in infants with upper airway obstruction. *Pediatrics* 1977; 60:742–744.
16. Weese-Mayer DE, Brouillette RT, Hunt C, et al: Assessing validity of infant monitor alarms with event recording. *J Pediatr* 1990; 117:568–574.
17. Krieger BP: Ventilatory pattern monitoring: Instrumentation and applications. *Respir Care* 1990; 35:697–708.
18. Krieger BP: Respiratory inductive plethysmography. *Problems Respir Care* 1989; 2:156–175.
19. Sackner MA, Krieger BP: Noninvasive respiratory monitoring, in Scharf SM, Cassidy SS (eds): *Heart-Lung Interaction in Health and Disease*. New York, Marcel Dekker, 1989, pp 663–805.
20. Konno K, Mead J: Measurement of the separate changes of rib cage and abdomen during breathing. *J Appl Physiol* 1967; 22:407.
21. Watson H: Technology of respiratory inductive plethysmography, in Stott FD, Raftery EB, Goulding L (eds): *ISAM Proceedings of the Third International Symposium on Ambulatory Monitoring*. London, Academic Press, 1980, pp 537–558.
22. Feinerman D, Krieger B, Belsito AS, et al: Calibration of respiratory inductive plethysmograph during natural breathing utilizing principles of isovolume maneuver procedure. *J Appl Physiol* 1989; 66:410.
23. Watson HL, Poole DA, Sackner MA: Accuracy of respiratory inductive plethysmographic measurement of cross-sectional area of models. *J Appl Physiol* 1988; 65:306.
24. Chadha TS, Watson H, Birch S, et al: Validation of respiratory inductive plethysmography using different calibration procedures. *Am Rev Respir Dis* 1982; 125:644–649.
25. Sackner MA, Watson H, Belsito AS, et al: Calibration of respiratory inductive plethysmography during natural breathing. *J Appl Physiol* 1989; 66:410–420.
26. Milic-Emili J: Recent advances in clinical assessment of control of breathing. *Lung* 1982; 160:1.
27. Gilbert R, Ashutosh K, Auchincloss JH, et al: Prospective study of controlled oxygen therapy; poor prognosis of patients with asynchronous breathing. *Chest* 1977; 71:456.
28. Higenbottom T, Allen D, Loh L, et al: Abdominal wall movement in normals and patients with hemidiaphragmatic and bilateral diaphragmatic palsy. *Thorax* 1977; 32:589.
29. Barrio JL, Feinerman D, Hesla PE, et al: Diaphragmatic flutter in a patient with lymphoma. *Mt. Sinai J Med (NY)* 1987; 54:188.
30. Krieger B, Feinerman D, Zaron A, et al: Continuous non-invasive monitoring of respiratory rate in critically ill patients. *Chest* 1986; 90:632.
31. Cohen CA, Zagelbaum G, Gross D, et al: Clinical manifestations of inspiratory muscle fatigue. *Am J Med* 1982; 73:308.
32. Tobin MJ, Chadha TS, Jenouri G, et al: Breathing patterns. 1. Normal subjects. *Chest* 1983; 84:202.
33. Tobin MJ, Mador JM, Guenther SM, et al: Variability of resting center drive and timing in healthy subjects. *J Appl Physiol* 1988; 65:309.
34. Tobin MJ, Chadha TS, Jenouri G, et al: Breathing patterns. 2. Disease subjects. *Chest* 1983; 84:286.
35. Tobin MJ, Perez W, Guenther SM, et al: The pattern of breathing during successful and unsuccessful trials of weaning from mechanical ventilation. *Am Rev Respir Dis* 1986; 134:111.

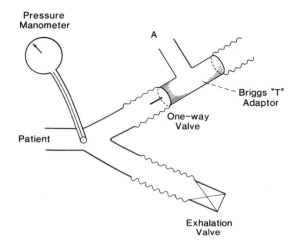

FIG 16–27.
Placement of the Braschi valve (Briggs adapter with one-way valve) in the inspiratory limb of the ventilator circuit. *Point A,* occlusion port to atmosphere. See text for details on use to determine auto-PEEP. (*From Kacmarek RM: Positive end-expiratory pressure, in Pierson D, Kacmarek RM (eds):* Foundations of Respiratory Care. *New York, Churchill Livingstone, 1992, pp 891–920. Used by permission.*)

on the inspiration side of the circuit; otherwise the auto-PEEP level is indicated on the ventilator manometer.

To use this valve, the port allowing gas to exit the circuit is opened once the patient begins exhalation. When the next controlled mechanical breath is delivered, the exhalation valve closes, the delivered volume exits the Braschi valve, and an end-expiratory hold is developed for the length of the inspiratory phase. Similar results can be obtained by the use of a three-way valve in the inspiratory limb, opened to the atmosphere once exhalation begins.[59] This technique functions well, provided the patient's mechanical respiratory rate is not excessive (greater than 25 breaths per minute) and the patient is not breathing spontaneously. Auto-PEEP may also be estimated by clamping the flex tube between the circuit "Y" and the artificial airway at precisely the moment of end expiration[57] (Fig 16–28). Provided a pressure tap is placed between the clamp and the airway, auto-PEEP can be read off a manometer taped into the system. Although this approach works, it requires exceptional coordination and ideally a recording of pressure waveform to ensure clamping is performed at the proper time. If the flex tube is clamped too soon or too late, excessive auto-PEEP levels are recorded.

Figure 16–29 illustrates the dynamic measurement of auto-PEEP during volume-targeted, square flow waveform controlled ventilation.[60] Since a pressure gradient exists within the lung at end expiration, maintaining expiratory flow at the point that the ventilator initiates a positive pressure breath, the ventilator must first match or counterbalance this pressure before gas can enter the airway. If simultaneous measurements of airway pressure and flow are made, the auto-PEEP level can be determined from the pressure waveform as the initial inspiratory pressure generated at the point where airway flow is zero. The major drawback associated

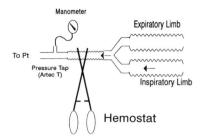

FIG 16–28.
Determination of auto-PEEP by the clamping of the flex tube between the circuit "Y" and the artificial airway at end expiration. Note a pressure tap and manometer must be placed at the airway distal to the point of clamping.

with this measurement is the need for a pressure transducer, pneumotachograph, and recording equipment.

Hoffman et al.[61] demonstrated that respiratory inductive plethysmography (Fig 16–30) could also be used to identify the level of auto-PEEP (see Chapter 15 for details). With this method, applied PEEP is slowly added until the baseline sum display begins to increase. The lowest level of applied PEEP not causing an increase in the baseline value approximates the auto-PEEP level.

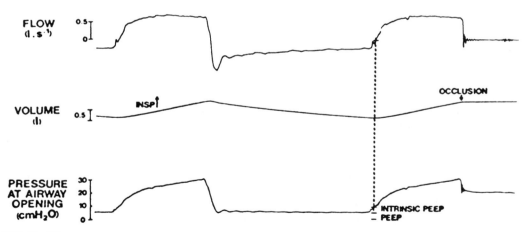

FIG 16–29.
Determination of auto-PEEP from the airway pressure and flow curve during volume-targeted, square waveform controlled ventilation (dynamic measurement technique). Waveforms are from a patient with COPD and 5.5 cm H_2O applied PEEP. Note expiratory flow continues through expiration and inspiratory flow starts only after a pressure change of 4.5 cm H_2O is applied by the ventilator as indicated by the broken line (point of zero gas flow). The 4.5 cm H_2O is equal to the auto-PEEP level. (*From Rossi A, Gottfried SB, Zocchi L, et al: Am Rev Resp Dis 1985; 131:672–677. Used by permission.*)

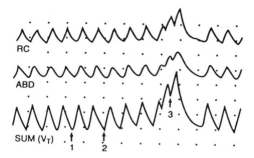

FIG 16–30.
Auto-PEEP as measured by respiratory inductive plethysmography. External PEEP was applied at *arrow 1* (4 cm H_2O), at *arrow 2* (6 cm H_2O), and at *arrow 3* (8 cm H_2O). The level of auto-PEEP is equal to the highest applied PEEP value without an increase in external thoracic/abdominal gas volume (6 cm H_2O). RC = Rib cage; ABD = Abdomen; Sum (VT) = Total rib cage plus abdomen. (*From Hoffman RA, Ershowsky P, Krieger BP: Chest 1989; 96:613–616. Used by permission.*)

The most accurate means of determining auto-PEEP during spontaneous breathing, whether or not ventilatory assistance is provided, requires insertion of an esophageal balloon and simultaneous measurement of esophageal pressure and pressure or flow at the airway opening.[54] Normally, there is only a minor nonmeasurable delay between the change in esophageal pressure and airway opening pressure or flow. However, if auto-PEEP is present, esophageal pressure may decrease significantly from baseline before flow or pressure change at the airway opening occurs. The difference between baseline esophageal pressure and the esophageal pressure required to alter flow or pressure at the airway is equal to the auto-PEEP level. Figure 16–31 depicts the determination of auto-PEEP by this method.

PRESSURE-VOLUME LOOPS

An illustration of an airway pressure-volume (P-V) loop during controlled ventilation, in a patient with normal compliance and resistance, is depicted in Figure 16–32. The line between 1 and 2 connects points of zero flow and the slope of this line equals the dynamic compliance. Area A represents the work to overcome nonelastic resistance to inspiration, while area B represents the work to overcome nonelastic resistance to exhalation. Figure 33 depicts an airway P-V loop on a patient with ARDS. Note the overall decrease in compliance, as well as areas representative of both inspiratory and expiratory resistance. The exact opposite changes are noted on the P-V loop of a patient with COPD (Fig 16–34). Here the loop is shifted upward and to the left (increased compliance) and the areas indicative of inspiratory and expiratory nonelastic work are larger. As observed in Figures 16–32, 16–33, and 16–34, airway P-V loops provide a rapid assessment of the overall impedance to gas movement and work required to inflate the lung-chest wall system. They are of characteristic shape, with specific disease states.

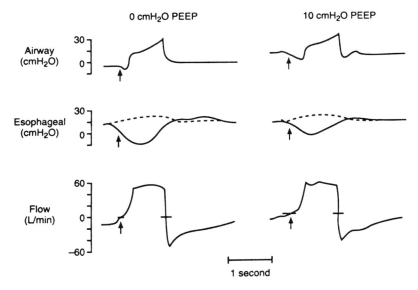

FIG 16–31.
Assessment of the level of auto-PEEP in a spontaneously breathing patient by the evaluation of esophageal pressure change relative to either airway opening pressure or flow at airway opening. Arrows indicate pressure and flow change at airway opening. The change in esophageal pressure between baseline and the level that allows change in airway opening pressure or in flow is equal to the auto-PEEP level. Note effect of 10 cm H₂O applied PEEP on the level of auto-PEEP (*left side*). (*From Smith TC, Marini JJ:* J Appl Physiol *1988; 65:1488–1499. Used by permission.*)

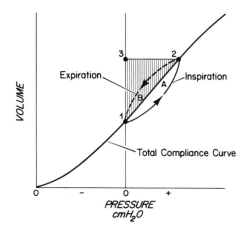

FIG 16–32.
Schematic airway pressure-volume loop during controlled mode, volume-targeted ventilation in a patient with normal compliance and resistance. The distance 1 to 3 equals tidal volume, while the distance 3 to 2 equals inspiratory pressure change. *Area A* represents nonelastic work and the area enclosed in the shaded triangle 1-2-3 represents elastic work, both performed by the ventilator. Area B represents nonelastic imposed work during exhalation. The line from 1 to 2, connecting points of zero flow, is the dynamic compliance curve. (*From Kacmarek RM:* Respir Care *1988; 33:99–120. Used by permission.*)

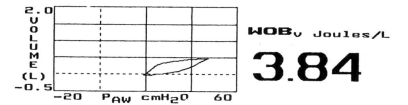

FIG 16–33.
Airway pressure-volume loop recorded on a patient with ARDS during controlled ventilation. Note the decrease in area representing nonelastic inspiratory and expiratory work and the shifting of the curve to right. Compliance is about 10 to 15 mL/cm H_2O.

During spontaneous breathing, very different configurations of the airway P-V loop are observed. Figure 16–35 depicts an idealized P-V loop during CPAP without pressure support (PS). The inspiratory phase is to the left of baseline (pressure below system baseline), indicating the ventilator system's imposed work. Since no positive airway pressure is applied at end inspiration, pressure returns to baseline. During exhalation, system pressure is more positive, indicating the imposed work of the exhalation/PEEP valve.[8, 11, 62] The greater the area to the left of baseline pressure during inspiration, the greater the imposed inspiratory work; while the greater the area to the right during exhalation, the greater the expiratory work.

Figure 16–36, A and B depict the addition of increasing levels of PS. Note that as PS is increased, less and less work is imposed on the patient and more and more work is performed by the ventilator. However, regardless of the PS level, the patient must still perform sufficient work to trigger each breath, as noted by the small area to the left of baseline at the onset of inspiration. The less sensitive the trigger setting, the greater the effort required to trigger (Fig 16–37).

The airway P-V loops during SIMV with PS are depicted in Figure 16–38. Note the difference in configuration as a result of the different ventilator delivery methodologies.

Airway P-V loops are of particular importance during volume-controlled ventilation of the patient with ARDS. As noted in Figure 16–39, A, hyperinflation can be easily identified by analyzing the P-V loop. At end inspiration a very small volume change results in an excessive pressure change. As a result of the overdistention, the compliance curve changes its slope at end inspiration, again documenting overdistention. Figure 16–39, B illustrates the change in the configuration of the P-V loop after a decrease in the tidal volume.

It is important to remember that airway P-V loops during spontaneous breathing only depict imposed work of breathing, which grossly underestimates actual patient work. Esophageal P-V loops are necessary to determine actual patient work during spontaneous breathing. In addition, airway P-V loops only represent work of breathing imposed by the ventilator system. To determine total imposed work of breathing (ventilator system plus artificial airway), tracheal P-V loops must be obtained.

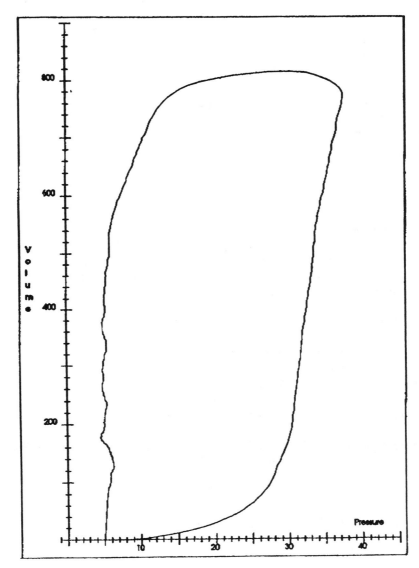

FIG 16–34.
Airway pressure-volume loop recorded on a patient with COPD during controlled ventilation. Note the increased nonelastic inspiratory and expiratory work (widening of the loop), as well as the shifting of the dynamic compliance curve upward and to the left.

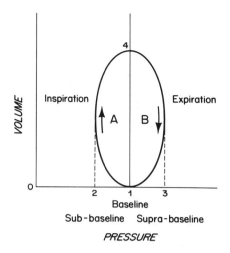

FIG 16–35.
Airway pressure-volume loop during spontaneous breathing. Area A represents imposed inspiratory work, and area B represents imposed expiratory work. The distance 1 to 4 represents VT, 1 to 2 represents pressure change during inspiration, and 1 to 3, pressure change during expiration. (*From Kacmarek RM: Respir Care 1989; 33:99–120. Used by permission.*)

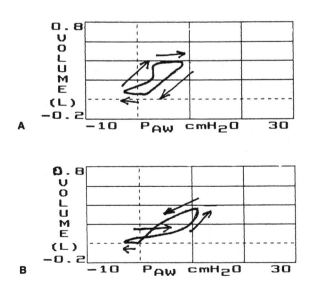

FIG 16–36.
Airway pressure-volume loops during two levels of pressure support in a given patient. **A,** Low level of pressure support approximately 5 cm H_2O. Insufficient to overcome imposed work of breathing. *Arrows* indicate inspiration and exhalation curves. **B,** Appropriate level of PS (12 cm H_2O). Note rapid establishment (*arrows*) of system positive pressure.

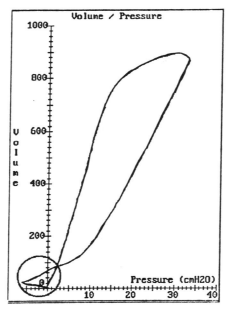

FIG 16–37.
Airway pressure-volume loop during assist control volume-targeted ventilation where sensitivity is inappropriately set. Note the large area in the circle indicative of patient effort to trigger the ventilator to inspiration.

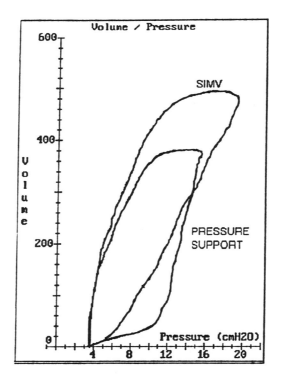

FIG 16–38.
Airway pressure-volume loops during a volume-targeted SIMV breath and a subsequent pressure support breath. Note the altered configuration of the P-V loops for each breath.

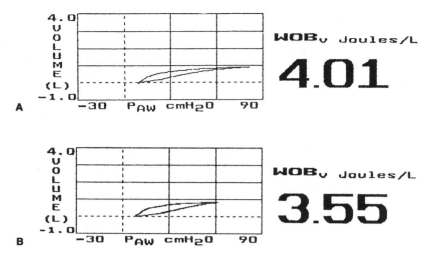

FIG 16–39.
Airway pressure-volume loops during volume-targeted ventilation demonstrating overinflation because of excessive tidal volumes. **A,** Tidal volume 950 mL PIP 82 cm H_2O. Note how little volume is delivered between the airway pressure increase from 60 to 82 cm H_2O. A change in the slope of the compliance curve as inspiration continues or a tail at the end of inspiration always indicates overinflation. **B,** Tidal volume was decreased to 900 mL, resulting in a PIP decrease of 22 cm H_2O. Overinflation is still present but not to the extent in **A.** VT should be decreased about 200 mL more to eliminate overdistension totally and establish PIP in the low 40 cm H_2O range.

FLOW-VOLUME LOOPS

Flow-volume (F-V) loops are normally produced in the pulmonary function laboratory to assist in the diagnosis of obstructive and restrictive lung disease. Similar types of loops can be measured in patients requiring mechanical ventilatory support. Figures 16–40, 16–41, and 16–42 depict F-V loops from patients with COPD, ARDS, and essentially normal lungs. The major differences between F-V loops produced during mechanical ventilation, as compared to spontaneous breathing, are the following:

1. The loop during ventilatory assistance is normally passively recorded, compared to active forced loops in the PFT laboratory.
2. The magnitude and shape of the inspiratory curve are a result of the ventilator's gas delivery pattern, not the patient.
3. The expiratory flow pattern, although similar to that generated during forced spontaneous breathing, has its peak expiratory flow limited by the size of the artificial airway.

In spite of these differences, it is easy to identify the differences between the F-V loop in Figures 16–40, 16–41, and 16–42. The primary uses of F-V loops during mechanical ventilation are (1) to establish response to bronchodilators (Fig 16–43, A and B); (2) to establish the presence,

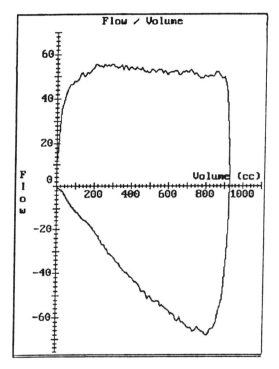

FIG 16–40.
Normal flow-volume loop during volume-controlled ventilation. Inspiratory curve is on top; expiratory curve on the bottom. Note the linear change in expiratory flow from peak to end exhalation. Also, end-expiratory flow is zero.

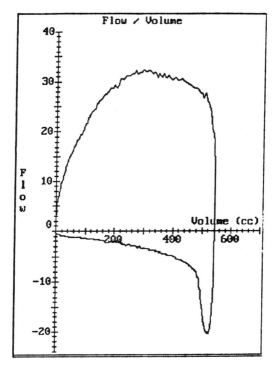

FIG 16–41.
Flow-volume loop during volume-controlled ventilation in a patient with COPD. Note the diminished peak expiratory flow (compared to Fig 16–40) and the scooped-out (concave) shape of the expiratory flow volume curve. Although no air trapping is noted, flow returns to zero at end exhalation. Inspiration (*top curve*); exhalation (*bottom curve*).

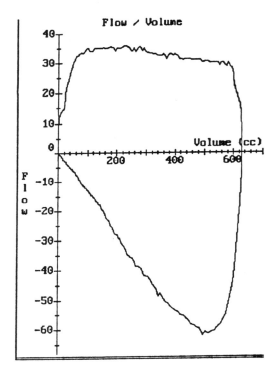

FIG 16–42.
Flow-volume loop during volume-controlled ventilation on a patient with ARDS. Note expiratory flow curve is similar to normal. Inspiration (*top curve*); exhalation (*bottom curve*).

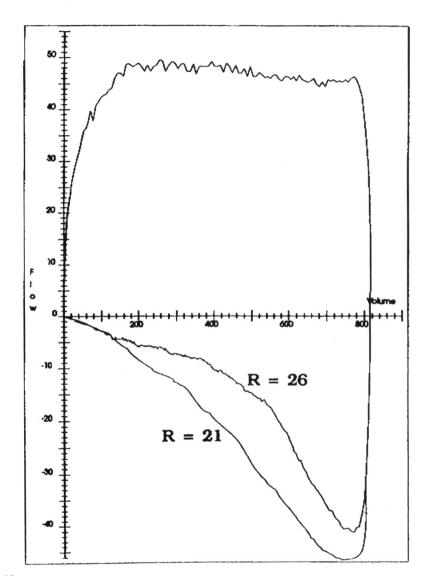

FIG 16–43.
Flow-volume loops before (*R* = 26) and after (*R* = 21) bronchodilator therapy in a patient with asthma. Note the alteration in the expiratory curve after therapy, high peak flow, less concave; however, no alteration occurs in the inspiratory flow pattern developed by the ventilator. Inspiration (*top curve*); exhalation (*bottom curve*).

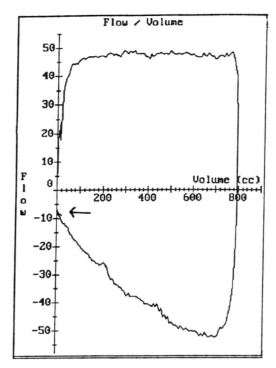

FIG 16–44.
Flow-volume loop on a patient where expiratory time is too short. Note that end-expiratory flow (*arrow*) does not return to baseline. This is always indicative of air trapping. Inspiration (*top curve*); exhalation (*bottom curve*).

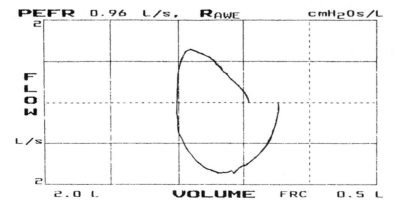

FIG 16–45.
Flow volume loop indicating large system leak (200 mL). Exhalation (*top curve*); inspiration (*bottom curve*).

but not the magnitude of auto-PEEP (Fig 16–44); and (3) to identify the presence and magnitude of a system leak (Fig 16–45). Of these three, establishing response to bronchodilator therapy represents the most important reason for performing bedside F-V loops. As noted in Figures 16–43, A and B, response to bronchodilator therapy can be rapidly established by simply visually comparing the pre- and post-bronchodilator curves.

REFERENCES

1. Kacmarek RM, Meklaus G: The new generation of mechanical ventilators. *Crit Care Clin* 1990; 6:551–578.
2. Sola A, Farina D, Rodriguez S, et al: Lack of relationship between the true airway pressure and the pressure displayed with an infant ventilator. *Crit Care Med* 1992; 20:778–781.
3. Kacmarek RM, Dimas S, Reynolds J, et al: Technical aspects of positive end-expiratory pressure: II. PEEP with positive pressure ventilation. *Respir Care* 1982; 27:1490–1504.
4. Christopher KL, Neff TA, Bowman JL, et al: Demand and continuous flow intermittent mandatory ventilation systems. *Chest* 1985; 87:625–630.
5. Kacmarek RM, Shimada Y, Ohmura A, et al: The second Nayoga conference: Triggering and optimizing mechanical ventilatory assist. *Respir Care* 1991; 26: 45–52.
6. Milic-Emili J, Tantucci C, Chasse M, et al: Introduction with special reference to ventilator-associated barotrauma, in Benito S, Net A (eds): *Pulmonary Function in Mechanically-Ventilated Patients*. Berlin, Springer-Verlag, 1991, pp 1–8.
7. Marini JJ. Lung mechanics determinations at the bedside: Instrumentation and clinical application. *Respir Care* 1990; 35:669–696.
8. Hirsh C, Kacmarek RM, Stanek I: Work of breathing during CPAP and PSV imposed by the new generation mechanical ventilators: A lung model study. *Respir Care* 1991; 36:815–828.
9. Truwit JD, Marini JJ: Evaluation of thoracic mechanics in the ventilated patient. part I: Primary measurements. *J Crit Care* 1988; 3:133–150.
10. Rossi A, Gottfried B, Zocchi L, et al: Measurement of static compliance of the total respiratory system in patients with acute respiratory failure during mechanical ventilation: The effect of intrinsic positive end-expiratory pressure. *Am Rev Resp Dis* 1985; 131:672–677.
11. Kacmarek RM, Goulet RL: PEEP devices. *Anesth Clin North Am* 1987; 5:757–770.
12. Sassoon CSH, Giron AE, Ely EA, et al: Inspiratory work of breathing on flow-by and demand flow continuous positive airway pressure. *Crit Care Med* 1989; 17:1108–1114.
13. Gurevitch MJ, Gelmont D: Importance of trigger sensitivity to ventilator response delay in advanced chronic obstructive pulmonary disease with respiratory failure. *Crit Care Med* 1989; 17:354–359.
14. Whilelaw WS, Derenne JP, Milic-Emili J: Occlusion pressure as a measure of respiratory center output in conscious man. *Respir Physiol* 1975; 23:181–199.
15. Sassoon CSH, Te TT, Mahutte CK, et al: Airway occlusion pressure. An important indicator for successful weaning in patients with chronic obstructive pulmonary disease. *Am Rev Respir Dis* 1987; 135:107–113.
16. Fernandez R, Benito S, Sanchis J, et al: Inspiratory effort and occlusion pressure in triggered mechanical ventilation. *Inten Care Med* 1988; 14:650–653.
17. Marini JJ, Rodriguez RM, Lamb VJ: The inspiratory workload of patient-initiated mechanical ventilation. *Am Rev Respir Dis* 1986; 134:902–909.
18. Kacmarek RM: Management of patient-mechanical ventilator system, in Pierson D, Kacmarek RM (eds): *Foundations of Respiratory Care*. New York, Churchill Livingstone, 1992, pp 973–998.

19. Truwit JD, Marini JJ: Evaluation of thoracic mechanics in the ventilated patient. part II. Applied mechanics. *J Crit Care* 1988; 3:199–213.
20. Marini JJ: Lung mechanics determinations at the bedside: Instrumentation and clinical application. *Respir Care* 1990; 35:669–696.
21. Pesenti A, Marolin R, Proto P, et al: Mean airway pressure vs. positive end-expiratory pressure during mechanical ventilation. *Crit Care Med* 1985; 13:34–37.
22. Primiano FP, Chatburn RL, Lough MD: Mean airway pressure: Theoretical considerations. *Crit Care Med* 1982; 10:378–383.
23. Gattioni L, Marolin R, Caspani M, et al: Constant mean airway pressure with different patterns of positive pressure breathing during the adult respiratory distress syndrome. *Bull Eur Physiopathol Respir* 1985; 21:275–279.
24. Ravenscraft SA, Burke WC, Marini JJ: Volume-cycled decelerating flow: An alternative form of mechanical ventilation. *Chest* 1992; 101:1342–1351.
25. Marcy TW, Marini JJ: Inverse ratio ventilation in ARDS: Rationale and implementation. *Chest* 1991; 100:494–504.
26. Hess D, Tabor T: Comparison of six methods to calculate airway resistance in adult mechanically ventilated patients (abstract). *Crit Care Med* 1992; 10:S27.
27. Mathews JG, Ingenito E, Davison B, et al: Endotracheal tube resistance: The effects of tube curvature, tube interfaces, gas-liquid interactions, and airflow direction (abstract). *Anesthesiol*, in press.
28. Milic-Emili J, Henderson JAM, Dolovich MB, et al: Regional distribution of inspired gas in the lung. *J Appl Physiol* 1966; 21:749–759.
29. Marini JJ, Culver BH, Butler J: Effect of positive end-expiratory pressure on canine ventricular function curves. *J Appl Physiol: Respirat Environ Exercise Physiol* 1981; 51:1367–1374.
30. Milic-Emili J, Mead J, Turner JM: Topography of esophageal pressure as a function of posture in man. *J Appl Physiol* 1964; 19:212–216.
31. Knowles JH, Henry SK, Rahn H: Possible errors using esophageal balloon in determination of pressure-volume characteristics of the lung and thoracic cage. *J Appl Physiol* 1959; 14:525–530.
32. Milic-Emili J, Mead J, Turner JM, et al: Improved technique for estimating pleural pressure from esophageal balloons. *J Appl Physiol* 1964; 19:207–211.
33. Baydur A, Behrakis K, Zin A, et al: A simple method for assessing the validity of esophageal balloon technique. *Am Rev Respir Dis* 1982; 126:788–791.
34. Lind FG, Truve AB, Lindborg BPO: Microcomputer-assisted on-line measurement of breathing pattern and occlusion pressure. *J Appl Physiol* 1984; 56:235–239.
35. Milic-Emili J: Recent advances in clinical assessment of control of breathing. *Lung* 1982; 160:1–17.
36. Tobin MJ: Respiratory monitoring in the intensive care unit. *Am Rev Resp Dis* 1988; 138:1625–1642.
37. Gottfried SB, Rossi A, Higgs BD, et al: Noninvasive determination of respiratory system mechanics during mechanical ventilation for acute respiratory failure. *Am Rev Resp Dis* 1985; 131:414–420.
38. Kacmarek RM: Noninvasive monitoring techniques in the ventilated patient, in Kacmarek RM, Stoller J (eds): *Current Respiratory Care*. Toronto, B.C. Decker, 1988, pp 182–187.
39. Hess D, McCurdy S, Simmons M: Compression volume in adult ventilator circuits: A comparison of five disposable circuits and a nondisposable circuit. *Respir Care* 1991; 36:1113–1118.
40. Suter PM, Fairley HB, Isenberg MD: Optimal end-expiratory airway pressure in patients with acute pulmonary failure. *New Eng J Med* 1975; 292:284–289.
41. Krieger I: Studies of mechanics of respiration in infancy. *Am J Dis Child* 1963; 105:439–448.
42. Jonson B, Nordstrom L, Olsson SG, et al: Monitoring of ventilation and lung mechanics during automatic ventilation. A new device. *Bull Physiopath Resp* 1975; 11:729–743.
43. Bergman NA: Properties of passive exhalations in anesthesized subjects. *Anesthesiol* 1969; 30:378–387.

44. Bergman NA, Waltermath CL: A comparison of some methods for measuring total respiratory resistance. *J Appl Phys* 1974; 36:131–134.
45. Comroe JH, Nisell OI, Nims RG: A simple method for concurrent measurement of compliance and resistance to breathing in anesthetized animals and man. *J Appl Phys* 1954; 7:225–228.
46. Hilberman M, Schill JP, Peters RM: On-line digital analysis of respiratory mechanics and automation of respirator control. *J Thoracic Cardiovascular Surg* 1969; 58:821–828.
47. Lavietes MH, Rochester DF: Assessment of airway function during assisted ventilation. *Lung* 1981; 159:219–229.
48. MacIntyre NR, Silver RM, Miller CW, et al: Aerosol delivery in intubated mechanically ventilated patients. *Crit Care Med* 1985; 13:81–85.
49. Fraser I, DaVall A, Dolovich M, et al: Therapeutic aerosol delivery in ventilator systems (abstract). *Am Rev Respir Dis* 1981; 123:107.
50. Pepe PE, Marini JJ: Occult positive end-expiratory pressure in mechanically ventilated patients with airflow obstruction: The auto-PEEP effect. *Am Rev Respir Dis* 1982; 126:166–170.
51. Rossi A, Gottfried SB, Zocchi L, et al: Measurement of static compliance of the total respiratory system in patients with acute respiratory failure during mechanical ventilation: The effect of intrinsic positive end-expiratory pressure. *Am Rev Respir Dis* 1985; 131:672–677.
52. Bergman NA: Intrapulmonary gas trapping during mechanical ventilation at rapid frequencies. *Anesthesiol* 1972; 37:626–633.
53. Marini JJ: Should PEEP be used in airflow obstruction? (editorial). *Am Rev Respir Dis* 1989; 140:1–3.
54. Smith TC, Marini JJ: Impact of PEEP on lung mechanics and work of breathing in severe airflow obstruction. *J Appl Physiol* 1988; 65:1488–1499.
55. Petrof BJ, Legare M, Goldberg P, et al: Continuous positive airway pressure reduces work of breathing and dyspnea during weaning from mechanical ventilation in severe COPD. *Am Rev Respir Dis* 1990; 141:281–289.
56. Kacmarek RM: Positive end-expiratory pressure, in Pierson D, Kacmarek RM (eds): *Foundations of Respiratory Care*. New York, Churchill Livingstone, 1992, pp 891–920.
57. Benson MS, Pierson DJ: Auto-PEEP during mechanical ventilation of adults. *Respir Care* 1988; 33:557–568.
58. Iotti G, Braschi A: Respiratory mechanics in chronic obstructive pulmonary disease, in Vincent JL (ed): *Critical Care Update*. Berlin, Springer-Verlag, 1990, pp 223–232.
59. Gottfried SB, Reissman H, Ranieri VM: A simple method for the measurement of intrinsic positive end-expiratory pressure during controlled and assisted modes of mechanical ventilation. *Crit Care Med* 1992; 20:621–629.
60. Rossi A, Gottfried SB, Zocchi L, et al: Measurement of static compliance of the total respiratory system in patients with acute respiratory failure during mechanical ventilation: The effect of intrinsic positive end-expiratory pressure. *Am Rev Resp Dis* 1985; 131:672–677.
61. Hoffman RA, Ershowsky P, Krieger BP: Determination of auto-PEEP during spontaneous and controlled ventilation by monitoring changes in end-expiratory thoracic gas volume. *Chest* 1989; 96:613–616.
62. Kacmarek RM: The role of pressure support ventilation in reducing the work of breathing. *Respir Care* 1980; 33:99–120.

Chapter 17

Measurement of Lung Volume at the Bedside

Thomas D. East, Ph.D.

INTRODUCTION

The total volume capacity of the lung can be divided into a variety of subdivisions (Fig 17–1). During mechanical ventilation, without full patient cooperation, only V_T, FRC, and TLC are reasonable to measure (Table 17–1). IRV and IC require a maximal inspiration, ERV requires a maximal exhalation, and VC requires both a maximal inspiration and expiration. V_T is routinely measured by a variety of different well-established techniques.[1] FRC is a parameter of interest in a variety of different pulmonary pathologies. In patients with obstructive lung disease, FRC may be increased above normal. FRC may also be elevated in patients with intrinsic positive end-expiratory pressure (PEEP). FRC is of particular importance in patients with acute restrictive pathologies such as ARDS. Patients with ARDS suffer from both refractory hypoxemia and decreased compliance in association with an acute lung volume loss and an acutely decreased FRC.[2, 3] In these patients PEEP returns FRC toward normal.[3] In an animal model of ARDS, titrating PEEP to normalize FRC has been shown to provide effective oxygenation without frequent blood gases.[4] Despite this goal of PEEP therapy, FRC is not routinely measured in these patients because standard techniques[5–20] for determination of FRC can require alteration of F_{IO_2}[5–20] and interruption of ventilatory therapy.[11, 18, 21–23] Any of these maneuvers may in themselves alter FRC and invalidate the measurement as well as endanger the patient. The purpose of this chapter is to summarize the techniques for measurement of FRC and TLC in mechanically ventilated patients and to discuss the potential efficacy of routine monitoring.

MEASUREMENT TECHNIQUES

FRC and TLC have been measured in many different ways. The measurement methods can be divided into gas dilution, radiographic, and thoracic dimension categories.

LUNG VOLUMES

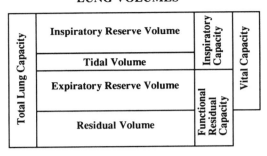

FIG 17–1.
Lung volumes typically measured and their subdivisions.

TABLE 17–1.
Definitions

ABD	Abdomen
ac	Alternating current
Ar	Argon
ARDS	Adult respiratory distress syndrome
CO_2	Carbon dioxide
COPD	Chronic obstructive pulmonary disease
CPPV	Controlled positive pressure ventilation
ERV	Expiratory reserve volume
FIO_2	Inspired oxygen fraction
FRC	Functional residual capacity
He	Helium
I : E	inspiratory : expiratory ratio
ICU	Intensive care unit
IRV	Inspiratory reserve volume
Kr	Krypton
N_2	Nitrogen
O_2	Oxygen
PA	Posterior-anterior
$PaCO_2$	arterial PCO_2 (mm Hg)
PaO_2	arterial PO_2 (mm Hg)
PC	Personal computer (IBM clone)
PEEP	Positive end-expiratory pressure (cm H_2O)
RC	Rib cage
RIP	Respiratory inductance plethysmography
SF_6	Sulfur hexafluoride
TLC	Total lung capacity
VC	Vital capacity
VR	ventilatory rate (breaths/min)
V_T	tidal volume (mL)
$\dot{V}$	Flow of gas (L/min)
$\dot{V}_A$	alveolar ventilation (L/min)
$\dot{V}_E$	expiratory minute ventilation (L/min)
Xe	Xenon

Gas Dilution FRC Measurement

In general, all gas dilution systems are similar. They all use an insoluble gas to do an indicator dilution measurement of FRC. The two broad classes of gas dilution techniques are open- and closed-circuit systems. The closed-circuit techniques require a closed, rebreathing, respiratory circuit into which a known volume of indicator gas is mixed. The open-circuit techniques provide a known concentration of indicator gas during inspiration but do not require rebreathing.

Closed-Circuit Gas Dilution FRC Measurement Systems

Closed-circuit gas dilution techniques consist of a reservoir of gas with a known volume that contains oxygen and a known concentration of the indicator gas (Fig 17–2). The patient rebreaths from this reservoir until the gas concentrations equilibrate. The FRC is then calculated as

$$C_1 \cdot V_1 = C_2 \cdot (V_1 + V_2) \tag{17–1}$$

where C_1 and C_2 are the starting and ending concentrations of the tracer gas in the spirometer, V_1 is the volume in the spirometer, and V_2 is the FRC.

There are two problems with this simple approach. The patient consumes oxygen from the reservoir during the rebreathing, thus reducing the volume (V_1), and he excretes CO_2, which accumulates in the reservoir and can stimulate ventilation as well as produce patient discomfort. To compensate for these problems, most systems in use today add oxygen to replace that which is consumed by the patient, to maintain V_1 constant, and include a soda lime CO_2 scrubber in the circuit (Fig 17–2).

Many different tracer gases can be used. The main criterion for the gas is that it be as insoluble as possible. In addition, the gas should have a viscosity that is similar to other respiratory gases to provide for uniform distribution throughout the lung. Helium, argon, neon, and SF_6 have been used. The most popular technique is He dilution.[5–12]

This measurement technique can be modified for use on patients who are being mechanically ventilated with PEEP (Fig 17–2, B). A "bag-in-box" or bellows system is used as the reservoir. The ventilator drives the bellows, which in turn ventilates the patient. An additional PEEP valve is placed on the expiratory limb to apply PEEP during the measurement. This technique has several problems that are summarized in Table 17–2.

Open-Circuit Gas Dilution FRC Measurement Systems

Open-circuit gas dilution techniques consist of a system to provide a known mixture of tracer gas during inspiration (Figs 17–3 and 17–4). The patient breathes from this mixture until the gas concentrations equilibrate. The tracer gas mixture is then turned off and washout occurs. The FRC is then calculated from the washout curve as:

$$\mathrm{FRC}_{\mathrm{STPD}} = \frac{\displaystyle\int_{t=0}^{T} C(t) \cdot \dot{V}_{\mathrm{STPD}}(t)\, dt}{C(0) - C(T)} \tag{17–2}$$

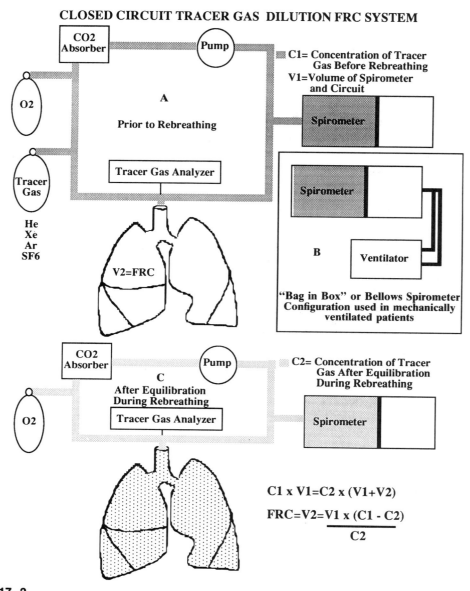

CLOSED CIRCUIT TRACER GAS DILUTION FRC SYSTEM

C1= Concentration of Tracer Gas Before Rebreathing
V1=Volume of Spirometer and Circuit

C2= Concentration of Tracer Gas After Equilibration During Rebreathing

$$C1 \times V1 = C2 \times (V1+V2)$$

$$FRC = V2 = \frac{V1 \times (C1 - C2)}{C2}$$

FIG 17–2.
Closed-circuit gas dilution FRC measurement system. **A,** The system prior to rebreathing. **B,** A modification of the system that allows it to be used with mechanically ventilated patients. **C,** The system after equilibration. (Some parts of this figure were reproduced with permission from MacAnatomy clip art.

TABLE 17–2.

Summary of Potential Problems with a Closed-Circuit He Dilution FRC Measurement System for Mechanically Ventilated Patients

Potential Problems	Possible Solutions
The delivered Vt is decreased by the large compressible volume.	Flow and pressure can be measured at the mouth and the ventilator adjusted to provide the desired Vt, PEEP, and pressure waveform.
The pressure and flow waveforms are distorted by the added system compliance and resistance.	
During the measurement there is no guarantee that the conditions (flow and pressure) are representative of the ventilatory pattern prior to measurement.	
The system can only be used with CPPV or PCIRV modes of mechanical ventilation.	
A complete parallel circuit, including a manifold with a PEEP valve, must be purchased and maintained.	
Most of these systems are large, cumbersome, difficult to operate, and require up to 30 minutes per measurement.	Some portions of the systems can be automated.
FIo$_2$ = 1.0 cannot be used because of the necessary dilution with the tracer gas.	
Some of the tracer gas is absorbed into the blood.	A correction of ≈100 mL can be subtracted for helium absorption.
Apparatus dead-space is included in the calculated FRC.	Apparatus dead-space volume can be measured and subtracted from measured FRC.

The tracer gas can be added by inspiring from a premixed tank of gas that contains the tracer gas (Fig 17–3) or by injecting the tracer gas into the inspiratory gas flow (Fig 17–4). The advantages and disadvantages of the open-circuit technique are outlined in Table 17–3.

Nitrogen Gas Dilution. — Several different open-circuit systems have been described. The most well-known systems use N_2 as the tracer gas.[7, 13–20] To wash out the lung, the patients are switched to 100% oxygen. The FRC calculations are the same as Equation (17–2). Flow is typically measured using a Fleisch pneumotach.

The N_2 concentration is measured either with mass spectrometry or emission spectroscopy. Emission spectroscopy involves placing a sample of gas in a vacuum chamber between two high-voltage (500- to 1500-V dc) electrodes and passing a current through it. The electrical discharge stimulates the atoms and causes rearrangement of outer electrons in atoms and molecules.[24] The electrons that are accelerated emit photons in well-defined frequency bands (310 to 480 nm) of ultraviolet light for N_2. The intensity of the light in these frequency bands is related to the concentration of the gas. The ultraviolet light is detected using a photoelectric tube that produces a current in proportion to the intensity of the light. For a fixed sample cell

**OPEN CIRCUIT TRACER GAS DILUTION FRC SYSTEM
USING PRE-MIXED TRACER GAS SUPPLIES**

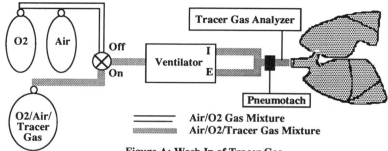

Figure A: Wash In of Tracer Gas

N2, Xe, Ar, SF6, or Kr

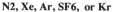

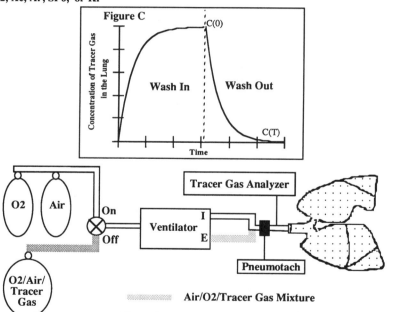

Figure B: Wash Out of Tracer Gas

FIG 17–3.
Open-circuit gas dilution FRC measurement system using premixed tanks of tracer gas. **A,** The system during wash in of tracer gas. **B,** The system during wash out of tracer gas. **C,** The concentration of the tracer gas in the lung during wash in and wash out. (Some parts of this figure were reproduced with permission from MacAnatomy clip art.)

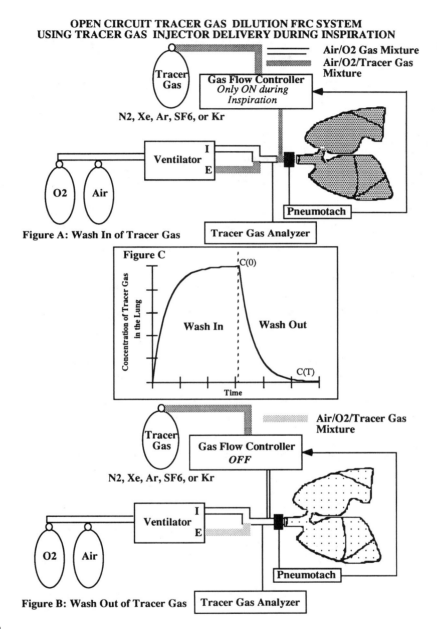

**OPEN CIRCUIT TRACER GAS DILUTION FRC SYSTEM
USING TRACER GAS INJECTOR DELIVERY DURING INSPIRATION**

FIG 17–4.

Open-circuit gas dilution FRC measurement system using tracer gas injected into the inspiratory flow. **A,** The system during wash in of tracer gas. **B,** The system during wash out of tracer gas. **C,** The concentration of the tracer gas in the lung during wash in and wash out. (Some parts of this figure were reproduced with permission from MacAnatomy clip art.)

TABLE 17–3.

Summary of Problems with an Open-Circuit Tracer Dilution FRC Measurement System for Mechanically Ventilated Patients

Potential Problems	Possible Solutions
If using premixed tracer gas supplies; only one F_{IO_2} is available during measurements. This may require an alteration in F_{IO_2} to make the measurements that can affect the measurement as well as potentially be harmful to the patient.	Use the tracer gas injector open-circuit systems; see SF_6 system.
If using premixed tracer gas supplies; cost of premixed tracer gas supplies.	Use the tracer gas injector open-circuit systems; see SF_6 system.
FRC measurement accuracy is sensitive to the accuracy of the flow transducer in the presence of humidity and changing gas mixtures.	1. Calibrate the flow transducer carefully. 2. Automatically correct for changes in viscosity related to gas composition changes. 3. Heat the pneumotach and add water traps to remove as much of the humidity as possible.
FRC measurement accuracy is sensitive to the time lag between the flow and tracer gas concentration signals.	Use an in-line tracer gas sensor with the smallest possible lag time and fastest response time. If a side-sampling system is used, then include a time shift correction to compensate for the lag time introduced by the sample line.
Most of these systems are large, cumbersome, difficult to operate, and require up to 30 minutes per measurement.	Many portions of the systems can be computerized and automated.
$F_{IO_2} = 1.0$ cannot be used because of the necessary dilution with the tracer gas.	Use a very small concentration of tracer gas (<1%). This requires a very sensitive tracer gas sensor.
Some of the tracer gas is absorbed into the blood.	Use as insoluble a tracer as possible or apply a correction for the estimated uptake.
Expired tracer gas in the trach tube and Y piece will be rebreathed, thus affecting the accuracy of FRC measurements.	Automatically include this rebreathed gas in the integral [Equation (17–2)]. The flow will be of the opposite sign, thus compensating for the rebreathed amount of tracer gas.
Apparatus dead-space is included in the calculated FRC.	Apparatus dead-space volume can be measured and subtracted from measured FRC.

geometry, vacuum, gas flow, and current, the output of the photoelectric tube is a nonlinear function of the molar fraction of N_2 in the expired gas.

Many of these N_2 washout systems will not work on patients who are mechanically ventilated with PEEP,[11, 18, 21–23] and those that do require modification of the ventilator and breathing circuit.[5–11, 14, 15, 18, 25, 26] With the exception of the system by Richardson et al.,[13, 16, 17] all of these systems require complex manual intervention to perform a measurement.

Argon Gas Dilution.—Imanaka et al.[27] reported an automated system using 10% argon as a tracer gas to measure FRC during high-frequency oscillatory ventilation. The argon concentration was measured with a mass spectrometer. To make the measurement, the supply gas of the ventilator was switched from 100% O_2 to 90% O_2 and 10% argon. Wash in of the tracer gas continued until the end-expired concentration reached equilibrium. At this point the ventilator supply gas was switched back to 100% O_2 to wash out the argon. The FRC calculations were the same as Equation (17–2).

Radioactive Tracer Gas Dilution.—Another technique for doing open-circuit tracer gas dilution is to use a radioactive gas such as xenon (^{127}Xe or ^{133}Xe)[23, 28, 29] or krypton (^{81m}Kr),[28] which is inhaled, and the concentration monitoring is accomplished by means of a scintillation counter or a gamma camera. The calculation of FRC is the same as that described for any other open-circuit washout technique. The disadvantage of these techniques is that they require the use and handling of radioactive materials. Expired gas must be collected in a trap to avoid radiation contamination. The gamma camera is large and expensive, which makes this technique an unlikely candidate for routine use at the bedside. The advantage of these techniques is that the radioactive gas and the gamma camera provide additional information about the regional distribution of ventilation throughout the chest during the respiratory cycle, which may be of importance.

SF_6 Gas Dilution.—SF_6 is a colorless, odorless, nontoxic tracer gas that is highly insoluble. It has been used in several automated computerized SF_6 washout FRC measurement systems for routinely measuring the FRC of patients being mechanically ventilated with PEEP using a nonmodified ICU ventilator and a standard breathing circuit.[15, 30–33] This system does not interrupt positive pressure therapy, require switching ventilators, or alter F_{IO_2} significantly. Measurements may be made automatically at specified intervals without manual intervention. Further development of these systems has produced a SF_6 washout FRC measurement system that will work with any mode of mechanical ventilation as well as with spontaneous respiration.[31, 33]

The SF_6 FRC measurement system is shown in Fig 17–5. The system consists of a fast SF_6 gas analyzer to determine SF_6 concentration, a pneumotachograph to measure flow, a gas metering system to deliver SF_6, and a computer to control the devices and make all the

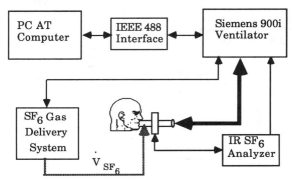

FIG 17–5.
Block diagram of the automated SF_6 washout FRC measurement system.

calculations. The SF_6 gas analyzer was a prototype fast, in-line, infrared analyzer developed by Siemens (Siemens-Elema, Solna, Sweden).[34] The pneumotachographs in the Siemens 900i Servo ventilator were used to measure flow. However, any pneumotachograph could be used. The 900i prototype ventilator was a 900c ventilator with a built-in small computer similar to an IBM-PC. The small computer in the 900i communicated with the IBM-PC/AT through a high-speed IEEE-488 communication bus. The IBM-PC/AT was used to collect all the information, control the measurement, and do all the calculations. All software was written in Lattice C.

The inspiratory and expiratory flow transducers in the servoventilator were used to measure airway flow. The pneumotachograph was calibrated using a room air, two-point volumetric calibration. Software-generated messages prompted the user to determine zero offset and then to push a 500-mL volume through the pneumotachograph using a calibrated super syringe. The super syringe was pushed with a reasonably constant flow; however, there was no attempt to guarantee the same flow at every calibration. After each calibration, the volume measurement system was tested by pushing the syringe through very rapidly and very slowly. The system was assumed to be adequately calibrated if the integrated volume was within 2% of 500 mL at the two extremes of flow. Errors in the pneumotachograph caused by viscosity changes of different gas compositions were corrected for in software as described previously.[30] The expiratory flow trasnducer was heated to reduce the effects of humidity and gas temperature. Bench tests indicate[30] that the accuracy of the pneumotachograph for volume measurements was within 2%.

The key to this system's ability to work with any mode of ventilation was the SF_6 delivery system. The SF_6 delivery system, shown in Figure 17–6, consisted of a small prototype Siemens piezoelectric valve that is switched on and off at a high frequency. The SF_6 delivery system guaranteed that the inspired concentration of SF_6 remained constant at 0.5% regardless of varying inspiratory flow. The cycle time of the valve was varied in direct proportion to the instantaneous inspiratory airway flow. The result was that the flow of SF_6 was in proportion to the inspiratory flow.

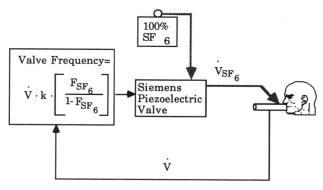

FIG 17–6.
Block diagram of the SF_6 gas delivery system. This system guarantees that the inspired concentration of SF_6 remains constant regardless of inspiratory flow profile.

The FRC measurement is made by washing in 0.5% SF_6 until steady state is achieved and then allowing washout to occur (see Fig 17–4). The FRC is calculated from the washout curve. The computer started the measurement by setting the SF_6 flow controller to meter the appropriate flow of 100% SF_6 into the breathing circuit to the patient. The expired gas was monitored during this wash-in period and the mixed-expired SF_6 concentration was calculated. The mixed expired SF_6 concentration was monitored until five sequential breaths had concentrations within 0.001% of one another. This guaranteed that even in cases where equilibration took more than the typical 1 to 3 minutes, a steady state was reached before washout was started. Once steady-state wash-in was achieved, the computer turned off the flow of SF_6, thereby starting washout. During washout, the flow signal was delayed 10 ms to correct for the response time of the SF_6 analyzer, and the airway flow times SF_6 concentration product was calculated. The SF_6 flow was then integrated. During the first part of inspiration, the SF_6 flow product was calculated before the SF_6 analyzer automatically rezeroed. This small amount of SF_6 was then subtracted from the integrated value to correct for rebreathed SF_6. Washout continued until the end-expiratory SF_6 concentration was below 0.005% SF_6. This normally took from 2 to 4 minutes. The FRC at STPD was determined using the following equation:

$$\text{FRC}_{\text{STPD}} = \frac{\sum_{i=0}^{n} F_S F_6(i) \cdot \text{flow}_{\text{STPD}}(i) \cdot \Delta t}{F_S F_6(0) - F_S F_6(n)} \tag{17–3}$$

where $\text{flow}_{\text{STPD}}(i)$ was the instantaneous flow signal corrected to STPD, $F_S F_6(i)$ was the instantaneous SF_6 fraction, and Δt was the time interval between digital samples ($\Delta t = 0.01$ second). The values for FRC were then corrected for the viscosity differences between the calibration gases (air) and the ventilation gases using the F_{IO_2} information given by the user.

The system can be programmed to make automatic measurements at a predetermined interval. This allows FRC measurements to be made over long periods of time without manual intervention. This system was evaluated in three different human studies.[31] In the first two studies, the accuracy of the system was compared with two conventional clinical techniques (a helium dilution system and a body plethysmograph) for measuring FRC in 12 spontaneously breathing normal volunteers and in 12 spontaneously breathing COPD patients. The absolute and percentage differences among the three FRC measurement techniques used in the 12 normal subjects and the 12 COPD patients are summarized in Table 17–4. In the normal volunteers, there was no significant difference among the three measurement techniques [$F(2,28) = 0.64$, $p = 0.53$]. Overall there was a significant difference between measurement techniques [$F(2,28) = 17.18$, $p < 0.0001$] in the COPD group. There was a significant difference in accuracy between the COPD and normal volunteer groups [$F(2,28) = 12.24$, $p = 0.0002$].

In the third human study, the reproducibility of the system and the efficacy of using this device on mechanically ventilated patients in an ICU environment was tested in 12 patients who had ARDS and were being mechanically ventilated with PEEP. All patient care proceeded normally with the exception that FRC was measured every 30 minutes. The patients were monitored for at least 24 hours and for no more than 96 hours. The patients were not paralyzed and had some spontaneous respiratory effort. As long as PEEP was unchanged, the patient

TABLE 17–4.

Absolute and Percentage Differences Among the Three FRC Measurement Techniques*†

Group	SF$_6$-Helium	SF$_6$-Body Pleth	Helium-Body Pleth	
Normal	-20 ± 60	-39 ± 100	-18 ± 108	mL
COPD	$-390 \pm 117\ddagger$	$-735 \pm 158\ddagger$	$-345 \pm 114\ddagger$	mL
Normal	0.2 ± 1.9	-1.1 ± 2.7	-1.3 ± 3.2	%
COPD	$-12 \pm 3\ddagger$	$-21 \pm 4\ddagger$	$-10 \pm 3\ddagger$	%

* From East TD, Wortelboer PJM, van Ark E, et al: *Crit Care Med* 1990; 18:84–91. Used by permission.
† Used in the 12 normal subjects and the 12 COPD patients (mean ± SEM). Shown are the three different pairings of the three techniques.
‡ Statistically significant difference, $p < 0.05$.

was considered to have a "stable" FRC for the purpose of this study. This assumption is not true because there are many other factors that effect the FRC; however, this measure of reproducibility gives a worst case measure of its usefulness in reflecting changes in FRC due to PEEP. The reproducibility in milliliters (p) and percent (p') were determined during these "stable" periods. There were a total of 1227 FRC measurements made on the 12 ARDS patients. Figure 17–7 is a representative sample from one patient of FRC measured at 30-minute intervals over 96 hours. The number of FRC measurements per patient was 102 ± 13 (mean ± SEM). The "stable" periods were 14 ± 2 hours long and ranged from 60 minutes to 63.5 hours. The reproducibility over all 12 patients was 188 ± 17 mL or $11.7 \pm 0.7\%$ (mean ± SEM).

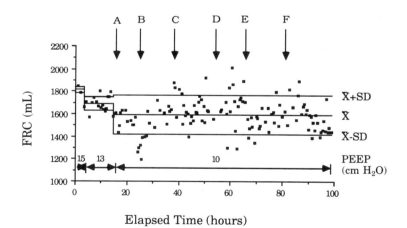

FIG 17–7.
FRC versus time for one representative ARDS patient. The PEEP levels and the corresponding mean and SD of the FRC values during these PEEP levels are shown. A = minor surgery on leg; B = patient very agitated, several doses of morphine given over next 8 hours; C = change bed and move patient; D = patient agitated, morphine and librium given over next 4 hours; E = change bed and move patient; F = morphine given over next 4 hours.

The automated SF_6 washout system was accurate in normal volunteers. There was no statistically significant difference between any of the three measurement techniques. The differences between the gas dilution techniques (SF_6 and helium) and body plethysmography shown in Table 17–4 agree well with the results of Dubois et al.[21] and Jonmarker.[32, 35] The difference is lower than that observed by Tierney and Nadel[19] (130 ± 110 mL)(mean ± SD), Reichel, Dannenberg, and Redecker[22] (218 ± 241 mL), and Schanning and Gulsvik[12] (306 ± 275 mL). Perhaps this was due to the lower age of our subjects and thus a more ideal distribution of ventilation. Our age distribution most closely matches that of Dubois and Jonmaker and is considerably lower than that of Schanning and Gulsvik[12] (20 to 68, mean = 43 years).

In the COPD group, there were differences among all three FRC measurement techniques. As shown in Table 17–4, body plethysmography gives the highest value followed by helium dilution and then SF_6 washout. The difference between body plethysmography and helium dilution agrees well with observations made in patients with obstructive lung disease by Schanning and Gulsvik[12] (mean difference = 530 mL). The major explanation for this difference is that there are areas of the lung with very poor ventilation. These regions do not completely equilibrate with the tracer gas. Consequently, the FRC calculated using the tracer gas is smaller. In addition, there are some potential small errors in body plethysmography. In patients with obstructive lung disease, mouth pressure may not accurately reflect alveolar pressure.[19, 36] This would result in an overestimation of the plethysmographic FRC.

Nieding et al.[37] have shown that the transport of SF_6 into the lung can be modeled by convective flow down to the 17th generation of the bronchi, and then diffuses into the lung periphery. The diffusion wash-in should be an exponential function over time with a time constant that is directly proportional to the square root of the mass of the gas. Comparing the theoretical diffusion of helium (mass = 4) and SF_6 (mass = 146), one would expect that the time constant for SF_6 would be the square root of (146/4) or 6.04 times that of helium. Nieding has shown that the washout time constant of SF_6 is about 2.16 times that of helium. This would indicate that convective flow does add a significant contribution. If the mixing time reported[12, 19] for helium is about 7 minutes, then this would indicate that a wash-in of 15.12 minutes would be required for SF_6. Our criteria for steady state were perhaps not stringent enough for the COPD patients since we did not see equilibration times that approached 15 minutes. If we used a prolonged wash-in and washout for the SF_6 FRC measurement, the difference between SF_6 washout and helium dilution should have become smaller. Despite the differences between SF_6 and the other two FRC measurement techniques, there was still a highly linear relationship between them. These regression equations could be used to predict FRC accurately even in patients with obstructive lung disease. SF_6 washout FRC measurements should certainly be able to provide accurate changes in FRC.

The reproducibility of the technique was excellent in patients with ARDS considering the assumption that the FRC was "stable" as long as the PEEP was constant. Figure 17–7 illustrates that there are many different factors such as drugs, body movements, and respiratory therapy interventions that also influence FRC. Previous studies have measured reproducibility by doing only 2 or 3 measurements within 15 minutes of one another in a carefully controlled situation. In this study we had more than 1000 measurements in 12 patients included in the calculation of reproducibility. This is a test of reproducibility under much harsher conditions than those that have been used previously. Despite this handicap, our reproducibility value of 11.7% is in the range of previously reported[6-8, 12, 15, 20, 23, 25, 32] reproducibility values (range = 2 to 12%) and exactly the same as that reported by Kauppinen-Walin et al.[23] for supine helium dilution measurements. We feel that calculation of reproducibility in this manner is more relevant because it gives the clinician a feel for the "real-world" reproducibility in the ICU setting. This calculation gives a worst case measure of the usefulness of the system for reflecting changes in FRC due to PEEP. If the changes in FRC due to PEEP are smaller than 11.7%, it would be highly unlikely that they could reliably be recognized in this type of clinical setting.

The SF_6 FRC measurement system that we used is built around the Siemens infrared SF_6 analyzer and the Siemens 900i ventilator.[30] There is nothing restricting the use of this technique to the Siemens ventilator. It could be used with any device that can provide flow information, such as a Fleisch pneumotachograph. The cost of such a system would include the initial expense of an IBM PC/AT, the SF_6 delivery system, the SF_6 analyzer, and the software to make the measurement. The SF_6 analyzer is not currently a regular Siemens product. The technology is similar to their 930 CO_2 analyzer; therefore, I would estimate the cost to be comparable to their CO_2 analyzer. The system could be constructed for approximately $10,000. The disposable costs would include the expense for SF_6 gas. We have been able to get about 2000 FRC measurements from one E cylinder of SF_6 (cost $200). This would result in a disposable cost of approximately 10 cents per FRC measurement. There is no need for a technician to operate the device. A rough estimate of the amortization of the equipment would be 15 cents per measurement. The estimated total cost, per FRC measurement, would be 25 cents.

Radiographic Measurement of FRC and TLC

If you have a chest radiograph of a patient and can measure the cross-sectional area of the lung with two different views (anteroposterior and lateral) then one can, theoretically, determine the volume of the lung. The assumptions inherent in this process are that the two views are taken under identical conditions and that the assumptions about the three-dimensional geometry of the lung are valid. This technique was first reported[38] in 1933. Barnhard et al.[39] evolved the technique to assume that the lung could be represented as a stack of elliptical cylindroids. Pratt and Klugh[40] introduced a technique known as a compensating polar planimeter, which measured the cross-sectional areas from the two different chest radiograph views and estimated the TLC. The general concept[41] of the technique is shown in Figure 17–8. The lung is divided into three main regions. The top two regions are further subdivided in two. These five regions are then modeled as stacked elliptical cylindroids. The volume of these cylindroids is summed and then corrections are made for the volume of the hemidiaphragm, heart, and pulmonary blood and tissue. This technique was found to be reasonably accurate in patients with obstructive and restrictive disease when compared to body plethysmography[42]; however, these were not mechanically ventilated patients in the ICU. Others have shown the technique to be effective in normal subjects in the supine position[43] and for measuring FRC in normal subjects during sleep.[44] Hedenstierna et al.[45] have used the CT scan to measure thoracoabdominal volumes in surgical patients.

PA Chest Radiograph   **Lateral Chest Radiograph**

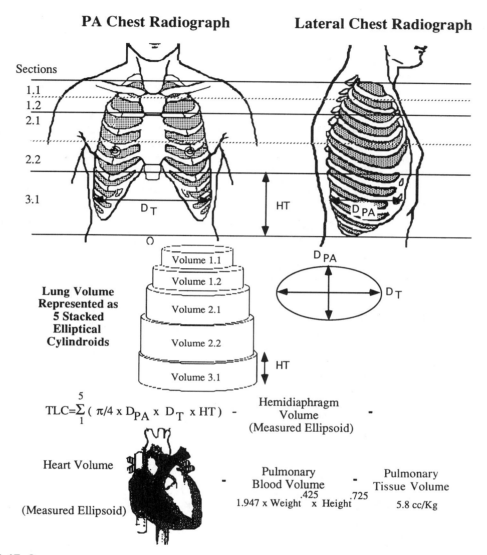

FIG 17–8.
Procedure for using chest radiographs to calculate TLC(41). (Some parts of this figure were reproduced with permission from MacAnatomy clip art.)

The major drawbacks to the radiographic techniques are that they require a large amount of complex equipment that is difficult or impossible (in the case of the CT scanner) to use effectively at the patient's bedside. The techniques require precise posterior-anterior alignment of the patient, the elimination of motion artifact[46] and ideally the two views would be taken simultaneously to avoid any possible change in lung volume between the two different radiographs. These requirements are just not realistic at the bedside of the complex critically ill patient.

Thoracic Dimension Measurement of Changes in FRC and TLC

In 1977 Cohn et al.[47] introduced a device known as an inductance plethysmograph that can accurately measure ventilation without interfering with the act of breathing. Respiratory inductance plethysmography (RIP) is a technique using two inductance transducers about the chest and abdomen to measure volume changes during breathing. The RIP allows noninvasive measurement of V_T, f, V_E, mean inspiratory flow, and inspiratory and expiratory time. Figure 17–9 is a block diagram of the RIP. The transducers are zigzag coil of wire attached to an elastic bandage. These coils are connected to a small oscillator module that is worn on the garment. The oscillators run at a frequency of approximately 300 kHz. They produce frequency-modulated signals around 20 kHz. The frequency of the oscillations is varied by changes in the inductance of the coils. The inductance of the coils changes in proportion to the cross-sectional area. A cylindrical model of lung volume (Fig 17–10) is used to translate the cross-sectional area into a volume. As the thoracic volume changes during respiration, the frequency of oscillations varies. All of these signals are low amplitude and are not radiated from the transducers or the wiring. The oscillators are connected to a demodulator/calibrator device with a wire approximately 5 to 10 m in length. The outputs of the optocouplers are sent to phase-locked loops that demodulate the signals from the oscillators and produce an electrical signal that is linearly related to the thoracic volume under the band. These signals are then fed through bandpass filters for an ac coupled option. Positioning of the coils is important. The rib cage (RC) coil should be worn over the sternum and as close to the armpits as possible. The abdominal (ABD) coil should be placed in the midregion below the lower ribs and the top of the hips. When the RIP is used on humans the model shown in Figure 17–10 is used. The upper cylinder represents RC cross-sectional area and the lower cylinder the

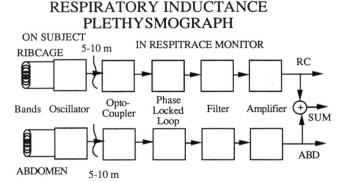

RESPIRATORY INDUCTANCE
PLETHYSMOGRAPH

FIG 17–9.
Block diagram of the respiratory inductance plethysmography unit.

RESPIRATION MODEL

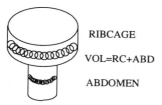

RIBCAGE

VOL=RC+ABD

ABDOMEN

FIG 17–10.
Model used with inductance plethysmography when calculating lung volumes.

ABD cross-sectional area. Using this model, the relationship between volume and flow and the RC and ABD signals is as follows:

$$V(t) = \alpha \cdot RC(t) + \beta \cdot ABD(t) \text{ and } \dot{V}(t) = \alpha \cdot \frac{d[RC(t)]}{dt} + \beta \cdot \frac{d[ABD(t)]}{dt} \qquad (17\text{–}4)$$

where α and β are the calibration coefficients, $RC(t)$ is the rib cage signal from the RIP, and $ABD(t)$ is the abdomen signal from the RIP.

Many different calibration techniques have been proposed; however, none of them provides an absolute measure of FRC or TLC. It is possible to measure the change in FRC accurately.[48] This technique has been used successfully to detect and measure intrinsic PEEP.[49] The advantage of the RIP technique is that it is relatively simple and inexpensive and it provides a breath-by-breath record of the changes in lung volume. The logistical problem of having bands around the chest of a critically ill patient with chest tubes, wound dressings, etc., is one of the primary disadvantages. Positional changes and changes in the location of the bands may alter the calibration and affect the accuracy. Motion artifacts are difficult to deal with. Despite these problems, if a record of the relative changes in FRC is important, then this system has been shown to do a reasonable job in an intensive care environment. This system has been shown to be effective outside of the ICU and it is commercially available.

SUMMARY

There are several different systems that can be used for measuring FRC in the mechanically ventilated patient. The most promising systems for routine clinical use at the bedside are the SF_6 washout FRC measurement system[15, 30–33] and the respiratory inductance plethysmography system.[47] The commercially available respiratory inductance plethysmography system is a good choice if measurement of relative changes in FRC is important. If absolute measurement of FRC is required then a system such as the SF_6 washout FRC system should be considered. The SF_6 washout FRC system does not require alteration of the breathing circuit or interruption in any way of ventilatory support. The system is simple to operate, fully automated, and can function independent of user intervention for many days. This system is relatively inexpensive to use but is not commercially available.

The ability to collect a large volume of information about temporal changes in FRC during mechanical ventilation is truly unique. FRC measurements such as those collected in our study using the SF_6 system[31] in 12 ARDS patients has rarely, if ever, been obtained in the past. This tool opens the door to future systematic evaluation of the effects of positive pressure, mechanical ventilation modalities, respiratory therapy maneuvers, drugs, etc., on FRC over time in the critically ill patient who is being mechanically ventilated. Only the results of systematic studies and randomized clinical trials will definitively determine the usefulness of FRC measurements in the treatment of mechanically ventilated patients. We anticipate that FRC may be used as a noninvasive guide to titration of PEEP, adjustment of expiratory times in pressure-controlled inverse ratio ventilation, and detection of gas trapping. This might reduce the costs and risks associated with the invasive monitoring currently required to perform these tasks.

REFERENCES

1. Marini JJ: Lung mechanics determinations at the bedside: Instrumentation and clinical application. *Respir Care* 1990; 35:669–693.
2. Shapiro BA: Airway pressure therapy for acute restrictive pulmonary pathology, in L SWCaTW (ed): *Critical Care State of the Art.* Fullerton, CA, Society of Critical Care Medicine, 1981, Vol 2, pp. 1–53.
3. Falke KJ, Pontoppidan H, Kumar A, et al: Ventilation with end-expiratory pressure in acute lung disease. *J Clin Invest* 1972; 51:2315–2323.
4. East TD, int Veen JCCM, Pace NL, McJames S: Functional residual capacity as a noninvasive indicator of optimal positive end-expiratory pressure. *J Clin Monit* 1988; 4:91–98.
5. Hylkema BS, Barkmeiger-Degenhart P, Van der Mark TW, et al: Measurement of functional residual capacity during mechanical ventilation for acute respiratory failure. *Chest* 1982; 81:27–30.
6. Weaver LJ, Pierson DJ, Kellie R, et al: A practical procedure for measuring functional residual capacity during mechanical ventilation with or without PEEP. *Crit Care Med* 1981; 9:873–877.
7. Ibanez J, Raurich JM, Moris SG: Measurement of functional residual capacity during mechanical ventilation. Comparison of a computerized open nitrogen washout method with a closed helium dilution method. *Int Care Med* 1983; 9:91–93.
8. Cooper KR, Boswell PA: Accurate measurement of functional residual capacity and oxygen consumption of patients on mechanical ventilation. *Anaesth Intens Care* 1983; 11:151–157.
9. Kondo T, Kurata T, Takasaki Y, et al: Measurement of functional residual capacity and pulmonary carbon monoxide diffusing capacity during mechanical ventilation with PEEP. *Tokai J Exp Clin Med* 1982; 7:561–573.
10. Suter PM, Schlobohm RM: Determination of functional residual capacity during mechanical ventilation. *Anesthesiol* 1974; 41:605–607.
11. Laws AK: Effects of anaesthesia and muscle paralysis on functional residual capacity of the lungs. *Can Anaesth Soc J* 1968; 15:325–331.
12. Schanning CG, Gulsvik A: Accuracy and precision of helium dilution technique and body plethysmography in measuring lung volumes. *J Clin Lab Invest* 1973; 32:271–277.
13. Richardson P, Anderson M: Automated nitrogen-washout methods for infants, evaluated using cats and a mechanical lung. *J Appl Physiol.* 1982; 52:1378–1382.

14. Saidel GM, Saniie J, Chester EH: Lung washout during spontaneous breathing. Parameter estimation with a time varying model. *Comp Biomed Res* 1980; 13:446–457.
15. Paloski WH, Newell JC, Gisser DG, et al: A system to measure functional residual capacity in critically ill patients. *Crit Care Med* 1981; 9:342–346.
16. Richardson P, Wyman M, Jung AL: A method of estimating the functional residual capacity of infants with respiratory distress syndrome. *Crit Care Med* 1980; 8:667–670.
17. Richardson P, Galway W, Olsen S, et al: Computerized estimates of functional residual capacity in infants. *Ann Biomed Eng* 1981; 9:243–255.
18. Weygandt GR: A sensitive five-breath N2 washout test of distribution of ventilation. *J Appl Phys* 1976; 40:464–467.
19. Tierney DF, Nadel JA: Concurrent measurements of functional residual capacity by three methods. *J Appl Physiol* 1962; 17:871–873.
20. Carlon GC, Miodownik S, Ray C, et al: A computerized technique to measure functional residual capacity in patients on mechanical ventilation. *Crit Care Med* 1984; 12:274.
21. Dubois AV, Botelho SY, Bedell GN, et al: A rapid plethysmographic method for measuring thoracic gas volume. A comparison with a nitrogen washout method for measuring functional residual capacity in normal subjects. *J Clin Invest* 1956; 35:322–329.
22. Reichel G, Dannenberg G, Redecker R: Bestimmung der funktionellen residualluft kapazitat mit dem Ganzkorperplethymographen und der Fremdgasmethode. Ein methodischer vergleich. *Arch Klin Med* 1968; 215:28–35.
23. Kauppinen-Walin K, Sovijarvi AR, Muittari A: Determination of functional residual capacity with 133-xenon radiospirometry. Comparison with body plethysmography and helium spirometry. Effect of body position. *Scand J Clin Lab Invest* 1980; 40:347–354.
24. Hecht E, Zajac A: Optics, in Reading, PA, Addison-Wesley, 1976, pp 456–457.
25. Stokke T, Hensel I, Burchardi H: A simple method for determination for the functional residual capacity during artificial ventilation. *Anaesthetist* 1981; 30:124–130.
26. Katz JA, Ozanne GM, Zinn SE, et al: Time course and mechanisms of lung-volume increase with PEEP in acute pulmonary failure. *Anesthesiol* 1981; 54:9–16.
27. Imanaka H, Takezawa J, Nishimura M, et al: Measurement of functional residual capacity during high-frequency oscillatory ventilation (HFOV) by argon washout method without interruption of HFOV. *Chest* 1990; 97:1152–1156.
28. Cinotti L, Susskind H, Zubal IG, et al: Measurement of lung volume with 81 Krm in a dynamic scintigram. *Nucl Med Comm* 1987; 8:479–488.
29. Sovijarvi ARA, Pajunen J, Turjanmaa V, et al: Reference values of regional ventilation, lung volumes and perfusion assessed by using an automated multidetector 133-Xe radiospirometer. *Ann Clin Res* 1986; 18:160–166.
30. East TD, Andriano KP, Pace NL: Automated measurement of functional residual capacity by sulfur hexafluoride washout. *J Clin Monit* 1987; 3:14–21.
31. East TD, Wortelboer PJM, van Ark E, et al: Automated sulfur hexafluoride washout functional residual capacity measurement system for any mode of mechanical ventilation as well as spontaneous respiration. *Crit Care Med* 1990; 18:84–91.
32. Jonmarker C, Jansson L, Jonson B, et al: Measurement of functional residual capacity by sulfur hexafluoride washout. *Anesthesiol* 1985; 63:89–95.
33. Larsson A, Linnarsson D, Jonmarker C, et al: Measurement of lung volume by sulfur hexaflouride washout during spontaneous and controlled ventilation: Further development of a method. *Anesthesiol* 1987; 67:543–550.
34. Jonmarker C, Castor R, Drefeldt B, et al: An analyzer for in-line measurement of expiratory sulfur hexafluoride concentration. *Anesthesiol* 1985; 63:84–88.

35. Larsson A, Malmkvist G, Werner O: Variations in lung volume and compliance during pulmonary surgery. *Br J Anaesth* 1987; 59:585–591.
36. Brown R, Ingram RH, McFadden ER: Problems in the plethysmographic assessment of changes in total lung capacity in asthma. *Am Rev Respir Dis* 1978; 118:685–692.
37. Nieding G, Lollgen H, Smidt U, et al: Simultaneous washout of helium and sulfur hexafluoride in healthy subjects and patients with chronic bronchitis, bronchial asthma, and emphysema. *Am Rev Respir Dis* 1977; 116:649–660.
38. Hutardo A, Fray WW: Studies of total pulmonary capacity and its subdivisions. II. Correlation with physical and radiologic measurements. *J Clin Invest* 1988; 12:807–823.
39. Barnhard HJ, Pierce JA, Joyce JW, et al: Roentgenographic determination of lung capacity. *Am J Med* 1960; 28:51.
40. Pratt PC, Klugh GA: A method for determination of total lung capacity from posteroanterior and lateral chest roentgenograms. *Am Rev Respir Dis* 1967; 96:548–552.
41. Rodgers RC: Instruction manual: SEC radiographic lung volume kit. Institute of Nuclear Medicine, Middlesex Hospital Medical School, London, England, 1977.
42. Wehr KL, Masferrer R: Clinical usefulness of planimetric estimation of total lung capacity. *Respir Care* 1975; 20:966–969.
43. Ries AL, Clausen JL, Friedman PJ: Measurement of lung volumes from supine portable chest radiographs. *J Appl Physiol* 1979; 47:1332–1335.
44. Block AJ, Bush CM, White C, et al: A radiographic method for measuring steady-state functional residual capacity in the supine patient: A method suitable for sleep studies. *Am Rev Respir Dis* 1981; 124:330–332.
45. Hedenstierna G, Strandberg A, Brismar B, et al: Functional residual capacity, thoracoabdominal dimensions, and central blood volume during general anesthesia with muscle paralysis and mechanical ventilation. *Anesthesiol* 1985; 62:247–254.
46. Pierson DJ: Measuring and monitoring lung volumes outside the pulmonary function laboratory. *Respir Care* 1990; 35:660–667.
47. Cohn MA, Rao ASV, Broudy M, et al: The respiratory inductive plethysmograph: A new non-invasive monitor of respiration. *Bull Europ Phsyiopath Resp* 1982; 18:643–658.
48. Cartwright DW, Willis MM, Gregory GA: Functional residual capacity and lung mechanics at different levels of mechanical ventilation. *Crit Care Med* 1984; 12:422–427.
49. Hoffman RA, Ershowsky P, Krieger BP: Determination of auto-PEEP during spontaneous and controlled ventilation by monitoring changes in end-expiratory thoracic gas volume. *Chest* 1989; 96:613–616.
50. Davis R: *MacAnatomy*. Houston, Macmedic Publications Inc. 1985, Vol 2.

Chapter 18

The Computer for Charting and Monitoring

Reed M. Gardner, Ph.D.

C. Gregory Elliott, M.D.

Loren Greenway, B.S., R.R.T.

INTRODUCTION

Frequent measurement of patient parameters such as heart rate, respiratory rate, blood pressure, and oxygen saturation have become a central feature in the care of acutely ill patients. When timely and accurate decisions are required for providing therapy, patient monitors frequently are used to collect and display physiological data. A patient monitor is usually thought of as a piece of equipment that watches for—and warns against—life-threatening events. Hudson has defined monitoring as: "Repeated or continuous observations or measurements of the patient, his or her physiological function, and the function of life support equipment, for the purpose of guiding therapeutic interventions, and assessment of those interventions."[1] Two decades ago, patient monitoring occurred only in the intensive care unit (ICU), but today it is not uncommon to have ECG telemetry transmitters and pulse oximeters attached to patients throughout the acute care areas of hospitals.

COMPUTERIZED PATIENT RECORDS

The medical record is the principal instrument for ensuring the continuity of patient care. There is a need to integrate and optimize medical data review and decision-making. The traditional handwritten medical record has several limitations:

1. It may be physically unavailable since it can only be used by one person at one location at a time.

2. It is often poorly organized, available only in the order and format in which it was recorded, and many times is illegible. As a result, information retrieval may be impossible, slow, and error prone.
3. Retrieval of data for research is time-consuming and cumbersome because it must be done manually.
4. Medical devices, such as pulse oximeters and ventilators, that present data in electronic form require their data to be captured by a human and written into the chart.

Thus, the medical record is a document that begs to be computerized.[2-4] Improvement in clinical information-management systems is frequently cited as one strategy for coping with the cost and inefficiency of our health care system.[2-4] Often information in a chart is written in illegible handwriting, has missing reports, and pages filed out of chronological order. Many times the data must be transcribed or rerecorded in another format for quality assurance reviews or billing purposes. Recently, the Institute of Medicine (IOM) undertook an 18-month study to examine the status of patient records and of computer-based approaches to their management.[2-4] The IOM called for an unequivocal adoption of computer-based medical records. They pointed out that informed patient-care decisions depend on timely access and management of patient information. The computer record provides an unusual opportunity to meet the objectives pointed out by the IOM.

The IOM made the following recommendations for the computerized medical record[4]:

1. Health care professionals and organizations should adopt the computer-based medical record as the standard for medical and all other records related to patient care.
2. The public and private sector should join in setting up a Computer-based Patient Record Institute (CPRI).
3. Both the public and private sectors should expand support for computerized records through research, development, and demonstration projects.
4. Uniform standards for data and security to facilitate implementation of computerized records and data bases should be developed.
5. Federal and state laws and regulations should be reviewed so that model legislation to facilitate computer records will be developed.
6. The cost of computerized record systems should be shared by public, private, and third-party payers.
7. Health care professional schools and organizations should enhance educational programs for students and practitioners in the use of computers.

In 1985, Andrews et al.[5] pointed out that an ideal computerized respiratory care charting and monitoring system would have the following characteristics:

1. No repetition of work or reporting.
2. Easy access to terminals for data entry and review.
3. Accurate, timely, and descriptive documentation.
4. Automatic performance of many functions from a singe data entry (for example, billing, management statistics, medical record generation, error checking, quality assurance, data interpretation, and computerized patient-care protocol generation).

5. Exact correlation between clinical charting and billing.
6. Integration of respiratory care information with that of other hospital departments (e.g., the blood gas laboratory, clinical laboratory, infectious disease department, and medical records).
7. Availability of information for diagnostic, treatment, and research purposes.
8. Easy implementation.
9. Reliable system operation (i.e., no downtime or loss of data).
10. Cost-effective—inexpensive equipment that pays for itself.
11. Electronic access to data from bedside data collection devices (e.g., pulse oximeters and ventilators).

Several of these ideals have been implemented at the LDS Hospital in Salt Lake City, Utah. Challenges and opportunities with this computerized hospital information system will be discussed to illustrate the feasibility of such systems.[5, 6]

LDS HOSPITAL AND THE HELP HOSPITAL INFORMATION SYSTEM

LDS Hospital is a 520-bed, university-affiliated, tertiary care center. The hospital serves as a referral center for trauma victims and maintains active programs in cardiovascular surgery and renal, liver, and cardiac transplantation, as well as other surgical services. The hospital has four adult ICUs with 60 beds and one 12-bed neonatal ICU.

The HELP Hospital Information System uses an integrated clinical patient data base and has decision-making capabilities.[6] Figure 18–1 shows the multitude of data collection sources used in the care of the acutely ill patient. As data flow into the data base, it activates (illustrated by the concentric circles in Fig 18–1) the medical decision-making capabilities of the computer system. The HELP computer runs on a highly reliable computer system that uses redundant processors and has "mirrored" disk volumes to provide the reliability and availability needed for clinical use. There are more than 1000 terminals, including terminals at all ICU bedsides, and more than 200 laser printers for generating reports.

Figures 18–1 and 18–2 illustrate how data flow into the integrated patient data base from multiple sources. The patient data base stores primarily coded data so that it can be used for computerized medical decision-making and report generation. Figure 18–2 shows that for respiratory care, the data entered into the system are used for a host of purposes. The left-hand side shows the more conventional uses of "charting" data and the right-hand side shows how the data are used by the computer for medical decision-making.

Charting

Charting by respiratory therapists and nurses is primarily initiated by entry through bedside terminals (note the computer terminal on the far left-hand side of Fig 18–3). Entries are made by selecting multiple-choice items from a menu, by number entry, or, in some limited situations, by typing in a free-text format. The menu entry format follows a logical sequence that corresponds with the charting requirements. Multiple entries at one time can be done

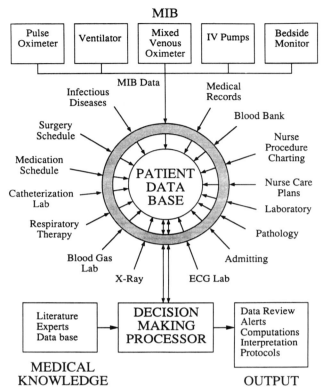

FIG 18–1.
Diagram of the HELP system computerized ICU data collection system. Shown are the large number of data sources required to take care of the ICU patient. The Medical Information Bus is used to collect data from the bedside noted. (*From Gardner RM, Hawley WH, East TD, Oriki T, Young HFW. Real Time Data Acquisition: Recommendations for the Medical Information Bus (MIB).* Intl J Clin Monit and Comput *1992; 8:251–258. Used by permission.*)

together. To speed the process, only questions pertinent to the specific procedure are asked. The only questions to which answers are required are those pertaining to medical, legal or billing issues. Therapists and nurses are responsible for complete and accurate charting. All entries are "tagged" with employee identifications numbers, which serve as an electronic "signature."

Patient Reports

Review of respiratory care charting is available from any of the more than 1000 terminals in the hospital or from phone-in capabilities from physicians' offices and homes. In addition, laser-printed hardcopy reports are available in the hospital (Fig 18–4). Physicians also have the

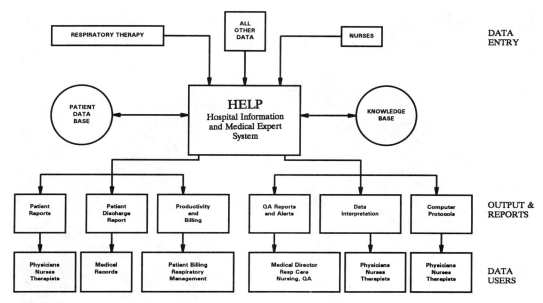

FIG 18–2.
Block diagram of the HELP Hospital Information System and how it integrated the patient data base and knowledge base used for medical decision-making. The system not only provides administrative support, but also uses the medical expert system capabilities of HELP to provide clinical decision support.

option of reviewing a summary of respiratory care data and a large variety of other patient data in a ROUNDS report as illustrated in Figure 18–5.

Administrative and Management Reports

Each night, just past midnight, the computer automatically generates two reports.

1. A patient discharge report for patients discharged the previous day. This report is sent to medical records as the final "official" report.
2. A respiratory therapy and hospital management report on productivity and billing. At the same time this report is generated, an "electronic" bill is automatically transmitted to the hospital's billing system.[5]

MEDICAL INFORMATION BUS: AUTOMATED DATA ACQUISITION

Care of the acutely ill patient requires rapid acquisition, recording, and communication of data. It is not unusual for a hospitalized patient to be connected to several monitoring and recording devices simultaneously (Fig 18–1).[7, 8]

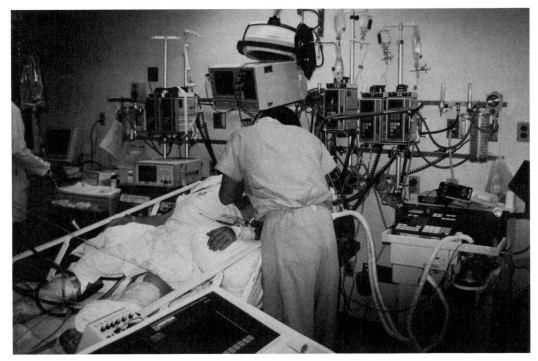

FIG 18–3.
Typical ICU setting. On the far left is a bedside computer terminal. Next is a mixed venous O_2 saturation monitor and four IV pumps. Above the patient's head is a bedside monitor that does ECG, arterial, and pulmonary artery pressure monitoring. To the right of the standing nurse is a Puritan-Bennett 7200 ventilator with a pulse oximeter on top. All of these electronic devices are connected to the HELP computer system through the Medical Information Bus.

Each of these devices is typically made by a different manufacturer who may specialize in one type of measurement (e.g., pulse oximetry). Most of the modern monitoring and recording devices are based on microcomputers and have communications capabilities. Unfortunately, as yet, no standard communications technology is available for all devices.[8] In addition, different clinical staff (physicians, nurses, or respiratory therapists) may be responsible for collection of data from these devices. As a result, the need exists to develop methods, standards, and strategies for automatic gathering of timely, accurate, and representative data from these devices.

To facilitate automatic data acquisition from the multitude of physiological devices located at the bedside, we have integrated data flowing from these devices with the Medical Information Bus (MIB).[7, 8] Experience with the prototype MIB we built gave us insight into the problems of using automated data collection. Problems arise around who owns the data. Should it be the nurses, therapists, blood gas technicians, or physicians who chart the inspired oxygen percentage? There also were problems with the timeliness of data entry as well as deciding

```
                    LDS HOSPITAL   RESPIRATORY CARE CHARTING
                                  DEC 26, 1991

                    AGE:  ██      SEX: M    E60█           PATIENT ID#:   12032██
LIVER CANCER                    DR. BELNAP, LEGRAND P.      ADMITTED:  DEC 12, 1991


12/26/91                                   VENTILATOR MONITORING

           VENT MODE  VR  Vt   O2  PF  IP TEMP IE RATIO PK  PL  MAP PP m-Vt c-Vt s-Vt  MR  SR  TR m-VE s-VE t-VE  Cth aOX vOX Pc  CF
26 07:29 B-II A/C     23 750  .49 65     35.0 1: 2.0 40  29      5 910  781         26      20.3           32.5 88  73 19 3.7
26 05:47 B-II A/C     22 750   50 65     35.0 1: 2.1 42  30      5 930  793         27      21.4           31.7 88  73    3.7
26 04:36 B-II A/C     23 750  .50 65     35.0 1: 2.2 40  30      5 940  811         26      21.1           32.4 88  75    3.7
26 04:36 B-II A/C               50

12/26/91  DUR/ENTRY                           OBSERVATIONS
26 07:29  20/07:35 - INTERFACE: ORALTRACH TUBE;  ALARMS CHECKED;  TEMP SETTING:  5.0;  POSITION: SEMI-FOWLER;  PATIENT CONDITION:
                    CALM;  SUCTIONED, 2 CC, AMBER, THICK;  COMMENT: CASCADE FILLED, TUBING DRAINED.  HR=116, BP=93/49  THERAPIST:
                    GORDON, LAYNE  RRT
26 05:47  15/05:48 - INTERFACE: ORALTRACH TUBE;  PEEP SETTING: 5 CM;  TEMP SETTING:  5.0;  POSITION: SEMI-FOWLER;  THERAPIST:
                    COOMBS, JOE  RRT
26 04:36  15/04:38 - INTERFACE: ORALTRACH TUBE;  BREATH SOUNDS: COARSE CRACKLES, BOTH LUNGS;  ALARMS CHECKED;  TEMP SETTING:  5.0;
                    POSITION: SEMI-FOWLER;  THERAPIST: COOMBS, JOE  RRT
26 04:36   0/04:36 - DISCUSSED THERAPY CHANGE WITH: JAY/PROTOCOLS  THERAPIST: COOMBS, JOE  RRT


12/26/91                                   VENTILATOR MONITORING

           VENT MODE  VR  Vt   O2  PF  IP TEMP IE RATIO PK  PL  MAP PP m-Vt c-Vt s-Vt  MR  SR  TR m-VE s-VE t-VE  Cth aOX vOX Pc  CF
26 01:47 B-II A/C     23 750   40 65     35.0 1: 2.1 40  30      5 940  811         26      21.1           32.4 88       3.7

12/26/91  DUR/ENTRY                           OBSERVATIONS
26 01:47  15/01:48 - INTERFACE: ORALTRACH TUBE;  PEEP SETTING: 5 CM;  PLACED TRACH CARE CATHETER IN CIRCUIT;  TEMP SETTING:  5.0;
                    POSITION: SEMI-FOWLER;  THERAPIST: COOMBS, JOE  RRT


12/26/91                                   VENTILATOR MONITORING

           VENT MODE  VR  Vt   O2  PF  IP TEMP IE RATIO PK  PL  MAP PP m-Vt c-Vt s-Vt  MR  SR  TR m-VE s-VE t-VE  Cth aOX vOX Pc  CF
25 23:49 B-II A/C     23 750   40 65     35.0 1: 2.4 40  30      5 950  821         24      19.7           32.8 88  72    3.7
25 21:43 B-II A/C     23 750   40 65     35.0 1: 1.8 40  30      5 1030 901        24      21.6           36.0 88  75    3.7

12/26/91  DUR/ENTRY                           OBSERVATIONS
25 23:49  15/23:50 - INTERFACE: ORALTRACH TUBE;  PEEP SETTING: 5 CM;  BREATH SOUNDS: COARSE CRACKLES, THROUGHOUT INSPIRATION, BOTH
                    LUNGS;  TEMP SETTING:  5.0;  POSITION: SEMI-FOWLER;  PATIENT CONDITION: QUIET;  SUCTIONED, 3 CC;  THERAPIST:
                    COOMBS, JOE  RRT
25 21:43  15/21:44 - INTERFACE: ORALTRACH TUBE;  TEMP SETTING:  5.0;  POSITION: SEMI-FOWLER;  THERAPIST: COOMBS, JOE  RRT

              ****** REPORT ONLY SHOWS CHARTING OF LAST 12 HOURS ******
              TO OBTAIN LONGER REPORTS, PLEASE USE OPTION #2 ON RT MENU
(END)                                                            #886 - pg1
```

FIG 18–4.
A typical 12-hour respiratory therapist's chart.

what was "representative" for a time frame. Figure 18–6 shows examples of these errors. The issues illustrated by Figure 18–6 are just the "tip of the iceberg." We must establish methods and strategies to decide how often and what data should be recorded. Once these issues are dealt with, automated data collection will be more accurate and efficient.

Figure 18–7 shows a closeup view of IV pump number 77. This pump is infusing lidocaine (see upper display window) at 3 mL/hour (see lower display window). Any time the physician or nurse changes the drip rate, the MIB and computer system automatically log the data. With the MIB connected to the IV pumps, we are able to record infusions in a much more timely and accurate manner than the manual charting methodology. Note in the ROUNDS report of Figure 18–5 that the patient was receiving dopamine at 2.00 mcg/kg/min and that the information was presented in the "Cardiovascular" section near the cardiac output determination since it will have a major effect on cardiac output production.

Figure 18–8 shows the MIB interface box and a pulse oximeter on top of a Puritan-Bennett 7200 ventilator. We store 20 different parameters from the ventilator into the patient's

```
                    L D S   H O S P I T A L   I C U   R O U N D S   R E P O R T
                              DATA WITHIN LAST 24 HOURS

NAME:                          NO.   12032      ROOM: E60         DATE: DEC 26 08:15
DR. BELNAP, LEGRAND P.    SEX: M   AGE:    HEIGHT: 187  WEIGHT: 98.70  BSA: 2.24  BEE: 2054  MOF:  0
ADMT DIAGNOSIS: LIVER CANCER              ADMIT DATE: 12 DEC 91
SURGERY: PANCREATIC-LIVER RESECTION
```

```
CARDIOVASCULAR:  0                                          EXAM: _____
TIME       CO    CI    HR   SV   SI   VP  MSP  MP  SVR LWI  PW   PA   PVR  RWI      _____
DEC 26 04:00 21.60 10.82  116  186  93 16.0M  80  65   2   78  18   26   .4  12.6
         DEC 26 02:42  DOPAMINE (INTROPIN)  2.00 MCG/KG/MIN
         LV PARAMETERS ARE WITHIN NORMAL LIMITS
              SP    DP    MP    HR  | LACT      CPK       CPK-MB     LDH-1      LDH-2
LAST VALUES   94    50    65   116  |
MAXIMUM      118    67    78   206  |  (    )   (    )    (    )     (    )     (    )
MINIMUM       67    28    44   104  |
```

```
RESPIRATORY:  0
          pH    PCO2  HCO3   BE   HB   CO/MT  PO2  SO2  O2CT  %O2  AVO2  VO2  C.O.  A-a  QS/QT  PK/ PL/PP  MR/SR
26 04:01 V 7.35  47.6  25.8   .5   9.7  3/ 1   44   71   9.8   40                                 0/ 0/ 5  25/ 0
26 04:00 A 7.36  44.7  24.9  -.2  10.3  2/ 1   58   85  12.3   40                                 0/ 0/ 5  25/ 0
         SAMPLE # 53, TEMP 37.9, BREATHING STATUS : ASSIST/CONTROL
         HB ERROR SUSPECTED, AV-O2, SHUNT,  O2 EXTRACT RATIO NOT CALCULATED
         MODERATE ACUTE RESPIRATORY ACIDOSIS
         MODERATE HYPOXEMIA
         SEVERELY REDUCED O2 CONTENT (12.3) DUE TO ANEMIA (LOW HB)
         HYPOVENTILATION NOT IMPROVED
25 22:09 A 7.34  46.3  24.5  -.9  10.3  3/ 1   64   87  12.7   40              120                0/ 0/ 5  25/ 0

      ------- machine settings -------|-------------------------- patient values ----------------------------
         VENT  MODE  VR  Vt   O2%  PF  IP   MAP  PK  PL  PP   m-Vt  c-Vt  s-Vt  MR   SR   TR  m-VE  s-VE  t-VE  Cth   Pc
26 07:29 B-II  A/C  23  750   49   65            40  29   5   910   781        20.3                   32.5  19
25 21:43 B-II  A/C  23  750   40   65            40  30   5  1030   901        24                     21.6        36.0
26 07:29 20/07:35  INTERFACE: ORALTRACH TUBE;  ALARMS CHECKED;  POSITION: SEMI-FOWLER;  PATIENT CONDITION: CALM;  SUCTIONED,
         2 CC, AMBER, THICK;  COMMENT: CASCADE FILLED, TUBING DRAINED.  HR=116, BP=93/49  THERAPIST: GORDON, LAYNE, RRT
25 21:43 15/21:44  .INTERFACE: ORALTRACH TUBE;  POSITION: SEMI-FOWLER;  THERAPIST: COOMBS, JOE, RRT
                                                                      EXAM: _____
    -- NO SPONTANEOUS PARAMETERS WITHIN THE LAST 24 HOURS --
```

```
NEURO AND PSYCH:  0
    GLASGOW  3 (08:00) VERBAL _____  EYELIDS _____  MOTOR _____  PUPILS _____  SENSORY _____

    DTR _____   BABIN. _____   ICP _____   PSYCH _____
```

```
COAGULATION:  0
    PT:   14.7  (05:30  ) PTT:  39 (05:30  ) PLATELETS:  90 (05:30  ) FIBRINOGEN:  (   ) EXAM: _____
    FSP-CON:  (   .   ) FSP-PT:  (        ) 3P: Neg       (24 20:17 )                      _____
```

```
RENAL, FLUIDS, LYTES:  0
    IN  13472 CRYST  2732  COLLOID  425  BLOOD    NG/PO   20  | NA  147 (05:30) K   4.3  (05:30) CL  107  (05:30)
    OUT  6945 URINE   923  NGOUT         DRAINS  5705 OTHER 1317 | CO2 26.0 (05:30) BUN  83  (05:30) CRE  3.3 (05:30)
    NET  6527 WT  98.70    WT-CHG  2.20  S.G.   1.017          | AGAP  18.3      UOSM           UNA       CRCL
```

```
METABOLIC --- NUTRITION:  0
    KCAL  2942 GLU  154(26 05:30) ALB   1.7 (26 05:30) | CA  6.8 (26 05:30) FE  (   ) TIBC  (      )
    KCAL/N2  446 UUN  (        ) N-BAL   .0             | PO4 6.6 (26 05:30) MG  (   ) CHOL  80 (26 05:30)
```

```
GI, LIVER, AND PANCREAS:  0                                                                      EXAM:
    HCT    30.7 (26 05:30) TOT BILI 35.0 (26 05:30) SGOT 741 (26 05:30) ALKPO4 970 (26 05:30) GGT 227 (26 05:30) ____
    GUAIAC  (   )  DIR BILI 28.0 (26 05:30) SGPT  87 (26 05:30) LDH 1330 (26 05:30) AMYL 311 (26 05:30)          ____
```

```
INFECTION:  0
    WBC 25.5(05:30 ) TEMP 38.0 (08:15)  DIFF  7 B, 73P, 14L,  6M,  E (05:30) GRAM STAIN: SPUTUM _____ OTHER _____
```

```
SKIN AND EXTREMITIES:
    PULSES _____  RASH _____  DECUBITI _____
```

```
TUBES:
    VEN _____  ART _____  SG _____  NG _____  FOLEY _____  ET _____  TRACH _____  DRAIN _____

    CHEST _____  RECTAL _____  JEJUNAL _____  DIALYSIS _____  OTHER _____
```

```
MEDICATIONS

ACETAMINOPHEN, SUPP          MGM  RECT    650   MAGNESIUM          MEQ  IV   10.000
METRONIDAZOLE (FLAGYL), INJ  MGM  IV     2000   ZINC               MGM  IV    6.000
NYSTATIN, SUSPENSION         ML   ORAL     20   COPPER             MGM  IV    1.200
CEFTAZIDIME (FORTAZ), INJ    MGM  IV     3000   MANGANESE          MGM  IV     .600
                                                                        #880 · pg1
```

FIG 18–5.
An ICU ROUNDS report used by medical staff during morning rounds in the Shock Trauma ICU. Note the respiratory care data summarized in the middle of the report.

AMPHOTERICIN B, INJ	MGM	IV	45	CHROMIUM		MCG	IV	12.000
DOPAMINE, INJ	MGM	IV	315	CHLORIDE		MEQ	IV	0
NOREPINEPHRINE (LEVOPHED), INJ	MGM	IV	27	SULFATE		MEQ	IV	10.000
FUROSEMIDE, INJ	MGM	IV	200	GLUCONATE		MEQ	IV	9.000
FAMOTIDINE (PEPCID), INJ	MGM	IV	40.000	ELECTROLYTE VOLUME		ML	IV	122.000
DIPHENHYDRAMINE (BENADRYL), INJ	MGM	IV	50	MVI-12 , INJ		ML	IV	10.400
POTASSIUM	MEQ	IV	0	PHYTONADIONE (AQUA-MEPHYTON), INJ		MGM	IV	10
CALCIUM	MEQ	IV	9.000					

```
-ANAER CULT-  **-PRELIMINARY REPORT-**      24DEC 18:50
     SOURCE:  OTHER, PELVIS
     SMEAR TYPE:  GRAM STAIN
     STAIN:  FEW WBCS.

-ROUTINE CULT-  **-PRELIMINARY REPORT-**     24DEC 18:50
     SOURCE:  OTHER, PELVIS
     SMEAR TYPE:  GRAM STAIN
     STAIN:  FEW WBCS.
     RESULT: NO GROWTH IN 24 HOURS.

-ANAER CULT-  **-PRELIMINARY REPORT-**      24DEC 18:40
     SOURCE:  OTHER,  PLEURA
     SMEAR TYPE:  GRAM STAIN
     STAIN:  NUMEROUS GRAM NEGATIVE BACILLI, MODERATE NUMBER OF WBCS, FEW
             YEAST.

-ROUTINE CULT-  **-PRELIMINARY REPORT-**     24DEC 18:40
     SOURCE:  OTHER,  PLEURA
     SMEAR TYPE:  GRAM STAIN
     STAIN:  NUMEROUS GRAM NEGATIVE BACILLI, MODERATE NUMBER OF WBCS, FEW
             YEAST.
     RESULT:  GRAM NEG. BACILLI    MODERATE GROWTH

-ANAER CULT-  **-PRELIMINARY REPORT-**      24DEC 18:15
     SOURCE:  FLUID  ABDOMEN
     SMEAR TYPE:  GRAM STAIN
     STAIN:  FEW WBCS, FEW YEAST.

-ROUTINE CULT-  **-PRELIMINARY REPORT-**     24DEC 18:15
     SOURCE:  FLUID  ABDOMEN
     SMEAR TYPE:  GRAM STAIN
     STAIN:  FEW WBCS, FEW YEAST.
     RESULT: NO GROWTH IN 24 HOURS.

-ANAER CULT-  **-PRELIMINARY REPORT-**      24DEC 18:00
     SOURCE:  FLUID  ABDOMEN
     SMEAR TYPE:  GRAM STAIN
     STAIN:  FEW WBCS, FEW YEAST.

-ROUTINE CULT-  **-PRELIMINARY REPORT-**     24DEC 18:00
     SOURCE:  FLUID  ABDOMEN
     SMEAR TYPE:  GRAM STAIN
     STAIN:  FEW WBCS, FEW YEAST.
     RESULT:  GRAM NEG. BACILLI    FEW

-ANAER CULT-  **-PRELIMINARY REPORT-**      24DEC 17:05
     SOURCE:  FLUID  ABDOMEN
     SMEAR TYPE:  GRAM STAIN
     STAIN:  MODERATE NUMBER OF WBCS.

-ROUTINE CULT-  **-PRELIMINARY REPORT-**     24DEC 17:05
     SOURCE:  FLUID  ABDOMEN
     SMEAR TYPE:  GRAM STAIN
     STAIN:  MODERATE NUMBER OF WBCS.
     RESULT:  GRAM NEG. BACILLI    FEW
(END)
```

#880 - pg2

FIG 18–5. Continued

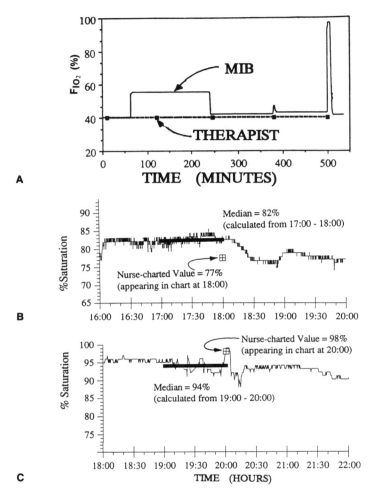

FIG 18–6.
Data recorded by the MIB. **A** shows MIB-recorded and therapist-charted F_{IO_2} data. Note the therapist *did not* chart the almost 3-hour increase in F_{IO_2}. **B** shows nurse- and MIB-charted O_2 saturations from a pulse oximeter. The nurse charted a saturation of 77% and said it occurred at 18:00. Most likely this was a "timeliness" error and the nurse made the measurement at 18:15. **C** shows that the nurse chose "atypical" for entry of saturation to put into the computer record. (*From Gardner RM, Hawley WH, East TD, et al: Real-time data acquisition: Recommendations for the Medical Information Bus.* Intl J Clin Monit Comput *1992; 8:251–258. Used by permission.*)

"electronic" medical record. Figure 18–9 shows a comparison of the data recorded by respiratory therapists and MIB for a 24-hour time interval. Therapists are instructed to record data at 2-hour intervals. As can be seen in Figure 18–9, the therapists have done an excellent job of data recording. However, at about 07:00 they increased the F_{IO_2} to 100% for a very short time interval and did not record it in the record. Later, at about 23:00 they increased the F_{IO_2}

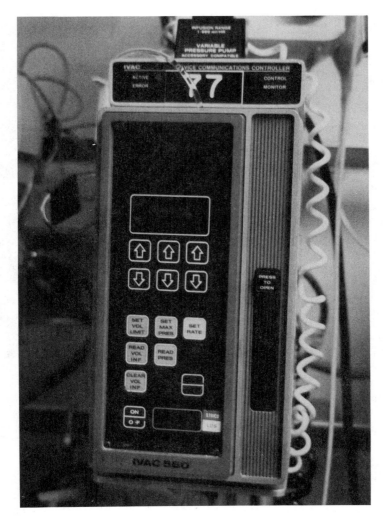

FIG 18–7.
Photograph of patient bedside IV pump indicating the medication lidocaine running at 3.0 mL/hour. Note the small MIB "box" with number 77 mounted on the top of the IV pump.

to 100% again and this time they did record the data. As can be seen from Figure 18–9, respiratory therapists record considerable "redundant" ventilator setting data. Nurses do not record the IV drip rates every hour or two, but only when they change the rate. Unlike IV drips, ventilators are commonly "played with" by physicians and others who *do not* record what they do, especially the change in ventilator settings. Therefore, there is a need to set up recording strategies to make sure these data are properly recorded. The MIB provides a method

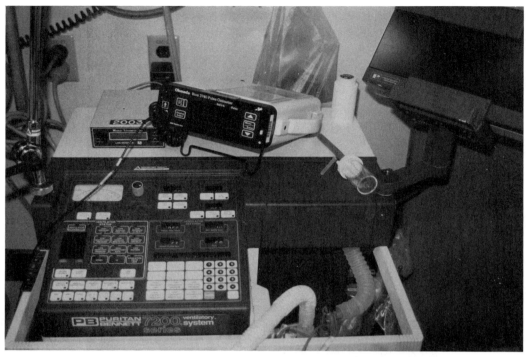

FIG 18–8.
Photograph of a Puritan-Bennett 7200 ventilator with an MIB data interface box number 2003 on top. Also a pulse oximeter located next to the MIB interface box.

for acquiring the data, but does not completely solve the problem of *who* made the ventilator setting change.

Figure 18–10 shows measured tidal volume data recorded by the MIB and that manually entered by respiratory therapists. As can be seen, the therapists faithfully recorded the data every 2 hours. Unfortunately, they did not always record "representative" data as can be seen by several of the data points. In an attempt to record more representative data with the MIB, we have experimentally used a moving median for a 3-minute interval to acquire data. The MIB collects data from the ventilator every 10 seconds and then records a median every 3 minutes only if there is greater than a 50-mL change in corrected tidal volume. The bold line in Figure 18–10 is the computer's selection of the "representative" values for the 24-hour time interval. Although this methodology for recording of values is not yet widely reviewed and accepted, it is likely to be useful in clinical practice.[7]

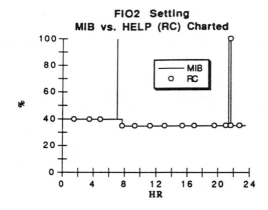

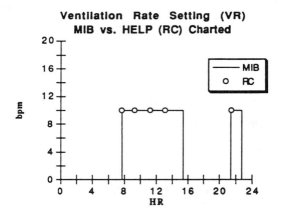

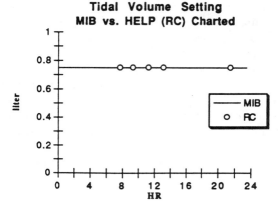

FIG 18–9.
MIB and respiratory care (RC) ventilator settings recorded for 24 hours from a Puritan-Bennett 7200 ventilator. Notice for the most part that the manually charted data follow the MIB data record (see text).

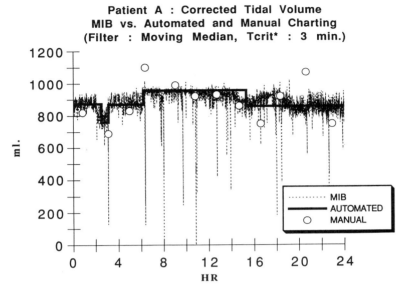

Patient A : Corrected Tidal Volume
MIB vs. Automated and Manual Charting
(Filter : Moving Median, Tcrit* : 3 min.)

FIG 18–10.
MIB and respiratory care (manual) measurement data recorded for 24 hours from a Puritan-Bennett 7200 ventilator. The open circles are the 2-hour respiratory therapists' recordings, the jaggy vertical lines are the breath-by-breath MIB data recordings. In addition a 3-minute median is plotted. The 3-minute median data plot is the recommended data recording method for recording data into the patient record.[7]

COMPUTER-ASSISTED QUALITY ASSURANCE

Webster defines quality as "The degree of excellence which a thing possesses."[9] Demming, a pioneer in producing high-quality products who helped the Japanese become the world leaders in producing quality products, points out that "Reliable service reduces costs. Delays and mistakes raise costs."[10] Berwick tells us that "Real improvement in quality depends, according to the Theory of Continuous Quality Improvement, on understanding and revising the production process on the basis of data about the processes themselves. Every process produces information on the basis of which the process can be improved."[11] James tell us that quality is roughly equivalent to medical outcomes.[12] He further states that quality is "one of those things that is difficult to define, but that anyone can recognize—I know it when I see it." These and others have shown that medicine, like any other process, can be improved and that among other things the transfer of information is key to improving health care systems.[13] In the late 1700s the great English writer Samuel Johnson said "Men more frequently need to be reminded than informed."

McDonald has stated that most adverse events in health care are preventable, particularly those due to errors or negligence.[14] He has shown that computers are able to help in the process of improving quality.

Medical decisions have traditionally been considered a scientific, as well as intuitive, process. In recent years, however, formal methods for decision-making have been applied to medical problem-solving and computer-assisted medical decision-making has gained wider acceptance.[3, 15–17] Computers can be used to interpret data (e.g., interpretation of the ventilatory status based on blood gas data). Computers can also be used to alert physicians, nurses or pharmacists that a medication may be contraindicated.[18, 19] Computers can also be used to provide physician guidance using patient treatment protocols. What follows is a brief description of several computerized activities using the HELP system.

Respiratory Care

The respiratory care charting and monitoring system was developed to be a computer-assisted quality assurance monitor.[5, 20, 21] The system addresses the immediate needs of patients through a daily medical director's alert report, which allows the medical director to intervene in acute situations as they arise.[20, 21] The department's quality assurance program monitors and evaluates clinical indicators of staff performance in terms of stated policies and procedures. The integrated data base of the HELP system is crucial to allow these functions, which would not be feasible using manual chart review.

Computerized, real-time quality assurance can be used to improve quality and reduce the cost of care. Most hospitals in the United States do quality assurance by defining a criteria for quality and then, via a random chart review, determine the compliance with this predetermined level. Then using educational or procedural mechanisms they attempt to improve the quality. Following that they study the problem with a second random chart review to determine the success rate. Using the computerized data base, criteria designated for quality care can be explicitly described and when breeches in that "standard" are found via computer surveillance an immediate report can be generated and the problem corrected immediately. This allows real-time improvement of care. Computerized quality monitoring can be used on every patient for every situation; thus, it is far superior to conventional quality assurance activities.

Computer monitoring also can dramatically improve the identification of problems. For example, when adverse drug reactions are detected by a continuous computer surveillance program, the rate of detecting adverse reactions was 80-fold higher than when reported by hand.[22] These types of audits are only achievable with an integrated computerized clinical decision-making data system.

Computerized respiratory care charting is efficient because it has streamlined the process of documentation while extracting the most "useful" information from the recording process. Without having to provide costly cumulative paper reports, the computer system provides better access for data entry and review. Overall, computer charting is preferred by therapists over manual charting, because it makes their jobs easier and improves the quality of information charted. Computer charting has added a high degree of confidence that there will be good correlation of clinical, administrative, and financial records. Such a system has demonstrated its value to the therapists, their department, the hospital, and most importantly to the patient.[5, 9]

COMPUTERIZED BLOOD GAS INTERPRETATION

Figure 18–11 illustrates the use of the computer to acquire and interpret a patient's blood gas results. With the increased sophistication of laboratory instruments, physicians, nurses, and respiratory therapists are being presented with large amounts of clinical data that they are expected to interpret and use to formulate therapeutic actions. Since this new information can be derived from blood gas instruments, we have connected blood gas machines to the HELP computer using the MIB. Error rates have decreased from 0.28% to *no* errors as a result of this electronic interface.[23] In addition, the computer uses its "knowledge base" to provide an interpretation of the results. Experience with the computerized blood gas interpretation system has shown that[24]:

1. The interpretation is accurate and appreciated by physicians and nurses.
2. The interpretations provide better care to a growing number of patients.
3. Quality control in the blood gas laboratory is enhanced.
4. Computerization has lead to standardization of classification criteria.
5. Terminology of blood gas interpretation has been standardized.
6. Computerization provides educational benefit to the medical staff, nurses, and others.
7. Turnaround time between sample taking and result reporting has decreased.

COMPUTERIZED PROTOCOLS DIRECT PATIENT CARE

Under the medical leadership of Drs. Alan H. Morris and Terry P. Clemmer of the pulmonary/ICU group at LDS Hospital, extensive computerized protocols have been developed.[25] Morris has said: "The explosion of medical information has found clear expression both in the proliferation of medical publications and in the staggering amount of information collected from critical care patients. A recent morning rounds review of a critically ill patient produced a list of 236 different variables."[25] With such a huge amount of data it is not surprising that Dr. David M. Eddy, in a recent JAMA commentary, stated " . . . all confirm what would be expected from common sense: The complexity of modern medicine exceeds the inherent limitations of the unaided human mind."[26]

With the able medical informatics assistance of Drs. Thomas D. East and Dean F. Sittig, the pulmonary division has developed, tested, and validated several computerized ventilatory care protocols.[27, 28] Computer protocols for the management of mechanical ventilation (respiratory evaluation, ventilation, oxygenation, weaning, and extubation) in patients with Adult Respiratory Distress Syndrome (ARDS) have been developed and validated at LDS Hospital.[27] These protocols use the bedside computer terminals (Fig 18–3) to prompt the clinical care team with therapeutic and diagnostic suggestions. The protocols, in both paper flow diagram and computer form, have been used for over 40,000 hours in more than 100 patients. The computerized protocols directed patient care 94% of the time. The remainder of the time, patient care was *not* protocol controlled because the current protocol logic did not include events such as transport for x-ray studies. The survival of these patients has been four times greater than was expected from historical controls.[27, 28]

NO. 12032███ DR. BELNAP, LEGRAND P.

	SEX M	AGE 44	ROOM E60█

DEC 26 91	pH	PCO2	HCO3	BE	HB	CO/MT	PO2	SO2	O2CT	%O2	AVO2	VO2	C.O.	A-a	Qs/Qt	PK/ PL/PP	MR/SR
NORMAL HI	7.45	40.6	26.0	2.5	17.7	2/ 1					5.5	300	7.30	22	5		
NORMAL LOW	7.35	27.2	15.8	-2.5	13.7	0/ 1	63	91	18.5		3.0	200	2.90		0		
26 04:01 V	7.35	47.6	25.8	.5	9.7	3/ 1	44	71	9.8	40						/ / 5	25/
26 04:00 A	7.36	44.7	24.9	-.2	10.3	2/ 1	58	85	12.3	40			21.60	127		/ / 5	25/

SAMPLE # 53, TEMP 37.9, BREATHING STATUS : ASSIST/CONTROL
HB ERROR SUSPECTED, AV-O2, SHUNT, O2 EXTRACT RATIO NOT CALCULATED
MODERATE ACUTE RESPIRATORY ACIDOSIS
MODERATE HYPOXEMIA
SEVERELY REDUCED O2 CONTENT (12.3) DUE TO ANEMIA (LOW HB)
HYPOVENTILATION NOT IMPROVED
PULSE OXIMETER SO2 87.0

| 25 22:09 A | 7.34 | 46.3 | 24.5 | -.9 | 10.3 | 3/ 1 | 64 | 87 | 12.7 | 40 | | | | 120 | | / / 5 | 25/ |

SAMPLE # 52, TEMP 37.8, BREATHING STATUS : ASSIST/CONTROL
MODERATE ACUTE RESPIRATORY ACIDOSIS
MILD HYPOXEMIA
SEVERELY REDUCED O2 CONTENT (12.7) DUE TO ANEMIA (LOW HB)
HYPOVENTILATION (PREVIOUSLY NORMAL)
PULSE OXIMETER SO2 88.0

| 25 17:43 V | 7.36 | 46.9 | 26.1 | .8 | 10.6 | 3/ 1 | 47 | 74 | 11.1 | 40 | | | | | | / / 5 | 24/ |
| 25 17:42 A | 7.38 | 43.9 | 25.6 | .9 | 10.9 | 2/ 1 | 63 | 88 | 13.4 | 40 | 2.03 | | | 124 | 46 | / / 5 | 24/ |

SAMPLE # 51, TEMP 37.9, BREATHING STATUS : ASSIST/CONTROL
MILD ACID-BASE DISORDER
MODERATE HYPOXEMIA
SEVERELY REDUCED O2 CONTENT (13.4) DUE TO ANEMIA (LOW HB)
HYPOVENTILATION CORRECTED
PULSE OXIMETER SO2 88.0

| 25 04:08 V | 7.39 | 44.3 | 26.5 | 1.8 | 11.3 | 1/ 1 | 44 | 78 | 12.4 | 40 | | | | | | / / 5 | 25/ |
| 25 04:07 A | 7.40 | 44.3 | 27.1 | 2.6 | 11.1 | 2/ 1 | 59 | 89 | 13.9 | 40 | 1.79 | 347 | 19.40 | 127 | 48 | / / 5 | 25/ |

SAMPLE # 50, TEMP 36.8, BREATHING STATUS : ASSIST/CONTROL
MODERATE CHRONIC RESPIRATORY ACIDOSIS
MODERATE HYPOXEMIA
SEVERELY REDUCED O2 CONTENT (13.9) DUE TO ANEMIA (LOW HB)
HYPOVENTILATION IMPROVED
PULSE OXIMETER SO2 89.0

| 24 21:51 V | 7.33 | 54.3 | 28.1 | 1.9 | 10.2 | 2/ 1 | 45 | 76 | 11.0 | 70 | | | | | | / / 5 | 24/ |
| 24 21:50 A | 7.36 | 48.2 | 26.8 | 1.5 | 10.3 | 2/ 1 | 67 | 91 | 13.2 | 70 | 2.12 | 332 | 15.70 | 296 | 46 | / / 5 | 24/ |

SAMPLE # 49, TEMP 36.6, BREATHING STATUS : ASSIST/CONTROL
MODERATE CHRONIC RESPIRATORY ACIDOSIS
MILD HYPOXEMIA
SEVERELY REDUCED O2 CONTENT (13.2) DUE TO ANEMIA (LOW HB)
HYPOVENTILATION MARKEDLY IMPROVED
PULSE OXIMETER SO2 91.0

| 24 20:25 A | 7.30 | 59.5 | 28.6 | 1.7 | 10.2 | 2/ 1 | 66 | 90 | 13.0 | 80 | | | | 346 | | / / 5 | 18/ |

SAMPLE # 48, TEMP 36.5, BREATHING STATUS : ASSIST/CONTROL
SEVERE MIXED CHRONIC AND ACUTE RESPIRATORY ACIDOSIS
MILD HYPOXEMIA
SEVERELY REDUCED O2 CONTENT (13.0) DUE TO ANEMIA (LOW HB)
HYPOVENTILATION MUCH WORSE
PULSE OXIMETER SO2 90.0

| 24 09:45 A | 7.47 | 45.4 | 32.9 | 9.2 | 9.2 | 2/ 1 | 58 | 88 | 11.5 | 40 | | | | 127 | | 48/ 32/ 5 | 23/ |

SAMPLE # 47, TEMP 36.9, BREATHING STATUS : ASSIST/CONTROL
MODERATE MIXED RESPIRATORY ACIDOSIS AND METABOLIC ALKALOSIS
MODERATE HYPOXEMIA
SEVERELY REDUCED O2 CONTENT (11.5) DUE TO ANEMIA (LOW HB)
HYPOVENTILATION (PREVIOUSLY NORMAL)
PULSE OXIMETER SO2 87.0

PRELIMINARY INTERPRETATION -- BASED ONLY ON BLOOD GAS DATA. ***(FINAL DIAGNOSIS REQUIRES CLINICAL CORRELATION)***
KEY: CO=CARBOXY HB, MT=MET HB, O2CT=O2 CONTENT, AVO2=ART VENOUS CONTENT DIFFERENCE (CALCULATED WITH AVERAGE OF A &V HB VALUES)
VO2=OXYGEN CONSUMPTION, C. O.=CARDIAC OUTPUT, A-a=ALVEOLAR arterial O2 DIFFERENCE, Qs/Qt=SHUNT, PK=PEAK, PL=PLATEAU, PP=PEEP
MR=MACHINE RATE, SR=SPONTANEOUS RATE.   *** SPECIMEN IDENTIFICATION: BLOOD (A=ARTERIAL, V=VENOUS, C=CAPILLARY, W=WEDGE)
FLUIDS (P=PLEURAL, J=JOINT, B=ABDOMINAL, S=ABSCESS); E=EXPIRED AIR;
ECCO2R (I=INFLOW, M=MIDFLOW, O=OUTFLOW)

KEEP FULL PAGE FOR RECORDS
(END)

FIG 18–11.

Blood gas report for a patient in the Shock Trauma ICU. Note the computerized interpretations following the reported data as well as the reporting of ventilator settings and F_{IO_2}. The arterial sample interpretation at 04:00 is interesting because there is a large (0.6) difference in the hemoglobin measures from the arterial (A) sample (9.7) and the venous (V) sample (10.3).

The success of these computer protocols and their acceptance by the clinical staff clearly establishes the feasibility of controlling the therapy of severely ill patients. We have now refined the process for generating computerized protocols. Six steps were found to be essential in developing these protocols[27]:

1. Develop protocol logic by consensus.
2. Test the logic at the bedside.
3. Computerize the protocol logic.
4. Validate the protocols with archival computerized data.
5. Clinically validate and refine the protocols.
6. Prepare to use the protocols in routine clinical applications by training the clinical staff and generating appropriate instructional material.

Figure 18–12 gives some examples of "expert system" computer output derived from the HELP system. The top line indicates a "weaning failure" from the ARDS protocol. The second line points out, based on laboratory data, that the patient may be having an adverse drug reaction (ADR). The line with time mark 04:16 is an indication from the ARDS protocol that the F_{IO_2} should be increased. The final line on the report indicates that the patient may have a nosocomial wound infection, based on data contained in the computerized data base, such as microbiology data.

THE FUTURE OF COMPUTER CHARTING AND MONITORING

The quantity of data available on any one patient in the ICU is phenomenal. With the ability to sample data continuously and automatically, it is possible to gather thousands of data points each day for each monitored parameter from each of the monitoring devices. This presents to the clinical and medical informatics team an enormous challenge of determining what data are needed, how often it is necessary to sample, and what data should be stored. If data are redundant, do we need to store the output from all the devices? If so, do we use the same codes for redundant data? If the redundant data are not identical, which data point takes priority? If we have redundant data, which should be used for decision-making, quality assurance, and alerts? These are fertile areas for research activities and crucial to future monitoring system development. Currently these decisions are arbitrarily made with little or no scientific validation.[29, 30]

We must discover what data are needed for decision-making.[31] Typically in the acute care setting we generate enormous volumes of data. However, Knaus and his associates, using the APACHE scoring system, have shown us that they can do very well at making patient prognosis using only a few key data items.[32, 33]

It is time for physicians and other health care professionals to interact with the computer. Any computer system used by clinical staff must be fast, reliable, and user friendly. With little or no training the user should be able to find the desired clinical information and generate reports.[29] The Stanford University Medical Informatics group has recently developed some

PATIENT IDENTIFICATION 12032XXX E60X

HELP DECISIONS

DATE	TIME	
26 DEC	07:38	WEANING ASSESSMENT FAILURE AT 7:30, BLOOD PRESSURE OUTSIDE LIMITS [90/50 < 200/120]. REMAIN IN POSITIVE PRESSURE VENTILATION.
26 DEC	06:59	***** PATIENT WITH POSSIBLE ADR (LAB) ***** 13 12/26/1991. 05:30
26 DEC	04:51	CONTINUE TO MONITOR AND DRAW AN ABG AT 6:36 FIO2 INCREASE AT 4:36, WITH 1 HOURS AND 45 MINUTES REMAINING IN A 2 HOUR WAIT.
26 DEC	04:16	INCREASE FiO2 BY 10%, FROM 40% TO 50%. DRAW AN ABG IN 15 MINUTES.
26 DEC	04:00	HYPOVENTILATION NOT IMPROVED SEVERELY REDUCED O2 CONTENT (12.3) DUE TO ANEMIA (LOW HB) MODERATE HYPOXEMIA MODERATE ACUTE RESPIRATORY ACIDOSIS HB ERROR SUSPECTED, AV-O2, SHUNT, O2 EXTRACT RATIO NOT CALCULATED SAMPLE #53, TEMP 37.9, BREATHING STATUS: ASSIST/CONTROL LV PARAMETERS ARE WITHIN NORMAL LIMITS
26 DEC	01:55	CONTINUE TO MONITOR PATIENT AND DRAW AN ABG IN 2 HOURS, AT 3:55 PATIENT CURRENTLY AT MINIMUM THERAPY.
25 DEC	22:18	CONTINUE TO MONITOR PATIENT AND DRAW AN ABG IN 2 HOURS, AT 24:18 PATIENT CURRENTLY AT MINIMUM THERAPY.
25 DEC	22:09	HYPOVENTILATION (PREVIOUSLY NORMAL) SEVERELY REDUCED O2 CONTENT (12.7) DUE TO ANEMIA (LOW HB) MILD HYPOXEMIA MODERATE ACUTE RESPIRATORY ACIDOSIS A-A GRADIENT 120 SAMPLE #52, TEMP 37.8, BREATHING STATUS: ASSIST/CONTROL
25 DEC	21:45	CONTINUE TO MONITOR PATIENT AND DRAW AN ABG IN 2 HOURS, AT 23:45 PATIENT CURRENTLY AT MINIMUM THERAPY.
25 DEC	18:00	LV PARAMETERS ARE WITHIN NORMAL LIMITS
25 DEC	17:56	TEST FOR VENTILATORY DRIVE (ALLOWED DURING WAIT TIMES): TITRATE VR (MAINTAIN CONSTANT Vt) DOWN TO 11 BR/MIN. ACTIVATE PROTOCOLS AFTER CHARTING. IF REASON NOT TO TEST, ENTER REASON USING OPT. #3 ON A
25 DEC	17:51	INCREASE FiO2 BY 20%, FROM 40% TO 60%. DRAW AN ABG IN 15 MINUTES.
25 DEC	14:11	CONTINUE TO MONITOR PATIENT AND DRAW AN ABG IN 2 HOURS, AT 16:11 PATIENT CURRENTLY AT MINIMUM THERAPY.
25 DEC	10:25	***** PATIENT WITH POSSIBLE NOSOCOMIAL WOUND ***** 83408 12/24/1991. 17:05

PATIENT IDENTIFICATION 12032XXX E60X
HELP DECISIONS #018 - pg1

FIG 18–12.
Printout of the computerized medical decisions made for an ICU patient on the ARDS protocol. Also shown are blood gas interpretations, adverse drug alerts (ADR), interpretations of hemodynamic (cardiac output) parameters, and infectious disease monitoring statements (nosocomial wound).

innovative methods for presenting ventilator advice.[34-36] They used "participatory design" as the method of developing the user interface.[35] Such methods are exciting and innovative, but must be "battle hardened" in the clinical setting to validate them (steps 4 to 6 in the protocol development process noted earlier).

It seems to us that advances in the use of computers in charting and monitoring will be evolutionary rather than revolutionary. Changes will be needed in the health care system, as pointed out by the IOM report on computerized patient records, before use of such computer systems will be widespread. The expectations of society for medical progress and increased use of computers in clinical practice is fueled by increased use of computers in everyday activities. We have made great progress in using computers in medicine, but the opportunities to do more and provide better and more efficient care are astounding!

REFERENCES

1. Hudson LD: Monitoring of critically ill patients: Conference summary. *Respir Care* 1985; 30:628–636.
2. Shortliffe EH, Tang PC, Detmer DE: Patient records and computers. *Ann Int Med* 1991; 115:979–981.
3. Rennels GD, Shortliffe EH: Advanced computing for medicine. *Sci Am* 1987; 257:154–161.
4. Dick RS, Steen EB (Eds): *The Computer-based Patient Record: An Essential Technology for Health Care.* Washington, DC, Institute of Medicine, National Academy of Sciences Press, 1991.
5. Andrews RD, Gardner RM, Metcalf SM, et al: Computer charting: An evaluation of a respiratory care computer system. *Respir Care* 1985; 30:695–707.
6. Kuperman GJ, Gardner RM, Pryor TA: *HELP: A Dynamic Hospital Information System.* New York, Springer-Verlag Inc, 1991.
7. Gardner RM, Hawley WH, East TD, et al: Real time data acquisition: Recommendations for the Medical Information Bus (MIB). *Intl J Clin Monit Comput* 1992; 8:251–258.
8. Shabot MM: Standardized acquisition of bedside data: The IEEE P1073 medical information bus. *Intl J Clin Monit Comput* 1989; 6:197–204.
9. Gardner RM: Computerization and quality control of monitoring techniques, in: *Contemporary Management in Critical Care #4: Respiratory Monitoring.* New York, Churchill Livingston Inc, 1991; pp 197–211.
10. Demming WE: Quality, productivity, and competitive position. Massachusetts Institute of Technology Center for Advanced Engineering Study, Cambridge, 1982.
11. Berwick DM: Continuous improvement as an ideal in health care. *N Engl J Med* 1989; 320:53.
12. James BC: Quality management for health care delivery. The Hospital Research and Education Trust of the American Hospital Association, Chicago, IL, 1989.
13. Kritchevsky BS, Simmons BP: Continuous quality improvement—concepts and application for physician care. *JAMA* 1991; 266:1817–1823.
14. McDonald CJ: Protocol-based computer reminders, the quality of care and the non-perfectibility of man. *N Engl J Med* 1976; 295:1351–1355.
15. Eddy DM: Clinical decision making: From theory to practice—the challenge. *JAMA* 1990; 263–287–290.
16. Eddy DM: Clinical decision making: From theory to practice—anatomy of a decision. *JAMA* 1990; 263:441–443.
17. Flanagin A, Lundberg GD: Clinical decision making: Prompting the jump from theory to practice (editorial). *JAMA* 1990; 263:279–180.

18. Hulse RK, Clark SJ, Jackson JC, et al: Computerized medication monitoring system. *Am J Hosp Pharm* 1976; 33:1061–1064.

19. Gardner RM, Hulse RK, Larsen KG: Assessing the effectiveness of a computerized pharmacy system. *SCAMC* 1990; 14:668–672.

20. Elliott CG, Simmons D, Schmidt CD, et al: Computer-assisted medical direction of respiratory care. *Resp Manage* 1989; 19:31–35.

21. Elliott CG: Computer-assisted quality assurance: Development and performance of a respiratory care program. *QRB* 1991; 17:85–90.

22. Classen DC, Pestotnik SL, Evans RS, et al: Computerized surveillance of adverse drug events in hospital patients. *JAMA* 1991; 266:2847–2851.

23. Howe S: Automated data acquisition from blood gas analyzers (MS thesis). University of Utah, 1991.

24. Gardner RM, Cannon GH, Morris AH, et al: Computerized blood gas interpretation and reporting system. *IEEE Comp* 1975; 8:39–45.

25. Morris AH: Use of monitoring information in decision making, in *Contemporary Management in Critical Care #4: Respiratory Monitoring.* New York, Churchill Livingston Inc, 1991; pp 213–229.

26. Eddy DM: Practice policies: Where do they come from? *JAMA* 1990; 263:1265–1275.

27. East TD, Morris AH, Wallace CJ, et al: A strategy for development of computerized critical care decision support systems. *Intl J Clin Monit Comput* 1992; 8:263–269.

28. Henderson S, Crapo RO, Wallace CJ, et al: Performance of computerized protocols for management of arterial oxygenation in an intensive care unit. *Intl J Clin Monit Comput* 1992; 8:271–280.

29. Clemmer TP, Gardner RM: Medical informatics in the intensive care unit: State of the art 1991. *Intl J Clin Monit Comput* 1992; 8:237–250.

30. Gardner RM, Shabot MM: Computerized ICU data management: Pitfalls and promises. *Intl J Clin Monit Comput* 1990; 7:99–105.

31. Bradshaw KE, Gardner RM, Clemmer TP, et al: Physician decision-making—evaluation of data used in a computerized ICU. *Intl J Clin Monit Comput* 1984; 1:81–91.

32. Knaus WA, Wagner DP, Lynn J: Short-term mortality predictions for critically ill hospitalized adults: Science and ethics. *Sci* 1991; 256:389–394.

33. Knaus WA, Wagner DP, Draper EA, et al: The APACHE III prognostic system: Risk prediction of hospital mortality for critically ill adults. *Chest* 1991; 100:1619–1636.

34. Rutledge GW, Thomsen G, Farr BA, et al: VentPlan: a ventilator-management advisor. *SCAMC* 1991; 15:869–871.

35. Tovar MA, Rutledge GW, Lenert LA, et al: The design of a user interface for a ventilator-management advisor. *SCAMC* 1991; 15:828–832.

36. Farr BR, Shacter RD: Representation of preferences in decision-support systems. *SCAMC* 1991; 15:1018–1024.

Chapter 19

Respiratory Monitoring in the Neonatal Intensive Care Unit

John W. Salyer, R.R.T.

"When technology is master
We shall reach disaster faster"

Piet Hein

INTRODUCTION

The bedside clinician in a neonatal intensive care unit (NICU) is typically faced with a vast array of information. Continuous bedside monitoring of a wide variety of neonatal physiologic variables is now ubiquitous. Yet, as recently as 10 years ago, continuous noninvasive monitoring of transcutaneous Po_2 was a novelty in many tertiary centers. It is now quite common to encounter a neonate with some combination of monitors that could include a continuous pulse oximeter, continuous electrocardiographic, blood pressure, respiration and body temperature monitoring, continuous transcutaneous Pao_2 and $Paco_2$ monitoring, continuous independent (separate from the ventilator) monitoring of airway pressures and temperatures, continuous invasive monitoring of intra-arterial or intravenous Pao_2 and intravenous $S\bar{v}o_2$, as well as continuous monitoring of Fio_2.

Aside from the question of what to do with all of these data now that we have them, one is led to wonder why this impressive edifice of continuous monitoring has been erected? In the NICU, an argument can certainly be made that the clinical instability that is inherent in this population makes continuous monitoring necessary. A single-point-in-time study, such as an arterial blood gas or a palpated or apical pulse determination, generally has little value in telling the clinician what happened an hour ago, or what might happen in 15 minutes. NICU patients are subject to rapid and profound changes in physiologic status. What might otherwise be a small insult to the larger pediatric or adult patient might well be cataclysmic to the neonate. Certain distinct features of neonatal physiology contribute to these concerns. Very brief periods of physiologic insult, such as profound hypoxemia, can cause neonates to revert to fetal circulatory pathways if not rapidly rectified. Lung immaturity often causes the neonate to have very little oxygen reserve in spite of frequent, agressive interventions. Thus even small drops in oxygenation can be serious.

These considerations lead one to believe that continuous noninvasive monitoring of oxygenation should have a significant impact on morbidity and mortality that are related to respiratory function. Unfortunately, having these monitors in place is of little value if the bedside clinicians are not rigorously trained in the application of the monitors and in the interpretation of the data they produce. This includes the use of high and low alarm limits on monitors such as pulse oximeters and F_{IO_2} analyzers. Clinicians can easily be led into a sense of false security by the presence of a wide array of noninvasive monitors, when in fact the monitors may be offering little utility if the alarms are not set properly or if clinicians are not responding to alarm conditions appropriately.

Another major contribution to the proliferation of continuous noninvasive monitoring of oxygenation in neonates is their predisposition toward the development of retinopathy of prematurity (ROP). There has historically been a widespread belief that scrupulous control of Pa_{O_2} could lead to the prevention of this disease.[1] It has now been recognized that ROP is probably not a preventable disease in very low birthweight infants.[2,3] Still, the clinicians caring for these infants must continue to play an important role. Careful monitoring (and control) or arterial oxygen levels is still considered by many to be a substantial part of reducing a neonate's risk of developing ROP.

The phenomenal growth of some of these noninvasive monitoring technologies can probably be attributed to the size of these patients. A relatively simple procedure such as obtaining a blood gas from very low birthweight infants can be very difficult if not impossible.[4] Intermittent percutaneous sampling is frought with difficulties.[5] Continuous invasive arterial lines also have considerable morbidity associated with them,[2] and can sometimes be very difficult to insert.

Frequent blood gas sampling from indwelling arterial lines can also deplete the patient's blood volume. With arterial lines, there is also a potential for increasing the risk for nosocomial infection.

The Goal of Respiratory Monitoring

The factors described above have contributed to the development and utilization of noninvasive respiratory monitoring in the NICU. These technologies are important, but it is also important that respiratory care practitioners, nurses, and physicians maintain a comprehensive understanding of precisely what is measured and how to respond to changes in these measurements.

This chapter will describe some of the basic technologies for monitoring various aspects of respiratory function in the neonatal intensive care unit. The application of any type of continuous or intermittent monitoring must be done with a clear understanding of the *goal* of the monitoring in mind. In a very broad sense, the goal of all types of continuous monitoring of respiratory function is the prevention of the morbidity and mortality associated with deterioration of respiratory function. Less broad definitions of the goals of such monitoring as pulse oximetry or transcutaneous gas monitoring in the NICU include (1) improved patient safety, (2) reducing the need for invasive procedures, and (3) better control of arterial oxygenation.

Unfortunately, there has been little controlled scientific investigation into the effect of these various monitoring modalities on morbidity and mortality, or indeed on whether or not the use of these monitors helps to achieves any of these stated goals.

Some would suggest that it is reasonable to assume that the use of respiratory monitors can improve patient safety. This possibility alone is enough for some to promote the widespread application of these monitors. Such *reasonable assumptions* were made for many years about the utilization of intermittent positive pressure breathing treatments in all postoperative surgical patients (and some preoperative ones!) who did not have pulmonary disease—practices that have for the most part been mercifully abandoned.

Clinicians must be critical in deciding which monitors to apply on which patients. These technologies are not benign. Transcutaneous monitoring can cause burns with permanent scarring, and erroneous data from any monitor can lead to inappropriate changes in therapy. There are also considerable costs associated with the application of these monitors. It was estimated that the capital costs alone for pulse oximetry in 1989 would approach $500 million.[6] Former Surgeon General C. Everett Koop points out that health care costs have continued to rise over the last decade without a concommitant rise in the quality of the care administered.[7] Clearly, continuous respiratory monitoring in the NICU has an important role. But, as the resources for funding health care become more limited (as they most certainly will), clinicians and managers are going to be forced to decide what forms of monitoring are absolutely essential. Are these monitors important enough that we would rather have them than clinicians?

Assessing the Utility of Respiratory Monitoring

Most noninvasive respiratory monitors attempt to measure some physiologic (as in the case of the pulse oximeter) or mechanical (as in the case of the FIO_2 analyzer) variable that can be accurately measured by other means (often invasively). Thus, in one sense, the accuracy of these instruments can be described as how closely their measurements approximate the standards against which they are compared. This is often referred to as *bias*.[8] As an example, the accuracy (or bias) of the pulse oximeter is usually described in terms of the mean difference between a series of paired samples of SpO_2 and SaO_2 as measured by a bench oximeter.

In addition, some of these instruments are described in terms of their sensitivity and specificity. In a broad sense, *sensitivity* is defined as the probability that a test will be positive when the condition of interest is present.[9] *Specificity* is described as the probability that a test will be negative when the condition of interest is not present. In the case of the pulse oximeter, for example, the condition of interest could be described as assuring that arterial PaO_2's remain between 60 to 80 mm Hg. If the pulse oximeter's low and high alarms were set at 85 and 95%, respectively, there would be a certain probability that any blood gas drawn while the oximeter's values were within this range would yield a PaO_2 within the desired range. This probability would be described by the oximeter's sensitivity. Conversely, the oximeter's probability of identifying PaO_2's outside this range would be described by its specificity.

In the following sections, various types of monitors will be discussed, as well as a brief history of the application of the monitor in the NICU, patient selection in the NICU, a description of utility (i.e., sensitivity, morbidity data) if any is available, and the limitations of each type of monitor.

As each modality is described, what scientific information is known about the utility of these devices and their relative accuracies (or lack thereof) will be reported.

CONTINUOUS PULSE OXIMETRY

History

Pulse oximetry as we know it today in ICUs was made possible when certain serendipitous discoveries of the absorption properties of a pulsating bed of tissue were combined with microprocessor technology for the processing of signals. More detailed descriptions of work that led to the theory of operation can be found elsewhere,[10-14] (see Chapter 10: Pulse Oximetry), as well as the history of the development of the pulse oximeter.[15] The first pulse oximeter manufactured and marketed was the Mochida Oximet (eventually Minolta),[15] which proved[16] to be accurate within ±5%. The first of the "modern" pulse oximeters was the Biox II (Ohmeda). The accuracy,[17, 18] convenience, relative economy, and general acceptance of this device was pivotal in the widespread utilization of pulse oximetry. The Nellcor N100 (one of the earliest widely sold pulse oximeters) solved one of the original problems with pulse oximeters by developing a small, disposable probe. Some authors[15] have described these probes as "inexpensive" ($15 to $20 each), but anyone who has had to manage a budget that includes the purchase of pulse oximeter probes can testify that these "inexpensive" items can grow to constitute a sizable expense!

Since the early to mid-1980s the presence of pulse oximeters has grown prodigiously. They can now be found in virtually every operating room, recovery room, and on most if not all mechanically ventilated intensive care patients. Unpublished data from a survey of more than 612 hospitals conducted in 1989 revealed that nearly 80% of all NICUs with more than 20 beds reported monitoring more than 80% of all their mechanically ventilated neonates continuously with a pulse oximeter.[19] This percentage has undoubtedly increased since then.

Patient Selection

Neonatal clinicians (as well as the anesthesiologists) were among the first to recognize the potential utility of continuous pulse oximetry. Indeed, pulse oximetry has been described as "arguably the most significant technological advance ever made in monitoring the well-being and safety of patients during anesthesia, recovery, and critical care."[20] At the time of its introduction into the NICU, most continuous monitoring of oxygenation (when it was done) was achieved with transcutaneous Po_2 ($Ptco_2$) monitors. These ingenious devices had considerable utility, but were also frought with technical and asthetic difficulties (see the section on transcutaneous monitors). Pulse oximeters did not have many of these problems, required no calibration, and were ostensibly very easy to apply (although we came to learn that getting a reliable reading on an active infant can sometimes be a rather protracted affair).

In fact, in many NICUs pulse oximeters rapidly replaced the Ptco$_2$ monitors. Unfortunately, this was done without a good scientific basis for their application (i.e., who would most benefit from them, how to interpret their readings, how well could they identify hypoxemia or hyperoxemia?). Nevertheless, continuous pulse oximetry on all mechanically ventilated neonates and on virtually all infants receiving oxygen therapy has become a *de facto* standard in the United States. In the litigious environment in which medicine is now practiced, it is unlikely that there will be any success in curbing the overutilization of pulse oximetry in the intensive care environment.

There is a conspicuous dirth of scientific data regarding patient selection for continuous monitoring with the pulse oximeter. Some of the most obvious considerations are listed in Table 19–1. Having many pulse oximeters in the NICU has led to frequent overutilization. The most obvious case is the infant who is not receiving oxygen and has no signs of respiratory distress. There is no reasonable justification for continuous pulse oximetry on this infant, and yet many such patients are monitored.

A frequent question is whether or not the pulse oximeter should be used in place of or in conjunction with Ptco$_2$ monitoring.[21-23] There do not appear to be any overwhelming advantages of one technology over the other. Table 19–2 is adapted from New[23] and describes the relative advantages and disadvantages of Ptco$_2$ versus Spo$_2$. Some authors have suggested that saturation measurements are intrinsically more meaningful clinically because they measure a more significant portion of the oxygen transport mechanism. This view is myopic. The mechanism of oxygen transport in the body is rather complex and all portions of it are interdependent on one another. The relative value of any estimate of oxygenation is well stated by Shapiro et al.[24] "No single measurement of oxygenation has any advantage over any other, they all require interpretation."

It is also possible to go into some NICUs and find concomitant Sao$_2$ and Ptco$_2$ monitoring. This amazing consumption of expensive resources seems to have little utility except possibly to reduce the level of anxiety of the bedside clinicians.

TABLE 19–1.
Selection Criteria for Neonatal Continuous
Pulse Oximetry

Continuous pulse oximetry may be indicated for:
    mechanically ventilated neonates
    neonates with an artificial airway
    neonates receiving oxygen
    neonates undergoing invasive procedures
    infants exhibiting signs and symptoms of
        respiratory distress
    neonates being transported within and
        between facilities
    neonates with feeding difficulties (monitored
        during feeding)
    neonates with (or suspected of having) central
        or obstructive apnea

TABLE 19–2.
Features and Benefits of Pulse Oximetry*

Features	Benefits	Alternative Technologies
Requires no heating; measurements made optically at extremely low light power	No risk of burns; sensor site need not be moved periodically	$PtcO_2$ monitors have internal heaters, causing risk of burns and/or patient discomfort, especially in premature neonates; sensor must be moved periodically, especially in neonates to avoid skin damage
Requires no skin preparation; skin may be dirty, burned, or pigmented, but not opaque (e.g., from synthetic fingernails)	No startup delays	$PtcO_2$ monitoring requires site and electrode preparation and warm-up period
Requires no calibration	Operation is instant, accurate	$PtcO_2$ monitors must be frequently calibrated due to intrinsic drift of electrodes
Measures true arterial oxygen (i.e., oxyghemoglobin as percentage of total hemoglobin available for oxygenation)	Accuracy is easily verified by drawing a simultaneous arterial sample for bench oximetry	$PtcO_2$ readings are intrinsically between arterial and venous PO_2 levels and cannot equal arterial PO_2 except under artificial conditions
	Gives a pure respiratory variable (i.e., separate from circulation)	$PtcO_2$ monitoring provides inseparably mixed respiratory/circulatory measurements; a drop in $PtcO_2$ may be caused by respiratory deficiency, circulatory deficiency, or both simultaneously; no separation is possible without independent measurement techniques
Measures arterial pulse wave	Indicates perfusion instantaneously; provides immediate verification of proper sensor operation; gives a pure circulatory variable (i.e., separate from respiration)	$PtcO_2$ monitors are intrinsically slower indicators of sudden circulatory arrest; evidence of proper operation is generally limited to the appearance of a "reasonable" oxygen, although some information can be gleaned from relative changes in perfusion power.
Displays continual pulse rate	Pulse rate is good indicator of change in cardiac output (i.e., circulation)	$PtcO_2$ provides no pulse rate
Displays continuous "real-time" hemoglobin saturation	Saturation is best indicator of change in arterial oxygen content (i.e., respiration)	$PtcO_2$ display skin PO_2, which may or may not agree well with arterial PO_2
Wide variety of sensor configurations available.	Broad clinical applications; patients of any size, disposable or nondisposable probes, ear, finger, toe, calf, wrist, glossal, nasal applications are all possible.	$PtcO_2$ monitors are limited to applications on smooth, flat surfaces that are covered by soft tissue; on VLBW neonates this can sometimes be hard to find

* Adapted from New W: *J Clin Monit* 1985; 1:126–129.

Scientific Data

The accuracy of pulse oximetry has been established in a wide variety of populations. Indeed, a great deal of literature has been published regarding pulse oximetry. A recent review of the literature revealed over 500 citations relating to pulse oximetry, of which more than 150 dealt with accuracy.[15]

One must be particularly careful when describing the accuracy of pulse oximeters in general. Considerable differences have been reported in the performance of different brands of oximeters. This has been demonstrated by Craig[25] who points out that published correlation coefficients of several pulse oximeters range from 0.57 to 0.99, while reported biases and precisions range from -4.5 ± 8.2 to 6.6 ± 10.2. This large reported range is probably related to differences between (1) design of devices, (2) patient populations, (3) levels of desaturation, (4) environmental conditions, and (5) study methodology.[25-27]

It is clear that in most populations the agreement between Spo_2 and Sao_2 is acceptable (biases and precisions from -0.31 ± 2.44 to 1.4 ± 3.1) during normoxemia and mild to moderate hypoxemia.[15, 28-30] During severe hypoxemia (e.g., $Spo_2 < 70\%$) it has been demonstrated that pulse oximeter accuracy deteriorates considerably.[26] However, it is unlikely that there is a need for pulse oximeters to be accurate in this range since clinicians generally attempt to keep their patient's $Spo_2 > 80$ to 90%.

There has been considerable investigation into the use of pulse oximetry in the neonatal population.[31-56] Its accuracy (ability to estimate Sao_2) has been well established (bias -0.2 to 1.4%)[47, 48] and not found to be appreciably different than that reported in adult populations. What is probably more important than its overall ability to estimate Sao_2 accurately is whether or not pulse oximetry can reliably identify periods of hyperoxemia as well as hypoxemia.

As the use of pulse oximetry began to proliferate in the NICU population, caveats were raised against its use.[40, 57, 58] These concerns were centered around the shape of the oxygen-dissociation curve that describes the relationship between oxygen and hemoglobin in blood. Oxygen exists in blood in two forms: dissolved in the plasma and chemically bound to hemoglobin molecules. As the partial pressure of oxygen in plasma increases, it binds to hemoglobin, forming oxyhemoglobin. However, the relationship is not linear. Small changes in the partial pressure can result in large changes in oxygen-hemoglobin bonding (saturation) on the lower or steeper portion of the curve and large changes in Pao_2 can result from small changes in the saturation on the upper or flat portion of the curve. The flat portion of the curve concerned clinicians considering the use of the pulse oximeter in neonates.

Tobin[59] summarized these concerns when he discussed the effect of the relative inaccuracy of oximeters on the ability to predict Pao_2. Describing the 95% confidence limits of oximeters (in general) as $\pm 4\%$, he then theorizes that an oximeter reading of 95% could represent a Pao_2 as low as 60 or as high as 160 mm Hg. This assumed that saturation could be as low as 91% or as high as 99%. Thus, many clinicians felt that the oximeter could not reliably identify periods of hyperoxemia.

However, recent investigations have apparently shown the oximeter to be capable of identifying hyperoxemia with reliability. In a series of 117 measurements on 58 infants, Hay and colleagues[32] reported that keeping Spo_2 at $92 \pm 3\%$ resulted in Pao_2s of more than 45 mm Hg but less than 100 mm Hg in all cases when an Ohmeda 3700 oximeter was used. Similar data have been reported by others and are recorded in Table 19-3. If the results of these findings

TABLE 19-3.

Studies Describing the Pulse Oximeter's Ability to Identify Periods of Hyperoxemia and Hypoxemia in Neonates

Investigators	Instrument Used	SaO_2 range(s)	PaO_2 range(s)	Sensitivity*
Ramanathan et al.[39]	Nellcor N100	87-96%	50-80%	90%
Hay et al.[32]	Ohmeda (Biox) 3700	89-95%	45-100 mm Hg	100%
Blanchette et al.[55]	Nellcor N100 & N200	92-96%	45-90 mm Hg	97%
Tzong et al.[38]	Nellcor N100	80-95%	40-80 mm Hg	88%
Deckardt and Steward[35]	Nellcor N100	80-95%	40-80 mm Hg[†]	94%
Southall et al.[37]	Nellcor N100	<90%	<50 mm Hg	87%
		≥98%	>100 mm Hg	92%
Wiswell[60]	Nellcor N100 Ohmeda 3700	85-94%	40-90 mm Hg	95%

* Sensitivity is defined here as the probability that the SpO_2 ranges listed would result in the PaO_2 ranges desired.
† Used transcutaneous PO_2 measurements, not PaO_2.

can be applied to general clinical use of these monitors, it seems to indicate that the use of the pulse oximeter can, in fact, reliably identify periods of hyperoxemia. Some authors have suggested some generic ranges for SpO_2 of (1) 92 to 96% for preterm infants < one week of age, (2) 90 to 96% for preterms infants > 1 week of age, and (3) 92 to 95% for infants with BPD.[61] However, practitioners must be careful when acting on such recommendations. Each manufacturer's models are different in some important ways including probe design and computer iteration. All models of pulse oximeters need to be studied in the fashion described earlier to establish machine specific ranges for neonates.

What we do not know is whether controlling PaO_2s in this fashion will have any impact on the overall outcome of the patients.[12] It is unlikely now that any prospective randomized trials will ever be conducted to answer such questions.

The Pulse Oximeter in the NICU

There is little value in having reliable pulse oximetry data at the bedside if clinicians do not respond to changes in SpO_2 in a consistent, systematic, and logical fashion. Early application of the pulse oximeter often resulted in nurses and respiratory care practitioners spending prohibitive amounts of time "chasing the pulse oximeter readings." This refers to the practice of setting limits for pulse oximeter values, and then anytime values fell outside these limits, responding by immediately changing FIO_2. One of the more stringent limitations of the pulse oximeter is the degree to which it is affected by motion artifact (see the section on limitations later in this section). This limitation requires that clinicians at the bedside not respond immediately to every change in saturation readings, but instead discriminate real changes in the patient's baseline condition from unreliable, transient readings, and then respond to such changes appropriately by adjusting levels of oxygen administration. One way to discriminate the reliability of pulse oximeter readings is to analyze the plethysmographic waveform that is available on some devices. The lack of display of this type is a serious limitation in oximeter design. A good plethysmographic representation of a strong pulsatile signal is the best way for a clinician to be confident that the displayed saturation in fact is representative. This is especially true in infants who tend to have enormous amounts of motion artifact.

Some published reports give detailed guidelines for the use of pulse oximetry.[62–65] Harbold describes a useful algorithm for responding to low and high saturation readings.[64] Figures 19–1 and 19–2 illustrate these algorithms.

Different facilities may well have differing philosophies regarding the goals of pulse oximetry. They may, in a broad sense, be used to identify periods of hyper- or hypoxemia, or they may be used more specifically to titrate oxygen therapy. However defined, these goals must be clearly described and communicated to the clinical staff. These should include detailed guidelines for use that define how clinicians should respond to changes in the pulse oximetry readings.

Motion Artifact During Pulse Oximetry

One of the most difficult issues concerning the application of the pulse oximeter in the NICU is the prevalence of motion artifact. The oximeter measures pulsatile changes in the absorption of light of certain wavelengths. If the measurement site changes shape (flexion or extension of a finger or hand, muscle contraction, limb rotation, etc.), the baseline absorption of the tissue bed changes. The pulse oximeter signal processors have difficulty distinguishing these changes in absorption from changes that are a result of pulsatile changes, or changes in the relative amounts of the different hemoglobin varieties.

The magnitude of this problem is often not realized by those who are not regularly at the bedside. It is common to hear pulse oximeters referred to as "random number generators" by more skeptical clinicians. Certainly this moniker is not entirely deserved, but it does illustrate the passion that surrounds this device.

Barrington and colleagues[53] investigated this issue and reported that in a neonatal series, pulse oximeter readings were found to be unreliable from 12 to 29% of the time depending on

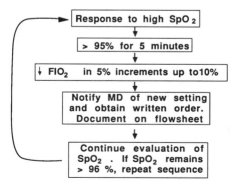

FIG 19–1.
The management of high pulse oximeter saturation readings.

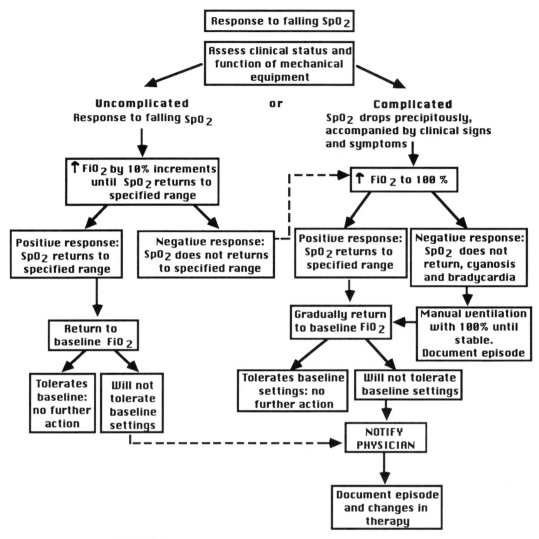

FIG 19–2.
The management of low pulse oximeter saturation readings.

the averaging mode used. They went on to summarize that the poor precision of oximeters ". . . suggests strongly that these devices should not be relied on as the sole means of estimating oxygenation." They are correct when they point out that "The use of pulse oximeters in active subjects must be approached cautiously and the results should be interpreted with an understanding of their limitations."

I found this to be most true during an attempt to obtain a "spot" oximeter reading on a one-month-old patient being mechanically ventilated for bronchopulmonary dysplasia. The patient was relatively montionless at the time I attempted to apply a hand-held oximeter (N-10, Nellcor Inc. Hayward, CA). There was, however, an occasional, small twitching motion of the extremeties. I did not initially anticipate difficulty obtaining a reliable reading. My first attempt resulted in a pulse oximeter reading of 76% and a heart rate that agreed very well with that displayed on the bedside ECG monitor. The problem, however, was that all the other aspects of my clinical evaluation of this patient led me to doubt that the saturation was really that low. Table 19–4 describes data obtained on this patient for 11 consecutive readings taken one immediately after the other on the same extremity with the hand-held oximeter. These data illustrate the need for discriminating analysis of the data from any monitor. The patient's true saturation was not determined because continuous vascular access was not available, and percutaneous sampling was so poorly tolerated that the information that could be obtained was not worth the insult to the patient. Thus, I was left with trying to determine which of the pulse oximeter values really represented the patient's condition. I finally gave up, and reported to the physician and nurse that I was unable to get a reliable pulse oximeter reading on this patient and that they should depend on their clinical assessment skills to determine if the patient was hypoxemic. It is most probable that these readings were unreliable due to motion artifact, because this oximeter and probe had worked well on other patients. Note, however, that there was no overt motion of this patient, only occasional, very small twitching motions. This episode does not necessarily represent the majority of experience with pulse oximeters, but does indicate how problematic data interpretation can be when using the pulse oximeter (or any other noninvasive monitor).

TABLE 19–4.

Serial Measurements (Spot Checks) of SpO_2 on a 1-month-old Infant Suffering from Bronchopulmonary Dysplasia Taken One Immediately after the Other. (Data gathered over a 12-minute period using the Nellcor N-10.)

Measurement Number	Saturation Measured by Pulse Oximeter (%)	Heart Rate as Measured by Pulse Oximeter (beats per minute)	Heart Rate as Measured by Electrocardiagram (beats per minute)
1	76	115	118
2	98	116	117
3	84	118	118
4	100	116	114
5	96	115	114
6	93	116	114
7	100	115	114
8	100	114	117
9	100	68	115
10	100	88	115
11	100	112	113

END-TIDAL CARBON DIOXIDE MONITORING

History

Noninvasive monitoring of ventilation by measuring exhaled carbon dioxide (CO_2) concentrations is a practice that is utilized in a wide variety of clinical settings including research laboratories, sleep study labs, adult ICUs, pulmonary function laboratories, and general care wards (see Chapter 12: Capnography).[66] It is probably most prevalent in the operating room where many anesthesiologists have been aware of the usefulness of this technology for some time. Recent improvements in technology have made these devices simpler and more convenient to operate. Yet the spread of exhaled CO_2 monitoring to patients in NICUs seems slower than one might have expected. Certain technical aspects of measuring exhaled CO_2 concentrations have led some to anticipate problems when monitoring the exhaled CO_2 of infants on mechanical ventilators.[66]

The measurement of exhaled CO_2 concentrations was attempted as early as the first half of the previous century.[67] The currently prevalent measuring techniques were first reported in the 1940s and 1950s.[68, 69]

While the measurement of exhaled CO_2 concentrations may potentially yield considerable information about a wide variety of physiologic conditions, one aspect of this type of monitoring has attracted the attention of clinicians more than any other: the relationship between the partial pressure of CO_2 in end-tidal gas ($Petco_2$) and alveolar gas ($Paco_2$). End-tidal gas is defined as the last portion of an exhaled breath and is assumed to be predominantly alveolar gas. Thus, $Petco_2$ is said[70] to closely approximate $Paco_2$. The normal gradient between alveolar and arterial Pco_2 is so small thay they are considered to be identical. Thus, a device that could accurately measure $Petco_2$ on a breath-by-breath basis could also closely estimate the $Paco_2$ and hence ventilation.

Scientific Data

A number of studies have established excellent agreement between end-tidal and arterial CO_2s ($Paco_2$ − $Petco_2$ ≤ 5 mm Hg) in certain populations.[71-73] However, a variety of conditions can occur under which the agreement between $Petco_2$ and $Paco_2$ deteriorates. Principal among these is any condition that causes an increase in physiologic dead-space (ventilation–perfusion mismatching) and obstructive airway disease.

The agreement between $Petco_2$ and $Paco_2$ has not been extensively studied in infants and children.[74-78] The measurement of exhaled CO_2 during anesthesia in infants and children has demonstrated generally excellent agreement. Unfortunately, agreement deteriorates in populations of critically ill infants, such as those neonates with respiratory distress syndrome (RDS). However, many infants with RDS who have acceptable agreement between $Petco_2$ and $Paco_2$ could benefit from the use of this monitor.

Under optimal conditions, capnometry yields fairly reliable results about the status of a patient's ventilation. It can be helpful in monitoring the status of many mechanically ventilated infants. However, the practitioner must be cautioned that a change in $Petco_2$ does not necessarily indicate a change in alveolar ventilation and thus $Paco_2$. Any change in the patient's physiologic dead-space will result in a change in $Petco_2$. The interpretation of exhaled CO_2 measurements requires an understanding of pulmonary physiology (which is dealt with in considerable detail elsewhere in this text, see Chapter 12).

Sampling Principles

Sampling and measuring techniques are discussed in detail elsewhere in this text. However, some controversy surrounds sampling techiques with regard to their application in the NICU. Two different sampling techniques are utilized in capnometry. *Mainstream sampling* places the measuring chamber in the patient's airway, usually between the ventilator tubing and the airway, thus allowing the exhaled gas to pass through it. *Sidestream sampling* aspirates gas from the patient's proximal airway into a nearby measuring chamber that is outside the airway.

Opinions about the superiority of one sampling technique versus another are divergent.[74, 75, 79, 80] Both techniques have certain limitations. Mainstream analyzers have sampling chambers that attach to the patient's endotracheal tube and add mechanical dead-space as well as resistance[81] (Fig 19–3). Earlier models had dead-space volumes as large as 10 mL, rendering them completely unsuitable for neonatal applications. Newer models have adapters with as little as 1.0- to 1.5-mL dead-space. While this is a significant improvement, 1.0 mL is still a considerable amount of dead-space to add to the airway of a 1000-g infant whose tidal volume may only be 8.0 to 10.0 mL. In fact, dead-space of this magnitude has been shown to cause CO_2 retention in neonates.[82] Also, mainstream sampling chambers can be bothersome because they are relatively heavy and may contribute to accidental extubation, especially if used in neonatal patients.

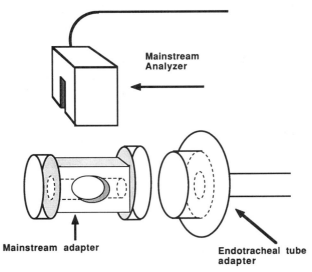

FIG 19–3.
Schematic of a mainstream end-tidal carbon dioxide adapter.

Sidestream analyzers can be prone to contamination and obstruction of the sampling line with fluids and secretions from the patient's airway. If these fluids are aspirated all the way into the instrument, they can render the device completely inoperative, although most sidestream instruments have water traps and filters that should prevent this. Sidestream sampling is usually performed by inserting an aspiration port as near the endotracheal tube connector as possible. In fact, it is possible to replace the normal endotracheal tube adapter with a special adapter with a built in aspiration port (Fig 19–4). This is an acceptable way to sample exhaled gases in infants and children. There is also a report of improved agreement between end-tidal and arterial CO_2 when the sample is aspirated from the endotracheal tube itself (in this case by means of a needle through the wall of the endotracheal tube) when compared to sampling from the proximal airway (between the ventilator circuit and the endotracheal tube).[83]

Another important consideration in sidestream sampling is the rate at which gas is aspirated from the airway. Rates between 30 and 300 mL/min have been reported.[66] Some authors have suggested that sampling rates of 150 to 300 mL/min are suitable for adults, and 50 to 100 mL/min are appropriate for pediatric patients.[66] The use of such generalizations is unfortunate. Factors known to influence the reliability of sidestream exhaled gas measurements include expiratory flow rate, sample flow rate, sample tube length, diameter, and materials, and ventilatory frequency.[80, 82, 84, 85] To suggest that pediatric sampling rates should be limited to 50 to 100 mL/min is an oversimplification. Higher (or lower) sampling rates might work very well on some pediatric and neonatal patients, depending on the ventilatory rate, expiratory flow rate, length of the sampling tube, etc. The broad range of patient sizes that fall under the general heading of pediatrics as well as a diversity of available technology renders the use of such generalized limitations inappropriate.

One report has suggested that mainstream analyzers are more appropriate for pediatrics

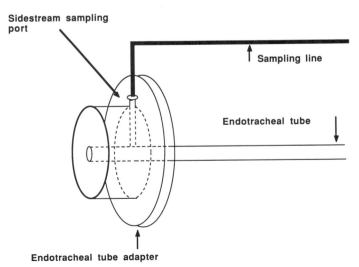

FIG 19–4.
Schematic of a sidestream end-tidal carbon dioxide adapter.

patients because the sidestream analyzer studied produced grossly distorted capnograms that had no plateau on the capnograph waveform.[74] The particular analyzer studied used a low (50 mL/min) sampling rate through a long (6-ft) sampling tube on patients with relatively high (24 to 54 breaths/min) ventilatory frequencies. No wonder capnograms were distorted! If the sampling flow rate is relatively low and the ventilator rate relatively high, the gas aspirated into the sampling tube will not have sufficient time to transit the sampling tube (especially if it is long) to the measurement chamber before the next breath has begun, thus never allowing a plateau to be achieved on the capnograph. It is interesting to note that while the capnogram was found to be distorted in the aforementioned study, there was no significant difference in the absolute value for peak exhaled CO_2 between sidestream and mainstream, and both agreed well with arterial CO_2. However, this study does demonstrate the need for waveform analysis to properly analyze capnometer performance. The detailed operational characteristics of capnometers are found in an ECRI *Health Devices* evaluation of 13 end-tidal carbon-dioxide monitors.[86]

The caveat against using higher sidestream sampling rates with pediatric and neonatal patients probably grew out of concerns related to the effect of aspirating gas out of the airway during inspiration. Patients with very small tidal volumes might have their tidal volume decreased by the use of these devices.[81] Neonatal practitioners have been known to express concerns that aspiration of gas from the airway on very low birthweight infants might severely affect ventilation.

The principle concern surrounding the use of sidestream sampling in pediatric volume ventilation is the effect of aspiration on delivered tidal volume. If the analyzer is aspirating during inspiration, then tidal volume is apt to be reduced. We tested this assumption by ventilating an infant test lung ($C = 1$ mL/cm) with a set tidal volume of 50 mL and an inspiratory time of one second while aspirating gas from the proximal airway using a sidestream CO_2 analyzer (Ohmeda Oxicap 4700).[87] We measured the affect of the insertion of this sidestream analyzer on the tidal volume and found that V_T decreased an average of $\approx 18\%$. This decrease is not surprising, since the Ohmeda device aspirates gas at 300 mL/min, even during inspiration. Since during the mechanical breath, the ventilator puts a fixed volume of gas into the circuit, any aspiration will reduce the delivered V_T. However, this decrease is easily compensated for by making an appropriate adjustment in the set V_T while the monitor is in use. The magnitude of this decrease was exaggerated by the very small set V_T used. As the set V_T increases, the sidestream analyzer's effect on delivered V_T will diminish. Also, the magnitude of the effect will be a function of the inspiratory time, with longer inspiratory times exaggerating the effect. A sidestream sampler can certainly be used with a pediatric application of a volume ventilator at small volumes, as long as care is taken to assure that the delivered V_T remains constant.

In theory, the use of sidestream sampling should have no effect on the delivered V_T in a continuous-flow, pressure-controlled ventilator. In neonatal applications the continuous flow output of such ventilators is customarily set between 4 to 14 L/min. Thus, during a mechanically delivered breath, the flow being delivered into the circuit is far in excess of both the peak flow rate of gas going through the endotracheal tube (typically 3 to 5 L/min in low birthweight infants) and the flow rate of gas being aspirated by the sidestream sampler (0.3 L/min) combined. In most such ventilators, the flow in excess of what is required to develop the desired pressure is vented from the circuit during inspiration. As the monitor aspirates gas, less excess gas will be vented from the circuit.

We tested the utility of sidestream exhaled CO_2 analysis in a neonatal population. In a series of 16 intubated patients we applied a combined sidestream CO_2 analyzer and pulse oximeter (Ohmeda 4700 Oxicap).[88] Weights ranged from 713 to 5110 g (mean 2338 g, SD = 1263 g). Simultaneous determinations of $Petco_2$ and $Paco_2$ were performed, and $Paco_2$ was compared before and after the monitor was applied to determine if, in fact, ventilation was affected by the monitor's aspiration rate. The mean difference between $Paco_2$ and $Petco_2$ was 7–8 mm Hg ($P = 0.0001$), with the $Petco_2$ always underestimating the $Paco_2$. Whether or not this magnitude of disagreement between these variables renders this monitor useful or not is a decision each clinician must make. We found the agreement between the $Petco_2$ and $Paco_2$ in some neonatal patients to be excellent. One is cautioned to assess this agreement by simultaneous determinations of $Petco_2$ and $Paco_2$ whenever possible when setting up the monitor. Even when agreement is poor, the device can be used to identify changes in ventilation (although the precise level of ventilation is sometimes not reliably demonstrated by the capnometer).

In this study,[88] the mean values for $Paco_2$ before and during the application of the capnometer were not significantly different (before = 39.6 mm Hg, during = 39.1 mm Hg, $P = 0.86$). During the study, no ventilator settings were changed. If the capnometer aspiration had reduced the patients' V_T (which we did not measure), then minute ventilation would have dropped because ventilator rate was unchanged. If minute ventilation had dropped, this would have been reflected in a rise in $Paco_2$. Thus it is reasonable to assume that the use of sidestream capnometry with an aspiration rate of 300 mL/min in this population had no effect on ventilation. In fact, we measured exhaled V_T on an infant lung model being ventilated with a pressure-limited ventilator, both before and during the aspiration of gas with the oxicap 4700 (Ohmeda Inc., Boulder, CO), and found no significant change in delivered V_T.

Some authors[77] have suggested that sidestream end-tidal CO_2 measurements are not as clinically useful as transcutaneous Pco_2 because they vary due to different ventilation-perfusion relationships in sick neonates. The investigators claim that capnometry does not currently appear to be of use in the routine monitoring of NICU patients because it seriously underestimates $Paco_2$. Unfortunately, they obtained 153 measurments from only 12 patients and then computed the correlation values to establish agreement. Correlation does not measure agreement, it measures instead association, and regression analysis is based on independent samples, not repeated samples on individual patients, thus the statistical analysis and hence the conclusions of the study may be invalid.[89] They also fail to discuss in detail the many practical problems associated with the use of transcutaneous CO_2 monitoring (remembraning, site burns, site rotation, frequent calibrations) that are not problems with the capnometer. It is not the purpose of this author to promote one technique over the other. However, it seems clear that the above-mentioned investigators drew broad conclusions that were unsupported by the study they conducted.

Patient Selection

Selecting patients who would benefit from continuous capnometry in the NICU remains somewhat intuitive. As with any intensive care population, patients with significant derangements of ventilation-perfusion will demonstrate poor agreement between $Paco_2$ and $Petco_2$.

There are, however, patients whom it would be reasonable to assume would be good candidates. Infants who are being mechanically ventilated but who do not have parenchymal lung disease (e.g., those with airway problems or central apnea) are good candidates. Of course, any patients in whom there is limited arterial vascular access might be considered for this technology, since it provides a noninvasive estimation of ventilation (when agreement is good). In my experience, it is difficult to predict reliably which patients will have good agreement.

No scientific evidence is available to support the broad application of capnometers on all or most mechanically ventilated NICU patients. However, there are clearly some patients who will have excellent agreement between $Paco_2$ and $Petco_2$ and thus would benefit from the application of this monitor.

TRANSCUTANEOUS GAS MONITORING

History

In the 1950s the discovery was made that by placing a finger in a beaker of heated phosphate buffer solution and then measuring the partial pressure of oxygen in the solution, it was possible to estimate accurately arterial oxygen tension through intact skin.[90] This discovery (and others) showed that the oxygen that diffuses through the skin could be measured under the proper hyperthermic and hyperemic conditions, and that the partial pressure of oxygen measured at the skin surface could closely approximate capillary and hence arterial Po_2s. In 1969 Huch, Huch and Lubbers[91] successfully measured skin Po_2 in newborns; hence was born the era of transcutaneous Po_2 monitoring of neonates. The development of transcutaneous Pco_2 electrodes closely followed those of Po_2 electrodes. Among the earliest reports of transcutaneous Pco_2 measurements were those of Severinghaus[92, 93] in 1960.

However, not until the late 1970s did these devices became commercially available. Some have speculated that their availability was delayed by the 1976 Amendment to the Federal Food, Drug, and Cosmetic Act.[94] This amendment required that medical devices be extensively evaluated for safety and effectiveness. In the early 1980s combined sensors that measure both Po_2 and Pco_2 transcutaneously became available.[95] Detailed discussions of the complex physiology surrounding the measurement of transcutaneous gases are found in the works of Huch and colleagues,[96] Cassidy,[97] Baumbach,[98] and Peabody and Emery.[99]

Indeed, in the early and mid-1980s it was not uncommon to find NICUs where most if not all mechanically ventilated patients were being continuously monitored with transcutaneous Po_2 and/or Pco_2 sensors. Many clinicians considered these devices invaluable, because they provided (when working) continuous monitoring of the patient's blood gases. This was thought to be an enormous advantage over intermittent blood gas sampling, because neonates tend to be very labile and can experience wide and potentially damaging swings in blood gases that might go undetected by intermittent blood gas sampling.[100]

Many also assumed that the use of these monitors would reduce the frequency of invasive blood gas sampling. Indeed, many managers and administrators were petitioned to purchase these instruments in part because they were told they would reduce blood gas laboratory operating costs. Alas, little investigation of this issue was ever done, and what *has* been published has been divergent. Indeed, Guilfoile[101] reported that at Children's Hospital in Cincinnati they did 0.98 hours of transcutaneous monitoring per patient day and 2.20 blood gases per patient day in 1981. By 1985, they were doing 3.94 hours of transcutaneous monitoring per patient day, while blood gas analyses per patient day remained essentially unchanged (2.08 per patient day). Conversely, Peevy and Hall[102] and Beachy and Whitfield[103] reported a reduction in the frequency of blood gas analyses attributable to the use of transcutaneous monitoring, while Kilbride and Merenstein[104] reported the opposite.

Scientific Data

The ability of the transcutaneous monitor to estimate reliably arterial blood gas levels in neonates under controlled conditions has been well documented (see Chapter 11: Transcutaneous Oxygen and Carbon Dioxide Measurements).[48, 104-123] However, arriving at a quantitative statement regarding the accuracy of transcutaneous monitors is somewhat difficult. Many of the published reports have used regression analyses with resultant correlation coefficients to describe the relationship between transcutaneous and arterial gas values. Unfortunately, this type of analysis is not always helpful, because data with poor agreement can yield fairly high correlation coefficients.[124]

In general, if perfusion is adequate, a properly operating transcutaneous Po_2 monitor, when used on a neonate, can reasonably be expected to yield results[125] that are within ± 10 mm Hg of the arterial Po_2. There are a number of exceptions to this statement which are discussed under limitations of the monitor.

The relationship between transcutaneous and arterial Pco_2 is more complicated and, in fact, transcutaneous Pco_2 is always higher than arterial Pco_2, for reasons that are beyond the scope of this discussion. Fortunately, this difference is fairly consistent and can be adjusted for in the calibration of the $Ptcco_2$ electrode.[126] Early models of $Ptcco_2$ monitors required the user to apply a correction factor to the readings the instrument produced. Newer models automatically correct for this adjustment during calibration. In clinical practice the $Ptcco_2$ monitors exhibit slightly better agreement with arterial values than do $Ptco_2$.

Limitations of Application

The basic principles that allow the transcutaneous monitors to work are hyperthermic-induced hyperemia and electrochemical measurement of the partial pressure of gases. Because of these, there are technical limitaions and inconveniences associated with the use of transcutaneous monitors. These are described in detail in Table 19–2, but can be summarized into two basic issues: (1) they are labor intensive, requiring frequent calibrations and site rotations and (2) they have the potential (not often realized in my experience) for burning the patient. Some of these disadvantages are offset by the device's ability to monitor active, moving infants without the degree of motion artifact that is so problematic with pulse oximeters. Other limitations include the potential for skin injury when monitoring very small premature infants. The adhesive disks that are used to affix the electrode to the patient can damage the very fragile skin of these patients, especially when superimposed on the heating of the skin incumbent with the use of these instruments.

The performance of transcutaneous monitors, especially Ptco$_2$, tends to deteriorate when applied to (1) patients with shock, (2) patients receiving tolazoline, (3) larger patients, (4) patients with considerable peripheral edema, and (5) patients with bronchopulmonary dysplasia.[110, 127–129]

Other limitations of transcutaneous Po$_2$ monitors include their deteriorating agreement with Po$_2$ under conditions of mild to moderate hyperoxemia.[121] When Po$_2$ exceeds 100 mm Hg, the Ptco$_2$ tends to underestimate the arterial Po$_2$ significantly. This, however, is also a significant liability of the pulse oximeter [e.g., its inability to identify varying magnitudes of hyperoxemia (Pao$_2$ 1100 mm Hg)].

Patient Selection

As previously stated, transcutaneous monitoring was nearly ubiquitous in some NICUs, only to be replaced by pulse oximetry. Some recommend monitoring both transcutaneous Po$_2$ and pulse oximetry.[21, 94] In some NICUs the decision about whether to use pulse oximetry or transcutaneous electrodes to monitor patients is reduced to the pragmatic simplicity of which device is available at the time monitoring is desired.

A growing trend (and one that seems reasonable) is the concomitant use of pulse oximetry and transcutaneous Pco$_2$ monitoring. This allows for both oxygenation and ventilation to be assessed noninvasively. Transcutaneous Po$_2$ monitoring continues to be very useful, especially in patients who are difficult to monitor with the pulse oximeter due to motion artifact.

Another useful application of the Ptco$_2$ monitors is the simultaneous estimation of pre- and postductal Pao$_2$. This is easily accomplished by placing one electrode on the patient's right upper thorax (preductal) and one on the patient's abdomen or left upper thorax (postductal). Differences in the Po$_2$ measured at these two sites (preductal being greater than postductal) can indicate significant right-to-left extrapulmonary cardiac shunting. This gradient can then be used to assess the efficacy of treatment of the shunting.[130] In fact, the existence of the transcutaneous monitor has helped to establish that significant right-to-left shunting at the level of the ductus arteriosis is rare in preterm infants with RDS.

Table 19–5 summarizes selection criteria for using transcutaneous monitors.

Temperature Selection for Electrodes

Because transcutaneous monitoring is based in part on an induced hyperemia, it is necessary to heat the skin under the electrode. But the selection of the best temperature for any given patient requires discriminating clinical judgment. Temperatures for P$_{tc}$o$_2$ electrodes have been reported[131] in the ranges of 42 to 45°C. The agreement between arterial and transcutaneous Po$_2$s is directly related to temperature, although this relationship is certainly not linear. As a rule of thumb, the higher the temperature used, the better the agreement. However, this must be balanced against skin damage from too much heat. Typical protocols in some NICUs recommend 42°C for infants weighing less than 1500 g and 43°C for infants weighing more than 1500 g.

TABLE 19–5.
Selection Criteria for
Transcutaneous Monitoring

$Ptco_2$
  Patients receiving supplemental oxygen
  Patients who have limited vascular access and
    have or are suspected of having respiratory
    insufficiency
  Patients who have a great deal of movement
    and activity
  Very labile patients in whom precise control of
    Pao_2 is desired
$Ptcco_2$
  Patients being mechanically ventilated
  Patients with dyspnea
  Patients with limited vascular access who have
    or are suspected of having respiratory
    insufficiency
  Patients with persistent pulmonary
    hypertension in whom hyperventilation is
    desired

Unlike $Ptco_2$ electrodes, good agreement can be obtained[132] with $Ptcco_2$ electrodes at 37°C. This is the result of carbon dioxide's greater diffusibility when compared to oxygen. However, agreement is even better when these electrodes are heated to ≈42°C. When combined O_2/CO_2 sensors are used, a temperature of 44°C has been recommended.[124]

The higher the temperature used, the more frequently the monitoring site needs to be rotated to avoid skin burns. Protocols vary from Q2 hour to Q6 hour schedules. It is advisable to check any site regardless of temperature within two hours of the initial application of the monitor or after any increase in electrode temperature.[133]

Transcutaneous Monitoring and Morbidity

For most forms of continuous monitoring, little if any investigations have been made into the ability of these monitors to affect respiratory morbidity. In the case of the transcutaneous monitor, the obvious question is whether or not the use of the transcutaneous monitor (or the pulse oximeter) can reduce one of the undesired side effects of oxygen administration to neonates, retinopathy of prematurity (ROP). Bancalari and colleagues[134] investigated this issue. They randomized patients to either have transcutaneous Po_2 monitoring or to be managed without it. They then looked at the incidence of retinopathy of prematurity in the two groups, stratified into different age groups. They found that under 1000 g there did not seem to be a difference in the incidence between the monitored and nonmonitored group. In the patients between 1000 and 1300 g, there was a significant reduction in the incidence of ROP. These findings seem to support the contention that in very low birthweight infants, ROP may not be preventable.

Whether or not these findings translate into a mandate to monitor all infants within certain weight groups at risk for ROP with transcutaneous monitors is unclear. It is, however, the only data in which the effect of such monitoring on neonatal morbidity has been studied.

CONTINUOUS MONITORING OF FIO_2

The measurement of the concentration of oxygen in inspired gases is practiced to some degree in nearly every NICU in North America, but there is considerable variation regarding exactly when, where, and how often these measurements should be made.

These instruments have enjoyed widespread utilization in the critical care environment for many years. Considering this, it is interesting to note that there are essentially no reports in the peer-reviewed medical literature describing the application and utility of oxygen analyzers.

In a survey[135] to which more than 320 hospitals providing specialized neonatal and pediatric care responded, it was discovered that 72% of all facilities reported measuring FIO_2 continuously in mechanical ventilator circuits, and 76% continuously in oxygen hoods (Table 19–6). This seems to indicate a *de facto* standard for the measurement of FIO_2 continuously in most, if not all, neonates receiving oxygen. Note, however, that nearly 25% of the facilities who provide specialized neonatal or pediatric care are not measuring FIO_2 continuously.

There are a number of types of oxygen analyzers: (1) physical analyzers, (2) electrical analyzers, (3) chemical analyzers, (4) electrochemical analyzers, and (5) mass spectrometry. The most widely used are the electrochemical types such as polarographic and galvanic cells.

Galvanic cells have proven to be very accurate and reliable. Most manufacturers report the accuracy of their analyzers at ±1 to 2% of full scale. This is a somewhat misleading statement. What these manufacturers are actually reporting is the *inaccuracy* of the instrument. The use of the word "accuracy" in the product literature is clearly a marketing decision.[136] To the practicing clinician, these numbers describe how much confidence can be placed in any given reading. A properly calibrated and functioning analyzer with a reported *inaccuracy* of ±2%

TABLE 19–6.
Survey Results of the Measurement of FIO_2 in 323 Neonatal Pediatric Facilities

	Measurement Site	
Measurement Frequency	In Ventilator Circuits (% of respondents)	In Oxygen Hoods (% of respondents)
Continuously	72%	76%
With ventilator checks	16%	—
Q1 hours	—	5%
Q2 hours	—	8%
Q4 hours	2%	8%
Q shift	—	3%
Not measured	2%	—

* From Salyer JW, Chatburn RL: *Respir Care* 1990; 35:879–888. Used by permission.

means that a reading of 80% implies that the true value may be as low as 78% and as high as 82%.[135]

Applying Oxygen Analyzers

As previously stated, decisions on how and when to apply any continuous monitor should be driven by a complete understanding of the *goals* of applying that particular monitor. In the case of oxygen analyzers, one of the most important considerations is the features of the analyzer, and whether or not these features will help to achieve the goals of the monitoring.

The most obvious goal of continuous oxygen concentration monitoring is to improve patient safety by ensuring the equipment used to deliver oxygen is functioning properly—but how to achieve this with an analyzer has some subtle distinctions.

Mechanical Ventilator Circuits

When applying analyzers to mechanical ventilators, the most widely accepted configuration for sensor placement is shown schematically in Figure 19–5, with the sensor being placed between the output of the ventilator and the input to the heat and humidification system. This kind of sensor placement avoids a number of problems that can affect the precision and accuracy of the analyzer. These include the effects of fluctuating temperature and high humidity. Fluctuating temperature (e.g., calibrating the sensor in the relative cool temperature of ambient gas and then placing in the warmed ventilator circuit) can adversely affect the galvanic cell, but this is avoided by analyzing the gas prior to it passing through the heated humidifier. A galvanic cell will generally give correct readings in any relative humidity. However, if it is

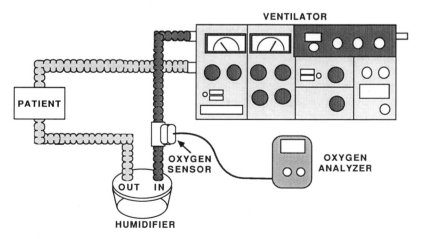

FIG 19–5.
Schematic of a typical oxygen analyzer placement in a ventilator circuit. Note that the sensor is placed in the gas stream before the gas has been humidified.

calibrated in a dry environment and then placed in gas with a high relative humidity, readings may be lower than expected.

Another problem with prolonged sensor exposure to humidified gas is that water tends to condense on the surface of the sensor, thereby restricting the diffusion of oxygen into the sensor to be measured, thus reducing measurement accuracy. If the sensor is calibrated in an ambient pressure environment and then placed in a positive pressure environment, there can be sightly higher than expected readings. This can be corrected by calibrating the sensor in the pressurized system. In practice, however, the effect of pressure is generally not enough to cause serious problems, and is simply accepted as an intrinsic part of the error in the measuring system.

Oxygen Hoods

When analyzing the oxygen concentration delivered by hoods, it is important to remember that the concentration of the gas delivered to the inlet of the hood may be significantly different than that inspired by the patient. Oxygen hoods are not airtight systems, and thus there is always some entrainment of the ambient gas to dilute the concentration of gas coming into the hood. A common mistake is to place an oxygen sensing probe in-line in the tubing delivering oxygen to the hood. This may serve to monitor the concentration of gas coming from the oxygen delivery device, but may say very little about what the patient is actually inspiring. A common practice in many NICUs is to place the oxygen sensor as close as practically possible to the patient's mouth, thus increasing the likelihood of measuring what the patient is actually inhaling.

If the gas being delivered to the hood is being heated and humidified, the same concerns about the effect of humidity and heat on the sensor are present when analyzing gas in the hood.

Alarms

If oxygen concentration is to be monitored continuously, it is recommended that the analyzer have both high and low alarms.[137] This makes intuitive sense if the goal of the monitoring is to avoid periods where the oxygen concentration is higher or lower than desired. Without audible alarms (that are properly set) such periods might go undetected, even by personnel at the immediate bedside if they are not looking directly at the analyzer display.

It is also recommended[137] that analyzers have alarms that cannot be disabled and that it not be possible to set the lower alarm limit below 18%. This last recommendation may need to be reconsidered in the near future. A new mode of oxygen therapy is emerging in some NICUs that has been termed *subambient oxygen therapy*. It is the intentional administration of levels of $F_{IO_2} < 0.21$ to patients who have ductal dependent cardiac defects. In these patients, pulmonary artery hypertension, and the resultant right-to-left shunting, is desired and must be maintained so that the patient can survive until the lesion can be corrected. If arterial oxygen levels are too high (approaching normal levels for other patients), pulmonary vascular resistance might decrease and the right-to-left shunting may diminish, thus placing the patient at increased risk, since somatic circulation in these patients is dependent entirely on shunting. Thus we have begun, on selected patients, to administer oxygen as low as an F_{IO_2} of 0.15 to 0.17. Clearly, oxygen analyzers as described above would not work for these patients.

Alarm limits should be set at ±2 to 3% of the desired F_{IO_2} level. Setting alarm ranges that are too narrow may result in analyzers alarming frequently when in fact the system is properly functioning. Oxygen analyzers will have some intrinsic "noise" in the readings (the most common cause being fluctuating pressure in the ventilator circuit). Alarms that are frequently a "nuisance" are generally ignored by the nursing and respiratory care staff, which is a good recipe for disaster.

Calibration

The calibration of oxygen analyzers is a fairly straightforward procedure and yet one that continues to be misunderstood by many practitioners. There are recommendations regarding the frequency of calibration of analyzers. These include the recommendation of the American Academy of Pediatrics (AAP) and the American College of Obstetrics and Gynecoloy (ACOG).[138] They recommend that neonates receiving supplemental oxygen have the oxygen concentration measured and recorded at least hourly, and that the oxygen analyzer be calibrated using both room air and 100% oxygen at least once every eight hours. This statement seems to imply that a galvanic oxygen analyzer can be "two-point calibrated." Many respiratory care practitioners continue to do what they believe is a "two-point calibration." A galvanic fuel cell type analyzer can be calibrated to either 100% oxygen or room air, but by its very nature cannot be "two-point calibrated." What clinicians can do is calibrate the device to 100% oxygen, and then expose it to room air and note that the readings should generally return to 21 ± 2%. If the readings do not return to these levels, it indicates that the cell is probably outside acceptable performance limits and should be replaced.

A practice in some NICUs is to calibrate the analyzer to 100% oxygen for those patients with a desired $F_{IO_2} > 0.50$, and to use room air for those with a desired $F_{IO_2} < 0.50$. This procedure seems sound because as a galvanic cell ages, it gradually loses its *linearity* (e.g., readings farthest from the calibration point begin to lose accuracy).[139] Thus, using calibration points closer to the levels the patient is receiving should improve accuracy.

NICUs wishing to follow manufacturers recommendations for calibrating oxygen analyzers will find some of these recommendations at odds with the AAP/ACOG recommendations. Some manufacturers recommend one-point calibration every 24 hours and a linearity check weekly,[140] while others[141] recommend a calibration only once every 1000 hours of operation, even though both devices use essentially identical cells. In such cases, it is probably advisable (from a risk-management point of view) to follow the AAP/ACOG recommendations.

The key to the successful use of oxygen analyzers (or any other monitoring device) is to train clinicians not only in the basic operation principles, but in the theoretical foundations of measurement science in general.[136]

AIRWAY PRESSURE MONITORING

All mechanical ventilators currently used in the United States incorporate some form of pressure monitoring device. These vary in complexity from simple mechanical pressure gauges to electronic pressure transducers interfaced with microprocessors that employ specialized software for monitoring a wide variety of pressure variables.

Nevertheless, there are many NICUs in which considerable money has been spent to purchase separate devices to monitor airway pressure. These are interfaced with the ventilator, usually in such a fashion as to allow for measuring pressure at the proximal airway. The variety in the ways these devices is applied is considerable. It is not uncommon to see a separate airway pressure monitor in use with a certain type of ventilator, only to travel down the street to another hospital and find the same ventilator employed without a seperate pressure monitor. The most immediate questions that arise are: (1) Why are these monitors used? (2) On whom should they be applied? (3) What is gained by using them?

Early and widely used airway pressure monitors included such features as displays of peak airway pressure (PiP), positive end-expiratory pressure (PEEP), mean airway pressure (MAP), airway temperature, and oxygen concentrations. Along with these displays, there are high and low alarms available for some of these parameters. A considerable number of such devices are now available with a wide variety of features.

How and when these devices should be applied or even what features such a monitor should have has not been defined in the literature. What few references there are to the practice of airway pressure monitoring[142-144] are nebulous. Most describe how such pressures are measured, and offer the clinician little help in making such decisions. There is, to my knowledge, no published literature describing the utility of such monitoring during mechanical ventilation in the neonatal or, for that matter, in any other population. And yet, clearly such monitors are widely used. It is reported that 67% of NICUs use auxillary continuous airway pressure monitors with time-cycled, pressure-controlled neonatal ventilators.[135]

Monitor Features

A single, comprehensive statement about what features an airway pressure monitor should have is not possible. It depends very much on with what kind of ventilator it will be used. Some ventilators have very sophisticated monitoring capabilities, coupled with excellent reliability, and the use of such a device in those cases would represent useless redundancy. The Infrasonics Infant Star (Infrasonics Inc, San Diego, CA) monitors both machine and patient pressures and uses a sophisticated software package to identify and alert the clinician to a wide variety of potentially undesirable pressure conditions. It is therefore unnecessary to employ a separate pressure monitor with the Star.

Some ventilators, in fact, are incompatible with auxiliary pressure monitors. The Bunnell Life-Pulse Jet ventilator (Bunnell Inc., Salt Lake City, UT) will not function properly if additional airway pressure monitoring lines are placed in-line with the airway pressure line of the triple lumen endotracheal tube. Also, the Bear Cub ventilator (Bear Inc., Riverside, CA) has long been known to be incompatible with the Pneumogard airway pressure monitor (Novametrix Inc., Wallingord, CT).[145]

Instead of attemping to describe the characteristics of an ideal airway pressure monitor, it is more useful to define what should be continuously monitored with mechanically ventilated patients. Table 19–7 defines these variables and describes the concommitant alarm requirements.

Peak inspiratory pressure should clearly be monitored continuously on all ventilated patients, and this is done by all ventilators intrinsically. But this may not be sufficient. Table 19–8 describes the relationship between proximal airway pressures displayed on the aneroid manometer on the front of a series of infant ventilators, the same pressure when measured by stand-alone airway pressure monitors, and the actual proximal airway pressures. These data were gathered while five time-cycled, pressure-controlled ventilators were in operation in an NICU. It was done at the request of the nursing staff, who asked the penetrating question: "Which pressure is more accurate, the one on the ventilator, or the one on the airway pressure monitor?" Clearly, the ventilator manometer was insufficiently accurate even though all of the ventilators tested had undergone the manufacturers' recommended six-month preventive maintenance procedures.

SUMMARY

Clearly, the setup and operation of noninvasive respiratory monitors currently constitute a considerable portion of the duties of neonatal respiratory care practitioners. The most demanding aspect of operating these devices is deciding who really needs them, and then critically evaluating the data received from them. What is not as clear is which patients will benefit the most from the different monitors.

TABLE 19–7.
Minimal Ventilatory Monitoring Standards for Patients Being Mechanically Ventilated with Pressure-controlled, Time-cycled Ventilators

Variable to be Continuously Monitored	Are Low Alarms Required?	Are High Alarms Required?
PiP	no	yes
PEEP	yes	yes
MAP	no	no
FiO$_2$	yes	yes
SpO$_2$/PtcO$_2$	yes	yes
PtcCO$_2$*	yes	yes
Airway temperature	yes	yes

* PtcCO$_2$ monitoring would only be considered as a minimal standard in patients who did not have vascular access for arterial blood gas sampling.

TABLE 19–8.
Comparison of Various Peak Airway Pressures on a Series
of Five Pressure-controlled, Neonatal Ventilators (all the
same brand)

Ventilator Number	PiP on Ventilator Manometer	PiP on Pressure Monitor*	Actual PiP†
1	8	14	14
2	6	18	18
3	9	11	11
4	16	22	23
5	14	18	19

* Peak inspiratory pressure as measured at the proximal airway by a stand-alone airway pressure monitor (Pneumogard 1230 A, Novametrix).
† Peak inspiratory pressure as measured at the proximal airway by the "standard" used by the hospital biomedical engineering department, the Timeter RT 200 calibration analyzer (Timeter Inc.).

Some *de facto* standards have developed that include (1) continuous monitoring with pulse oximetry for mechanically ventilated neonates, (2) continuous monitoring of FIO_2 (with high and low alarms) in all neonatal ventilator circuits and all oxygen hood setups, and (3) continuous monitoring (with high and low alarms) of PiP, PEEP, and MAP on all mechanically ventilated neonates.

Whether any of these *standards* have any real impact on patient saftey or respiratory morbidity and mortality has not been established and probably never will be tested because of the litigious environment in which critical care medicine is now practiced.

We can, however, learn from our experience. Let us hope that as new monitoring technologies become available, we rigorously investigate their utility before we commit enormous resources to procure them. There is now sufficient evidence to assure us that the physiologic variables described in this chapter can be measured with an acceptable degree of reliability under many conditions. However, there remains the unanswered question, *have these monitors made any real difference?*

REFERENCES

1. Korones SB: High-risk Newborn Infants: The basis for Intensive Nursing Care, ed 4. St Louis, CV Mosby, 1986; pp 265–268.
2. Korones SB: Complications, in Goldsmith JP, Karotkin EH (eds): *Assisted Ventilation of the Neonate*, ed 2. Philadelphia, WB Saunders, 1989, pp 245–271.
3. Martin RJ, Fanaroff AA: Complications of neonatal respiratory care, in Carlo W, Chatmar RL (eds): *Neonatal Respiratory Care*, ed 2. Chicago, Yearbook Medical Publishers, 1988, pp 347–364.
4. Burgess WR, Chernick V: *Respiratory Therapy in Newborn Infants and Children*, ed 2. New York, Thieme, 1986, pp 274–281.
5. Aloan CA: *Respiratory Care of the Newborn: A Clinical Manual*. Philadelphia, JB Lippincott, 1987, pp 65–66.

6. Berlin SL, et al: Pulse oximetry: A technology that needs direction. *Resp Care* 1988; 33:243–244.

7. Koop CE: The health care mess. *Newsweek* Aug 28, 1989; p 10.

8. Chatburn RL: Metrology; the science of measurement. *Respir Care* 1990; 35:520–545.

9. Chatburn RL, Lough MD: *Handbook of Respiratory Care*, ed 2. Chicago, Yearbook Medical, 1990, p 353.

10. Kelleher JF: Pulse oximetry. *J Clin Monit* 1989; 5:37–62.

11. Severinghaus JW, Astrup P: *The History of Blood Gases, Acids and Bases*. Copenhagen, Munksgaard, 1986.

12. Peabody JL: Historical perspective of noninvasive monitoring. *J Perinatol* 1987; 7:306–308.

13. Pologe JA: Pulse oximetry: Technical aspects of machine design, in *Advances in Oxygen Monitoring*. Boston, Little, Brown, and Co, 1987; 25;1–20.

14. Finnerup E, Miller MA: Understanding pulse oximetry measurements. Cleveland, Radiometer Copenhagen, 1987.

15. Wukitsch MW, Petterson MT, Tobler DR, et al: Pulse oximetry: Analysis of theory, technology, and practice. *J Clin Monit* 1988; 4:290–301.

16. Yoshiya I, Shimada Y, Tanaka K: Spectrophotometric monitoring of arterial oxygen saturation in the fingertip. *Med Biol Eng Comput* 1980; 18:27–32.

17. Cecil WT, Petterson MT, Lamoonpun S, et al: Clinical evaluation of the Biox II A ear oximeter in the critical care environment. *Respir Care* 1985; 30:179–183.

18. Chapman KR, D'Urso B, Rebuck AS: The accuracy and response of a simplified ear oximeter. *Chest* 1983; 83:860–864.

19. Salyer JW: Pulse oximetry in the neonatal intensive care unit (editorial). *Respir Care* 1991; 36:17–22.

20. Severinghaus JW, Astrup PB: History of blood gas analysis: VI. pulse oximetry. *J Clin Monit* 1986; 2:270–288.

21. Dear PRF: Monitoring oxygen in the newborn: Saturation or partial pressure? *Arch Dis Child* 1987; 62:879–881.

22. Smith NT: Pulse oximetry versus measurement of transcutaneous oxygen (editorial). *J Clin Monit* 1985; 1:126.

23. New W: Pulse oximetry. *J Clin Monit* 1985; 1:126–129.

24. Shapiro BA, Harrison RA, Cane RD, et al: *Clinical Application of Blood Gases*, ed 4. Chicago, Yearbook Medical Publishers, 1989, p 229.

25. Craig KC: Clinical application of pulse oximetry, in *Problems in Respiratory Care: Applied Noninvasive Respiratory Monitoring*. Philadelphia, JB Lippincott, 1989; vol 2, pp 255–273.

26. Severinhaus JW, Naifeh KH, Koh SO: Errors in 14 pulse oximeters during profound hyposia. *J Clin Monit* 1989; 5:72–81.

27. Tremper KK, Barker SJ: Pulse oximetry. *Anesthesiol* 1989; 70:98–108.

28. Yeldermen M, New W: Evaluation of pulse oximetry. *Anesthesiol* 1983; 59:349–352.

29. Chapman KR, Liu FLW, Watson RM, et al: Range of accuracy of two wavelength oximetry. *Chest* 1986; 4:540–542.

30. Kagle DM, Alexander CM, Berko RS, et al: Evaluation of the Ohmeda 3700 pulse oximeter: Steady state and transient response characteristics. *Anesthesiol* 1987; 66:376–380.

31. Jennis MS, Peabody JL: Pulse oximetry: An alternative method for the assessment of oxygenation in newborn infants. *Pediatrics* 1987; 79:524–528.

32. Hay WW, Brockway JM, Eyzaguirre M: Neonatal pulse oximetry: Accuracy and reliability. *Pediatrics* 1989; 83:717–722.

33. Fanconi S. Reliability of pulse oximetry in hypoxic infants. *J Pediatr* 1988; 112:424–427.

34. Solimano AJ, Smyth JA, Mann TK, et al: Pulse oximetry advantages in infants with bronchopulmonary dysplasia. *Pediatrics* 1986; 78:798–803.

35. Deckardt R, Steward DJ: Noninvasive arterial hemoglobin oxygen saturation versus transcutaneous oxygen tension monitoring in the preterm infant. *Crit Care Med* 1984; 12:935–939.
36. Wilkinson AR, Phibbs RH, Heilbron DC, et al: In vivo oxygen dissociation curves in transfused and untransfused newborns with cardiopulmonary disease. *Am Rev Respir Dis* 1980; 122:629–634.
37. Southall DP, Bignall S, Stebbens VA, et al: Pulse oximeter and transcutaneous arterial oxygen measurements in neonatal and paeditric intensive care. *Arch Dis Child* 1987; 62:882–888.
38. Tzong JW, Bautista A, Ko SH et al: Pulse oximetry-its reliability in predicting arterial oxygenation (abstract). *Pediatr Res* 1987; 1:208A.
39. Ramanathan R, Durand M, Larrazabal C: Pulse oximetry in very low birth weight infants with acute and chronic lung disease. *Pediatrics* 1987; 79:612–617.
40. Walsh MC, Noble LM, Carlo WA, et al: Relationship of pulse oximetry to arterial oxygen tension in infants. *Crit Care Med* 1987; 15:1102–1105.
41. Praud JP, Carofilis A, Bridey F, et al: Accuracy of two wavelength pulse oximetry in neonates and infants. *Pediatr Pulm* 1989; 6:180–182.
42. Anderson JV: The accuracy of pulse oximetry in neonates: Effects of fetal hemoglobin and bilirubin. *J Perinatol* 1987; 7:323.
43. Pologe JA, Raley DM: Effects of fetal hemoglobin on pulse oximetry. *J Perinatol* 1987; 7:324–326.
44. Emery JR: Skin pigmentation as an influence on the accuracy of pulse oximetry. *J Perinatol* 1987; 7:329–330.
45. Cunningham MD, Shook LA, Tomazic T: Clinical experience with pulse oximetry in managing oxygen therapy in neonatal intensive care. *J Perinatol* 1987; 7:333–335.
46. Kopotic RJ, Mannino FL, Colley CD, et al: Display variability, false alarms, probe cautions, and recorder use in neonatal pulse oximetry. *J Perinatol* 1987; 7:340–342.
47. Durand M, Ramanathan R: Pulse oximetry for continuous oxygen monitoring in sick newborn infants. *J Pediatr* 1986; 109:1052–1056.
48. Mok J, Pintar M, Benson L, et al: Evaluation of noninvasive measurements of oxygenation in stable infants. *Crit Care Med* 1986; 14:960–963.
49. Lafeber HN: Reliability of transcutaneous oxygen tension and pulse oximetry in normocemic and hypoxemic newborns, in *Proceedings of the Third International Conference on Cutaneous Transcutaneous Monitoring*, Zurich, Switzerland, October 1–4, 1986.
50. Baeckert P, Bucher HU, Fallenstein F, et al: Is pulse oximetry reliable in detecting hyperoxemia?, in *Proceedings of the Third International Conference on Cutaneous Transcutaneous Monitoring*, Zurich, Switzerland, October 1–4, 1986.
51. Hodgson A, Horbar J, Sharp G, et al: The accuracy of the pulse oximeter in neonates, in *Proceedings of the Third International Conference on Cutaneous Transcutaneous Monitoring*, Zurich, Switzerland, October 1–4, 1986.
52. Fait CD, Wetzel RC, Dean JM, et al: Pulse oximetry in critically ill children. *J Clin Monit* 1985; 1:232–235.
53. Barrington KJ, Finer NN, Ryan CA: Evaluation of pulse oximetry as a continuous monitoring technique in the neonatal intensive care unit. *Crit Care Med* 1988; 16:1147.
54. Ryan CA, Barrington KJ, Vaughan D, et al: Directly measured arterial oxygen saturation in the newborn infant. *J Pediatr* 1986; 109:526.
55. Blanchette T, Dziodzio J, Harris K: Pulse oximetry and normoxemia in neonatal intensive care. *Respir Care* 1991; 36:25–31.
56. Boxer RA, Gottesfeld I, Singh S, et al: Noninvasive pulse oximetry in children with cyanotic congenital heart disease. *Crit Care Med* 1987; 15:1062–1064.
57. Stern L: in Thibeault DW, Gregory GA (eds): *Neonatal Pulmonary Care*, ed 2. Norwalk, Appleton-Century-Crofts, 1986; p 373.

58. Duc G, In Klaus MH, Fanaroff AA (eds): *Care of the High Risk Neonate*, ed 3. Philadelphia, WB Saunders, 1986; p 177.

59. Tobin MJ: Respiratory monitoring in the intensive care unit. *Am Rev Respir Dis* 1988; 138:1625–1642.

60. Wiswell TE: Pulse oximetry versus transcutaneous oxygen monitoring in perinatology applications. *J Perinatol* 1987; 7:331–332.

61. Uhing M, Dziedzic K: Pulse oximetry in neonatal management. *Respir Manage* 1990; 20:116–120.

62. Reynolds G, Yu V: Guidelines for the use of pulse oximetry in the noninvasive estimation of oxygen saturation in oxygen dependent newborn infants. *Aust Paediatr J* 1988; 24:346–350.

63. Dziedzic K, Vidyasagar D: Pulse oximetry in neonatal intensive care. *Clin Perinatol* 1989; 16:177–197.

64. Harbold LA: A protocol for neonatal use of pulse oximetry. *Neonat Network* 1989; 8:41–57.

65. Hay WW: Physiology of oxygenation and its relation to pulse oximetry in neonates. *J Perinatol* 1987; 7:309–319.

66. Hicks GH, Jung RC: Monitoring respiratory gases, in: *Problems in Respiratory Care: Applied Noninvasive Respiratory Monitoring.* Philadelphia, JB Lippincott, 1989, vol 2, p 216.

67. Shapiro BA, Cane RD: Blood gas monitoring: Yesterday, today, and tomorrow. *Crit Care Med* 1989; 17:573.

68. Luft K: Uber einie neue Methode der registrierenden gasanalyse mit hilfe der absorbition ultraroter strahlen ohne spektrale zerlegung. *Ztschr f Techn Phys* 1943; 24:97.

69. Fowler RC: A rapid infra-red gas analyzer. *Rev Sci Instrum* 1949; 20:175.

70. Pilbeam SP: *Mechanical Ventilation: Physiological and Clinical Applications.* St Louis, CV Mosby/Multi-Media, 1986, p 187.

71. Takki S, Aromaa U, Kauste A: The validity and usefulness of the end-tidal PCO_2 during anesthesia. *Ann Clin Res* 1972; 4:278.

72. Whitesell R, Asiddao C, Gollman D, et al: Relationship between arterial and peak expired carbon dioxide pressure during anesthesia and factors influencing the difference. *Anesth Analg* 1981; 60:508.

73. Mackersie RC, Karagianes TG, York J, et al: End-tidal PCO_2 monitoring during resuscitation of severe head injuries (abstract). *Crit Care Med* 1989; 17:S45.

74. Pascucci RC, Schena JA, Thompson JE: Comparison of a sidestream and mainstream capnometer in infants. *Crit Care Med* 1989; 17:560–562.

75. Badgwell JM, McLeod ME, Creighton RE: End-tidal PCO_2 measurement sampled at the distal and proximal ends of the endotracheal tube in infants and children. *Anesth Analg* 1987; 66:959.

76. Bissonnette B, Lerman J: Single breath end-tidal CO_2 estimates of arterial PCO_2 in infants and children. *Can J Anaesth* 1989; 36:110.

77. Hand IL, Shepard EK, Krauss AN, et al: Discrepancies between transcutaneous and end-tidal carbon dioxide monitoring in the critically ill neonate with respiratory distress syndrome. *Crit Care Med* 1989; 17:556.

78. Badgwell JM, Heavner JE, May WS, et al: End-tidal PCO_2 monitoring in infants and children ventilated with either a partial rebreathing or a non-rebreathing circuit. *Anesthesiol* 1987; 66:405.

79. Nuzzo PF: Capnometry in infants and children. *Perinat Neonat* 1978; 2(May/Jun): 30–31.

80. From RP, Scamman FL: Ventilatory frequency influences accuracy of end-tidal CO_2 measurements: Analysis of seven capnometers. *Anesth Analg* 1988; 67:884–886.

81. McPhearson SP: *Respiratory Therapy Equipment*, ed 4. St Louis, CV Mosby, 1990, p 145.

82. Epstein RA, Reznik AM, Epstein MAF: Determinants of distortions in CO_2 catheter sampling systems: A mathematical model. *Respir Physiol* 1980; 41:127.

83. Rich GF, Sconzo JM: Continuous end-tidal CO_2 sampling within the proximal endotracheal tube estimates arterial CO_2 tension in infants. *Can J Anaesth* 1991; 38:201–203.

84. Scamman FL: Accuracy of a central mass spectrometer system as high respiratory frequencies (abstract). *Anesthesiol* 1986; 65:A136.

85. Scamman FL, Fishbaugh JK: Frequency response of long mass-spectrometer sampling catheters. *Anesthesiol* 1986; 65:422.

86. ECRI: Evaluation: Carbon dioxide monitors. *Health Dev* 1986; 15:255–285.

87. Salyer JW, Henry W, Christie H: The effect of Oxicap 4700 endi-tidal CO2 analyzer sampling rate on tidal volume delivered by a volume ventilator to an infant lung model (abstract). *Respir Care* 1990; 35:1121.

88. Salyer JW, Rogers M, Myers T: An evaluation of the accuracy of the Ohmeda Oxicap 4700 in a neonatal population (abstract). *Respir Care* 1990; 35:1128–1129.

89. Altman DG, Bland JM: Measurement in medicine: The analysis of method comparison studies. *Statistician* 1983; 32:307–317.

90. Baumberger JP, Goodfrien RB: Determination of arterial oxygen tension in man by equilibration through intact skin. *Fed Proc Fed Am Soc Exper Biol* 1951; 10:10.

91. Huch A, Huch R, Lubbers DW: Quantitative polarographische Sauerstoffdruckmessung auf der Kopfhaut des Neugeborenen. *Arch Gynakol* 1969; 207:443–451.

92. Severinghaus JW: Spannung und Perfusion in Gewebe. *Anaesthetist* 1960; 9:50.

93. Severinghaus JW: Methods of measurement of blood and gas carbon dioxide during anesthesia. *Anesthesiol* 1960; 21:717.

94. Harris K: Noninvasive monitoring of gas exchange. *Respir Care* 1987; 32:544–555.

95. Beran AV, Huxtable RF, Black KS, et al: Investigation of transcutaneous O2-CO2 sensors and their application in human adults and newborns. *Birth Defects: Original Articles Series* 1979; 15:421.

96. Huch R, Huch A, Lubbers DW: *Transcutaneous PO2.* New York, Thieme-Stratton Inc, 1981.

97. Cassidy G: Transcutaneous monitoring in the newborn infant. *J Pediatr* 1983; 103:837–848.

98. Baumbach P: Understanding transcutaneous PO2 and PCO2 measurements. *Radiometer Copenhagen* 1986; TC 100.

99. Peabody JL, Emery JR: Noninvasive monitoring of blood gases in the newborn, in Peabody JL, Emery JR (eds): *Clinics in Perinatology*, 1985; 12:147–160.

100. Lucy JF, Peabody JL, Philip AGS: Recurrent undetected hypoxia and hyperoxia, a newly recognized iatrogenic problem of "intensive care" (abstract). *Pediatr Res* 1977; 11:537.

101. Guilfoile TD: Bedside monitoring of the acutely ill neonate: The impact of transcutaneous monitoring on neonatal intensive care. *Respir Care* 1986; 31:507–512.

102. Peevy KJ, Hall MW: Transcutaneous oxygen monitoring; economic impact on neonatal care. *Pediatrics* 1985; 75:1065–1067.

103. Beachy P, Whitfield JM: The effect of transcutaneous PO2 monitoring on the frequency of arterial blood gas analysis in the newborn with respiratory disease. *Crit Care Med* 1981; 9:584–586.

104. Kilbride HW, Merenstein GB: Continuous transcutaneous oxygen monitoring in acutely ill preterm infants. *Crit Care Med* 1984; 12:121–124.

105. Huch R, Lubbers DW, Huch A: Quantitative continuous measurement of parital oxygen pressure on the skin of adults and newborn babies. *Pfluegers Arch* 1972; 337:185.

106. Hansen TN, Tooley WH: Skin surface carbon dioxide tension in sick infants. *Pediatrics* 1979; 64:942–945.

107. Cabal LA, Hodgman J, Siassi B, et al: Factors affecting heated transcutaneous PO2 and unheated transcutaneous PCO2 in preterm infants. *Crit Care Med* 1981; 9:298–304.

108. Yahav J, Mindorff C, Levison J: The validity of the transcutaneous oxygen tension method in infants and children with cardiorespiratory problems. *Am Rev Respir Dis* 1981; 124:586–587.

109. Fenner A, Muller R, Busse HG, et al: Transcutaneous determination of arterial oxygen tension. *Pediatrics* 1975; 55:224.

110. Huch R, Hutch A, Alboni M, et al: Transcutaneous PO2 monitoring in routine management of infants and children with cardiorespiratory problems. *Pediatrics* 1976; 57:681.

111. Peabody JL, Gregory GA, Willis MM: Transcutaneous oxygen tension in sick infants. *Am Rev Respir Dis* 1978; 118:83–85.

112. Rohe MI, Weinberg G: Transcutaneous oxygen monitoring in shock and resuscitation. *J Pediatr Surg* 1979; 14:773–775.

113. Eickhoff JH, Wimberly PD: The influence of changes in arterial blood pressure on transcutaneous oxygen tension in the newborn. *Acta Paediatr Scand* 1982; 365–368.

114. LeSouef PN, Soutter LP, Reynolds EOR: Comparison of transcutaneous and arterial oxygen tension during prolonged continuous monitoring of infants with respiratory illnesses. *Pediatr Res* 1977; 11:1029–1031.

115. Riegel KP, Versmold HT: Intra-arterial versus transcutaneous PO2 monitoring in newborn infants. *Biotelem Pat Mon* 1979; 6:32–43.

116. Huch R, Lubbers DW, Huch A: Reliability of transcutaneous monitoring of arterial PO2 in newborn infants. *Arch Dis Child* 1974; 49:213–218.

117. Swanstrom S, et al: Transcutaneous PO2 measurements in seriously ill newborn infants. *Arch Dis Child* 1975; 50:913–919.

118. Lofgren O, Anderson D: Simultaneous transcutaneous carbon dioxide and transcutaneous oxygen monitoring in neonatal intensive care. *J Perinat Med* 1983: 11;1983.

119. Wimberley PD, Friis-Hansen B: The use of TC-PO2 monitoring in neonatal intensiv care. *Danish Med Bull* 1981; 28:37–40.

120. Bucher HU, Fanconi S, Fallenstein F, et al: Transcutaneous carbon dioxide tension in newborn infants: Reliability and safety of continuous 24 hour measurement at 42° C. *Pediatrics* 1986; 78:631–635.

121. Martin RJ, Robertson SS, Hopple MM: Relationship between transcutaneous and arterial oxygen tension in sick neonates during mild hyperoxemia. *Crit Care Med* 1982; 10:670–672.

122. Herrell N, Martin RJ, Pultusker M, et al: Optimal temperature for the measurement of transcutaneous carbon dioxide tension in sick infants. *J Pediatr* 1980; 97:114–117.

123. Brustler I, Enders A, Versmold HT: Skin surface PCO2 monitoring in newborn infants in shock: Effects of hypotension and electrode temperature. *J Pediatr* 1982; 100:454–457.

124. Martin RJ: Transcutaneous monitoring: Instrumentation and clinical applications. *Respir Care* 1990; 35:577–583.

125. Phillips BL, McQuitty J, Durand DJ: Blood gases: Technical aspects and interpretation, in Goldsmith JP, Karotkin EH (eds): *Assisted Ventilation of the Neonate*, ed 2. Philadelphia, WB Saunders, 1988; pp 221–222.

126. Monaco R, McQuitty JC, Nickerson BG: Calibration of a heated transcutaneous carbon dioxide electrode to reflect arterial carbon dioxide. *Am Rev Respir Dis* 1983; 127:322–324.

127. Paxson CL, Clayton BR: Effect of parenteral medication on tcPO2/PaO2 ratios. *J Pediatr* 1984; 104:426–428.

128. Rome ES, Stork EK, Carlo WA et al: Limitations of transcutaneous PO2 and PCO2 in infants with bronchopulmonary dysplasia. *Pediatrics* 1984; 74:217–220.

129. Hamilton PA, Whitehead MD, Reynolds EOR: Underestimation of arterial oxygen tension by transcutaneous electrode with increasing age in infants. *Arch Dis Child* 1985; 60:1162–1165.

130. Pearlman SA, Maisels MJ: Preductal and postductal transcutaneous oxygen tension measurements in newborns with hyaline membrane disease. *Pediatrics* 1989; 83:98–100.

131. Rooth G, Huch A, Huch R: Commentaries: Transcutaneous oxygen monitors are reliable indicators of arterial oxygen tension (if used correctly). *Pediatrics* 1987; 79:283–286.

132. American Academy of Pediatrics. Task force on transcutaneous oxygen monitors. Report of consensus meeting. *Pediatrics* 1989; 83:122–126.

133. Taylor W: Transcutaneous and transconjunctival blood gas monitoring, in Hicks GH (ed): *Problems*

in Respiratory Care: Applied Noninvasive Respiratory Monitoring. Philadelphia, JB Lippincott, 1989; Vol 2, pp 240–254.

134. Bancalari E, Flynn J, Goldberg RN, et al: Influence of transcutaneous oxygen monitoring on the incidence of retinopathy of prematurity. *Pediatrics* 1987; 79:663–669.

135. Salyer JW, Chatburn RL: Patterns of practice in neonatal and pediatric respiratory care. *Respir Care* 1990; 35:879–888.

136. Chatburn RL: Fundamentals of metrology: Evaluation of instrument error and method agreement. *Respir Care* 1990; 35:520–545.

137. ECRI: Oxygen analyzers for breathing circuits. *Health Dev* 1983; 12:183–197.

138. Frigoletto FD, Little GA, Freeman RK, et al: *Guidelines for Perinatal Care*, ed 2. American Academy of Pediatrics, American College of Obstetrics and Gynecologists, 1988; pp 244–248.

139. Operating manual for updated galvanic oxygen analyzers, Ventronics Inc, 1981.

140. Operating manual for Mini-Ox II. Catalyst Research Corporation.

141. Servo 900C operating manual. Siemenes-Elema Inc.

142. Fallat RJ, Osborn JJ: Patient monitoring techniques, in Burton GC, Hodgkin JE (eds): Respiratory Care: A Guide to Clinical Practice, ed 2. Philadelphia, JB Lippincott, 1984; pp 940–954.

143. Day S, MacIntyre NR: Ventilator alarms systems, in Fulkerson WJ, MacIntyre NR (eds): *Problems in Respiratory Care: Complications of Mechanical Ventilation*, Philadelphia, JB Lippincott, 1991; Vol 4, pp 118–126.

144. Wilkins R, Hicks GH: Gas volume, flow, pressure and temperature monitoring, in Hicks GH (ed): *Problems in Respiratory Care: Applied Noninvasive Respiratory Monitoring.* Philadelphia, JB Lippincott, 1989; Vol 2, pp 126–155.

145. ECRI. Hazard alert: Ventilation monitor/ventilator incompatibility. *Health Dev* 1982; 328–329.

Chapter 20 _____

Monitoring in Pediatric Care

Daniel P. Brutocao, M.D.

P. Pearl O'Rourke, M.D.

INTRODUCTION

Methods of monitoring the cardiac and respiratory function of the pediatric patient must encompass a wide range of ages, sizes, developmental physiology, and diseases. Many of the routine monitoring techniques used for adults can be difficult to use and/or inappropriate for the child. This chapter will discuss the application of current respiratory and cardiac monitoring techniques to the spectrum of pediatric illness.

An understanding of the profound anatomic and physiologic differences between the neonate, toddler, adolescent, and adult is essential to the discussion of respiratory monitoring. The neonate is not born with a small but fully developed adult lung; rather, he is born early on the continuum of pulmonary maturation. The first part of this chapter discusses some of these developmental changes and the impact they have on the pulmonary system in health and in disease.

ANATOMY AND PHYSIOLOGY

The neonatal and infant pulmonary system is characterized by a poorly compliant lung within a very compliant thorax, resulting in a tendency toward lung collapse. This effectively decreases functional residual capacity (FRC), thereby reducing the margin of safety for adequate oxygenation. Activity and crying in the normal baby serve to routinely reestablish FRC (Fig 20–1). The decreased lung compliance reflects alveolar as well as airway immaturity. Gestational airway development is complete by 16 weeks, but the airway caliber is very small, increasing proportionately with lung growth.[1] Young infants are therefore more vulnerable to airway diseases with associated edema and/or infection (Fig 20–2). The infant's lung is also character-

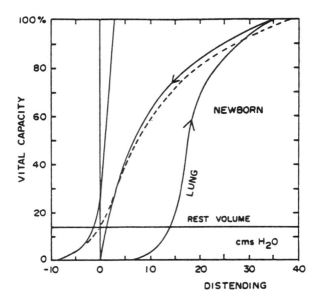

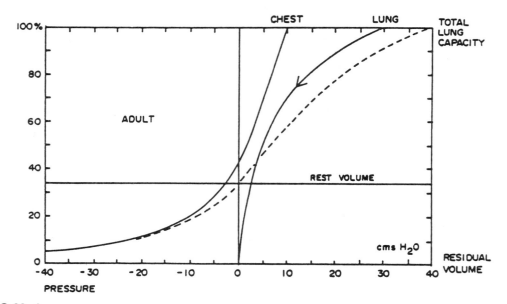

FIG 20–1.
Pressure-volume curves for newborn and adult. Total respiratory system represented by dashed line. Note tendency toward lung collapse as shown by decreased FRC (resting volume) in newborn. (*From Smith CA, Nelson NM: The Physiology of the Newborn Infant. ed 4. Springfield, Charles C Thomas, p 205. Used by permission.*)

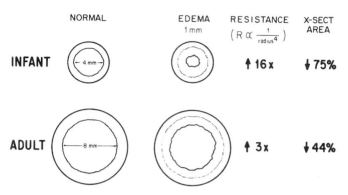

FIG 20–2.
Effect of 1-mm airway edema shown in infant and adult. Greater increased resistance to air flow make infants more vulnerable to diseases associated with airway edema (*From Ryan JF, Todres ID, Cote CJ, et al:* A Practice of Anesthesia for Infants and Children. *Philadelphia, WB Saunders Co, 1986. Used by permission.*)

ized by a decreased amount of elastin. Not only does elastin contribute to lung compliance, it also provides tone to the small airway. The proportion of elastin increases slowly with lung growth, peaking in adolescence.[2] The infant and small child are therefore more prone than the adult to airway collapse at relatively large closing volumes. At birth the full-term neonate has mature, as well as immature, thick-walled alveoli. After birth, alveoli continue to develop and increase in number at the rate of one per second until eight years of age, at which point adult numbers are reached.[3] Subsequent lung growth then occurs by increase in alveolar size.[4]

In contrast to this relatively stiff lung, the child's thorac is very compliant. One of the main reasons is the presence of cartilagenous, rather than bony ribs, which have a mechanical disadvantage with a more horizontal arrangement than in adults. Additionally the child has relatively decreased intercostal and diaphragmatic muscle strength.[5]

The child's upper airway is different from that of the adult, having a more cephalad and anteriorly placed larynx (Fig 20–3). Patency of the airway is therefore better maintained with the head in the sniffing position, as opposed to hyperextension in the adult. The narrowest part of the adult airway is at the vocal cords, while the child's airway is narrowest at the level of the cricoid cartilage, which is a subglottic location. It is therefore not uncommon to be able to place an endotracheal tube through the larynx, yet be unable to advance it further into the airway. In addition, the relative subglottic narrowing produces a good seal around the endotracheal tube in children under six to seven years of age, obviating the need for cuffed endotracheal tubes.

Other physiologic characteristics of the child affect the respiratory system, such as a higher metabolic rate, resulting in an increased indexed oxygen consumption. Also, in the first months of life, a normal physiologic anemia diminishes the oxygen-carrying capacity.

The differences are significant in the diseases that affect children and adults. In general, the child is more likely to have single-organ system failure rather than the multiple-organ system failure (MOSF) seen in the adult. Congenital anomalies usually present clinically in

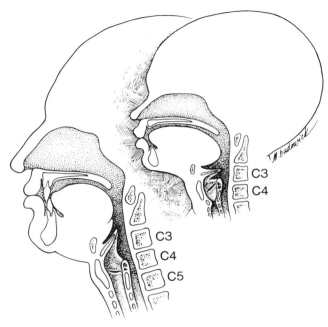

FIG 20–3.
Position of larynx: Anterior and cephalad in infant (C3-4) versus adult (C4-5). Also, note narrowest point of airway at cricoid in infant. (*From Finncane BT, Santora AH:* Principles of Airway Management. *Philadelphia, FA Davis Co, 1985. Used by permission.*)

the first months of life. Congenital pulmonary anomalies are listed in Table 20–1. The control of breathing is incompletely developed at birth, especially in the premature infant. Through early infancy, even in term neonates, apnea can result form various stresses such as anesthesia and sepsis.[6] The relationship of apnea to sudden infant death syndrome (SIDS) and the effectiveness of home monitoring is discussed later in this chapter.

Infection and its complications comprise the majority of pediatric diseases. This is partly because the young child has difficulty isolating infection, leading to an increased chance of bacteremia and sepsis. Hence, children with bacterial penumonia, for instance, are more likely than adults to have positive blood cultures. Children are also prone to a slightly different spectrum of pathogens than adults. Their response to them may also vary with age. A good example is respiratory syncytial virus (RSV), which infects 95% of children by five years of age.[7] In the child, this usually causes small airway disease, which can potentially lead to severe airway obstruction and pneumonia. In the adult, it usually manifests as mild rhinorrhea.

Upper airway diseases are more common in children than adults. Epiglottitis is mainly a pediatric disease, with Haemophilus influenzae type b (HIB) as the usual bacterial pathogen. Epiglottitis can be seen in the adult, but its propensity for the child most likely reflects the increased occurrence of HIB disease in the younger age group. Croup, or laryngotracheobronchitis (LTB), is a much more common pediatric disease than epiglottitis, resulting from a

TABLE 20–1.
Congenital Pulmonary Anomalies Seen in the Newborn

EXTRATHORACIC

Choanal atresia
Pierre Robin syndrome
Macroglossia—congenital tumors or primary
Laryngeal webs
Vocal cord paralysis
Laryngocoele
Laryngeal stenosis
Laryngomalacia
Cervical masses causing compresson of airway (cystic hygroma, teratoma)
Tracheoesophageal fistula
Esophageal atresia

INTRATHORACIC

Anterior mediastinal masses causing compression (cystic hygroma, congenital
   goiter, thymic teratoma)
Posterior mediastinal masses causing compression (neuroblastoma,
   bronchogenic cyst, esophageal duplication)
Vascular rings
Pneumothorax
Chylothorax
Congenital diaphragmatic hernia
Congenital lobar emphysema
Congenital lung cysts
Cystic adenomastoid malformation

viral infection of the subglottic region. Seemingly small amounts of edema can significantly compromise the child's already narrow airway (Fig 20–2).

PHYSICAL EXAMINATION

The physical examination is of primary importance in the evaluation of the pediatric patient. Both the physical and neurological development of the child must be addressed in the assessment of the pulmonary system. For example, when noting the child's position of comfort, it is important to remember that small, weak, or very sick children will often be found in a position imposed on them by their caretakers, rather than in a self-selected position.

The initial exam should include heart rate, respiratory rate, temperature, and an assessment of perfusion. High respiratory rates by adult standards may be normal in children (Table 20–2). More important than a specific rate is the child's degree of comfort or discomfort. A general assessment of the work of breathing should be made. Evidence of increased work of breathing includes nasal flaring, expiratory grunting, and retractions. Because the chest wall is so flexible and compliant, impressive intercostal, suprasternal, and subcostal retractions can be seen.

TABLE 20–2.
Respiratory Rate Variation with Age

Age	Respiratory Rate
Term newborn	50 ± 10
6 month old	30 ± 5
12 month old	24 ± 6
3 year old	24 ± 6
5 year old	23 ± 5
12 year old	18 ± 5
Adult	12 ± 3

From Crone RK: The respiratory system, in Gregory G (ed): *Pediatric Anesthesia*. New York, Churchill Livingstone, 1983, p 84. Used by permission.

Breath sounds are readily transmitted through the small, thin chest wall making auscultation quite easy, but the increased referral of sound can make localization of abnormalities problematic. In fact, a pneumothorax may be difficult to diagnose by auscultation. Examination should always include visual inspection for symmetric chest wall movement (Table 20–3). Because of the child's compliant chest wall, diaphragmatic movement plays a major role in the generation of negative intrathoracic pressure. Any abdominal distension, such as that caused by ascites, hepatosplenomegaly, or ileus, can limit adequate chest inflation, potentially resulting in respiratory decompensation.

TABLE 20–3.
Anatomic and Physiologic Differences in Pediatric Versus Adult Patients

Pulmonary
Decreased lung compliance
Increased thoracic compliance
Decreased FRC
Decreased elastin
Decreased alveolar size and number
Decreased intercostal and diaphragmatic muscle strength
Smaller diameter of conducting airways
Elevated "normal" respiratory rates (see Table 20–2)
Increased referral of breath sounds

Airway
Larynx cephalad and anterior
Narrowest at cricoid instead of vocal cords

Other
Higher metabolic rate
Increased indexed O_2 consumption
Decreased "normal" hematocrit
Propensity to single-organ failure versus MOSF
Prone to different spectrum of pathogens

The neurological assessment is also important. The exam should include a comparison to age-appropriate and neurodevelopment. Evidence of neurologic disability should prompt evaluation of muscle tone, strength, and airway reflexes.

OXYGENATION

Visual inspection to assess the degree of oxygenation is quite poor. Studies have shown that examiners are clinically unable to differentiate between large variations in oxyhemoglobin saturation.[8-10] As mentioned previously, children tend to desaturate more quickly than adults. This reflects less oxygen reserve from a lower FRC, as well as a higher rate of oxygen consumption. The need for monitoring of oxygenation in children is therefore greater than in adults.

In addition to the child with acute respiratory disease, there are a number of specific pediatric indications for oxygenation monitoring. Infants with a congenital heart disease characterized by right-to-left shunt and oxygen desaturation can have profound changes in shunt, resulting from a number of physiologic insults. Monitoring of oxygenation is mandatory in these children during any illness or stress. It is also important to identify any oxygen desaturation during sedation for procedures or during airway manipulation. Additionally, oxygenation monitoring is utilized as an important adjunct to apnea monitoring.[11, 12]

Pulse Oximetry

Continuous pulse oximetry has gained clinical acceptance, with reasonable accuracy for trending documented[13, 14] to saturations as low as 70%. Pulse oximetry is routinely used in the operating room, pediatric intensive care unit (ICU), emergency room, and during inter- and intrahospital transport for any patient requiring supplemental oxygen or with the potential for cardiorespiratory decompensation.[10, 15] A recent study by Cote et al.[10] demonstrated that children under two years of age were at greater risk of suffering a major hypoxic event during anesthesia when continuous O_2 saturation monitoring was unavailable. Nineteen of 32 unmonitored children had hypoxic events, compared to 7 of 33 monitored children.[10] Pulse oximetry can be helpful for diagnosis, as well as for therapeutic decision-making, and is often used to help wean patients from mechanical ventilation.[16] The short warm-up time (10 seconds) and lack of calibration requirement make it ideal for "spot checks." Placement of the probe must be tailored to patient size, using the entire hand or foot in small infants. Thermal injury is rare, but prevention may require probe site changes, especially in the newborn with thin skin.

It is imperative that the physician and nursing staff be well acquainted with the relationship between saturation and Pao_2. They must appreciate that a small drop in oxygen saturation, even in the mid-90th percentile, corresponds to a much greater decline in the Pao_2. Also, they must recognize that a reading of greater than 98% could correspond to Pao_2 of 100, 200, 300 mm Hg, or more. A decline in Pao_2 of 300 to 100 mm Hg, representing significant deterioration of gas exchange, would be masked by a persistent saturation of greater than 98% (Fig 20–4) (see Chapter 10 for details on pulse oximetry).

Transcutaneous Oxygen Monitoring

Transcutaneous O_2 ($Ptco_2$) monitoring can also be used for continuous evaluation of oxygenation. The technology and requisite warm-up time make it less useful for "spot checks" than oximetry. The $Ptco_2$ monitor works very well in small children whose thin skin allows reliable sampling, but may be compromised when perfusion is decreased (i.e., shock states). An inverse relationship between $Ptco_2$ and cardiac index (CI) has been shown[17] in adults when CI is less than 1.5 L/min/m². It is not known whether this relationship exists in children as well. Because the probe requires a relatively large area of flat skin, placement is usually limited to the trunk. The probe must be repositioned frequently (every 2 to 6 hours) to avoid thermal injury.[18] Pulse oximetry has now essentially replaced $Ptco_2$ monitoring. A few situations do exist in which continuous assessment of the Pao_2 is preferable to assessment of saturation [i.e., pre- and postductal monitoring in neonates with persistent pulmonary hypertension of the newborn (PPHN)] (see Chapter 11 for further details).

Blood Gas Analysis

Measurement of arterial blood gases (ABGs) remains the gold standard for assessment of oxygenation; however, continuous monitoring is not yet available. Sampling of arterial blood can be done via an indwelling catheter or isolated arterial punctures. Needless to say, the

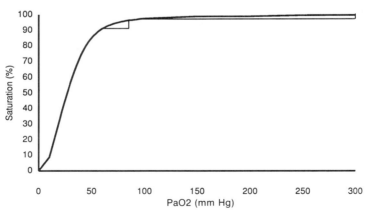

FIG 20–4.
Oxygen-hemoglobin dissociation curve. A decrease in Pao_2 from 300 to 100 mm Hg corresponds to a decrease in oxygen saturation from 99% to only 98%, a difference that cannot be reliably distinguished by pulse oximetry. Note, however, that the small decrease in oxygen saturation from 96% to 91% corresponds to a much larger decrease in Pao_2 from 80 to 60 mm Hg.

arteries in a child are smaller than in an adult; therefore, increased technical difficulty results when obtaining blood from a child. This usually warrants placement of an indwelling arterial catheter earlier than in the adult. Indwelling Po_2 and Pco_2 sensing devices inserted through the arterial catheter are currently under evaluation for continuous blood gas determination.[19, 20] Their use in the pediatric population may well be limited by catheter size.

Capillary blood gases (CBGs) have also been used in children. An extremity is warmed and "stabbed." The "arterialized" capillary blood is allowed to flow freely into a capillary tube for evaluation. This procedure is used more commonly in children in whom arterial access is problematic. The CBG provides a reliable measure of the $Paco_2$ and pH, but the Pao_2 is usually much higher than indicated by the CBG.

VENTILATION

The assessment of ventilation can likewise be determined on an intermittent basis using arterial or capillary blood gas analysis to evaluate Pco_2 and pH. Venous sampling is also used. Though this is less exact than arterial or capillary sampling, the ease with which venous blood can be obtained through indwelling central catheters at times makes it more desirable.

Transcutaneous CO_2

For continuous evaluation of ventilation, two methods have emerged: transcutaneous CO_2 ($Ptcco_2$) and end-tidal CO2 ($Petco_2$) monitoring. Using similar technology to the $Ptco_2$, the $Ptcco_2$ monitor provides a continuous estimation of $Paco_2$. The correlation is 0.8 to 0.9 under hemodynamically stable conditions with the $Ptcco_2$ generally overestimating[21] the actual $Paco_2$ by 5 to 20 mm Hg. (Fig 20–5). Frequent calibration with blood samples is necessary, thus

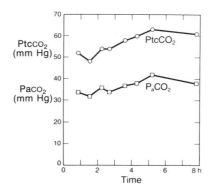

FIG 20–5.
Comparison of $Ptcco_2$ and $Paco_2$ values from a single neonate. Correlation is shown, though up to 20 mm Hg difference between the two can be seen. (*From Monaco F, McQuitty JC: Transcutaneous measurements of carbon dioxide partial pressure in sick neonates.* Crit Care Med 1981, 9:757. Used by permission.)

negating some of its perceived effect of decreasing the need for blood gases. As with $Ptco_2$ monitoring, current $Ptcco_2$ technology presents the potential for thermal injury, requirement of frequent calibration, expense, and relatively slow response time. $Ptcco_2$ is rarely used, but may be useful for infants and small children in whom CO_2 trends should be documented and for whom $Petco_2$ is unavailable or impractical. This could include nonintubated children with neuromuscular disease, patients undergoing bronchoscopy, and infants with extreme tachypnea (>70/min) for whom $Petco_2$ may be inaccurate[22] (see Chapter 11 for details).

End-Tidal CO_2

Another noninvasive method of estimating $Paco_2$ is analysis of expired gas concentration of CO_2, or end-tidal CO_2 ($Petco_2$). The usefulness of this measurement is increased when it is displayed graphically versus time throughout the respiratory cycle. This is termed *capnography*.

Airway gas is continuously sampled and monitored through either a mainstream or a sidestream analyzer, placed at the patient end of the endotracheal tube. The Pco_2 is determined by infrared absorption analysis or, less commonly, mass spectrometry. The sidestream system draws gas from the airway through small bore tubing to the analyzer, while the mainstream is placed in-line at the end of the endotracheal tube (ETT). There are problems with both of these systems in pediatrics. The mainstream analyzer adds weight to the end of the ETT and, if not properly supported, increases the risk of accidental extubation, especially in the infant or small child.[23] These also contribute a potentially significant degree of dead-space to the smaller child. The sidestream sampling systems do not add dead-space but they draw air at such rapid speed that fresh inhaled gas can be entrained. This can dilute the amount of CO_2 and result in falsely low values. Most capnography is done with an endotracheal tube, although nasal sampling has recently been used in adults.[24]

As mentioned, $Petco_2$ can be displayed versus time and a characteristic waveform generated (Fig 20–6). There are four phases on the ideal capnograph, based on the sequential sampling of dead-space to alveolar gas. The baseline inspiratory Pco_2 extends into the beginning of expiration, as gas is delivered from the pure anatomical dead-space. The second phase is a gradual upslope, corresponding to proportionately increasing alveolar gas concentration mixed with dead-space gas. The plateau phase follows, representative at its peak of "pure" alveolar gas. Fourth, there is an abrupt return to baseline at end-expiration, signaling the beginning of inspiration. The $Petco_2$ value usually underestimates[21, 25] the true arterial Pco_2 by as much as 1 to 5 mm Hg. For this reason, $Petco_2$ should never be interpreted alone, except for the confirmation of ETT placement into the airway.[26]

Information about the patient, the ventilator circuit, or the sampling system can be derived from analysis of the capnograph. For example, the initial upslope can provide information about air movement in the small airways, while the slope of the plateau can be indicative of alveolar emptying time. The height of the plateau may vary with the proximity of the sampling port to the patient, the amount of fresh gas entrained, especially in pediatric patients, or, of course, the actual alveolar Pco_2. A disconnection between patient and sampling port, dislodgement of the ETT, or an apneic episode would result in a dramatically and abruptly depressed series of plateaus. Many other alterations can exist that correspond to either patient

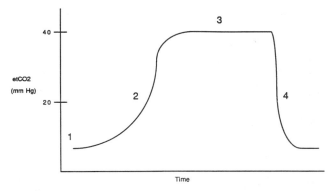

FIG 20–6.
Typical capnograph of a single respiratory cycle: 1 = End of inspiration—beginning of expiration; 2 = Increasing alveolar gas concentration; 3 = Plateau phase ("pure" alveolar gas); and 4 = End-expiration return to baseline.

or equipment malfunction. It is imperative for clinicians who use capnography to be comfortable with its interpretation (see Chapter 12).

Capnography is commonly used as a continuous monitor of cardiorespiratory function and support in the operating room, ICU, and during patient transport. It is used primarily as a safety device to monitor any interruption of respiration, such as a dislodged endotracheal tube or a ventilator circuit break, and for rapid assessment of unexpected, abrupt physiologic changes such as pneumothorax or pulmonary embolus. It has also been used to wean patients from mechanical ventilation, though caution must be exercised in the interpretation of $Petco_2$ values alone. A patient with progressive hypopnea, for instance, would have an increasing proportion of dead-space contribution (low $Petco_2$) resulting in a potentially unrecognized underestimation of the true $Paco_2$. Confirmation via blood gas analysis is mandated if the patient's clinical cardiorespiratory exam changes or if $Petco_2$ increases significantly (>5 mm Hg).[27, 28] Its main advantages remain the constant on-line, noninvasive monitoring of ventilation and decrease in frequency of required ABG measurements (see Chapter 12 for details).

OXYGEN DELIVERY

Evaluation of the efficiency of oxygen delivery from the lungs to the arterial circulation is best quantified as the measurement of shunt, or venous admixture,[2, 21, 29] that is, the fraction of blood that is returned to the left ventricle without participating in gas exchange. This can result from intracardiac right-to-left shunt, from deoxygenated blood returning from the thebesian or bronchial veins, or from intrapulmonary shunting through lung segments having a low ventilation to perfusion ratio, such as occurs with atelectasis or pneumonia. It should be reemphasized that a number of children have congenital heart disease with associated intracardiac shunt. In addition, many children can have a right-to-left shunt through a patent foramen ovale, resulting from an acutely elevated pulmonary arterial pressure.

Shunt percentage can be determined by the amount of venous blood that would need to be added to a given quantity of fully oxygenated pulmonary capillary blood in order to result in the actual obtained Pao_2. This percent shunt can be calculated: $Qs/Qt = (Cco_2 - Cao_2)/(Cco_2 - C\bar{v}o_2)$, where Qs = shunted blood, Qt = total cardiac output, Cco_2 = pulmonary capillary O_2 content, Cao_2 = arterial O_2 content, and $C\bar{v}o_2$ = mixed venous O_2 content.

Mixed venous O_2 can only accurately be sampled from the right ventricle or pulmonary artery. All other values can be obtained noninvasively. The Cco_2 is assumed to be equal to alveolar oxygen content (Cao_2), which can be estimated from the alveolar-air equation; Cao_2 is determined from an ABG sample.

The intrapulmonary shunt can be calculated by determining the O_2 content in the arterial, the pulmonary capillary, and the mixed venous blood. For example, assume a child with pneumonia has an arterial oxygen saturation of 95%, while breathing 100% oxygen with 12 g% Hb and a mixed venous oxygen saturation of 75%, and pulmonary capillary O_2 saturation of 100%. The shunt fraction is calculated:

$$Qs/Qt = \frac{Cco_2 - Cao_2}{Cco_2 - Cvo_2} = \frac{16.0 - 15.2}{16.0 - 12.0} = 0.2 \text{ or } 20\% \text{ shunt fraction}$$

The normal shunt fraction is less than 5%.

Fiber-optic and oximetric technology have been combined in a flow-directed pulmonary artery catheter that can provide continuous measurement of mixed venous oxygen saturation. This allows rapid detection of changes in oxygen delivery and/or consumption.[30, 31] When used in combination with pulse oximetry (termed dual oximetry) a continuous estimate of shunt fraction can be computed.[32, 33] While this technology allows rapid recognition of changes in clinical status, the effect on patient outcome has yet to be demonstrated.

The relationship of Fio_2 and Pao_2 can be used to estimate shunt, using an isoshunt diagram (Fig 20–7). This assumes normal ranges of hemoglobin, $Paco_2$, and cardiac output, which makes it less accurate in critically ill patients. Another clinical method used to estimate shunt that avoids the need for central venous cannulation is the alveolar to arterial oxygen tension difference, or $P(A-a)o_2$, which is calculated:

$$(Fio_2 \times (P_B - P_{H_2O})) - Paco_2/RQ - Pao_2$$

where P_B = barometric pressure, P_{H_2O} = water vapor pressure, and RQ = respiratory quotient. The ratio of arterial to alveolar oxygen tension (Pao_2/PAo_2), and the Pao_2/Fio_2 ratio can also be used. These are adequate when the shunt fraction is small, but become less helpful as shunt increases.

INDIRECT CALORIMETRY

The need for proper nutritional support of the critically ill patient is becoming increasingly evident, especially for the child who needs calories for growth, as well as recovery. Assessment of increased nutritional requirements is aided by an estimation of energy expenditure. This

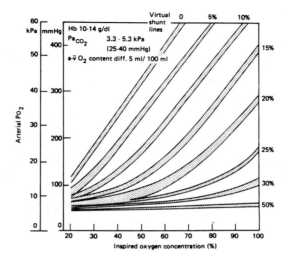

FIG 20–7.

The isoshunt diagram. (*From Benatar SR, Hewlett AM, Nunn JR: The use of iso-shunt lines for control of oxygen therapy.* Br J Anaesth 1973; 45:711–718. Used by permission.)

can be obtained through the use of indirect calorimetry. The two general techniques used to determine nutritional support by indirect calorimetry are the open and closed systems. The most commonly used approach is the open-circuit technique, in which inspired and expired gases are separated by a valved system. The volume and concentration of CO_2 and O_2 are measured in each, allowing calculation of CO_2 production and O_2 consumption. From this, the resting energy expenditure is determined.

The child who has sustained severe burns or trauma may benefit from indirect calorimetry, since there is as much as a 100% increase in energy expenditure after major burns, and 40% after multisystem trauma.[34] Frequent, accurate assessment, beginning with this early postinjury stress, will facilitate appropriate nutritional management as the child recovers, although there are many technical factors that limit the use of indirect calorimetry in this group (see Chapter 13 for details).

Calculation of resting energy expenditure of the child demands accurate equipment. Significant error is introduced when there are minor variations in F_{IO_2} or tidal volume over the collection period.[34, 35] The F_{IO_2} measurements at concentrations greater than 0.50 to 0.60 are inherently inaccurate, precluding the use of the metabolic cart in many critically ill patients.[36, 37] Also, the leak around uncuffed endotracheal tubes leads to an additional source of error in volume calculations. The need for patient stability must also be emphasized, because the amount of expired CO_2 measured will be affected by both CO_2 production and its equilibrium within the body. Alteration of CO_2 equilibrium is caused by variation in acid-base status, body temperature, activity, or ventilatory pattern. This is another limitation of its use in critically ill patients.

PULMONARY FUNCTION TESTING

Pulmonary function testing (PFT) is used in the diagnosis and management of children with acute and chronic respiratory disease. Cooperative children over five years of age generally can be tested in the same way as adults. Unfortunately, testing has been suboptimal in children between one month and five years of age, yet the increasing survival of critically ill neonates has created a significant pediatric population with both chronic and acute pulmonary disease. Recently, imaginative playful methods to maximize the child's cooperation for effort-dependent portions of PFTs have been developed. Also, equipment adaptations that provide better sensitivity at low volumes have improved the accuracy of measurements.[1]

Normal PFT reference ranges for children have been based on regression analysis of adult values.[38] While lung function is also affected by sex and race, the best predictor of lung function is the child's body size, rather than age.[39] As children track along percentile growth curves, so too does their lung function.[40] Monitoring these trends is useful in clinically assessing children with chronic lung disease such as cystic fibrosis.

In the nonintubated patient, PFTs are commonly used to evaluate small airway disease, neuromuscular disease, and cystic fibrosis. Peak expiratory flow and forced expiratory volume (FEV) are routine methods of evaluation of small airway (or obstructive) disease. This can be easily performed using spirometry or peak flow meters in the office, emergency room, ward, or ICU. A comparison to previously obtained values may provide insight into the slow progression of an underlying condition or the severity of an acute exacerbation. Immediate response to bronchodilator therapy can also be determined.

Flow volume loops can be used at the bedside to evaluate the mechanics of lung function.[41] Older children can use a mouthpiece, while infants need a tight-fitting mask. Older infants and toddlers usually require sedation for mask placement, which may alter the results. Though the tidal flow volume loops are not quantifiable, they may display characteristic patterns in infants, which are useful in detecting airway obstruction, as well as the response to medical or surgical therapy. A technique of rapid chest compression, using rapidly inflatable jackets to augment passive exhalation, has been used in children under three years of age to evaluate expiratory flow and volume[42, 43] (Fig 20–8).

The child with neuromuscular disease, whether acute, like Guillain-Barre, or a chronic myopathy, requires reliable, objective documentation of respiratory strength and reserve.[44] Vital capacity (VC) and maximum inspiratory pressure (MIP) are most commonly used, but necessitate some cooperation during mask or mouthpiece placement, as noted earlier. The younger child may need numerous attempts to obtain three acceptable curves, which could compromise accuracy by increasing fatigue and/or boredom.[38, 45] Crying vital capacity (CVC) can be used in uncooperative younger children. Exhaled volume is measured while the child is allowed or encouraged to cry through a mask. Two to four maximal breaths within 4 mL of each other are necessary to establish reliability[46] (see Chapters 9 and 17 for details).

Children with restrictive lung disease resulting from respiratory muscle weakness, chest wall skeletal abnormalities like scoliosis, or interstitial fibrosis are monitored by periodic assessment of their total lung capacity and functional residual capacity (FRC). This is accomplished through the use of body plethysmography or gas dilution techniques. The latter is preferred in uncooperative children, but is less accurate when small airway disease is present,

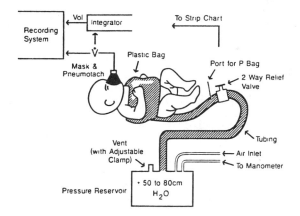

FIG 20–8.
Rapid chest compression device. Inflatable jacket positioned around thorax is used to augment passive exhalation in determining expiratory flow volume relationships in a child under three years of age. (*From Morgan WJ, et al: Partial expiratory flow-volume curves in infants and young children.* Pediatr Pulmonol *1988; 5:236. Used by permission.*)

because of unequal gas distribution. Plethysmography is limited to cooperative children who can safely be placed in the "box." This excludes most ICU patients (see Chapter 17 for details).

Tidal volume (VT) is measured in several ways in children, depending on their age and the acuity of their disease.[41] Chest wall impedance pneumography is often used in infants for apnea monitoring. If calibrated by another method, termed *respiratory induction plethysmography*, it can be used to monitor VT continuously and quantitatively.[47, 48] Pneumotachography (the use of flow resistors) and hot wire anemometers are other common methods for measuring VT in infants. Body plethysmography and simple collection of expired gas divided by respiratory frequency are used in the older child and infant.

Lung volume and mechanics must be frequently evaluated in the mechanically ventilated child. This enables caregivers to assess and respond to changes in pulmonary function through the child's disease course, as well as help identify causes of acute respiratory distress. For example, MIP and VC are used to assess the probability of successful extubation of the child with resolving acute neuromuscular disease or a prolonged course of mechanical ventilation.

Some of the newer generation ventilators provide constant monitoring of inspiratory and expiratory VT, which is helpful in assessing the child's clinical status as well as providing ongoing monitoring of mechanical ventilation. In clinical reviews, 26 to 60% of recognized complications were secondary to mechanical failure.[49, 50] Forty percent of these were related to circuit leaks, disconnects, or exhalation valve dysfunction, all of which could have been diagnosed by in-line monitoring.

Compliance (change in volume divided by the change in pressure) is usually measured for the entire respiratory system. This includes the compliance of both the lungs and the chest wall in the relationship:

$$1/C_T = 1/C_L + 1/C_{Th}$$

where C_T = respiratory system compliance, C_L = lung compliance, and C_{Th} = chest wall compliance.

Compliance of the lung is affected by a number of factors (i.e., surfactant, presence of alveolar or interstitial disease, FRC, amount of lung water). It is calculated as the change in volume divided by the change in alveolar transmural pressure (alveolar-pleural pressure) over the respiratory cycle. The pressure at the airway is assumed to be alveolar and P_{pl} is assumed to be esophageal.

Bedside estimates of compliance, without the aid of an esophageal balloon during mechanical ventilation, determine C_T. This is done by determining the amount of inspiratory pressure required to deliver a tidal volume. Both static and dynamic compliance can be measured. The measurement of dynamic compliance is done when airflow has stopped at the airway, but active airflow within the lungs may still be occurring;[51] that is the tidal volume divided by the difference between the peak inspiratory and end-expiratory airway pressures. Computer-based methods using least-squares regression analysis from constant sampling are often used to measure dynamic compliance at the bedside.

Static compliance is calculated as the change in volume divided by the pressure required to maintain a static volume in the lung. This pressure is determined as the plateau pressure when an inspiratory hold is activated during mechanical ventilation. If the child is not paralyzed, and is spontaneously breathing but cooperative, this value can be obtained by voluntary holding inspiration. The infant's static compliance can be measured by taking advantage of the Hering-Breuer reflex. When an infant's lung volumes are greater than FRC, airway occlusion leads to transient relaxation of respiratory muscles, maintaining lung expansion. A technique has been developed that can actually be adapted to children up to two years old, in which plateau pressures at various lung volumes are determined, and static compliance then calculated[52] (Fig. 20–9).

A leak around the endotracheal tube can produce a declining, rather than a sustained, plateau pressure when an inspiratory hold is applied. An accurate plateau pressure may therefore be unobtainable when a patient has an uncuffed endotracheal tube.

Decreased total respiratory system compliance may be noted during IRDS, ARDS, hyperinflation (asthma and bronchiolitis), or when excessive positive end-expiratory pressure (PEEP) is applied. Excessive PEEP or hyperinflation causes decreased chest wall compliance and does not necessarily imply more severe lung disease. In these cases, it may be prognostically important to delineate the respective contributions of the lung and chest wall to the total respiratory system compliance, using an esophageal balloon to estimate pleural pressure. Anything that serves to limit the expansion of the lungs effectively decreases chest wall compliance. This may be from intrathoracic pathology (i.e., pneumothorax or pleural effusion), or from impaired diaphragmatic movement (phrenic nerve paralysis or increased abdominal pressure), or structural anomalies (scoliosis). Compliance measurements in children are often corrected for lung volume (referenced to FRC), termed *specific compliance* (Table 20–4). (For a complete discussion of lung mechanics, see Chapters 9 and 16).

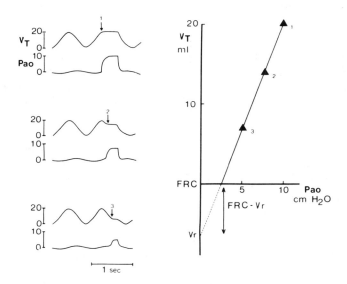

FIG 20–9.

Determination of static compliance using multiple expiratory occlusion technique. At left, arrows indicate the time during expiration when occlusion was performed, with resultant airway pressure plateaus Pao = airway pressure, V_T = tidal volume). At right, change in lung volume is plotted against corresponding airway pressure plateau. The slope of the line equals total respiratory system compliance, while the intercept on the volume axis indicates the resting volume of the respiratory system. (*From Mortola JP, Saetta M: Measurement of respiratory mechanics in the newborn: A simple approach.* Pediatr Pulmonol 1987; 3:123. *Used by permission.*)

TABLE 20–4.

Pulmonary Function Tests

Obstructive Diseases

Peak expiratory flow

Forced expiratory volume

Flow volume loops (infants and small children only)

Functional residual capacity (may be increased)

Restrictive Diseases (including neuromuscular disease, weakness)

Vital capacity

Maximal inspiratory pressure

(Crying) vital capacity

Total lung capacity

Functional residual capacity

APNEA

Apnea is the cessation of respiratory airflow. It can be classified as central (no respiratory effort), obstructive (no air movement despite effort), or mixed (both central and obstructive components). While short (<15 seconds) central apnea can be normal at all ages, apnea is considered pathologic if it lasts 20 seconds or more.[12, 53] It is also abnormal if it is accompanied by cyanosis, pallor, hypotonia, or bradycardia as a manifestation of the resultant hypoxemia.

An understanding of the multiple causes of apnea is essential when attempting to decide which patients need monitoring. Apnea must be recognized as a potential manifestation of serious, systemic diseases in infants, such as sepsis, meningitis, pneumonia, or bronchiolitis.[12, 54] In these cases, it resolves with resolution of the primary disease. However, apnea occurs most commonly in the premature neonate in the absence of underlying disease; this is termed *apnea of prematurity*. It is attributed to immaturity of the respiratory control centers and usually resolves by 37 weeks gestational age, after which persistence is considered pathologic.[53] Other children at risk for apnea include those with neuromuscular diseases, encephalopathies, tracheostomies, or obstructive sleep apnea (commonly resulting from tonsilar and adenoidal hypertrophy).

Most apnea monitors utilize thoracic bioimpedance technology. This allows detection of both rate and depth of respiration. It must be emphasized that this method is most useful for the infant with central apnea, as those with obstructive apnea still exhibit chest wall motion, though it may be erratic or exaggerated. Additional information can be obtained by monitoring ECG for heart rate. In this way the bradycardia that can accompany apnea may also be detected. These monitors are equipped with an alarm system that can be variably set for duration of apnea (usually 15 to 20 seconds) and a high/low heart rate; the latter must be adjusted for age. Determination of the appropriateness of the alarm is an important component in interpretation of its effectiveness. Substantiating data such as recorded bradycardia are helpful. Some advocate the addition of pulse oximetry as a more specific indication of hypoxia to better evaluate the significance of an apneic episode.[11, 12]

The decision of "who to monitor for apnea" is easy to make for the hospitalized patient. All patients in the ICU have cardiorespiratory monitors. Those undergoing mechanical ventilation often have transcutaneous devices, capnography, or airflow detection devices built into their ventilator circuit to detect disconnection or apnea. Children at risk for acute airway obstruction should have both cardiorespiratory monitoring and pulse oximetry while hospitalized. It must be remembered that clinical observation cannot be supplanted by monitoring and these patients often require 1:1 nursing care, such as is available in an ICU setting. Children with acute neuromuscular diseases that may compromise respiratory effort such as botulism and Guillain-Barre should also be continuously monitored. As noted above, newborns with other systemic diseases may also become apneic and should be monitored. The difficult and often controversial decisions regarding appropriateness of apnea monitoring await the physician at the child's discharge. The association of apnea with SIDS and apparent life threatening event (ALTE) ("near miss SIDS," "aborted SIDS") is controversial.[53, 55, 56, 57] Epidemiologic data are accumulating to help clarify the relationship in an effort to delineate those infants and children at risk who therefore require some form of home monitoring.[53, 58, 59] All infants and children admitted after an ALTE should be monitored for their entire hospitalization. If a cause for the ALTE is determined and treated, monitoring may be discontinued. Those for whom no cause has been ascertained usually have monitoring continued at home. If the ATLE required vigorous resuscitation, the infant or child may have up to a 60% chance of recurrence.[57]

Inherent in the discussion of home monitoring is the concept that monitoring, in and of itself, does not prevent death—it merely warns of a potential event. Parents and caregivers must be educated regarding their response to, and assessment of, alarms. While home monitoring is largely thought to help allay parental anxiety, it is often the cause of increased stress. Consideration of these effects on the home environment is necessary in deciding if home apnea monitoring is warranted. In an effort to clarify the appropriateness of home monitoring, the NIH Consensus Conference on Infantile Apnea and Home Monitoring convened in 1986. They recommend four specific groups of infants for whom home monitoring is indicated[53]: (1) those who have had ALTE severe enough to require resuscitation; (2) symptomatic premature infants who are otherwise ready to be discharged before resolution of their apnea; (3) siblings of two or more SIDS victims; and (4) infants with certain diseases or conditions such as central hypoventilation syndrome. Others include infants with tracheostomies and those with bronchopulmonary dysplasia (BPD) on home oxygen therapy. Infants of drug-addicted mothers, siblings of a single SIDS victim, and those who had less severe ALTE must also be considered for home monitoring on an individualized basis.

The time to discontinue monitoring is based on the event that initiated it and the frequency of real alarms. For the child who has had an ALTE, monitoring is generally continued for two months following the last alarm, and until the child is at least six months old and has been stressed by a URI. Siblings of SIDS victims often continue home monitoring until one to two months beyond the age at which the previous sibling died. Infants requiring respiratory stimulants such as caffeine or theophylline are usually monitored for one to two months after the medication has been discontinued.[54, 57]

Current investigation with simultaneous use of multiple and reliable sensors of apnea and hypoxia, with "hardcopy" event recording, will hopefully better characterize the severity of the apneic episodes. These new techniques of home apnea monitoring may more clearly delineate the population at risk. Further study regarding the ability of home apnea monitoring to reduce infant mortality is needed since this is its primary purpose.

CARDIOVASCULAR MONITORING

The goals of hemodynamic monitoring of the pediatric patient are to provide accurate diagnostic information, evaluation of ongoing therapy, and warning of unexpected events or changes in clinical condition.

Anatomy and Physiology

The physical examination remains the most important and reliable method of assessing and monitoring the hemodynamic status of the pediatric patient. Before considering cardiovascular monitoring, it is important to discuss the causes of hemodynamic compromise in the child and adult and how they differ. Cardiovascular decompensation at any age can result from a number of physiologic states. These can be divided into two general categories: intravascular hypovolemia and intravascular normovolemia. Intravascular hypovolemia is caused by either a true loss of volume or by a loss of vascular resistance. Decompensation with intravascular normovolemia is secondary to myocardial dysfunction or outflow obstruction (i.e., aortic stenosis, coarctation of the aorta) (Fig. 20–10). It is important to recognize these distinct causes in that the clinical signs and symptoms, as well as therapy, differ.

By far the most common pediatric etiology is intravascular hypovolemia, usually resulting from vomiting and diarrhea. The physiologic response to hypovolemia differs in the child and adult. In infants and children the initial compensatory response to hypovolemia is increased heart rate and increased systemic vascular resistance with decreased perfusion of skin, splanchnic, and renal vascular beds.[60] The blood pressure in the central circulation is maintained until there is extreme hypovolemia, at which point abrupt hypotension occurs. With this in mind, the early detection of hypovolemic compromise is best accomplished by assessment of end organ perfusion and heart rate, rather than blood pressure. The adult with a similar degree of hypovolemia would demonstrate systemic hypotension much earlier.

Physical Examination

End organ perfusion can be monitored by evaluating urine output, mental status, and skin perfusion. Skin perfusion is assessed by temperature and capillary refill. Capillary refill is performed by applying firm fingertip pressure to a nail bed or the skin overlying a bony

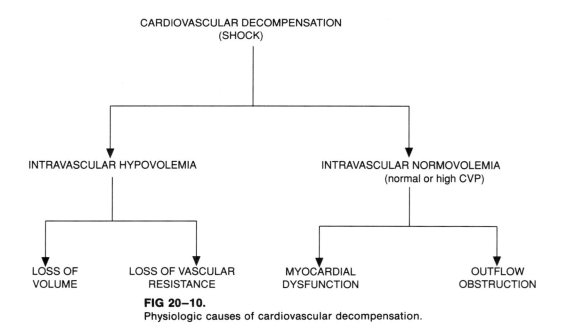

FIG 20–10.
Physiologic causes of cardiovascular decompensation.

prominence, such as the anterior tibia. After the initial blanch, color should return completely within two seconds. Prolongation to greater than five seconds implies significant hypoperfusion. Temperature is assessed by simply feeling the extremity and documenting the peripheral level of coolness. The difference between central (esophageal or foley catheter) temperature and skin temperature can also be used to quantitate perfusion.

Heart rate is determined by auscultation or pulse palpation. Electrical activity of the heart is easily and rapidly determined by ECG, which can be correlated to palpable heart rate (except in cases of electromechanical dissociation). All children, upon admission to the ICU, have continuous ECG monitoring at the bedside, with digital heart rate readout and high/low alarms set appropriate to age (Table 20–5).

Blood Pressure

Blood pressure measurements are important in any disease state with potential hemodynamic decompensation. Manual sphygmomanometry is routinely used in the ER and ward settings but has become increasingly rare in the ICU setting. Doppler probes can be used instead of a stethoscope for infants and children in whom Korotkoff sounds are difficult to auscultate.[61] ICUs are more routinely employing an automatically inflated cuff with oscillometric determination of blood pressure, such as the Dinamapp 845 (Applied Medical Research Corp). This can have regular, timed cycles, with digital display of systolic, diastolic, and mean pressures.

Transducing an arterial catheter is the gold standard of blood pressure measurement. Not only can systolic, diastolic, and mean pressures be directly and continuously monitored, but the tracing itself can provide diagnostic information. For instance, a variation in the baseline with positive pressure ventilation is suggestive of hypovolemia. The position of the dicrotic notch on the arterial waveform tracing can also be used to estimate intravascular volume status, though it is also affected by other factors, such as the length and compliance of the tubing.

TABLE 20–5.
Heart Rate Variation with Age

Age	Heart Rate
Term newborn	133 ± 18
6 month old	120 ± 20
12 month old	120 ± 20
2 year old	105 ± 25
5 year old	90 ± 10
12 year old	70 ± 17
Adult	75 ± 5

From Crone RK: *Pediatric Intensive Care.* ASA Refresher Courses in Anesthesiology. Vol. 9 Philadelphia, JB Lippincott, 1981. Used by permission.

Central Venous Pressure

To evaluate and monitor adequately the cardiovascular status of the critically ill infant or child, a central venous pressure (CVP) catheter is often necessary.[62] However, before placing a CVP catheter, the child should be evaluated. If hypovolemia is suspected, the child's volume status is further assessed by the response to crystalloid (or colloid) infusions of 10 to 20 m/kg. If, after 40 to 60 m/kg of rapid volume resuscitation there is little improvement, a CVP catheter should be considered. While the absolute CVP obtained may be helpful, the trend noted over successive volume infusions is much more relevant.[63] A rising CVP would indicate adequate intravascular volume with a cardiogenic etiology of the shock state, whereas a persistently low CVP (less than 3 to 4 mm Hg) would imply relative hypovolemia. The CVP must always be evaluated in conjunction with clinical assessment.

CVP catheters can be placed via the internal and external jugular, femoral, subclavian, and brachiocephalic veins. There are a variety of lengths and diameters designed for pediatric use. Specific indications and risks, as well as insertion techniques, are discussed elsewhere.[64, 65] It is important to remember that the catheter tip must be intrathoracic, in the inferior vena cava (IVC) or superior vena cava (SVC) at the entrance to the right atrium (RA). The latter placement correlates best with RA pressure, which is reflective of right ventricular end-diastolic pressure (RVEDP), or preload.[65] X-ray confirmation is mandatory. If the tip is in the RA the catheter should be repositioned into the SVC or IVC to avoid any potential risk of myocardial perforation.[66, 67]

Pulmonary Artery Catheter

Because children more often have biventricular dysfunction, rather than isolated left ventricular dysfunction like adults, the CVP is usually adequate for assessment of intravascular volume and cardiac function. Pulmonary artery (PA) catheters are infrequently needed in children, but the ability to monitor left ventricular function, cardiac output, or vascular resistance can be important in some situations; children after surgery for congenital heart disease, children requiring high levels of PEEP (>15 cm H_2O), children with myocarditis/cardiomyopathy, and children with sepsis.[63, 68–70]

The triple lumen PA catheter allows continuous measurement of pressures in the pulmonary artery and right atrium (or vena cava) and when intermittently wedged (balloon inflated), a pulmonary capillary wedge pressure (PCWP). PCWP is considered to be equivalent to left atrial pressure and thus reflects left ventricular end-diastolic pressure.[71] The thermistor tip makes it possible to determine cardiac output (CO) using the thermodilution technique.[72] True mixed venous blood can be drawn from the PA. With the information obtained, systemic and pulmonary vascular resistances, cardiac output, and shunt fraction can be calculated. Evaluation of left and right ventricular function is possible as well.[68, 73] Determination of cardiac output by thermodilution has been found to be accurate for a wide range of patient sizes.[74, 75]

The catheter has three lumens, two for infusions and pressure transducing and one for the balloon inflation. The pressure ports are placed such that the proximal port is in the RA and the distal port in the PA, distal to the balloon. A "fourth" lumen is for the thermistor, located at the distal tip of the catheter.

Placement is accomplished through the same access sites as for the CVP, dictated by physician experience and other clinical indicators. Catheter sizes currently available are 5 and 7 French (Fr) for patients less than and greater than 18 kg, respectively. The main difference between these catheters is the distance between CVP and PA ports (15 cm in 5 Fr and 30 cm in 7 Fr). Smaller PA catheters with no CVP (proximal) lumen are available in 2 to 4 Fr, which require a separate right atrial catheter for injection of cold saline.[70] In infants and small children (<10 kg), it is necessary to use the femoral venous approach, so that the proximal infusion port is within the central circulation so that cardiac output determinations remain accurate, even with the infusion port outside the right atrium.[76]

Placement of the PA catheter includes all of the risks and limitations of central venous catheter insertion. Its location in the pulmonary artery, passing through the tricuspid and pulmonic valves, makes myocardial and valvular damage more likely, and it can cause arrhythmias.[70, 77]

Air embolus from rupture of the balloon during catheter insertion is usually insignificant as it passes into the pulmonary vascular system. In pediatric patients with potential right-to-left intracardiac shunt, balloon rupture can have devastating consequences. For this reason the balloon should be inflated with CO_2 in patients at risk.[63, 68] In infants, the inflated balloon may obstruct the pulmonary artery, leading to acute decompensation. The balloon should never remain inflated for longer than 15 seconds. Because of smaller vessel size and shorter distances, spontaneous wedging is also more likely to occur in infants and children than in adults.[62, 63] Other life-threatening complications can include rupture of the pulmonary artery or peripheral vessel.[63, 68]

Left Atrial Catheter

A left atrial catheter can provide a more reliable reflection of LVEDP than the PCWP, especially when there is mitral valve regurgitation.[78] The obvious need for a thoracotomy limits its use almost entirely to infants having repair of congenital heart defects.[64] Blood sampling and administration of medications through an LA catheter are avoided to minimize the chance of systemic emboli[62, 64] (see Chapter 8 for details).

Noninvasive Methods

Noninvasive methods of hemodynamic monitoring are beginning to emerge. These include the use of echocardiography, Doppler ultrasound, and thoracic bioimpedance.[79-81] The latter has been used to determine CO, and its correlation with traditional thermodilution methods has recently improved.[82-84]

Echocardiography provides information pertaining to intracardiac and great vessel anatomy, as well as valvular function. With the addition of Doppler ultrasound, estimation of CO, intracardiac shunting, and PA pressures are now available.[80] Estimates of CO, determined by the pulsed Doppler technique, correlate with those obtained by thermodilution in children undergoing elective cardiac catheterization, but not in critically ill children.[85, 86] Further development may make these noninvasive methods of cardiac function evaluation more easily interpretable and economically accessible (see Chapter 14 for details).

SUMMARY

Anatomic and physiologic differences between the child and adult and their response to disease help tailor the application of current cardiac and respiratory monitoring. The risk of data acquisition must always be weighed against potential clinical benefit. This risk/benefit ratio is a function not only of the intensity or severity of disease, but also of age and size of the patient. Most invasive monitoring has high risk in the small child, which has encouraged development of more noninvasive techniques. Monitoring technology in adults as well as pediatric patients is a rapidly evolving field that requires ongoing reevaluation and assessment.

REFERENCES

1. Fisher BJ, Waldemar AC, Doershuk CF: Pulmonary function testing from infancy through adolescence, in Scarpelli EM (ed): *Pulmonary Physiology: Fetus, Newborn, Child, and Adolescent*, ed. 2. Philadelphia, Lea and Febiger, 1990, pp 421–445.
2. O'Rourke PP, Crone RK: The respiratory system, in Gregory GA (ed): *Pediatric Anesthesia*, ed. 2. New York, Churchill Livingstone, 1989, pp 63–91.
3. Bucher U, Reid L: Development of the intrasegmental bronchial tree: The pattern of branching and development of cartilage at various states of intra-uterine life. *Thorax* 1961; 16:207–218.
4. Dunnill MS: Postnatal growth of the lung. *Thorax* 1962; 17:329–333.
5. Muller NL, Bryan AC: Chest wall mechanics and respiratory muscles in infants. *Pediatr Clin North Am* 1979; 26:503–516.
6. Gross I: Apnea, in Oski FA (ed): *Principles and Practice of Pediatrics*. Philadelphia, JB Lippincott Co, 1990; pp 343–344.
7. Hall CB: Respiratory synctial virus, in Feigin RD, Cherry JD (eds): Philadelphia, WB Saunders Co, 1987; p 1656.
8. Comroe JH Jr., Botelho S: Unreliability of cyanosis in the recognition of arterial anoxemia. *Am J M Sc* 1947; 214:1–6.
9. Pullerits J, Burrows FA, Roy WL: Arterial desaturation in healthy children during transfer to the recovery room. *Can J Anesth* 1987; 34:470–472.
10. Cote CJ, Goldstein EA, Cote MA, et al: A single-blind study of pulse oximetry in children. *Anesthesiol* 1988; 68:184–188.
11. Poets CF, Southall DP: Control of breathing, apnea, and sudden infant death. *Curren Op Pediatr* 1991; 3:413–417.
12. Brooks JG: Abnormalities of control ventilation, in Rudolph AM (ed): *Rudolph's Pediatrics*, ed 19. Norwalk, CT, Appleton and Lange, 1991, pp 1478–1483.
13. Francone S: Reliability of pulse oximetry in hypoxic infants. *J Pediatr* 1988; 112:424–427.
14. Yelderman M, New W: Evaluation of pulse oximetry. *Anesthesiol* 1983; 59:349–352.
15. Taylor MB, Whitwarn JG: The current status of pulse oximetry. *Anesthesia* 1986; 41:943–949.
16. Fanconi S, Doherty P, Edmonds JF, et al: Pulse oximetry in pediatric intensive care: Comparison with measured saturations and transcutaneous oxygen tension. *J Pediatr* 1985; 107:362–366.
17. Tremper KK, Shoemaker WC: Transcutaneous oxygen monitoring of critically ill adults, with and without low flow shock. *Crit Care Med* 1981; 9:706–709.
18. Hicks DA, Anas NG: Transcutaneous oxygen monitoring, in Levin DL, Morriss FC (eds): *Essentials of Pediatric Intensive Care*, St. Louis, Quality Medical Publishing, Inc, 1990, pp 858–861.
19. Barker SJ, Hyatt J, Tremper KK, et al: Continuous fiberoptic blood-gas monitoring: A comparison of 18 and 20 gauge arterial cannulas. *Anesthesiol* 1989; 71:A377.

20. Bratanow N, Polk K, Bland R, et al: Continuous polarographic monitoring of intra-arterial oxygen in the peri-operative period. *Crit Care Med* 1985; 13:859–860.
21. Marini JJ: Monitoring during mechanical ventilation. *Clin Chest Med* 1988; 9:73–100.
22. McEvedy BAB, McLeod ME, Mulera M, et al: End-tidal, transcutaneous, and arterial PCO2 measurements in critically ill neonates: A comparison study. *Anesthesiol* 1988; 69:112–119.
23. Anas N: End tidal carbon dioxide monitoring (capnography), in Levin DL, Morriss FC (eds): *Essentials of Pediatric Intensive Care* St. Louis, Quality Medical Publishing, 1990; pp 869–873.
24. Roy J, Mc Nulty SE, Torjman MC: An improved nasal prong apparatus for end-tidal carbon dioxide monitoring in awake, sedated patients. *J Clin Monit* 1991; 7:249–252.
25. Ledingham IM, Hanning CD: Monitoring of ventilation, in Shoemaker WC, Thompson WL, Holbrook PR (eds): *Textbook of Critical Care*, ed 2. Philadelphia, WB Saunders Co, 1989, pp 201–215.
26. Murray JP, Modell JM: Early detection of endotracheal tube accidents by monitoring carbon dioxide concentration in respiratory gas. *Anesthesiol* 1983; 59:344–346.
27. Healey CJ, Fedullo AJ, Swinburn AJ, et al: Comparison of noninvasive measurements of carbon dioxide tension during withdrawal from mechanical ventilation. *Crit Care Med* 1987; 15:764–768.
28. Carroll GC: A continuous monitoring technique for management of acute pulmonary failure. *Chest* 1987; 92:467–469.
29. Nunn JF (ed): *Oxygen in Applied Respiratory Physiology*, ed 3. Cambridge, UK, Butterworth and Co, 1987, pp 235–283.
30. Fahey PJ, Harris K, Vanderward C: Clinical experience with continuous monitoring of mixed venous oxygen saturation in respiratory failure. *Chest* 1984; 86:748–752.
31. Prough DS, Scuderi PE: Monitoring considerations in 1990, in Lumb PD, Shoemaker WC (eds): *Critical Care: State of the Art*, ed 11. Fullerton, CA, Society of Critical Care Medicine, 1990, pp 271–300.
32. Rasanen J, Downs JB, Hodges MR: Continuous monitoring of gas exchange and oxygen use with dual oximetry. *J Clin Anesth* 1988; 1:3–8.
33. Scuderi PE, Harris LC, Brockschmidt JK: Clinical trial of a prototype dual oximeter. *Anesthesiol* 1989; 71:A374.
34. Moore EE: Nutritional considerations in critical care medicine: Observations from postinjury total enteral nutrition versus total parenteral nutrition, in Lumb PD, Shoemaker WC (eds): *Critical Care: State of the Art*, ed 11. Fullerton, CA, Society for Critical Care Medicine, 1990, pp 33–57.
35. Ultman JS, Bursztein S: Analysis of error in the determination of respiratory gas exchange at varying FiO2. *J Appl Physiol* 1981; 50:210–216.
36. Shayevitz JR, Weissman C: Nutrition and metabolism in the critically ill child, in Rogers MC (ed): *Textbook of Pediatric Intensive Care*. Baltimore, Williams and Wilkins, 1987, pp 943–978.
37. Bartlett RH, Dechert RE, Mault JR, et al: Measurement of metabolism and multiple organ failure. *Surgery* 1982; 92:771–779.
38. Eisenberg JD, Wall MA: Pulmonary function testing in children. *Clin Chest Med* 1987; 8:661–667.
39. Hsu KHK, Jenkins DE, Hsi BP, et al: Ventilatory functions of normal children and young adults: Mexican-American, white and black. I. Spirometry. *J Pediatr* 1979; 95:14–23.
40. Dockery D, Berkey C, Ware J, et al: Distribution of forced vital capacity and forced expiratory volume in 1 second in children 6 to 11 years of age. *Am Rev Respir Dis* 1983; 128:405–412.
41. Antonio-Santiago MT, Clutario BC: Pulmonary function testing, in Scarpelli EM (ed): *Pulmonary Physiology: Fetus, Newborn, Child, and Adolescent*, ed 2. Philadelphia, Lea and Febiger, 1990, pp 446–472.
42. Godfrey S, Bar-Yishay E, Arad I, et al: Flow-volume curves in infants with lung disease. *Pediatr* 1982; 72:517–522.
43. Taussig LM, Landau LI, Godfrey S: Determinants of forced expiratory flows in newborn infants. *J Appl Physiol* 1982; 53:1220—1227.
44. McBride JT, Wohl MEB: Pulmonary function tests. *Ped Clin North Am* 1979; 26:537—551.

45. GAP Conference Committee, Cystic Fibrosis Foundation. Standardization of lung function testing in children. *J Pediatr* 1980; 97:668–676.
46. Andreou A, Keh E, Bhat R, et al: Critical care problems in the newborn: CVC in infants on assisted ventilation. *Crit Care Med* 1980; 8:291–293.
47. Dolfin T, Duffty P, Wilkes DL, et al: Calibration of respiratory induction plethysmography in infants. *Am Rev Respir Dis* 1982; 126:577–579.
48. Tabachnik E, Muller N, Toye B, et al: Measurement of ventilation in children using the respiratory inductive plethysmograph. *J Pediatr* 1981; 99:895–899.
49. Streiter RM, Lynch JP: Complications in the ventilated patient. *Clin Chest Med* 1988; 9:127–139.
50. Zwillich CW, Pierson DJ, Creagh CE, et al: Complications of assisted ventilation. *Am J Med* 1974; 57:161–170.
51. Chatburn RL: Evaluation of pediatric pulmonary function: Theory and application. *Respir Care* 1989; 34:597–608.
52. Stocks J, Nothen U, Sutherland P, et al: Improved accuracy of the occlusion technique for assessing total respiratory compliance in infants. *Pediatr Pulmonol* 1987; 3:71–77.
53. National Institutes of Health Consensus Development Conference on Infantile Apnea and Home Monitoring. September 29 to October 1, 1986: Consensus Statement. *Pediatrics* 1987; 79:292–299.
54. Brooks JG: Sudden infant death syndrome and apparent life threatening events, in Levin DL, Morriss FC (eds): *Essentials of Pediatric Intensive Care*, St. Louis, Quality Medical Publishing, Inc, 1990, pp 262–266.
55. Southall DP, Richards JM, DeSwiet M, et al: Infancy: Evaluation of predictive importance of prolonged apnoea and disorders of cardiac rhythm or conduction. *BMJ* 1983; 286:1092–1096.
56. Weese-Mayer DE, Morrow AS, Conway LP, et al: Assessing clinical significance of apnea exceeding fifteen seconds with event recording. *J Pediatr* 1990; 117:568–574.
57. Loughlin GM, Carroll JL: Sudden unexplained death and apparent life threatening events, in: Frank Oski (ed): *Principles and Practice of Pediatrics*. Philadelphia, JB Lippincott Co, 1990, pp 972–981.
58. Guntheroth WG, Lohmann R, Spiers PS: Risk of sudden infant death syndrome in subsequent siblings. *J Pediatr* 1990; 116:520–524.
59. Waggener TB, Southall DP, Scott LA: Analysis of breathing patterns in a prospective population of term infants does not predict susceptibility to sudden infant death syndrome. *Pediatr Res* 1990; 27:113–117.
60. Wetzel RC: Shock, in Rogers MC (ed): *Textbook of Pediatric Intensive Care*. Baltimore, Williams and Wilkins, 1987, pp 483–524.
61. Chinuanga HM, Smith JM: Modified Doppler flow detector probe: An aid to percutaneous radial artery cannulation in infants and small children. *Anaesthesia* 1979; 50:256–258.
62. Wetzel RC, Rogers MC: Pediatric monitoring, in Shoemaker WC, Thompson WL, Holbrook PR (eds): *Textbook of Critical Care*, ed 2. Philadelphia, WB Saunders Co, 1989, pp 215–222.
63. Fields AI: Invasive hemodynamic monitoring in children. *Clin Chest Med* 1987; 4:611–633.
64. Lake CL: Monitoring of the pediatric cardiac patient, in Lake CL (ed): *Pediatric Cardiac Anesthesia*. Norwalk, CT, Appleton and Lange, 1988, pp 87–120.
65. Toro-Figueroa LO, Hammond KA: Venous access, in Levin DL, Morriss FC (eds): *Essentials of Pediatric Intensive Care*. St. Louis, Quality Medical Publishing, Inc, 1990, pp 800–817.
66. Aldridge HE, Jay AWL: Central venous catheters and heart perforation. *Can Med Assoc J* 1986; 135:1082–1084.
67. Agarwal KC, Ali Khan MA, Falla A, et al: Cardiac perforation from central venous catheters: Survival after cardiac tamponade in an infant. *Pediatrics* 1984; 73:333–338.
68. Katz RW, Pollack MM, Weibley RE: Pulmonary artery catheterization in pediatric intensive care. *Adv Pediatr* 1984; 30:169–190.

69. Moodie DS, Feldt RH, Kaye MP, et al: Measurement of post operative cardiac output by thermodilution in pediatric and adult patients. *J Thorac Cardiovasc Surg* 1979; 78:796–798.

70. Tabata BK, Kirsch JR, Rogers MC: Diagnostic tests and technology for pediatric intensive care, in Rogers MC (ed): *Textbook of Pediatric Intensive Care.* Baltimore, Williams and Wilkins, 1987, pp 1401–1431.

71. Falicov RE, Resnekov L: Relationship of the pulmonary artery end-diastolic and mean filling pressures in patients with and without left ventricular dysfunction. *Circulation* 1970; 42:65–73.

72. Forrester JS, Ganz W, et al: Thermodilution cardiac output determination with a single flow-directed catheter. *Am Heart J* 1972; 83:306–311.

73. Swan HJ, Ganz W: Measurement of right atrial and pulmonary arterial pressures and cardiac output: Clinical application of hemodynamic monitoring. *Adv Intern Med* 1982; 27:453–473.

74. Moodie DS, Feldt RH, Kaye MP, et al: Measurement of cardiac output by thermodilution: Development of accurate measurements at flow applicable to the pediatric patient. *J Surg Res* 1978; 25:305–311.

75. Freed MD, Keane JF: Cardiac output measured by thermodilution in infants and children. *J Pediatr* 1978; 92:39–42.

76. Light JK, Pollack MM, Rivera O, et al: Effect of malposition of catheter site in cardiac output determination (abstract). *Crit Care Med* 1981; 9:286.

77. Elliot CG, Zimmermann GA, Clemmer TP: Complications of pulmonary artery catherization in the care of critically ill patients: A prospective study. *Chest* 1979; 76:647–652.

78. Toro-Figueroa LO, Craft M, Morris-Copeland M, et al: Swan-Ganz pulmonary artery catheters and left atrial catheters, in Levin DL, Morriss FC (eds): *Essentials of Pediatric Intensive Care.* St. Louis, Quality Medical Publishing, Inc, 1990, pp 834–844.

79. Kumar A, Minagoe S, Thangathurai D, et al: Noninvasive measurement of cardiac output during surgery using a new continuous-wave Doppler esophageal probe. *Am J Cardiol* 1989; 64:793–798.

80. Fripp RR, Berman W: Noninvasive assessment of cardiopulmonary function in critically ill infants and children. *Clin Chest Med* 1987; 619–633.

81. Tremper KK: Continuous noninvasive cardiac output: Are we getting there? *Crit Care Med* 1987; 15:278–279.

82. Introna RPS, Pruett JK, Crumrine RC, et al: Use of transthoracic bioimpedance to determine cardiac output in pediatric patients. *Crit Care Med* 1988; 16:1101–1105.

83. Bernstein DP: Continuous noninvasive real-time monitoring of stroke volume and cardiac output by thoracic electrical bioimpedance. *Crit Care Med* 1986; 14:898–901.

84. Appel PL, Kram HB, Mackabee J, et al: Comparison of measurements of cardiac output by bioimpedance and thermodilution in severely ill surgical patients. *Crit Care Med* 1986; 14:380.

85. Alverson DC, Eldridge M, Dillon T, et al: Noninvasive pulsed Doppler determination of cardiac output in neonates and children. *J Pediatr* 1982; 101:46–50.

86. Notterman DA, Castello FV, Steinberg C, et al: A comparison of thermodilution and pulsed Doppler cardiac output measurement in critically ill children. *J Pediatr* 1989; 115:554–560.

Chapter 21

Monitoring in Adult Critical Care

Carlos A. Vaz Fragoso, M.D.

INTRODUCTION

Attainment of an appropriate acid-base status and oxygen delivery (Do_2) is the hallmark of patient management in adult critical care. Reaching these goals ensures aerobic cellular metabolism and, thereby, prevents organ system dysfunction. The respiratory system, by virtue of its capacity to oxygenate mixed venous blood and to eliminate carbon dioxide (CO_2), plays an integral role in maintaining euphemia and adequate tissue oxygenation. Any significant derangement in the respiratory system will, therefore, potentially interfere with life-sustaining cellular metabolism and requires early intervention.

The two major types of respiratory system dysfunction in the adult critical care unit are hypercapneic respiratory failure and hypoxemic respiratory failure.[1] These are directly or indirectly associated with acidotic states and/or diminished Do_2. By directly assessing a patient's ventilatory and oxygenation capacity, respiratory monitoring will allow the identification of the various features of hypercapneic and hypoxemic respiratory failure. This, in turn, provides a rational basis for intervention and for the determination of subsequent clinical responses. This chapter outlines the relationships between the pathophysiology of respiratory failure and available, clinically applicable respiratory monitoring. Special emphasis is placed on the mechanically ventilated patient.

HYPERCAPNEIC RESPIRATORY FAILURE

By regulating the arterial CO_2 tension ($Paco_2$), the respiratory system contributes to the maintenance of a physiologic acid-base status and, indirectly, arterial O_2 tensions. Disease states that are associated with a rise in the $Paco_2$ will lead to tissue acidemia and hypoxemia.

Likewise, inappropriate ventilatory compensation for either a metabolic acidosis or alkalosis will result in disproportionate changes in pH relative to conditions where there is only an isolated metabolic derangement. Utimately, the $Paco_2$ level is a consequence of the level of alveolar ventilation ($\dot{V}_A$; minute ventilation, which is involved in actual gas exchange) relative to CO_2 production ($\dot{V}co_2$)[2]:

$$Paco_2 = K\ \dot{V}co_2/\dot{V}_A \qquad (21-1)$$

$$K = Constant$$

Equation (1) suggests that in order to maintain an appropriate CO_2 homeostasis, $\dot{V}co_2$ at any absolute level must necessarily be matched by changes in $\dot{V}_A$. The latter, in turn, is limited by the absolute levels of minute ventilation ($\dot{V}_E$) and the dead-space ratio (V_D/V_T; reflects the fraction of the tidal volume that does not participate in gas exchange). This is outlined in the derivation[3] of Equation (3):

$$
\begin{aligned}
\dot{V}_E &= \dot{V}_A + \dot{V}_D & (21-2)\\
\dot{V}_A &= \dot{V}_E - \dot{V}_D \\
\dot{V}_A &= \dot{V}_E\ (1 - \dot{V}_D/\dot{V}_E) \\
\dot{V}_A &= \dot{V}_E\ (1 - [V_D \times f]/[V_T \times f]) \\
\dot{V}_A &= \dot{V}_E\ (1 - V_D/V_T) \\
Paco_2 &= K\ \dot{V}co_2/\dot{V}_E(1 - V_D/V_T) & (21-3)
\end{aligned}
$$

The argument is thus put forth that in hypercapneic respiratory failure an understanding of the factors that influence CO_2 homeostasis, namely, $\dot{V}co_2$, $\dot{V}_E$, and V_D/V_T, will by and large determine the respiratory monitoring needs. The physiologic basis of this is summarized in Table 21–1.

$Paco_2$

Pathophysiology

The goal of the ventilatory pump is to maintain an appropriate $Paco_2$. Derangements in ventilatory function may reveal themselves as an elevation in the $Paco_2$. Identifying such a rise, therefore, is crucial to the diagnosis and management of hypercapneic respiratory failure. The population at risk would be any patient presenting with a significant degree of dyspnea and/or progressive lethargy.

It needs to be emphasized, however, that an abnormal $Paco_2$ may be a late phenomenon in the events that lead to hypercapneic respiratory failure. That is, a normal $Paco_2$ would not necessarily exclude the presence of a potentially limiting V_D/V_T, $\dot{V}co_2$, and/or $\dot{V}_E$. This is especially true in the mechanically ventilated patient. For this reason, other indicators are available that can reflect early deterioration without necessarily having an abnormal $Paco_2$.

TABLE 21–1.
Physiologic Basis of Hypercapneic Respiratory Failure

Parameter	Clinical Setting
I. Increased V_{CO_2}	Excessive CHO supplementation, metabolic acidosis, increased metabolism (e.g., sepsis, trauma, burns)
II. Increased V_D/V_T	COPD, PPH, PE, pulmonary vasculitis, PPV, shallow breathing pattern (e.g., muscle weakness)
III. V_E (reduced or nonsustainable) a. Reduced central drive	Obesity-hypoventilation syndrome, CNS disorders (see text), metabolic alkalosis, hypothyroidism, CO_2 narcosis, severe hypoxemia, malnutrition, myopathies, respiratory muscle and central fatigue, sedating drugs, hypothermia
b. Increased central drive	Hyperventilation syndrome, fever, pain, drugs, hyperthyroidism, myopathies, hypoxemia, metabolic acidosis, CNS disorders (see text), increased respiratory impedance
c. Increased respiratory impedance	Resistance . . . . . . COPD, asthma, secretions, tracheal stenosis, foreign body, extrinsic airway compression, small-sized endotracheal tube
	Elastance . . . . chest wall trauma or burns, pleural effusions, pulmonary edema, pneumonia, interstitial lung disease
d. Reduced respiratory muscle capacity	Malnutrition, neuromyopathies, metabolic disorders (see text), muscle fatigue

Monitoring

Table 21–2 summarizes the available monitoring systems for the evaluation of $Paco_2$ levels. These include direct measurements of arterial CO_2 tension, transcutaneous CO_2, and capnometry. The most accurate is arterial blood gases (ABGs), either by a single stick or through an indwelling arterial catheter. The latter is recommended if more than four ABGs are anticipated over a 24-hour period. The disadvantage of such a monitoring system is its invasiveness, potential for vascular damage, lack of continuous data, and the possibility of catheter contamination, colonization, and/or sepsis.

Transcutaneous CO_2 ($Ptcco_2$) measurements utilize a miniaturized blood gas electrode, which is placed on the skin. Although continuous and noninvasive, they are technically problematic (warm-up time, elaborate setup, surface burns, limited in low perfusion states) and do not provide a real-time sequence. These are usually not employed in the adult intensive care unit (ICU).

Capnometry involves the measurement of end-tidal CO_2 ($Petco_2$) by the spectrophotometric analysis of exhaled gas.[4] It is achieved in one of two ways—*mainstream analysis* describes the analysis of exhaled gas at the airway while *sidestream* utilizes a capillary tube to extract a small sample of the exhaled gas. Although technically less demanding than the $Ptcco_2$, these systems also have some significant limitations. Sidestream analysis is limited by the delay in actual sampling relative to data presentation and by its capillary tube being easily occluded by

TABLE 21–2.
Monitoring Basis of Hypercapnic Respiratory Failure—Pa_{CO_2}, V_{CO_2}, V_D/V_T

Parameter	Monitor	Patient Population	Advantages	Disadvantages
I. Pa_{CO_2}	ABGs	Respiratory distress	Most accurate	Invasive
	$V_E \times Pa_{CO_2}$	Change in mental status	Assess severity	Possible vessel damage
	Pet_{CO_2} (main or sidestream)	Abnormal central drive but stable cardiopulmonary status	Noninvasive; Continuous data	May underestimate Pa_{CO_2}; Misleading in lung disease
	Ptc_{CO_2}	Abnormal central drive but stable cardiopulmonary status	Noninvasive; Continuous data	Technically problematic; Not real time
II. V_{CO_2}	Indirect calorimetry	Catabolic states (e.g., trauma, burns); Poor respiratory reserve (COPD); Long-term nutritional support	Substrate utilization; Metabolic stress; V_D/V_T	Expensive; Requires skill; Requires F_{IO_2} <60%; Requires steady state
	Harris-Benedict	Catabolic states (e.g., trauma, burns); Poor respiratory reserve (COPD); Long-term nutritional support	Inexpensive; No instrumentation	? accuracy in the ICU; No V_D/V_T; No substrate patterns
	PA line derived data	Catabolic states (e.g., trauma, burns); Poor respiratory reserve (COPD); Long-term nutritional support	F_{IO_2} not a limitation; Steady state not required	No V_D/V_T; No substrate patterns; Invasive
	24-hr UUN	Catabolic states (e.g., trauma, burns); Poor respiratory reserve (COPD); Long-term nutritional support	Nitrogen balance; F_{IO_2} not a limitation; Steady state not required; No instrumentation	? accuracy in the ICU
III. V_D/V_T	Indirect calorimetry	Ventilator dependence	Measures Pet_{CO_2}	See above
	Douglas bag	Ventilator dependence	Measures Pet_{CO_2}	Requires mass spectrometer
	Pet_{CO_2}	Ventilator dependence	Not time-consuming	Variable accuracy

moisture. Mainstream analysis avoids some of these difficulties but requires bulky equipment and some degree of tourque being applied on the artificial airway. The technical quality of these systems can be substantially improved with capnography. This device not only measures the $Petco_2$ but also displays a waveform. This allows one to assess the validity of the $Petco_2$ by inspecting the quality of the waveform.

Regardless of the method employed, the major difficulty with capnometry is that it may be an inaccurate estimate of $Paco_2$ trends, even after determining a baseline $Paco_2$ − $Petco_2$ (Fig 21–1).[5] This may be due to changes in the level of $\dot{V}E$ and/or VD/VT. Unfortunately, in most adult critical care units, this is a frequent problem. There may be, however, a role for such monitoring in the neurosurgical ICU or in the perioperative period. These situations lend themselves to the occurrence of an abnormal central drive with a stable cardiopulmonary status and/or a need for continuous data analysis.

Other putative roles for capnometry include monitoring during cardiac arrest ($Petco_2$ may be proportionate to cardiac output if ventilation remains constant) and in the detection of esophageal intubation. Such an efficacy in the clinical setting remains to be proven.

CO_2 Production

Pathophysiology

Under steady-state conditions, changes in the level of $\dot{V}co_2$ will predominantly reflect changes in cellular respiration and bicarbonate buffering. The former varies with the degree of metabolic stress and/or substrate utilization, while the latter varies with the rate of acid production and/or clearance. These issues are summarized in Table 21–1.

In the ICU, there is considerable variation in the degree of metabolic stress to which a given patient may be exposed. In those with burns, trauma, or sepsis, extremely high levels of metabolic rates and, therefore, CO_2 flux, are often achieved.[6] This is particularly significant when these patients are in the flow or catabolic phase of injury.

Inappropriate nutritional supplementation in the critically ill patient may result in severe ventilatory problems.[7,8] When excessive, for example, it is often associated with a marked change in cellular metabolism that results in a characteristic pattern of substrate utilization. This includes a predominance of carbohydrate utilization with gas exchange evidence of a net lipogenic state. The result is a potentially ventilatory limiting increase in CO_2 flux and metabolic derangements. Figure 21–2 details such an example.[7] In contrast, when nutrition is inadequate, it may be associated with progressive decline in respiratory muscle function due to a loss of diaphragmatic mass.[9] The result is a potential decline in the ability of the respiratory muscles to generate appropriate levels of $\dot{V}E$.

Increased acid accumulation requiring bicarbonate buffering is a common complication in the ICU. The lactic acidosis of the sepsis syndrome is such an example, with its increased level of bicarbonate buffering leading to large increases in the CO_2 flux. Magnifying the problem is the direct stimulus of the central and peripheral chemoreceptors by an acidotic pH. The latter being not only a result of an increase in acid production but also due to a reduction in acid clearance. which is primarily due to the frequent occurrence of impaired renal function in this type of a patient population.

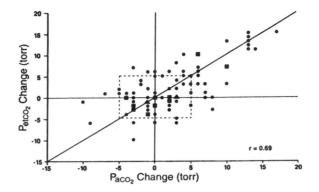

FIG 21–1.

The relationship between the change in Petco$_2$ and the change in Paco$_2$ in 113 data sets. The diagonal line is the line of identity. Solid squares represent two data points with the same value. Those values within the data box represent a change of ±5 mm Hg. Note that data points in the left upper and right lower quadrants represent data sets in which Paco$_2$ and Petco$_2$ changed opposite directions. (*From Hess D, Schlotlag A, Levin B, et al: An evaluation of the usefulness of end-tidal PCO2 to aid weaning from mechanical ventilation following cardiac surgery. Respir Care 1991; 36:837–843. Used by permission.*)

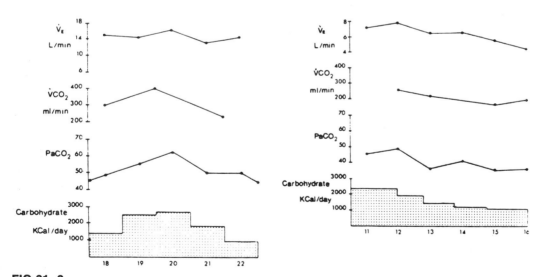

FIG 21–2.

Physiologic data from two patients showing the relation of carbohydrate loading in kilocalories per day and changes in minute ventilation (V̇E), carbon dioxide production (V̇co$_2$), and arterial carbon dioxide (Paco$_2$). All patients had an increase in carbon dioxide production and arterial Pco$_2$ with increasing carbohydrate load, despite no change or an increase in minute ventilation. The opposite was true when carbohydrate calories were decreased. (*From Covelli HD, Black JW, Olsen MS, Beekman JF. Respiratory failure precipitated by high carbohydrate loads. Annals of Internal Medicine 1981; 95:579–581. Used by permission.*)

The common denominator in these various processes is that increases in $\dot{V}_{CO_2}$ will lead to proportional increases in $\dot{V}_A$ such that appropriate CO_2 homeostasis is maintained. This, however, may have far reaching consequences. This is based on the clinical observation that levels of $\dot{V}_E$ exceeding 10 L/min are often associated with a poor outcome when weaning patients from mechanical ventilation.[10] Since an increase in CO_2 flux leads to an increase in ventilatory needs, it follows that the $\dot{V}_{CO_2}$ may become a limiting factor in ventilator weaning, as well as precipitating hypercapneic respiratory failure. Patients especially at risk are those unable to increase proportionally or maintain the elevation in $\dot{V}_A$. These include those with a blunted central neuroinspiratory drive, elevated V_D/V_T, increased respiratory system impedance, and/or diminished respiratory muscle capacity. By measuring $\dot{V}_{CO_2}$ levels, one may intervene to prevent such a scenario. This may include treating the underlying metabolic stress, appropriate adjustment of nutritional support, and promotion of adequate Do_2—all of which could result in a decrease in $\dot{V}_{CO_2}$ and the level of acidosis, thereby lowering the levels of $\dot{V}_A$.

Monitoring

A variety of methods may be employed to assess some of the issues related to CO_2 production (Table 21–2). At the present time, $\dot{V}_{CO_2}$ is most often measured by indirect calorimetry.[11] (see Chapter 13). This utilizes analysis of inspired and expired CO_2 fractions together with pneumotachygraph measurements of $\dot{V}_E$. Most modern metabolic carts will reliably and accurately measure $\dot{V}_{CO_2}$ and have made the Douglas bag method largely obsolete. Certain technical limitations, however, must be understood. These would include the following[11–13]: A stable fractional inspired oxygen concentration of less than 60%; appropriate analysis and calibration of standard gas mixtures; avoidance of leaks and mixing of inspired and expired gases; and at least a 10-minute period of steady-state conditions such that the $\dot{V}_{CO_2}$ measured at the mouth corresponds to cellular respiration and not to abrupt changes in $\dot{V}_E$ or *pro re nata* ICU analgesia/sedation. [Steady-state conditions refer to less than 5% variation in the respiratory quotient (RQ) and $\dot{V}_{CO_2}$ and less than 10% variation in the $\dot{V}_{O_2}$.] A normal level of $\dot{V}_{CO_2}$ under resting, nonstressed, and steady-state conditions is in the range of 200 cc/min.

Given that the $\dot{V}_{O_2}$ is concurrently measured with the $\dot{V}_{CO_2}$, indirect calorimetry also allows the determination of the respiratory exchange ratio (RQ = $\dot{V}_{CO_2}/\dot{V}_{O_2}$) and the resting energy expenditure (REE; as determined by the Weir formula)[11]:

$$RQ = (3.9\ \dot{V}_{O_2} + 1.1\ \dot{V}_{CO_2})\ 1.44 \tag{21–4}$$

if a 24-hour urine urea nitrogen is available:

$$RQ = (3.9\ \dot{V}_{O_2} + 1.1\ \dot{V}_{CO_2})\ 1.44 - 2.17\ (24\text{-HrUN}) \tag{21–5}$$

When measured under steady-state conditions, these will also reflect substrate utilization. For example, an RQ value greater than 1.0 when associated with an actual total caloric intake to REE ratio greater than 1.0 is very suggestive of a net lipogenic state, i.e., excessive CHO supplementation.[14] Such an analysis adds diagnostic depth to interpretations of $\dot{V}co_2$ levels without any added testing.

As described later in this chapter, a measurement of the patient's Vd/Vt may also be accomplished by indirect calorimetry when the $Paco_2$ is concurrently determined. Since the Vd/Vt is an important factor in determining the degree to which $\dot{V}a$ may augment, this broadens the utility of indirect calorimetry without necessarily complicating its monitoring requirements.

No widely accepted recommendations are available as to the frequency and patient population that should undergo indirect calorimetry. Clinical experience would dictate that in those patients who have borderline ventilatory capacity, either from preexisting chronic lung disease and/or subsequent to an acute injury, and who require levels of $\dot{V}e$ greater than or equal to 10 L/min, an indirect calorimetry study should be performed to assess the $\dot{V}co_2$, RQ, REE, and Vd/Vt. These will allow a determination of the extent to which there may be a metabolic stress, inappropriate substrate utilization, confirmation of significant increases in the bicarbonate buffering of acid, and the degree of wasted ventilation (Vd/Vt). As to the frequency of testing, it is proposed that unexpected deteriorations in the ventilatory capacity or major changes in the nutritional prescription be the determinants as to when indirect calorimetry should be performed.

Alternatives to indirect calorimetry are few and limited. For monitoring energy expenditure (EE), these include pulmonary arterial (PA) line derived data,[15] 24-hour urine urea nitrogen (24-HrUN) determinations, and the Harris-Benedict (HB) predictive equations. The advantage of a PA line is that EE may be reliably determined at Fio_2 levels greater than 50%. The disadvantages are that it is an invasive procedure that also requires arterial and mixed venous blood sampling and that it assumes an RER of 0.85:

$$EE = (CO)(Hb)(Sao_2 - Svo_2) \tag{21-6}$$

where CO = cardiac output, Hb = hemoglobin, and Sao_2, Svo_2 = arterial and mixed venous O_2 saturations, respectively.

The 24-HrUN is of importance in determining whether a patient is in positive nitrogen balance, but it only roughly estimates the EE. This is in part due to assumptions that protein-related kilocalories represent 12% of the total required amount, that 24-hr urine collections are accurate, that insensible nitrogen losses are equivalent to 4 g/day, and that the urine urea nitrogen is representative of the total nitrogen excretion:

$$EE = [(24\text{-}HrUN + 4)(6.25)(4)]/0.12 \tag{21-7}$$

$$6.25 \text{ g protein/nitrogen}$$

$$4 \text{ kcal/g protein}$$

The HB predictive equations in the ICU are not accurate since they rely on assigned stress factors, which are subjectively determined and which have been shown to correlate poorly with the REE[16:]

$$\text{BEE (males)} = 13.7 \text{ Wt} + 5.0 \text{ Ht} + 66 - 6.8 \text{ Age} \tag{21-8}$$

$$\text{BEE (females)} = 9.6 \text{ Wt} + 1.7 \text{ Ht} + 655 - 4.7 \text{ Age} \tag{21-9}$$

where BEE = basal energy expenditure, Wt = weight, and Ht = height. Regardless of the alternative to indirect calorimetry, direct measurements of the $\dot{V}_{CO_2}$, $\dot{V}_{O_2}$, RQ, and V_D/V_T are not determined with these methods. These may be crucial in assessing the degree of CO_2 flux, pattern of substrate utilization, and the effectiveness of gas exchange.

Dead-Space Ratio

Pathophysiology
A second factor affecting the physiological relationship between CO_2 homeostasis and alveolar ventilation is what amount of a given tidal breath does not participate in gas exchange, i.e., dead-space (ventilation without perfusion).[2] Under normal conditions, most of the dead-space is due to anatomic dead-space, which accounts for approximately 150 cc in the average 70-kg man. This includes all the airways proximal to, and including, the terminal bronchioles. In conditions that cause progressive reductions in the pulmonary capillary bed,[2] the amount of dead-space will far exceed that which is ascribed to the anatomic dead-space and is termed the physiologic dead-space, V_D/V_T.

It is understood that for any given level of $\dot{V}_E$, the higher the V_D/V_T, the lower the $\dot{V}_A$ and, subsequently, the higher the CO_2 tension. This is on the basis that a component of the $\dot{V}_E$, the dead-space ventilation ($\dot{V}_D$), does not participate in gas exchange. The subsequent physiologic response to the elevated V_D/V_T may take two distinct paths. One is an elevation in the ventilatory output in order to restore the appropriate level of $\dot{V}_A$ for that degree of CO_2 flux and, thereby, avoid a respiratory acidosis. The trade-off is that the patient who has a blunted central respiratory drive or respiratory muscle dysfunction, with or without limiting respiratory impedance, will not be able either to generate or sustain such an increase in $\dot{V}_E$. As previously discussed, this is especially problematic in levels of $\dot{V}_E$ greater than 10 L/min and in clinical situations associated with an elevated $\dot{V}_{CO_2}$.

The second path is characterized by a resetting of the CO_2 setpoint to higher tensions, i.e., central fatigue. This may be due to the central respiratory controller responding to feedback input from peripheral respiratory muscle receptors that indicate a fatiguing ventilatory pump. By accepting higher CO_2 tensions, the need for further increases in $\dot{V}_E$ is minimized. The end result may be a permissive level of respiratory acidosis but with levels of $\dot{V}_E$ that may be more sustainable due to a reduction in respiratory muscle load.

Regardless of the chosen path, the ultimate physiologic consequences of an increase in dead-space will be some degree of respiratory-induced acidosis and respiratory muscle fatigue. This may become limiting if the cause of the elevated V_D/V_T is progressive or magnified by increases in $\dot{V}_{CO_2}$. Note that dead-space ratios that exceed 0.60 are predictive of a failure to wean from mechanical ventilation.[10] This is for reasons similar to those outlined earlier.

Clinically significant causes of elevated V_D/V_T are by and large due to reductions in the pulmonary vascular bed, which are considered disproportionate to any coexisting reductions in alveolar volume. These include the following; chronic obstructive pulmonary disease (COPD) with or without hypoxemia; primary pulmonary hypertension (PPH); pulmonary thromboembolism (PE); pulmonary vasculitis; chronic alveolar hypoxia secondary to sleep apnea, interstitial lung disease, or COPD; congenital heart disease with Eisenmenger physiology; acidosis, especially when in combination with hypoxemia; and positive pressure ventilation (PPV) with or without auto-PEEP in a patient with coexisting lung disease such as COPD. These lead to reductions in pulmonary perfusion by a combination of an increase in pulmonary vascular resistance, destruction, or remodeling, and/or by a decreae in right ventricular systolic function.

An increase in V_D/V_T may also be achieved through a patient's breathing pattern. Shallow breaths with a high respiratory rate (f) but small V_T will increase the V_D/V_T ratio without any absolute increases in the physiologic or anatomic dead-space. It is unlikely that by itself this will lead to a respiratory acidosis but in the setting of severe respiratory muscle dysfunction, reduced static compliance, or an elevation in $\dot{V}_{CO_2}$, an increase in CO_2 tension may develop.

In summary, increases in V_D/V_T will result in an increase in $\dot{V}_E$ in order to preserve an adequate $\dot{V}_A$. By monitoring the V_D/V_T, its contribution to a patient's elevated $\dot{V}_E$ may be assessed. Both interventional and prognostic decisions may then be subsequently determined. These will certainly be affected by the etiology underlying the increase in V_D/V_T. Unfortunately, when established, most are irreversibly or poorly responsive to therapy.

Monitoring

Several approaches may be undertaken to determine the level of dead-space ventilation (Table 21–2). The most clinically accurate technique is by the modified Bohr method[2]:

$$V_D/V_T = (Pa_{CO_2} - P_{\overline{E}CO_2})/Pa_{CO_2} \qquad (21-10)$$

This requires arterial sampling (ideally with an arterial line in place) for the Pa_{CO_2} and either indirect calorimetry or a Douglas bag for the mean expired CO_2 tension ($P_{\overline{E}CO_2}$).

Noninvasive estimates of V_D/V_T rely on the diference between the end-tidal CO_2 (Pet_{CO_2}) and the P_{CO_2}. The basis for this is that the Pet_{CO_2} approximates the alveolar CO_2 tension, which, in turn, is assumed to approximate the Pa_{CO_2}. This may be relatively accurate in patients without significant lung disease, but in those with such a disease this noninvasive method becomes inaccurate either as an absolute value or as a reflection of a trend in dead-space changes, i.e., the Pet_{CO_2} will not be equivalent to the Pa_{CO_2}.

It may be argued that if an elevation in $\dot{V}_E$ is required to maintain appropriate CO_2 homeostasis and if there is no clinical predisposition to an increase in $\dot{V}_{CO_2}$, it can be safely deduced that the patient has an abnormal V_D/V_T without necessarily relying on the above monitoring. This may be true, but, often enough, problems in the medical ICU tend to be multifactorial and require an assessment of the predominant factor. This is of special importance in the patient at risk for hypercapneic respiratory failure.

Total Minute Ventilation (V_e)

Pathophysiology

To this point our discussion has been limited to the two major causes of an elevated $\dot{V}_E$, namely, the $\dot{V}_{CO_2}$ and V_D/V_T. These factors are important in that they assign the level of stress under which the ventilatory pump must operate. Brief references have already been made to the consequences of excessive levels of $\dot{V}_{CO_2}$ and V_D/V_T driving $\dot{V}_E$ beyond that of 10 L/min. Such levels of $\dot{V}_E$ may not be achievable or sustainable due to abnormalities in respiratory muscle capacity, respiratory impedance, and/or central respiratory drive. The following section discusses such issues.

Central Respiratory Drive

Pathophysiology

An appropriate response to increases in CO_2 flux or V_D/V_T is in part dependent on an intact central respiratory controller. If the central controller has a blunted response, the $\dot{V}_A$ may be inadequate and the result is a respiratory acidosis. Likewise, an accentuated respiratory drive yields levels of $\dot{V}_A$ that may be adequate but which could result in an overburdened ventilatory pump.

A blunted central respiratory drive may be associated with a variety of factors. These would include the following: obesity-hypoventilation syndrome; CNS-associated disorders such as encephalitis, cerebrovascular disease, and structural lesions; hypothyroidism; metabolic alkalosis; CO_2 narcosis; severe hypoxemia; malnutrition; myopathies; respiratory muscle fatigue; hypothermia; and a variety of sedating drugs such as opioids, benzodiazepenes, and barbiturates. It may also reflect the phenomenon of central fatigue. This is discussed at length in the section on respiratory muscle capacity. Briefly, it describes a reduction in central drive as a direct response to feedback input from a potentially fatiguing ventilatory pump. It results in permissive hypercapnia with a potential improvement in the sense of dyspnea, as well as lower levels of respiratory muscle load.

An accentuated central respiratory drive can occur in the following settings; hyperventilation syndrome, fever, pain, drugs (aspirin overdose, amphetamines, cocaine), hyperthyroidism, neuromyopathic disorders, hypoxemia, metabolic acidosis, and CNS-related disorders. It may also reflect the degree of inspiratory impedance, that is, when an elveated central drive is accompanied by a low muscle power output, it may be reflecting the degree of inspiratory impedance. The clinical significance of this type of elevation in central respiratory drive has not been overlooked. Recent work has suggested that levels of respiratory drive can be predictive of who will fail to wean from mechanical ventilation. These studies have shown that an elevation in central drive is strongly correlated with respiratory impedance and failure to wean[17–19] (Table 21–3).

In summary, the level of $\dot{V}_E$ that may be achieved or sustained by the ventilatory pump is partially dependent on the central respiratory controller. More often than not it reflects the effects of other limiting factors to the ventilatory response rather than being an isolated limiting abnormality. By monitoring central respiratory drive, important diagnostic and therapeutic information regarding hypercapneic respiratory failure may be obtained.

TABLE 21–3.
Clinical Efficacy of P100s and the OCB

Reference	Patient Population	Conclusion
17	$n = 11$; acute respiratory failure, marginal weaning candidates COPD (3), ARDS (2), drug OD (3), flail chest (2), sepsis (1)	P_{100} (CO_2)/P100 predicts weaning success 1.17 ± 0.03 (fail) vs 2.04 ± 0.25 (success)
18	$n = 12$; respiratory failure, COPD	P_{100} >6.0 predicts failure to wean V_T/T_I, T_I/T_{tot}, and HR—also of predictive value
19	$n = 16$; respiratory failure, COPD	P_{100} may reflect the likelihood of muscle fatigue P_{100} >6.0 in those who failed to wean $P_{100}/V_T/T_I$ ratio also useful as a predictor
26	$n = 20$; ventilator dependent	OCB correlated positively with total wean time; when the OCB as a fraction of V_{O_2} exceeded 10%, there was a prolonged weaning time
27	$n = 13$; cardiorespiratory disease	Inverse relationship between the FEV1 and the OCB
28	Case report—COPD with respiratory failure	Effect of mode of ventilation on the OCB

Monitoring

Few alternatives are available for the measurement of central respiratory drive (Table 21–4). Mouth occlusion pressures (P_{100}'s) have been shown to correlate with phrenic nerve activity and are thus considered to be a measure of central drive.[20–22] Monitors are currently available that are able to measure P_{100}s in a user-friendly and patient-comfortable setting. The pressure reported is the change in pressure during the first 100 ms of inspiration in response to a transient occlusion. The minimal latency period required for the patient to be aware of such an occlusion is 150 ms. A normal level for the P_{100}s at rest is in the 2 to 4 cm H_2O range.

The method of occlusion as well as the type of pressure measured varies depending on the protocol. The occlusion may be achieved by either an actual occlusion of the inspiratory limb or through the resistance generated by the opening of the demand valve of a ventilator (quasi-occlusive method.)[23] It has been my observation that patients appear more comfortable with the demand valve being the source of the transient occlusion rather than an actual occlusion of the inspiratory limb. This method, however, requires insertion of an esophageal balloon, but it also provides data to determine work of breathing. An alternative to the esophageal balloon in the determination of the P_{100}s involves the measurement of airway pressure. This may be achieved by a computer-based program that analyzes digitized airway pressures obtained subsequent to an occlusion of the inspiratory limb.[24] On the Servo ventilator, the latter is achieved by depressing the expiratory pause button, which leads to a closure of the inspiratory valve.[24]

The interpretation of P_{100}s must be tempered with the notion that several variables may secondarily affect central drive. Some of these include changes in functional residual capacity (FRC), positive end-expiratory pressure (PEEP), work of breathing (WOB), chemoreceptor input (CO_2 and O_2), and baseline, predisease levels of central drive.[18] Additionally, one should also be cognizant that to assess the clinical utility of the P_{100}s fully larger trials need to be undertaken to confirm their predictive value.

There are really no other clinically available alternatives to P_{100} measurements as indices of central drive. Direct measurement of phrenic nerve activity is cumbersome and is primarily a research tool. Although easily obtained, monitoring the $Petco_2$ or the level of $\dot{V}E$ relative to CO_2 flux will not necessarily reflect central drive. Peripheral problems would also affect such parameters and these would include respiratory muscle weakness and/or increases in VD/VT. In settings where the likelihood of lung disease is low but the risk of central hypoventilation is high, e.g., a neurosurgical unit, monitoring of the $Petco_2$ may be of some utility as an index of changes in respiratory drive and $Paco_2$. Transcutaneous measurements of Pco_2 have likewise been proposed but are technically inferior to the $Petco_2$ measurements even in this patient population. Regardless of the monitoring system employed, the limitations of these units must always be kept in mind when interpreting their data.

Respiratory Impedance

Pathophysiology

Respiratory impedance will to a significant extent determine whether or not the ventilatory pump will achieve and maintain a level of $\dot{V}E$ appropriate for CO_2 homeostasis. This is based on the evidence that the output and endurance of the respiratory muscles may be reduced

TABLE 21–4.
Monitoring Basis of Hypercapneic Respiratory Failure—V_E

Parameter	Monitor	Patient Population	Advantages	Disadvantages
IV. V_E				
a. Central drive	P_{100}	Ventilator dependence	Reflects impedanceReflects central drive	Expensive instrumentation
b. Impedance	C_{dyn}, C_{ES} (pressure-time curves)	Any ventilated patient	Reflects resistance Reflects elastance Easily obtained Noninvasive	None
	Raw	Any ventilated patient	Reflects resistance Noninvasive	None
	WOB	Ventilator dependence	Quantifies actual WOB Relatively noninvasive	May need balloons (WOBp)
	$P_{100}/V_T/T_I$	Ventilator dependence	Reflects impedance Relatively noninvasive	Requires instrumentation Doesn't distinguish impedance
	V_E/P_{100}	Ventilator dependence	Reflects impedance Relatively noninvasive	Requires instrumentation Doesn't distinguish impedance
	OCB	Ventilator dependence	Reflects impedance Relatively noninvasive	Requires instrumentation Doesn't distinguish impedance Affected by other variables

depending on the amount of impedance against which they must contract. This carries important clinical implications because hypercapneic respiratory failure is often accompanied by increases in respiratory system impedance, specifically elastance or resistance. The detection and treatment of such changes in impedance will thus play a major role in ensuring that the input of central drive equals the output of the respiratory muscles.

Impedance due to an increase in resistance may be due to several factors. These include bronchospasm, airway inflammation, secretions, foreign body in the airway, tracheal stenosis, extrinsic airway compression, and/or an inappropriately small endotracheal tube. In contrast, increases in elastance may be the result of such factors as chest wall trauma or burn (especially circumferential), pleural effusion or thickening, cardiogenic or noncardiogenic pulmonary edema, pneumonia, interstitial lung disease, and/or hyperinflation associated with air-trapping. By identifying and, subsequently, treating the specific type of impedance, the respiratory muscles may achieve and sustain the required level of $\dot{V}E$.

Monitoring

Markers of respiratory impedance include central respiratory drive, oxygen cost of breathing, and pressure-volume and pressure-flow relationships. Central respiratory drive as an index of impedance is determined by the level of the P_{100} relative to the respiratory muscle output. The latter is reflected by the VT/TI (inspiratory flow) and the $\dot{V}E$. The VT/TI is the major determinant of $\dot{V}E$, and, in essence, both are considered to be equivalent;

$$\dot{V}E = VT/TI \times TI/TTOT \qquad (21-11)$$

where $TI/Ttot$ = duty cycle, TI = inspiratory time, and $Ttot$ = total respiratory cycle time. Changes in the VT/TI or $\dot{V}E$ that are proportionate to changes in the P_{100} will, therefore, suggest that the inspiratory impedance is normal. In contrast, the higher the P_{100} relative to the VT/TI or $\dot{V}E$, the greater the impedance.[18, 25] [$\dot{V}E/P_{100}$ values <7 suggest a mechanical abnormality[25]; a $P_{100}/VT/TI$ ratio exceeding 11.7 during a T-piece wean are predictive of a failure to wean[18] (Fig 21–3).] Respiratory muscle weakness may similarly lead to higher P_{100} values relative to the VT/TI or $\dot{V}E$. By evaluating respiratory muscle strength, this factor can be accounted for easily. Unfortunately, what specific type of impedance is involved cannot be determined by this type of analysis.

Oxygen cost of breathing (OCB) has also been utilized as an index of respiratory impedance.[26–28] The principle behind this approach is that under steady-state conditions the level of oxygen consumption ($\dot{V}O_2$) reflects, in part, the energy expenditure and efficiency of all the forms of work performed by the respiratory muscles. Measurements of the work of breathing (WOB), for example, fail to include the isometric contraction component of the respiratory muscles. If all else remains stable, changes in $\dot{V}O_2$ may, therefore, reflect increases in all the various types of the WOB. Technically, the OCB is determined by comparing the $\dot{V}O_2$ during controlled mechanical ventilation versus the $\dot{V}O_2$ during spontaneous breaths. The difference is the OCB—a normal value corresponds to <5% of the $\dot{V}O_2$. When in excess of 15%, it becomes predictive of a failure to wean[10] (see also Table 21–3). Unfortunately, the critically ill patient is often unstable and, as a result, the $\dot{V}O_2$ is affected by several other factors unrelated to the WOB. Among these are oxygen delivery, oxygen extraction, and nutritionally related

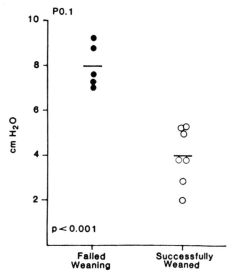

FIG 21–3.
Airway occlusion pressure ($P_{0.1}$ or P_{100}) during the immediate weaning period without assisted ventilation in patients who failed to wean and in those who were successfully weaned. (*Sassoon CSH, Te TT, Mahutte CK, et al: Airway occlusion pressure. An important indicator for successful weaning in patients with chronic obstructive pulmonary disease. Am Rev Respir Dis 1987; 135:107–113. Used by permission.*)

metabolic changes. This type of analysis is also unable to distinguish the specific type of impedance.

Identification of the specific type of respiratory impedance can only be determined by a pressure-volume analysis. The two major approaches to this analysis are compliance and WOB. Compliance refers to changes in volume relative to changes in pressure:

$$\text{Compliance} = \Delta V / \Delta P \qquad (21\text{--}12)$$

The change in volume being the expired V_T and the change in pressure depending on whether the measurements are being made under static (flow absent) or dynamic conditions (flow present), as well as on the level of total PEEP:

$$C_{dyn} = V_T / (P_{I}P - PEEP_t) \qquad (21\text{--}13)$$

$$C_{ES} = V_T / (P_{plat} - PEEP_t) \qquad (21\text{--}14)$$

where $P_{I}P$ = peak inspiratory pressure, P_{plat} = plateau pressure, and $PEEP_t$ = extrinsic PEEP + intrinsic PEEP. Dynamic compliance (C_{dyn}) will reflect both resistance as well as elastance related problems, i.e., the pressure changes being measured under conditions of active inspiratory flow. Static compliance (C_{ES}) will only identify problems in elastance since the measured pressure changes are in the absence of active flow. By comparing C_{dyn} and C_{st} values, certain conclusions may be made as to the specific type of impedance. Reductions in C_{dyn} and C_{ES} that are proportionate suggest an increase in elastance, while a reduced C_{dyn} that is accompanied by a normal C_{ES} suggests an increase in resistance. Furthermore, C_{dyn} values that are less than 25 mL/cm H_2O describe a level of impedance that may result in a failure to wean from mechanical ventilation[8] (see Chapter 16).

Compliance may also be measured during spontaneous breathing. This, however, requires placement of an esophageal balloon. Most often such measurements are not required in the clinical setting because the compliance values obtained during mechanical ventilation suffice.

WOB is accomplished by determining the pressure-volume product;

$$WOB = V_T \times \Delta P \qquad (21-15)$$

Depending on the pressures recorded, such an evaluation will provide information on both patient-related and ventilator-related WOB (WOB_p and WOB_v, respectively). For WOB_v, measuring the change in airway pressures will suffice, while for WOB_p the transpulmonary pressure is required.[23] The latter describes the pressure difference between the pleural cavity (as measured by an esophageal balloon) and mouth. [Certain technical considerations must be adhered to in the placement of an esophageal balloon to ensure that the measured pressure truly reflects intrapleural pressure (see Chapter 9)]. As to some possible uses of WOB_p values, it has been found that when in excess of 1.8 kg/min/m, there is a high likelihood of a limiting level of impedance and subsequent failure to wean from mechanical ventilation.[10] Additionally, when respiratory muscle weakness is associated with such high levels of respiratory impedance, it would suggest that muscle fatigue may be a potentially reversible cause of such weakness.

Pressure-flow analysis allows the determination of airway resistance as a reflection of changes in resistive impedance. By measuring the change in pressure relative to an inspiratory flow rate, airway resistance (R_{aw}) may be calculated;

$$R_{aw} = (P_{aw} - P_{alv})/\dot{V}_I \qquad (21-16)$$

or

$$R_{aw} = (P_IP - P_{plat})/\dot{V}_I \qquad (21-17)$$

where $\dot{V}_I$ = inspiratory flow rate. Values exceeding 15 cm H_2O/L/sec are associated with a failure to wean. Although not as broad in evaluation as compliance or WOB, airway resistance is an easily obtained value that provides the intensivist with important impedance-related data.

In summary, respiratory impedance may reduce the response of the respiratory muscles to a given level of central neuroinspiratory drive. This may result in hypercapnic respiratory failure, particularly if there are associated increases in $\dot{V}CO_2$ and V_D/V_T. Analysis of central respiratory drive, OCB, compliance, WOB, and airway resistance may provide in various degrees an evaluation of the severity of the respiratory impedance. In clinical practice, most of the necessary data may be obtained by simply monitoring the various types of airway pressures.

Respiratory Muscle Capacity

Pathophysiology

The ability to ventilate appropriately is dependent on the power output of the respiratory muscles. It is analogous to a never-ending marathon that is characterized by intermittent uphill struggles. Strength and endurance are requisites. The respiratory muscles, of which the diaphragm is the most important, may at times exhibit a loss of strength and endurance as part of the events that lead up to hypercapneic respiratory failure. This is especially true when the level of respiratory muscle strength is reduced to levels below -20 cm H_2O. At this level, there may be significant reductions in $\dot{V}E$ relative to any other ongoing stresses, e.g., increases in $\dot{V}CO_2$ or VD/VT. Therefore, early detection of respiratory muscle deterioration is crucial in the adult critical care unit. This would lead to early intervention and, hopefully, avoidance of hypercapneic respiratory failure.

Clinically, failure of the respiratory muscles may be due to a variety of factors. These would include malnutrition (chronic disease), neuromyopathic disorders, and systemic metabolic changes such as hypoxemia, acidosis, hypokalemia, hypomagnesemia, hypophosphatemia, and hypocalcemia. The result would be respiratory muscle weakness, some of which may be reversible depending on the myopathic factor.

Respiratory muscle weakness may also be a result of respiratory muscle fatigue (RMF). The latter refers to the inability of the respiratory muscles to sustain a power output relative to a given workload but which may be significantly improved by resting that muscle and/or relieving the work load.[29] This implies that in RMF there may be reversibility to the loss of strength, if respiratory impedance is reduced and muscle rest is provided. In essence, RMF reflects the level of endurance.

Evaluation and treatment of RMF requires an understanding of its various forms—high- and low-frequency fatigue.[30] The defining parameter is the ability of the diaphragm to generate transdiaphragmatic pressures in response to various frequencies of supramaximal, unilateral phrenic nerve stimulation.[30] Recovery from high-frequency fatigue may occur within minutes. It is demonstrated by a normalization of the transdiaphragmatic pressures in response to a high frequency range (50 to 100 Hz) of phrenic nerve stimulation. The cause of this type of RMF is most likely metabolic, e.g., inadequate ATP levels, lactic acid, and/or changes in intracellular electrolytes. In comparison, recovery from low-frequency fatigue may persist for hours. It is demonstrated by depressed transdiaphragmatic pressures in response to a low frequency range (10 to 20 Hz) of phrenic nerve stimulation. Also characteristic of low-frequency fatigue is that the maximal inspiratory pressure (MIP) and the maximal voluntary ventilation (MVV) maneuver may be normal. This is in contrast with high-frequency fatigue where both are abnormal. The cause of low-frequency fatigue is most likely due to a damage of the muscle by toxic by-products such as free radicals. The clinical implications of these two forms of fatigue are that the length of time required to rest the muscles may vary and that the MIP may not always be an adequate reflection of RMF.

It should be noted that fatigue, in general, is not exclusive to the respiratory muscles but may also involve other components of the respiratory system.[30] (This is an important consideration in the patient who fails a weaning trial.) Specifically, these other components include transmission (neuronal) and central fatigue. The latter refers to a depressed level of central drive, which is accompanied by both a normal diaphragmatic EMG activity and transdiaphragmatic pressure in response to maximal phrenic nerve stimulation. In contrast, the former refers to an abnormal diaphragmatic EMG activity and transdiphragmatic pressure in response to maximal phrenic nerve stimulation. The clinical implication is that a depressed respiratory muscle output relative to changes in V_{CO_2} or V_D/V_T may be due to fatigue at one of three different levels—central, transmission, or contractile. Excluding the presence of one does not necessarily preclude the possibility of fatigue at the other levels.

In summary, reduced respiratory muscle capacity in hypercapneic respiratory failure may be the result of myopathic factors and fatigue. When in combination with increases in V_{CO_2} or V_D/V_T, it will be most often this milieu that ultimately is responsible for the loss of strength and endurance of the respiratory muscles and their subsequent failure.

Monitoring

A variety of monitoring options are available (Table 21–5). These include an assessment of the patient's breathing pattern, vital capacity (VC), MVV, maximal inspiratory pressures, tension time index, and electromyographic patterns. Clinical applicability is affected by the degree of technical complexity and invasiveness, as well as by the etiology underlying the loss of the respiratory muscle capacity.

The breathing pattern may be clinically evaluated by the physical examination, pneumotachygraph-related data, and by an impedance plethysmograph (IP) (see Chapter 15). The physical examination includes the following: determination of the RR (>25/min or a net increase in the baseline f >10/min); increases in heart rate (HR) or blood pressure; and the notation of any verbal dyspnea, posturing, accessory muscle use, respiratory alternans, and/ or abdominal paradox. The pneumotachygraph (within the ventilator or through the metabolic cart) provides respiratory times, e.g., T_I/T_{tot}, and the V_T. A duty cycle of less than 0.4 or increases by more than 0.1 during a spontaneous breathing trial reflects both respiratory muscle fatigue and the subsequent response of the central respiratory controller.[18, 31] The V_T, especially when indexed to f, has also been found to be predictive of a failure to wean, i.e., f/V_T >100 (Fig 21–4).[32] The pathophysiologic basis of this ratio is not completely understood but may reflect the response of the central respiratory controller to an imbalance between respiratory impedance and respiratory muscle capacity. IP may provide a more reliable means of clinically detecting respiratory alternans and abdominal paradox.[33–35] It may do this in a continuous fashion as opposed to intermmitent observations by medical personnel (especially advantageous when staffing levels are low). Likewise, it will also monitor for any changes in V_T without the need for a pneumotachygraph. It should be emphasized, however, that regardless of the method employed to determine the breathing pattern, there is no single measurement that is 100% predictive of a failure to wean unless it is markedly abnormal. A case in point is that respiratory alternans or abdominal paradox, although indicative of an increase in the respiratory impedance, are not necessarily associated with RMF nor predictive of a failure to wean.[36]

TABLE 21–5.
Monitoring Basis of Hypercapneic Respiratory Failure—$\dot{V}_E$ (muscles)

Parameter	Monitor	Patient Population	Advantages	Disadvantages
IV. $\dot{V}_E$				
c. Respiratory muscles	Physical exam; e.g., f, HR, BP, speech, posturing, breathing patterns.	Any presenting patient	Simplicity of evaluation	Lacks 100% sensitivity
	VC	Any ventilated patient	Noninvasive	Effort dependent Affected by other variables Lacks 100% sensitivity
	MIP	Any ventilated patient	Noninvasive	Effort dependent Lacks 100% sensitivity
	Raw/MIP	Any ventilated patient	Noninvasive Reflects fatigue	Lacks 100% sensitivity
	Pneumotachograph; e.g., T_I/T_{tot}, f/V_T	Any ventilated patient	Simplicity of evaluation	Lacks 100% sensitivity
	MVV maneuver	Ventilator dependence	Noninvasive	Effort dependent
	IP	Ventilator dependence	Continuous data Potential for central monitoring	Expensive
	Ppl or Pdi	Ventilator dependence	Tension time index More accurate assessment of strength	Relatively invasive Time-consuming
	EMG analysis	Ventilator dependence	Evaluate fatigue	Invasive Time-consuming Skill required

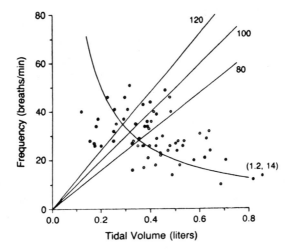

FIG 21–4.
Isopleths for the breathing frequency/Vт (f/Vт) ratio representing different degrees of rapid shallow breathing. For the patients indicated by the points to the left of the isopleth, representing 100 breaths/min/L, the likelihood that a weaning trial would fail was 95% whereas for the patients indicated by the points to the right of this isopleth, the likelihood of a successful weaning outcome was 80%. The hyperbola represents a minute ventilation of 10 L/min, a criterion commonly used to predict weaning outcome. Apparently, this criterion was of little value in discriminating between successfully weaned patients (*open circles*) and the patients in whom weaning failed (*solid circles*). Values for one patient (Vт 1.2 L and respiratory frequency of 14 breaths per minute) lay outside the graph. (*From Yang KL, Tobin MJ: A prospective study of indexes predicting the outcome of trials of weaning from mechanical ventilation.* N Engl J Med *1991; 324:1445–1450. Used by permission.*)

Measurement of the vital capacity will also reflect the capacity of the respiratory muscles such that values <10 cc/kg are predictive of a failure to wean.[10] Interpretation of the VC must be cautious, however, for a variety of factors, including the following: restrictive lung diseases may cause reductions in the VC independent of the respiratory muscle capacity; considerable respiratory muscle weakness may exist prior to major changes in the VC; and, technically, measurements may be limited by the effort of the patient as well as that of the respiratory therapist.

The MVV maneuver also demands a significant level of patient cooperation. It requires that the patient attempt a doubling of the resting $\dot{V}_E$. If such a doubling is not achieved, it suggests that the level of the resting $\dot{V}_E$ may not be sustainable and that weaning will be unsuccessful.[10] This is, in part, based on the knowledge that the maximal sustainable ventilatory capacity, i.e., the level of $\dot{V}_E$ that can be sustained for 15 minutes or longer, corresponds to at least 60% of the MVV.[36]

The maximal inspiratory pressure (MIP) may reflect both the level of respiratory muscle strength as well as its endurance, especially if serial measurements are followed. MIP levels less negative than -20 cm H_2O are predictive of a failure to wean from mechanical ventilation and of subsequent hypercapneic respiratory failure.[37] The MIP is measured at the mouth during a Mueller maneuver from RV and is relatively simple to obtain (Fig 21–5). It may, however, have a large degree of variation depending on the efforts of the respiratory therapist[38] and the patient's state of sedation. Alternatively, maximal inspiratory strength may be evaluated by more invasive techniques that utilize an esophageal balloon, either alone or in combination with a gastric balloon. The esophageal balloon by itself generates the esophageal equivalent of pleural pressures, and when done as a sniff, expulsive, or Mueller maneuver will generate the equivalent of the MIP, the P_{plmax}. Placement of both an esophageal and gastric balloon is the most invasive and technically demanding of the three methods. It, however, provides the most sensitive evaluation of diaphragmatic strength, pattern of respiratory muscle recruitment, and early detection of abdominal paradox (decreasing or negative gastric pressures).

Regardless of the method employed, however, all of these have a role in assessing respiratory muscle strength and in relating the latter to a tension-time index.

The tension-time index is described as follows[31]:

$$TTi = P_{di}/P_{dimax} \times TI/Ttot \qquad (21–18)$$

This may be approximated by the following equations:

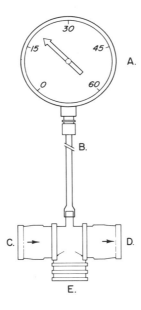

FIG 21–5.
Apparatus used to determine MIP in patients with artificial airways. **A**, manometer; **B**, connecting tubing; **C**, inspiratory one-way valve with port for thumb occlusion; **D**, expiratory one-way port; **E**, 22-mm-ID port for attachment to artificial airway. (*From Kacmarek RM, Cycyk-Chapman MC, Young-Palazzo PL, et al: Determination of maximal inspiratory pressure: A clinical study and literature review. Respir Care 1989; 34:868–878. Used by permission.*)

$$TTi = PIP/MIP \times T_I/Ttot \qquad (21-19)$$

$$Tti = P_{pl}/P_{plmax} \times T_I/Ttot \qquad (21-20)$$

These relate that if the pressure load of the diaphragm is excessive ($P_{di}/P_{dimax} > 0.40$) and its product with the duty cycle exceeds a value of 0.15, the WOB is such that respiratory muscle fatigue will ensue.[30] Similar information may be suggested by monitoring serial changes in the R_{aw}/MIP ratio.[39] A decreasing value would suggest an improvement in resistive impedance and/or respiratory muscle capacity and, consequently, a less fatiguing work load (Fig 21–6).

Diaphragmatic electromyographic (EMG) analyses may be utilized to specifically evaluate ventilatory fatigue.[30, 36] These would include EMG Hi/Lo ratios, EMG and P_{dimax} responses to phrenic nerve stimulation, and EMG/P_{di} ratios. The diaphragmatic EMG Hi/Lo ratio describes the power spectrum of the diaphragm at high frequencies relative to low frequencies. A reduction in the ratio suggests a fall in the power of the diaphragm at high frequencies but with an increase at low frequencies. It is associated with eventual respiratory muscle fatigue, but as with the MIP, this may not be present with the low-frequency form of fatigue. The physiologic mechanisms underlying these power spectral changes are not clearly understood. Likewise, although predictive of RMF, a reduced ratio may occur as an isolated value without other direct evidence of ongoing RMF.

EMG and transdiaphragmatic pressure responses to phrenic nerve stimulation allow the determination of the type of fatigue—central, transmission, or contractile fatigue.[30] Theoretically, this could be especially useful in excluding the possibilities of central or low-frequency contractile fatigue. These are the two forms of fatigue that are difficult to assess with standard respiratory monitoring.

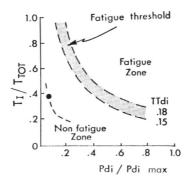

FIG 21–6.

Tension-time index for the human diaphragm (TT_{di}). The inspiratory time/total ventilatory cycle time ratio ($T_I/Ttot$) plotted against the ratio of transdiaphragmatic pressure during normal breathing to the maximum P_{di} possible (P_{di}/P_{di}max). The fatigue threshold represents a TT_{di} that can be sustained for one hour or longer and has a value of 0.15 to 0.18 in the normal human diaphragm. The TT_{di} threshold can be achieved with a large variety of P_{di} and $T_I/Ttot$ values. Patterns in the "fatigue zone" will result in fatigue in less than one hour; patterns in the nonfatigue zone can be sustained indefinitely. The circle represents TT_{di} during resting breathing in normal subjects. (*From Grassino A, Bellemare F, LaPorta D: Diaphragm fatigue and the strategy of breathing in COPD. Chest 1984; 85:51S–54S. Used by permission.*)

EMG/P_{di} ratios reflect the degree of neuronal input relative to the required transdiaphragmatic tension for a given tidal breath.[30] An increasing ratio would suggest a high risk for respiratory muscle fatigue. It is, in some ways, analagous to the P_{100} to V_T/T_I and $\dot{V}_E$ to P_{100} ratios discussed previously.

The technique of diaphragmatic EMG analysis, however, is often limited to research and not to clinical practice. It requires a significant level of expertise, invasiveness, and the ability to discriminate whether the recorded data actually respresent diaphragmatic activity. Hopefully, as technology improves, such data may be obtained in a more user-friendly and patient-comfortable type of setting. It would certainly add to the clinical understanding of hypercapneic respiratory failure.

Summary

Hypercapneic respiratory failure may be the result of several factors. These include $\dot{V}_{CO_2}$ (RQ, REE), V_D/V_T, and $\dot{V}_E$. The latter is a complex product of interactive balances that include central respiratory drive, respiratory impedance, and respiratory muscle capacity. Respiratory monitoring is currently available to assess each of these factors. At what level each is utilized will depend on the patient population and hospital economics. Table 21–6 outlines what may be considered necessary or supplemental. The stratification is based on the previous discussion. A proposed scheme may also be outlined on the basis of what pathophysiologic problem the patient's clinical status presents. It could be as follows:

Patient population; hypercapneic respiratory failure
Respiratory monitoring;
- Any patient requiring mechanical ventilation:
  Level 1—achieved by standard ventilator measurements:
      Serial analysis of airway pressures to assess MIP, R_{aw}, C_{dyn}, C_{st}, P_{breath}/MIP, R_{aw}/MIP, WOB_v
      Serial analysis of VC
      Serial analysis of breathing pattern response to spontaneous breathing to assess V_T/f, f, V_T/T_I, T_I/T_{tot}, TTi (P_{breath}/MIP).
- If diagnosis unclear or ventilator dependence is an issue:
  Level 2—achieved by indirect calorimetry
      $\dot{V}_{CO_2}$, RQ, REE, V_D/V_T, OCB
- If respiratory impedance remains an issue despite above studies:
  Level 3a—requires esophageal balloon
      WOB_p (pressure–volume curves)
  Level 3b—requires insertion of esophageal and gastric balloons
      P_{di}, P_{dimax}, TTi (P_{di}/P_{dimax})
- If central drive is an issue:
  Level 3c—requires special monitors or an esophageal balloon
      P_{100}

TABLE 21–6.
Monitoring Basis of Hypercapneic Respiratory Failure—Prioritizing Tests

Monitor	Necessary	Supplemental	Comments
Physical exam	X		f, HR, BP, speech, posturing, patterns
ABGs	X		
$Petco_2$		X	May be necessary in the OR and neuro ICU
$Ptcco_2$		X	
Indirect calorimetry	X		When clinically indicated
Harris-Benedict	X		
PA line	X		When clinically indicated
24-HrUN	X		When clinically indicated
Douglas bag	X		If indirect calorimetry not available
P100		X	
C_{dyn}, C_{st}	X		
R_{aw}		X	
WOB		X	
$P_{100}/V_T/T_I$		X	
V_E/P_{100}		X	
OCB		X	
VC	X		
MIP	X		
R_{aw}/MIP		X	
Pneumotachograph	X		$T_I/Ttot$ and V_T derived data
MVV		X	
IP		X	
P_{pl}, P_{di}		X	
EMG		X	

- If diagnosis remains unclear:
    Level 4a—requires EMG analyses and balloon placement
            EMG/P_{di}, EMG Hi/Lo ratio
    Level 4b—requires EMG analyses, balloon placement, and phrenic nerve stimulation
            Diaphragmatic EMG activity and transdiaphragmatic pressure responses

Levels 1 and 2 should be available in most adult critical care units. If a hospital's fiscal situation allows, levels 3a and 3c should also be available. Levels 3b, 4a, and 4b are primarily research tools and would not, in general, be required. Cost savings could be realized by ensuring appropriate nutritional plans[8] and by having a sound data base for the diagnosis and treatment of hypercapneic respiratory failure.

HYPOXEMIC RESPIRATORY FAILURE

Adequate levels of oxygen delivery (Do_2) are dependent on three main factors: cardiac output (CO), hemoglobin concentration (Hb), and oxygen saturation (O_2Sat);

$$Do_2 = CO\{[(1.34) \, (Hb) \, (SaO_2)] + (0.003 \, Pao_2)\} \qquad (21-21)$$

The contribution of the Pao_2 is minimal and may be simplified to

$$Do_2 = CO[(1.34) \, (Hb) \, (SaO_2)] \qquad (21-22)$$

Correcting for unit differences,

$$Do_2 = CO[(1.34) \, (Hb) \, (SaO_2 \, (10)] \qquad (21-23)$$

$$Do_2 = ml \, O_2/min$$

Hypoxemia becomes a critically limiting factor in Do_2 when the Pao_2 reaches levels below 60 mm Hg. This is due in part to the morphology of the oxygen-hemoglobin dissociation curve, which shows that, as hypoxemia progresses beyond such a level there will be steep reductions in the arterial O_2 saturation and, consequently, arterial O_2 content. Respiratory diseases that lead to hypoxemic respiratory failure, therefore, will lead to a significant reduction in the Do_2 and to a greater need for compensatory increases in the cardiac output (i.e., to maintain adequate levels of Do_2).

Hypoxic states are pathophysiologically associated with a variety of gas exchange abnormalities (Table 21–7). These include alveolar hypoventilation, ventilation/perfusion ($\dot{V}/Q$) mismatching, shunting, and/or a low mixed venous Po_2 ($P\bar{v}o_2$). (Diffusion-related abnormalities are not usually the primary mechanism behind hypoxemia in the adult critical care unit.) Respiratory monitoring—by assessing the oxygen saturation, alveolar-arterial O_2 difference [$P(A - 2)o_2$], shunt fraction, and the $P\bar{v}o_2$—provides an evaluation of the respiratory component of Do_2 and its possible pathophysiologic basis (Tables 21–8 and 21–9). The following

TABLE 21–7.
Physiologic Basis of Hypoxemic Respiratory Failure

Parameter	Clinical Setting
I. Alveolar hypoventilation	
a. Central	Reduced central drive (see Table 21–1)
b. Peripheral	Increased VD/VT (see Table 21–1)
	Reduced respiratory muscle capacity (see Table 21–1)
II. V/Q mismatch	Atelectasis, pneumonia, PE, pulmonary edema
III. Shunt	ARDS (see text), av malformations, PFO (see text)
IV. Low $P\bar{v}o_2$	Low cardiac output, severe anemia, severe hypoxemia, disproportionate Vo_2 relative to Do_2

TABLE 21–8.
Monitoring Basis of Hypoxemic Respiratory Failure—Oxygenation and Alveolar Hypoventilation

Parameter	Monitor	Patient Population	Advantages	Disadvantages
I. SaO_2	ABGs PaO_2/FiO_2	Respiratory distress Change in mental status	Most accurate Most complete	Invasive Possible vessel damage
	$P(a/A)O_2$ Pulse oximetry	Respiratory distress Change in mental status	Assess severity Noninvasive Continuous data	Affected by external light, cardiovascular instability, presence of HbCO or hypothermia, degree of hypoxemia; PaO_2 can only be estimated
	Transcutaneous	Respiratory distress	Noninvasive	Changes are not specific to oxygenation; but rather to DO_2; Dependent on adequate perfusion and skin thickness; Limited in adults
		Change in mental status	Continuous	
			Reflects DO_2	
II. Alveolar Hypoventilation	$P(A - a)O_2$	CO_2 retention Abnormal PaO_2	Simplicity	Invasive Possible vessel damage Cannot distinguish central vs peripheral
	P_{100}	See Table 21–4	See Table 21–4	See Table 21–4
	V_D/V_T	See Table 21–2	See Table 21–2	See Table 21–2
	Respiratory muscles	See Table 21–5	See Table 21–5	See Table 21–5

TABLE 21–9.
Monitoring Basis of Hypoxemic Respiratory Failure—V/Q, Shunt, Pv_{O_2}

Parameter	Monitor	Patient Population	Advantages	Disadvantages
III. V/Q	None DX by exclusion	Abnormal Pa_{O_2}	—	—
IV. Shunt	Qs/Q % Shunt	Limiting level of hypoxemia	Prognostic value Potentially reversible	Relatively invasive May be time-consuming Pv_{O_2} may be needed
V. Low Pv_{O_2}	Pv_{O_2}	Refractory hypoxemia	Cause of hypoxemia	Invasive May be nonspecific

discussion describes monitoring as it relates to the pathophysiology and management of hypoxemic respiratory failure.

Oxygenation

Pathophysiology

The diagnosis and management of hypoxemic respiratory failure requires the determination of the arterial oxygen saturation (Sa_{O_2}). As discussed above, this is critical given that Do_2 is in part dependent on the arterial content of oxygen. As a consequence, monitoring of the Sa_{O_2} takes on a principal role in the adult critical care unit.

Monitoring

Table 21–8 summarizes the available options for monitoring the Sa_{O_2}. The most accurate and complete method remains the ABG. As previously described, this method has its advantages and disadvantages. One especially significant defect is the absence of continuous data. As a result, two alternatives have been developed that provide such a sequence of data. One is transcutaneous O_2 (Ptc_{O_2}), but it is rarely used in the adult ICU (see Chapter 11). This is related to problems with skin thickness as well as many of the same issues noted with the Ptc_{CO_2} (see Chapter 12). Due to its greater technical simplicity, pulse oximetry remains the noninvasive, continuous monitoring system of choice in the ICU (see Chapter 10). It analyzes spectrophotometrically the differential absorption of light by oxyhemoglobin relative to deoxy-hemoglobin.[40] It achieves a measurement of the Sa_{O_2} without a need for local arterialization (e.g., heat) by measuring only the pulsatile change in light transmission. Ideally, any unstable patient who is in respiratory distress, has a change in mental status, and/or is being mechani-cally ventilated is a good candidate for intermittent or continuous pulse oximetry. Significant limitations remain, however, and are listed in Table 21–8. The most important limitations are low perfusion states, bright ambient light, and/or an elevated carboxyhemoglobin (Hbco).

Additionally, it must be emphasized that simply determining if there is a correlation between the pulse on the oximeter and the EKG HR does not ensure that an accurate Sao_2 has been obtained. This is due to the high sensitivity of such instruments to the pulse even when blood flow is reduced to as low as 4% of normal.[41]

Alveolar Hypoventilation

Pathophysiology

CO_2 retention will lead to hypoxemia by reducing the alveolar oxygen tension (Pao_2). This is explained by the alveolar gas equation[42]:

$$Pao_2 = [Fio_2(Pb - Ph_2o)] - [Paco_2(Fio_2 + (1 - Fio_2)/RQ))] \qquad (21-24)$$

where Fio_2 = inspired fraction of O_2, Pb = barometric pressure, and Ph_2o = vapor pressure. It follows then that that higher the $Paco_2$, the lower the Pao_2 and, consequently, the lower the Pao_2. Since the reductions in the alveolar and arterial O_2 tensions are proportionate, the *sine qua non* of alveolar hypoventilation is the absence of a widened $P(A-a)o_2$ and a relative facility in reversing the hypoxemia with oxygen supplementation.

The section on hypercapneic respiratory failure discussed at length the most common abnormalities associated with CO_2 retention. Briefly, this implied that $\dot{V}co_2$, Vd/Vt, central respiratory drive, respiratory impedance, and respiratory muscle capacity have major roles in determining the adequacy of the alveolar ventilation. It should be emphasized that some of these factors can also be associated with $\dot{V}/Q$ mismatch, shunting, and/or a low $P\bar{v}o_2$. This is due to the multifactorial nature of respiratory failure pathology and to the high prevalence of multisystem organ dysfunction in the ICU.

Monitoring

Alveolar hypoventilation in its pure form is associated with a preserved $P(A-a)o_2$. This analysis is determined by obtaining arterial blood gases and employing the alveolar gas equation. Monitoring approaches to CO_2 retention were discussed earlier in this chapter and summarized in Tables 21–2, 21–3, and 21–5.

Ventilation/Perfusion Mismatching

Pathophysiology

The most common etiology of hypoxemia in the ICU is $\dot{V}/Q$ mismatch—specifically, areas with a low ventilation-to-perfusion ratio. Diseases such as atelectasis, pneumonia, pulmonary embolism, and noncardiogenic and cardiogenic pulmonary edema are associated with various degrees of $\dot{V}/Q$ mismatch. Most of these disease states are also associated with elevated levels of respiratory impedance, which may lead to hypercapneic respiratory failure especially during excessively prolonged weaning trials.

Monitoring

Two options are available that may be used to assess the $\dot{V}/\dot{Q}$ balance in the lung. However, these are not clinically applicable given the lack of a need for such approaches and the labor intensiveness/technical skill/invasiveness required of these techniques. The multiple inert gas elimination technique is one such option but it is used mostly as a research tool. The second possibility involves a substantial amount of invasive data and is summarized in the following formula[43]:

$$\dot{V}/\dot{Q} = [(RER)\,(P_B - P_{H_2O})\,(Ca_{O_2} - Cv_{O_2})]/(Pa_{CO_2} \times 100) \qquad (21\text{–}25)$$

where P_B = barometric pressure and P_{H_2O} = partial pressure of water in alveolar gas (47 mm Hg at 37°C). Instead, $\dot{V}/\dot{Q}$ imbalance is most often a diagnosis of exclusion and is indirectly determined by evaluating the $P(A\text{-}a)_{O_2}$, Pa_{O_2}/F_{IO_2}, or $P(a/A)_{O_2}$, and shunt fraction. If the $P(A\text{-}a)_{O_2}$, Pa_{O_2}/F_{IO_2} or $P(a/A)_{O_2}$ is abnormal but the shunt fraction is relatively preserved, the most likely cause of the hypoxemia is $\dot{V}/\dot{Q}$ mismatch. The severity of $\dot{V}/\dot{Q}$ mismatch may be also nonspecifically assessed by the Pa_{O_2}/F_{IO_2} or $P(a/A)_{O_2}$ ratios, as well as by the Sa_{O_2} via pulse oximetry. Qualitatively, reductions in the Sa_{O_2} may be approached in a similar fashion as one does with the Pa_{O_2}/F_{IO_2} and $P(a/A)_{O_2}$ ratios. That is, Sa_{O_2} levels below 90% while on an $F_{IO_2} > 40\%$, a Pa_{O_2}/F_{IO_2} ratio < 238, or an $P(a/A)_{O_2}$ ratio <0.47 are all indicative of severe levels of $\dot{V}/\dot{Q}$ imbalance (see Chapter 7 for details).

Shunt

Pathophysiology

An intrapulmonary shunt describes that fraction of pulmonary perfusion which is not ventilated. Clinically, it is most commonly seen in the adult respiratory distress syndrome (ARDS). It ultimately leads to profound levels of hypoxemia manifested by severe reductions in the Pa_{O_2}/F_{IO_2} and $P(a/A)_{O_2}$ ratios. Mechanical ventilation with high levels of PEEP support is almost always required.

The most common diseases associated with ARDS include pneumonia, aspiration syndromes, trauma, transfusion-related reactions, drug overdose, pancreatitis, prolonged shock, and the sepsis syndrome. One alternative diagnostic possibility that may also present with refractory levels of hypoxemia is an intracardiac shunt through a patent foramen ovale (PFO). When anatomically present, a right-to-left shunt through a PFO may result when right-sided pressures exceed that of the left. Such may be seen with a massive pulmonary embolism or in the setting of a right ventricular infarct. The diagnosis would be suggested by refractory hypoxemia in the setting of a relatively normal chest roentengram and confirmed with a bubble study utilizing either a transthoracic or transesophageal echocardiography. Other diagnostic possibilities are uncommon and may include pulmonary arteriovenous (av) fistulas and cirrhosis-associated av malformations.

Monitoring

Direct assessment of the degree of physiologic shunting may be determined by having the patient inspire 100% F_{IO_2} until there is adequate nitrogen washout ($P_{N_2} < 15$ mm Hg or after a 15-minute period of 100% F_{IO_2}). The resulting high P_{AO_2} allows one to assume that the end-capillary blood contains an amount of oxygen equal to the oxygen capacity of hemoglobin plus 2.0 cc of dissolved $O_2/100$ mL. The following equation is then utilized[42]:

$$Q_S/Q_T = (C_{aO_2} - C_{cO_2})/(C_{vO_2} - C_{cO_2}) \qquad (21-26)$$

where

C_{aO_2}	= arterial O_2 content
C_{cO_2}	= end-pulmonary blood O_2 content
C_{vO_2}	= mixed venous blood O_2 content
Q_S	= blood flow through shunt
Q_T	= total blood flow
O_2 content	= (1.34) (Hb) (O_2Sat)

This method requires sampling of mixed venous blood through the distal port of a pulmonary arterial line as well as an arterial blood gas. In cases where a low mixed venous P_{O_2} is unlikely, Equation (21–26) may be simplified to the following[44]:

$$Q_S/Q_T = (P_{AO_2} - P_{aO_2})/17 \qquad (21-27)$$

The reader is referred to Equation (21–18) for the calculation of the alveolar P_{O_2}.

Once the %Shunt is obtained, two issues need to be resolved. One is to determine if the shunt is at a level that could be limiting to weaning from mechanical ventilation. If it exceeds 20%, it is predictive of a failure to wean.[1, 10, 37] The second issue is whether the %Shunt will totally account for the patient's hypoxemia. This is arrived at by the following formulas[44]:

$$\text{amount of desaturation} = 0.01 (S_{vO_2} - S_{cO_2}) (Q_S/Q_T) \qquad (21-28)$$

S_{vO_2} = mixed venous saturation and is equal the S_{aO_2} less 25% (assuming normal O_2 extraction)

S_{cO_2} = pulmonary capillary saturation and is equal to 100% on room air (if the P_{aCO_2} is normal).

If the s_{aO_2} is 90% and there is a normal P_{aCO_2} and O_2 extraction, equation (28) becomes:

$$\text{amount of desaturation} = 0.01 (65 - 100) (Q_S/Q_T)$$

$$\text{amount of desaturation} = 0.35 (Q_S/Q_T)$$

As an example, a 20% Shunt would cause the S_{aO_2} to decrease from 100% to 93% while breathing room air. Since the patient's actual S_{aO_2} is below 93%, there must be an additional etiology to the desaturation. Such an analysis permits the identification of the etiology behind a patient's hypoxemia (see Chapter 7 for details).

TABLE 21–10.
Monitoring Basis of Hypoxemic Respiratory Failure—Response to Therapy

Therapy	Monitor	Patient Population	Advantages	Disadvantages
I. PEEP				
a. extrinsic	PaO_2/FIO_2, SaO_2	Any ventilated patient	Simplicity Therapeutic endpoint	Relates to lung only
	PCWP	Hemodynamic instability with PEEP	Therapeutic risk	Estimates transmural pressure Invasive
	Pes	Hemodynamic instability with PEEP and elevated airway pressures	Transmural pressure	Relatively invasive
	Stroke volume	Hemodynamic instability with PEEP	Cardiac portion of Do_2	Invasive
	Pvo_2	Hemodynamic instability with PEEP	Adequacy of Do_2 may be continuous	May be nonspecific Invasive
b. intrinsic	Same as above			
	Expiratory hold	PCV High levels of V_E CO_2 retention Hemodynamic instability	auto-PEEP	May be inaccurate at high RR
	Volume-time curves	PCV High levels of V_E CO_2 retention Hemodynamic instability	Air trapping	None
	Flow-time curves	PCV High levels of V_E CO_2 retention Hemodynamic instability	auto-PEEP Adequacy of Ti in PCV	None

Mixed Venous Oxygen

Pathophysiology

A low mixed venous Po_2 will magnify the effects of $\dot{V}/\dot{Q}$ mismatch and shunting on a patient's level of oxygenation. The cause of a low $P\bar{v}o_2$ is most often due to an imbalance between Do_2 and Vo_2. It reflects greater oxygen extraction as a compensation for inadequate Do_2 relative to ongoing cellular metabolism. Low cardiac output states, severe anemia, and hypoxemia all contribute to an inadequate Do_2. Increases in Vo_2 due to metabolic stresses will likewise render a given level of Do_2 inadequate if there isn't an appropriate compensatory increase in the cardiac output.

It follows then that the detection and treatment of a low $P\bar{v}o_2$ may result in an improvement in the patient's level of arterial oxygenation. The reasoning may seem a bit circuitous but it emphasizes the interactive relationships between the Vo_2, Do_2, and the level of arterial oxygenation.

Monitoring

There are only invasive alternatives to mixed venous oxygen monitoring. These may be intermittent as in the sampling of mixed venous blood from the distal port of a PA line or continuously by utilizing specially designed PA lines that measure directly the mixed venous oxygen saturation.

Summary

Respiratory monitoring in hypoxemic respiratory failure can lead to greater accuracy in diagnosis as well as in determining the patient's response to therapy. (A proposed scheme to guide the use of such monitoring is suggested in Table 21–11). The level of priority is based on the previous discussions.

The approach to monitoring may also be based on the suspected pathophysiologic etiology of hypoxemia. This could be as follows:

Patient population; hypoxemic respiratory failure:
Respiratory Monitoring:
- All patients suspected of having hypoxemic respiratory failure:
  Level 1—requires pulse oximetry and arterial sampling
  Sao_2 (intermittent or continuous)
  pH, $Paco_2$, Pao_2, Pao_2/Fio_2, $P(a/A)O_2$, $P(A-a)o_2$
- If hypoxemia is severe ($Fio_2 > 0.70$) and its etiology is unclear
  Level 2—requires arterial sampling and 100% O_2 study
  Qs/Qt [Equation (21–26)]
- If a low $P\bar{v}o_2$ is suspected and hypoxemia is severe ($Fio_2 > 0.70$)
  Level 3—requires a PA line
  $P\bar{v}o_2$, Qs/Qt [Equation (21–27)]

TABLE 21–11.
Monitoring Basis of Hypoxemic Respiratory Failure—Prioritizing Tests

Monitor	Necessary	Supplemental	Comments
Physical exam	X		See Table 21–6
ABGs	X		
Pulse oximetry	X		
Transcutaneous O_2		X	Not useful in the adult ICU
P100		X	
V_D/V_T (ind calorimetry)	X		When clinically indicated
Respiratory muscles			See Table 21–6
Qs/Q		X	
PA line	X		When clinically indicated
PCWP	X		
SV	X		
Pv_{O_2}	X		
Pes		X	
Expiratory hold	X		When clinically indicated
Volume-time curves	X		
Flow-time curves	X		

Almost all standard ICUs have the capacity to determine the above measurements. Most of the data are obtained as part of routine ICU management of the critically ill patient.

MONITORING NEEDS RELATED TO THE THERAPY OF RESPIRATORY FAILURE

Central to the treatment of hypercapneic or hypoxemic respiratory failure is the modality of positive pressure ventilation (PPV). Although of tremendous value, it utilizes a mode of ventilation that is totally contrary to what evolution has dictated, namely, negative pressure ventilation. As such, PPV has brought on the significant problems of barotrauma and negative cardiopulmonary interactions. These can lead to further lung injury unrelated to the actual clinical insult, as well as a reduction in oxygen delivery.

The following section outlines two major areas of monitoring related to the above listed problems of PPV: positive end-expiratory pressure (PEEP) and the various inspiratory airway pressures, i.e., the peak inspiratory pressure (PIP) and the mean airway pressure (MAP).

PEEP

Pathophysiology
The treatment of hypercapneic respiratory failure may require the administration of high levels of ventilatory support. However, this support may have undesirable side effects. For example, a $\dot{V}_E$ that exceeds 20 L/min will often result in inadequate exhalation times. This may lead to

significant levels of auto-PEEP (intrinsic PEEP) resulting in a reduction in venous return and cardiac output. Subsequently, hemodynamic instability may develop, resulting in a decrease in Do_2 and an increase in VD/VT. The latter is especially counterproductive in hypercapneic respiratory failure because it may be associated with further CO_2 retention.

The same pathophysiology is seen with Fio_2-related problems in patients with hypoxemic respiratory failure. PEEP, applied either extrinsically or intrinsically (e.g., via ventilatory manipulations such as inverse-ratio ventilation) is often used to improve arterial oxygenation and/or minimize Fio_2 toxicity. The basis of this therapy is to improve alveolar recruitment and, thereby, $\dot{V}/\dot{Q}$ balance and shunt. The result is an improvement in the Sao_2 at more acceptable levels of Fio_2 and, it is hoped, an increase in the Do_2. However, in the same scenario as outlined above, there may be negative hemodynamic and Do_2 consequences to such an intervention. This is especially prevalent when PEEP levels exceed the 10 to 15 cm H_2O range, when the patient is hypovolemic, and/or when there is baseline inotropic dysfunction. The risk is that an improvement in the Sao_2 may be paradoxically associated with a reduction in Do_2 as a result of a PEEP-induced decrease in stroke volume and cardiac output.

Monitoring

As a result of these issues, PEEP in its various forms has necessitated diagnostic monitoring, which is intended to maximize the therapeutic effect while minimizing the risks. Table 21–10 summarizes the monitoring approach to both extrinsic and intrinsic PEEP. It is primarily based on the evaluation of the components of Do_2 and techniques to identify the presence of intrinsic PEEP.

As previously described, Do_2 is dependent on cardiac output (CO), hemoglobin concentration (Hb), and the Sao_2. Monitoring issues related to the Sao_2 were discussed earlier in this chapter. The Hb concentration is simply obtained by venous sampling and, ideally, it should be at least 8 g/dL in the critically ill patient. The cardiac output is dependent on the heart rate (HR) and stroke volume (SV), i.e., CO = HR × SV. Given that intrinsic or extrinsic PEEP may have a deleterious effect on the Do_2, it is critical that the SV be determined, especially if despite an Sao_2 of 90% and a Hb of 8 g/dL clinical evidence of ongoing anaerobic cellular metabolism remains (e.g., lactic acidosis, unexplained metabolic acidosis with a widened anion gap, a low $P\overline{v}o_2$), and/or hemodynamic instability. SV monitoring may be accomplished in a variety of ways (see Chapter 8). The most widely used employs the Swan-Ganz catheter. It applies a thermodilution technique and the Fick principle to determine the cardiac output. It additionally provides by far the most complete assessment of the cardiovascular status. It does so by evaluating the right (RV) and left (LV) ventricular preload reserve [the right atrial pressure and the pulmonary capillary wedge pressure (PCWP), respectively], the RV and LV afterload state (the pulmonary and systemic vascular resistances, respectively), the level of inotropy (SV), and the $P\overline{v}o_2$. Of special importance relative to the effects of PEEP is the changes in the PCWP, SV, and the $P\overline{v}o_2$. These allow an evaluation of the consequences of PEEP-induced reductions in venous return, as well as a guide to subsequent interventions should those parameters necessitate such.

The PCWP as obtained by the Swan-Ganz catheter is of special importance in the evaluation of patients with hypoxemic respiratory failure and diffuse pulmonary infiltrates. It allows the distinction of cardiogenic (PCWP > 12 to 18 mm Hg) versus noncardiogenic (PCWP < 12 to

18 mm Hg) pulmonary edema. This has diagnostic and therapeutic implications because it separates cardiac causes of alveolar flooding from capillary leak states as seen in ARDS. It should be emphasized, however, that the PCWP is only an estimate of the transmural left atrial pressure (left atrial transmural pressure = PCWP − P_{pl}). Most often the P_{pl} is not of any significant value when the PCWP is measured at end-expiration; as a result, the PCWP will approximate the transmural pressure. However, in situations where the PEEP level exceeds 10 to 15 cm H_2O or when there is significant respiratory variation precluding end-expiratory measurements of the PCWP, it is recommended that an esophageal balloon be placed to determine the P_{pl}, and, thereby, the transmural pressure. This is especially true in critically ill patients where accurate knowledge of the left atrial filling pressure is crucial in the attempts to establish hemodynamic stability and appropriate levels of O_2D.

There are several alternatives to the evaluation of the SV, but these do not provide any additional data other than an estimate of SV. These include radioisotopic-derived ejection fractions [SV = end-systolic counts − end-diastolic counts) (EF)], right ventricular ejection fraction catheters, echocardiographic estimates of the EF, and other indicator-dilution techniques such as the indocyanine green dye (also utilizes the Fick principle but requires a central venous line injection and an indwelling peripheral arterial line for sampling). These have their relative merits but, in general, are not as complete as the Swan-Ganz catheter measurements. It should be mentioned that with the Swan-Ganz catheter the SV may be determined by an additional method. This employs the Fick equation but also requires an indirect calorimetry study to measure the $\dot{V}o_2$, i.e., CO = $\dot{V}o_2/(Cao_2 − Cvo_2)$. It is not appropriate simply to estimate the $\dot{V}o_2$ in the critically ill patient because the values can show a wide ranged based on the patient's status and therapeutic regimen. On occasion, however, this particular method may be of benefit when there is tricuspid regurgitation or a low flow state. In the latter two situations, the CO by thermodilution is inaccurate.

The measurement of auto-PEEP is critical in determining the iatrogenic effects of postive-pressure ventilation on the V_D/V_T and on the cardiovascular status. An expiratory hold as outlined by Pepe and Marini[45] allows such a quantitation but is limited in patients requiring high mechanical rates and/or spontaneously ventilating over the set mechanical rate. A qualitative approach that is more sensitive is the analysis of pressure-time, volume-time, or flow-time curves. This is illustrated in Figure 21–7. When clinically appropriate, identification of auto-PEEP may allow for effective intervention. This would include efforts primarily directed at prolonging the exhalation time and/or decreasing airway resistance. Additional benefits derived from the analysis of pressure-time, volume-time, or flow-time curves are outlined in Table 21–10 and in Chapter 16.

PiP and MAP

Pathophysiology

Depending on the level of ventilatory support, PEEP, inspiratory flow pattern, and/or compliance characteristics of the respiratory system, PPV may be associated with a high enough level of pressure that it could conceivably lead to further lung injury, as well as hemodynamic instability. There is evidence to suggest that it is the mean alveolar pressure (MalvP) that

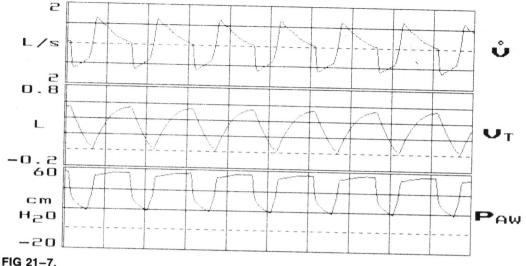

FIG 21–7.
Volume-time and pressure-time curves demonstrating auto-PEEP in a patient on pressure control ventilation of 42 cm H_2O. Note that the flow (V) waveform does not fully return to baseline at the end of expiration.

physiologically determines the likelihood of such events. Levels exceeding 35 cm H_2O may be associated with hemodynamic instability and injury to the alveolar-capillary unit.[46, 47] The latter could include pneumothorax, interstitial emphysema, tension cyst formation, and/or pulmonary edema. Since it cannot be directly measured, the MAP has been used to estimate the MalvP by the following relationship[46]:

$$MalvP = MAP + V_E (R_E - R_I) \qquad (21-29)$$

where R_E = expiratory resistance and R_I = inspiratory resistance. It would thus appear that the most clinically applicable monitor of barotrauma and hemodynamic-related problems might be the MAP. Efforts at accepting certain levels of permissive hypercapnea and/or minimizing R_E would serve to maintain MalvP levels at an acceptable range.

The role of the PIP as an index of barotrauma or hemodynamic instability has recently been deemphasized given the relationship between the MAP and the MalvP. However, it has previously been shown to correlate with barotrauma-related lung injury and its importance should, therefore, remain intact. PiP levels above 35 to 50 cm H_2O may be associated with significant levels of lung injury.[48, 49]

An additional parameter that may be used to monitor lung injury is the use of static compliance measurements in the management of severe ARDS unresponsive to conventional treatment.[49] Gattinoni et al.[49] have outlined such a protocol and it is characterized by the interaction between C_{ES}, level of CO_2 elimination, and responses to various modes of ventilation. The endpoint is the achievement of adequate gas exchange but without the iatrogenic barotrauma of PPV.

Monitoring

The MAP is measured and can be continuously displayed by the most recent generation of ventilators. It reflects the average pressure applied by the ventilator over the entire respiratory cycle and is measured at the airway opening.[47] The clinical need to determine the R_E and R_I, and hence the MalvP, is open to some debate given that it should be the patient's ventilatory support requirements that determine settings rather than the goal of aiming for an artifactual MAP level. Considerations such as an appropriate machine set tidal volume relative to the patient's lung disease, e.g., $V_T < 10$ cc/kg in ARDS, or acceptance of levels of permissive hypercapnia that do not interfere with Do_2, would serve to improve the risk-benefit profile of PPV. The alternative role for the MAP would thus be to determine the wisdom of a specified ventilator setting, i.e., can the V_T, mechanical rate, inspiratory flow pattern, or level of PEEP be modulated to fit the pathophysiology of the respiratory disease.

The utility of the PiP is dealt with in the same manner as the MAP. It, too, is ideally measured at the airway opening at peak inspiration and may be visualized via an inspiratory pressure-time curve (see Chapter 16).

SUMMARY

It was the purpose of this chapter to establish the needs of respiratory monitoring out of an understanding of the pathophysiology of respiratory failure. Recognizing the various complexities integral to CO_2 elimination and oxygen delivery forms the very foundation of critical care. Respiratory monitoring plays a crucial role by providing the data base for diagnosis and intervention. This may be done in a cost-effective manner by targeting its utilization on the basis of physiologic principles and specific patient populations.

REFERENCES

1. Hall JB, Wood LDH: Liberation of the patient from mechanical ventilation. *JAMA* 1987; 257:1621–1628.
2. West JB: *Respiratory Physiology—The Essentials*, ed 4. Baltimore, Williams & Wilkins Co, 1990.
3. Roussos C, Macklem PT: Inspiratory muscle fatigue, in *Handbook of Physiology—The Respiratory System III*, pp 511–527, Oxford University Press, 1986.
4. Hess D: Capnometry and capnography: Technical aspects, physiologic aspects, and clinical applications. *Resp Care* 1990; 35:557–576,
5. Hoffman RA, Krieger BP, Kramer MR, et al: End-tidal carbon dioxide in critically ill patients during changes in mechanical ventilation. *Am Rev Respir Dis* 1989; 140:1265–1268.
6. Bassili HR, Dietel M: Nutritional support in long term intensive care with special reference to ventilator patients: A review. *Can Anaesth Soc J* 1981; 28:17–21.
7. Covelli HD, Black JW, Olsen MS, et al: Respiratory failure precipitated by high carbohydrate loads. *Ann Intern Med* 1981; 95:579–581.
8. Dark DS, Pingleton SK, Kerby GR: Hypercapnia during weaning—a complication of nutritional support. *Chest* 1985; 88:141–143.
9. Arora NS, Rochester DF: Respiratory muscle strength and maximal voluntary ventilation in undernourished patients. *Am Rev Respir Dis* 1982; 126:5–8.

10. Stoller JK: Establishing clinical unweanability. *Resp Care* 1991; 36:186–198.
11. Branson RD: The measurement of energy expenditure: Instrumentation, practical considerations, and clinical application. *Resp Care* 1990; 35:640–656.
12. Browning JA, Linberg SE, Turney SZ, et al: The effects of a fluctuating FIO2 on metabolic measurements in mechanically ventilated patients. *Crit Care Med* 1982; 10:82–85.
13. Swinamer DL, Phang PT, Jones RL, et al: Effect of routine administration of analgesia on energy expenditure in critically ill patients. *Chest* 1988; 92:4–10.
14. Anderson CF, Loosbrock LM, Moxness KE: Nutrient intake in critically ill patients: Too many or too few calories? *Mayo Clin Proc* 1986; 61:853–858.
15. Liggett SB, Renfro AD: Energy expenditures of mechanically ventilated nonsurgical patients. *Chest* 1990; 98:682–686.
16. Weissman C, Kemper M, Askanazi J, et al: Resting metabolic rate of the critically ill patient: Measured versus predicted. *Anesthesiol* 1986; 64:673–679.
17. Montgomery AB, Holle RHO, Neagley SR, et al: Prediction of successful ventilator weaning using airway occlusion pressure and hypercapnic challenge. *Chest* 1987; 91:496–499.
18. Sassoon CSH, Te TT, Mahutte CK, et al: Airway occlusion pressure—an important indicator for successful weaning in patients with chronic obstructive pulmonary disease. *Am Rev Respir Dis* 1987; 135:107–113.
19. Murciano D, Boczkowski J, Lecocguic Y, et al: Tracheal occlusion pressure: A simple index to monitor respiratory muscle fatigue during acute respiratory failure in patients with chronic obstructive pulmonary disease. *Ann Intern Med* 1988; 108:800–805.
20. Eldridge FL: Relationship between respiratory nerve and muscle activity and muscle force output. *J Appl Physiol* 1975; 39:567–574.
21. Whitelaw WA, Derenne J-P, Milic-Emili J: Occlusion pressure as a measure of respiratory center output in conscious man. *Resp Physiol* 1975; 23:181–199.
22. Milic-Emili J, Whitelaw WA, Derenne JPh: Occlusion pressure—a simple measure of the respiratory center's output. *N Engl J Med* 1975; 203:1029–1030.
23. Marini JJ: Lung mechanics determinations at the bed side: Instrumentation and clinical application. *Resp Care* 1990; 35:669–693.
24. Brenner M, Mukai DS, Russell JE, et al: A new method for measurement of airway occlusion pressure. *Chest* 1990; 98:421–427.
25. Scott GC, Burki NK: The relationship of resting ventilation to mouth occlusion pressure—an index of resting respiratory function. *Chest* 1990; 98:900–906.
26. Harpin RP, Baker JP, Downer JP, et al: Correlation of the oxygen cost of breathing and length of weaning from mechanical ventilation. *Crit Care Med* 1987; 15:807–812.
27. Field S, Kelly SM, Macklem PT: The oxygen cost of breathing in patients with cardiorespiratory disease. *Am Rev Respir Dis* 1982; 126:9–13.
28. Kanak R, Fahey PJ, Vanderwarf C: Oxygen cost of breathing—changes dependent upon mode of mechanical ventilation. *Chest* 1985; 87:126–127.
29. NHLBI Workshop Summary: Respiratory muscle fatigue—report of the respiratory muscle fatigue workshop group. *Am Rev Respir Dis* 1990; 142:474–480.
30. Aldrich TK: Respiratory muscle fatigue. *Clin Chest Med* 1988; 9:225–236.
31. Marini JJ: Monitoring during mechanical ventilation. *Clin Chest Med* 1988; 9:73–107.
32. Yang KL, Tobin MJ: A prospective study of indexes predicting the outcome of trials of weaning from mechanical ventilation. *N Engl J Med* 1991; 324:1445–1450.
33. Krieger BP, Ershowsky P: Noninvasive detection of respiratory failure in the intensive care unit. *Chest* 1988; 94:254—260.
34. Tobin MJ, Perz W, Guenther SM, et al: The pattern of breathing during successful and unsuccessful trials of weaning from mechanical ventilation. *Am Rev Respir Dis* 1986; 134: 1111–1118.

35. Krieger BP, Chediak A, Gazeroglu HB, et al: Variability of the breathing pattern before and after extubation. *Chest* 1988; 93:767–771.

36. Rochester DF: Tests of respiratory muscle function. *Clin Chest Med* 1988; 9:249–261.

37. Sahn SA, Lakshminarayan S, Petty TL: Weaning from mechanical ventilation. *JAMA* 1976; 235:2208–2212.

38. Multz AS, Aldrich TK, Prezant DJ, et al: Maximal inspiratory pressure is not a reliable test of inspiratory muscle strength in mechanically ventilated patients. *Am Rev Respir Dis* 1990; 142:529–532.

39. Begin P, Grassino A: Inspiratory muscle dysfunction and chronic hypercapnia in chronic obstructive pulmonary disease. *Am Rev Respir Dis* 1991; 143:905–912.

40. Wiedmann HP, McCarthy K: Noninvasive monitoring of oxygen and carbon dioxide. *Clin Chest Med* 1989; 10:239–254.

41. Lawson D, Norley I, Korbon G, et al: Blood flow limits and pulse oximeter signal detection. *Anesthesiol* 1987; 67:599–603.

42. Forster III RF, Dubois AB, Briscoe WA, et al: in Appendix: *The Lung—Physiologic Basis of Pulmonary Function Tests*, ed 3. Chicago, Year Book Medical Publishers, 1986.

43. Chatburn RL, Lough MD. in: Chapter 3: Physiologic Monitoring: *Handbook of Respiratory Care*, ed 2. Chicago, Year Book Medical Publishers, 1990.

44. Johnson D: Massachusetts General Hospital/Pulmonary and Critical Care Unit laboratory manual, 1985.

45. Pepe PE, Marini JJ: Occult positive end-expiratory pressure in mechanically ventilated patients with airflow obstruction—the autopeep effect. *Am Rev Respir Dis* 1982; 126:166–170.

46. Marcy TW, Marini JJ: Inverse ratio ventilation in ARDS—rationale and implementation. *Chest* 1991; 100:494–504.

47. Marini JJ: Lung mechanics in the adult respiratory distress syndrome—recent conceptual advances and implications for management. *Clin Chest Med* 1990; 11:673–690.

48. Kolobow T, Moretti MP, Fumagalli R, et al: Severe impairment in lung function induced by high peak airway pressure during mechanical ventilation. *Am Rev Respir Dis* 1987; 135:312–315.

49. Gattinoni L, Pesenti A, Caspani ML, et al: The role of total static lung compliance in the management of severe ARDS unresponsive to conventional treatment. *Int Care Med* 1984; 10:121–126.

Chapter 22

Monitoring in Adult General Care

Kathy Harris, M.P.H., R.R.T.

Tim Blanchette, M.S., R.R.T.

INTRODUCTION

The emergence of critical care units in the 1960s spurred the development of invasive and, later, noninvasive monitoring techniques and equipment. Some of these monitoring technologies have found their way to general non-ICU floors. This diffusion is enhanced by equipment that is easy to use and requires little effort to learn. Physicians accustomed to having oximeters in the ICU often want one to stand watch against hypoxemia on the general floors. Monitoring, which is important and appropriate in critical care areas, may not be necessary or justifiable in other settings. There are also complex monitors that are underutilized in this patient population. However, in order to determine the usefulness of these monitoring techniques in general care areas, many factors must be considered and evaluated (Table 22–1).

TECHNOLOGY AND MEDICAL COSTS

Medical technology is expensive, and careless unjustified proliferation is indefensible. Monitoring and diagnostic technology have contributed substantially to rising medical costs, and estimates report that 33 to 75% of the per diem hospital cost increases are due to new technology.[1] It is not just the big ticket items, such as magnetic resonance imaging and lithotriptors, that are the source of escalating costs. Relatively inexpensive technologies often escape close scrutiny and slowly drive up health care costs. Other areas of public spending have been forced to make tough choices. We do not equip school buses with seat belts because it has been determined the price to save a life is too high. This country currently spends two-thirds of a trillion dollars on health care.[2] Sooner or later we will have to answer such difficult questions as "What is it worth to identify a hypoxic event that may or may not be clinically significant?"

It may be that certain monitoring techniques are cost-effective. King and Simon[3] reported

TABLE 22–1.
Considerations When Assessing Usefulness of
Monitoring in General Care Areas

Cost
Evaluating technology
Logistical problems
Current practices
Complexity of equipment
Knowledge level required
Failure to try
Importance of measurement

that using pulse oximetry to taper oxygen saved money by reducing arterial blood gases and shortening the number of days on oxygen, and Joseph et al.[4] found a reduced number of blood gas analyses with the use of pulse oximetry in emergency ward patients. However, some studies on cost effectiveness are flawed by the use of charges instead of cost. Finkler[5] emphasizes that we must measure resource consumption and not what we charge. Though we have not conducted a formal study, our data indicate no decrease in the number of arterial blood gases since the advent of pulse oximetry, but we have seen a rapid rise in pulse oximetry usage over the past three years, which is just beginning to plateau (Fig 22–1). Patient monitoring may lead to cost savings in specific areas with well-established protocols; however, we have not found a beneficial impact of monitoring on the general hospital budget.

EVALUATION

There is no unified central system for evaluating technology in the United States. Nevertheless, there are some fundamental questions that should be raised by all users of medical technology. Is the service or device efficacious, effective, appropriately utilized, and cost-effective? Efficacy addresses the question "Does it work in the laboratory?" Effectiveness addresses the question "Does it work in the real world?" Appropriateness addresses the question "Is it the right monitor for this patient?"

A cost-benefit analysis is rarely done because of the inherent difficulties of putting a price on a life. However, cost analysis can address specific questions, such as "What is the best way to monitor carbon dioxide levels in general floor patients?" A comparison can be made of the costs of alternate approaches. After a comprehensive description of the end-tidal CO_2 and transcutaneous CO_2 monitoring is developed, analysis of the relative effectiveness of both methods can be made when all relevant costs are detailed.

Because cost is not the only factor involved, all the issues that concern the users must be identified. Such issues include: Why monitor? Which patient should be monitored? What parameter should be monitored? Which brand of monitor? When do we want to monitor? Who will perform the monitoring? This process can identify problems and address conflicts,

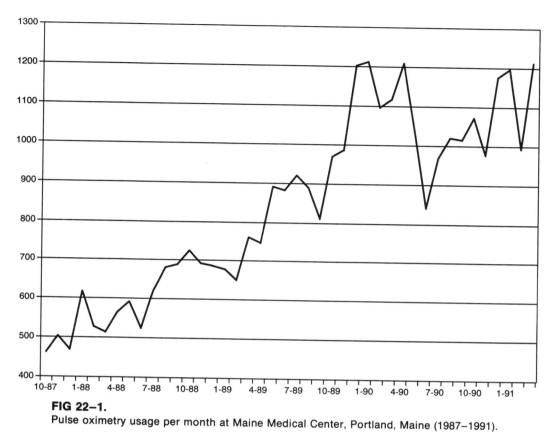

FIG 22–1.
Pulse oximetry usage per month at Maine Medical Center, Portland, Maine (1987–1991).

as well as detail what a given technology is likely to cost to both purchase and operate. It provides information for informed discussion prior to purchase.

LOGISTICAL PROBLEMS ON THE GENERAL FLOORS

Monitoring in the general care areas presents unique logistical and clinical problems. Continuous monitoring in noncritical areas must be limited by time constraints placed on the clinician. Patients in critical care units generally can be monitored intensely because of nurse, physician, and therapist/patient ratios. General floor care usually necessitates setting priorities for monitoring. If continuous respiratory monitoring is required, or requested, for a patient on the general floors, who is responsible for the monitor/monitoring (e.g., nurse, therapist)? Does the need for monitoring justify the cost of transferring a patient to intensive care? On the other hand, is the answer a noninvasive, intermediate respiratory care unit similar to the one described by Bone and Balk,[6] or a pulmonary noninvasive monitoring unit, utilizing respiratory inductive plethysmography and pulse oximetry as described by Krieger?[7]

What is Going on Now?

Currently a number of approaches have been taken to monitor the noncritically ill patient. Typically, hospitals use individual oximeters and other monitors as the need arises. Some hospitals use networks, such as Nellcor's OXINET oximeter system, which can continuously monitor many patients from a central station. This type of system is expensive, but may be appropriate for cardiopulmonary step-down units where patients are at risk for hypoxemia. Other hospitals use intermediate units, which rely heavily on noninvasive monitoring. Maine Medical Center has recently opened a transitional rehabilitation unit (TRU) for stable patients with multiple system problems, including respiratory/upper airway dysfunction, requiring multidisciplinary management. Patients in this unit may be on portable ventilators, but all have well-defined rehabilitation goals requiring aggressive intervention to improve mobility, self-care skills, nutritional status, and cognitive function. This unit is new, but we anticipate it to be an ideal setting for evaluation of respiratory monitors.

COMPLEXITY OF EQUIPMENT

Every manufacturer wants to develop a monitor like the pulse oximeter. The pulse oximeter exemplifies many desirable features of a monitoring device: no calibration, ease of use, relative accuracy. However, most monitors are more complex and time-consuming to operate than pulse oximeters, although many manufacturers have done much to make equipment easier to operate. For example, the Novametrix expired CO_2 monitor has hermetically sealed calibration gases and creative help screens. Nellcor has attempted to make their CO_2 monitor look as simple as their oximeters. Still, these are not instruments one can just pick up and use like pulse oximeters. It is perhaps unfortunate that the pulse oximeter has set the standard for ease of use. Practitioners used to pride themselves on "jury-rigging" equipment and making do with what was available.[4] Manufacturers have made significant strides in developing user-friendly equipment; however, practitioners must still invest time to ensure mastery of the equipment.

KNOWLEDGE LEVEL REQUIRED

Even the apparently simple pulse oximeter requires significant knowledge and judgment when positioning and evaluating signal strength, pulse bars, waveforms, artifacts, and alarms. Besides understanding the technology, the clinician must be aware of the physiologic principles that can affect the accuracy and usefulness of monitors in specific settings. For example, what are the effects of dyshemoglobins on pulse oximetry, or increased dead-space on expired CO_2

measurement? Knowledge of monitor accuracy and bias, as well as a working knowledge of oxygen saturation versus Po_2 and the oxygen dissociation curve, is necessary for accurate interpretation of pulse oximetry results. The uninformed clinician is at risk of gaining a false sense of security or a false sense of urgency by using and relying on monitors before sufficient expertise has been developed.

WHICH MONITORS ARE ESSENTIAL?

Monitoring oxygenation is widely considered useful. As Kelleher[8] states in his review on pulse oximetry, "hypoxia is the common final pathway of many medical mishaps." However, for the respiratory patient there is also concern about arterial carbon dioxide, as well as airway mechanics and the function of the respiratory muscles. Though a large variety of monitors is available (Fig 22–2), as well as many studies on monitoring in the ICU, there is a lack of research about patient monitoring techniques on general floor patients. The available scientific

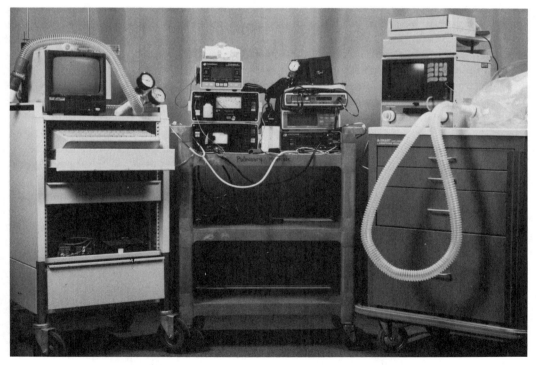

FIG 22–2.
Examples of monitoring equipment used in general care.

investigation provides little evidence to make conclusions about what monitors are necessary for which patients.

Which patients are at enough risk to justify the use of continuous (or intermittent) monitoring in the general care areas? The questions of "what is too much" or "what is too little" monitoring on the general floors has not been answered, although the debate has begun.[9, 10]

With these problems and concerns in mind, let us examine monitoring technologies with demonstrated or perceived usefulness in the adult noncritical care areas. In this chapter we present our (and others') clinical experience with monitoring, and hope that we can contribute to the dialogue concerning the appropriate use of technologies on the general adult care floor.

BASIC MONITORING IN GENERAL CARE

Unlike the ICU patient for whom monitoring is often continuous (Chapter 21), the noncritically ill patient is typically evaluated intermittently. Monitoring technology would be misguided if it were to supplant basic clinical patient assessment and evaluation on general care units, since "hands-on" clinical assessment is simpler, more compassionate, and more direct.[11] Indeed, regular and basic clinical patient evaluation is the cornerstone of monitoring in the hospital's general care areas. The time-honored methods of physical exam that we use to evaluate respiratory disease have changed little from those described by Laennec[12] in his *Treatise on Diseases of the Chest* in 1819. We still use the human senses to evaluate the chest by means of inspection, palpation, percussion, and auscultation, as well as to evaluate vital signs with the aid of simple equipment, such as the sphygmomanometer and the thermometer.

There are significant advantages to monitoring by physical exam in the general care areas ("clinical" monitoring) as opposed to more "high-technology" electronic monitoring often required in critical care. Advantages of "clinical" monitoring include the following:

1. Clinical monitoring is readily available (i.e., the clinician does not have to locate specialized equipment but generally carries the necessary tools, in the form of eyes, ears, and hands, at all times).
2. Clinical assessment is quick and easy for the experienced clinician and does not involve setting up, plugging in, calibrating, and troubleshooting equipment.
3. Clinical observations are more direct, can be qualitatively judgmental, and provide a wider range of information than technical monitors. For example, it is not yet practical for machines to monitor everything or to evaluate what they are monitoring—the monitor can display an exhaled CO_2 value or respiratory rate, but cannot indicate to the clinician whether the chest is expanding symmetrically, the lung sounds are equal, the patient is using accessory muscles of respiration, or exhaling through pursed lips. Nor can the machine ask the appropriate questions, such as "Where does it hurt?"

Before presenting the use of various pieces of machinery in general care monitoring, a brief evaluation of the simple clinical monitoring techniques most frequently used in general care areas is appropriate.

Hands-on monitoring by the clinician is the mainstay of patient surveillance and in some ways these "tough" techniques, as described by MacIntyre,[11] require a more skillful clinician than the "high-tech" methods that are so often espoused. Looking at the different methods of information processing involved in MacIntyre's "touch versus tech" (Table 22–2), it is evident that it is easier to read numbers off a monitor than to develop good clinical judgment. Furthermore, it is often unfortunate that an objective number (which could be wrong) is given more weight than an experienced subjective judgment. For example, the simple monitoring of vital signs usually provides the first clue that something has gone awry.

VITAL SIGNS

Vital signs consist of respiratory rate, temperature, pulse, and blood pressure, each of which is considered in the following.

Respiratory rate is a very simple and sensitive indicator of respiratory distress in all age groups[13] but is nonspecific. However, measuring respiratory rate has been called "an expensive tribute to tradition," which can be highly inaccurate and of little clinical value.[14] Gravelyn and Weg[15] more recently depicted respiratory rate as a sensitive and reasonably specific marker of acute respiratory dysfunction. Tachypnea is seen in a variety of cardiac, pulmonary, metabolic, central nervous system, and infectious diseases, and an elevated respiratory rate needs to be treated much the same way as an elevated temperature, i.e., investigated and explained.

An elevated temperature is frequently the first indication of an infectious or inflammatory process. Although it may result from a variety of other conditions, an elevated (or subnormal) temperature may provide evidence that further evaluation or monitoring is needed. Since oral temperatures are generally about 1°F (0.55°C) lower than rectal temperatures, Tandberg and Sklar[16] have demonstrated that the difference averages 1.67°F (0.93°C) in tachypneic patients and that this difference increases with respiratory rate and is independent of whether the patient is mouth breathing.[16] Others have found that sublingual temperatures are not affected

TABLE 22–2.
Information Gathering and Processing: "Tech Versus Touch"*

	Monitors ("Tech")	Clinical Observation ("Touch")
Power	Electrical	Clinical skills
Calibration/maintenance	Engineering principles	Clinical skills
Sensors	Electrical-mechanical	Eyes, hands, ears
Processors	Focus on specific parameter	Broad and clinically integrated, clinician designed
Displays	Engineering or marketing design Analog, digital	Inherent observation
Clinical decision results	Engineering or marketing design Needs understanding of monitor, then clinical picture	Direct incorporation into clinical picture

* From MacIntyre NR: *Respir Care* 1990; 35:546. Used by permission.

by increased respiratory rate or depth of breathing, but are affected by open mouth breathing.[17] With respiratory distress, there may be a tendency toward mouth breathing and changes in sublingual temperatures. Rectal temperatures are thus the most accurate monitors of body temperature in this group of patients.

Pulse rate is often increased as a compensatory mechanism, with respiratory distress or hypoxemia, while tachycardia and tachypnea are the usual consequences of hyperthermia.

Indirect blood pressure measurements are subject to much variability, depending on the time of day, cuff location, patient position, and anxiety level, as well as the technique, expertise, and bias of the clinician taking the measurement. The reader is referred to Chapter 14 for a discussion of noninvasive methods of blood pressure measurement, although a full description of the diagnostic interpretation of blood pressure changes is beyond the scope of this chapter.[18]

PHYSICAL EXAM

Inspection

Any physical exam should begin with patient observation and inspection. If questions are raised by the history or initial inspection, the physical exam can proceed with a heightened awareness of possible causes for abnormal findings. Evaluation of the depth and rhythm of respirations, as well as the rate, can provide valuable diagnostic clues. Critical clinical observation of the patient provides the first impression upon which future monitoring needs are based, and looking at the patient is the simplest and often most important of all patient monitoring techniques.

Palpitations

"Hands-on" evaluation can be useful in evaluating chest symmetry and the presence of decreased chest movement, which may be the earliest evidence of reduced lung distensibility.

Percussion

When performed with good technique by an experienced clinician, percussion sounds of various pitch can be of value in evaluating a consolidation or effusion (dullness), emphysema, or pneumothorax (hyper-resonance) and other pulmonary anomalies.

Auscultation

Assessment of breath sounds with a stethoscope is one of the most common diagnostic respiratory procedures performed by clinicians. As with the former techniques, auscultation can be said to be a monitoring tool when frequent, serial evaluations are utilized to quantitate changes in lung sounds and help explain changes in the clinical condition. Adventitious lung sounds (e.g., crackles, wheezes, rhonchi) or abnormally located bronchial breath sounds are frequently present in the respiratory patient. In conjunction with other physical findings, a chest x ray, and laboratory tests, auscultation may frequently be the only evaluation and monitoring necessary for the respiratory patient in the general ward.

INVASIVE MONITORING IN GENERAL CARE

Clinical examination and the monitoring of vital signs are the cornerstone of general clinician evaluation and monitoring, while arterial blood gases (ABGs) frequently supply additional critical information in assessing the patient with respiratory system compromise.

Analysis of Po_2, Pco_2, and pH, via ABG sampling, provides information on the gas exchange characteristics of the lung, as well as the acid-base status of the body's internal milieu. Arterial blood gases are the gold standard for evaluating oxygenation and ventilation, but they do have limitations. An adequate arterial Po_2 alone is no guarantee of adequate tissue oxygenation. Oxygen content, primarily determined by the oxyhemoglobin saturation and the hemoglobin level, is of critical importance when evaluating oxygenation. Shifts in the oxygen dissociation curve, based on patient temperature and pH, and the presence of carbon monoxide and other dyshemoglobinemias may diminish the usefulness of Pao_2 monitoring. Pao_2 may not provide for optimal monitoring of oxygenation in all circumstances, and CO-oximetry measurements of Sao_2, hemoglobin and dyshemoglobins must be obtained in patients suspected of having dysfunctional hemoglobin.

Monitoring alveolar ventilation is most accurately accomplished through measurement of $Paco_2$, which describes the relationship of alveolar ventilation to CO_2 production. The monitoring of $Paco_2$ can indicate if a patient has increased dead-space or CO_2 production and whether the patient is hypo- or hyperventilating. However, $Paco_2$ must be evaluated in light of the whole clinical picture. The asthmatic patient with an acute attack, for example, may have a "normal" $Paco_2$ of 40 mm Hg, but be working extremely hard to overcome the resistive forces of constricted airways. This "normal" $Paco_2$ may actually be an indication of severe airway obstruction and impending respiratory failure, based on an inability to hyperventilate despite tremendous respiratory effort. The $Paco_2$ values must be integrated with clinical observations in order to be useful. A low $Paco_2$ may indicate compensatory hyperventilation in diabetic ketoacidosis, but measuring and monitoring of pH is critical to elucidate the primary cause of the abnormality. Determining a patient's acid-base status by measuring pH, along with $Paco_2$, is necessary to determine the existence of a primary metabolic disorder, an acute or chronic respiratory disorder, or a mixed acid-base disturbance. The pH is necessary to determine the acuity of a respiratory problem and is therefore a critical part of ABG analysis. Though Pao_2 and $Paco_2$ can both be estimated by noninvasive means, pH cannot at this time be measured noninvasively.

Although continuous indwelling devices are forthcoming, arterial blood gas samples are intermittent and invasive and are indicative of only a single point in time. Despite these shortcomings, currently there is no single or combination of noninvasive monitors that provides the information that is obtained from an arterial blood gas!

NONINVASIVE MONITORING

Monitoring of the general care patient most frequently involves intermittent clinical assessment, based on physical findings. With the development and proliferation of easy-to-use noninvasive monitoring equipment (which may be more accurate than physical evaluation), continuous monitoring of physiologic or functional status in the general care areas is becoming more commonplace. However, the rate and impact of this noninvasive monitoring in general clinical care is controversial.

Relatively few studies have attempted to evaluate the clinical usefulness of various noninvasive monitoring techniques in the general care areas. Furthermore, studies that are available suggest that monitoring may be overused in general medical wards. For example, Bowton et al.[19] examined the impact of pulse oximetry measurements in general ward patients and found that although 75% of patients periodically desaturated (i.e., oxygen saturation <90%), these desaturations frequently went unrecognized by doctors and nurses and rarely led to corrective changes.

Currently available noninvasive respiratory monitoring that may be of use in general care includes monitoring of oxygenation, ventilation, respiratory mechanics, and metabolic function. To develop current recommendations for the use of monitors, we must examine each in more detail. Severinghaus[20] has summed it up by saying, "For life, nothing is more important than oxygen supply." Although it is difficult to determine what oxygen saturation or Po_2 limit is clinically damaging, it is generally accepted that $Sao_2 \geq 90\%$ or a $Pao_2 \geq 60$ mm Hg is adequate to prevent tissue damage in the adult patient.

Transcutaneous Po₂ Monitoring

In adults, transcutaneous Po_2 ($Ptco_2$) is lower than arterial Po_2. In older children and adults, the skin creates an increased barrier to O_2 diffusion.[21] Low blood flow states also increase the difference between transcutaneous Po_2 and arterial Po_2 values ($Pao_2 \neq Ptco_2$) especially in adults.

Though there is some evidence that $Ptco_2$ can trend and follow Pao_2 values in adults, the large and sometimes variable ($Pao_2 - Ptco_2$) difference limits its value in clinical medicine, as has been well demonstrated by Palmisano and Severinghaus[22] and shown in Figure 22–3. Also, transcutaneous monitoring requires time-consuming instrument calibration, changing of membranes, site preparation, warm-up time, and periodic rotation of the sensor site. Transcutaneous Po_2 monitoring has been used successfully by vascular surgeons to evaluate perfusion and healing potential of wounds.[23] However, the lack of accuracy of transcutaneous Po_2 monitoring in adults, along with the training and understanding necessary to maintain, calibrate, apply, and understand the measurements (along with the advent of pulse oximetry), has limited the appeal and popularity of $Ptco_2$ monitoring for adult care in most hospitals (see Chapter 11 for details).

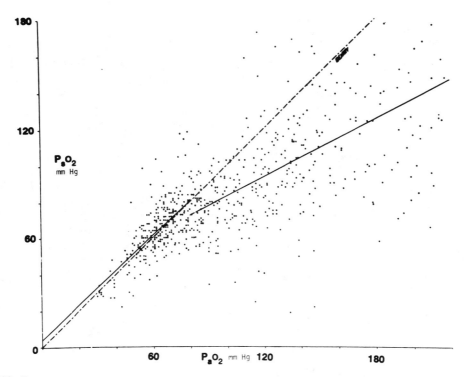

FIG 22–3.
The relationship of Ptco$_2$ (Pso$_2$) to Pao$_2$, *n* = 723. Regression lines are shown for Pao$_2$ below and above 80 mm Hg. (*From Palmisano BW, Severinghaus JW: J. Clin Monit 1990; 6:189–195. Used by permission.*)

Pulse Oximetry

Clinicians may not be able to detect cyanosis and oxygen desaturation until saturations fall to near 70%.[24] It is little wonder that Severinghaus referred to pulse oximetry as arguably the most significant technological advance in the history of monitoring patients' well being during anesthesia and critical care.[20] The question is, does the same statement apply in noncritical care patients?

Many hospital patient care units and respiratory care departments are attempting to justify the purchase of pulse oximeters (Fig 22–4). Clinicians in these same units and departments are asking questions about the accuracy and reliability of the numbers displayed on their pulse oximeters. Is this actual and impending proliferation warranted, based on the current scientific evidence? Relatively scant data exist to verify the clinical usefulness of pulse oximetry in the general care area. Pulse oximetry is accepted as a useful continuous monitor for maintaining surveillance of patients' oxygenation status, though the study by Bowton et al.[19] suggests overuse. Moreover, other problems are encountered when the pulse oximeter is utilized for

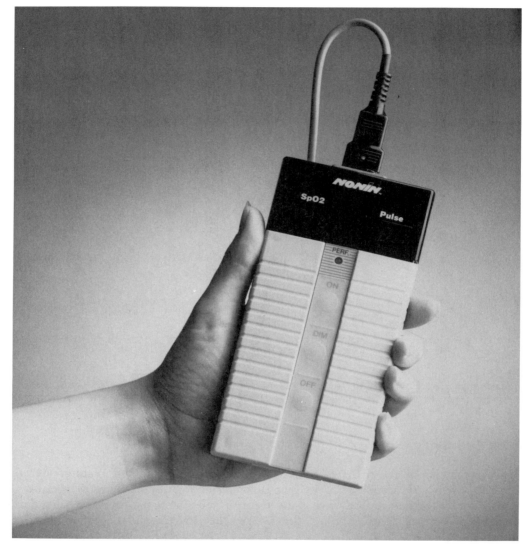

FIG 22–4.
The Nonin portable pulse oximeter.

one-time or intermittent spot checks. The question is, do pulse oximeters have sufficient accuracy to guide clinical and therapeutic changes?

Many pulse oximeter manufacturers mislead the user by reporting one standard deviation accuracy at ±2%.[25] One standard deviation tells us that 68% of the pulse oximeter readings will be within ±2% of the saturation calculated from CO-oximeter values. Studies generally report accuracy (actually inaccuracy) at two standard deviations, telling us that 95% of the pulse oximeter readings should be within the stated range. In our example, 95% of the time pulse oximeter readings would be within ±4% of the calibration standard or CO-oximeter. In clinical practice, even a 4% inaccuracy at a borderline saturation of 88 or 90% could be very important and might lead to changes in clinical decisions. Most clinical studies actually report slightly poorer accuracy than manufacturer specifications: 95% of pulse oximeter saturations (Spo_2) are usually within ±5% of measured arterial saturations in these studies.[2] In regular use, oximeters may produce far greater inaccuracy than those obtained from clinical trials under controlled conditions.

It is clear to manufacturers and clinicians alike, that as oxygen saturations decrease, pulse oximetry inaccuracy increases—finally to a point where accuracy can no longer be specified.[25] Severinghaus and Naifeh[26] have demonstrated significant inaccuracy in response to profound hypoxemia, with saturations less than 70%. Knowing the actual saturation when major desaturation events (<70%) occur is less important once it has been recognized that oxygenation has deteriorated below acceptable levels and therapeutic intervention must begin. However, the gray zone between adequate and not quite enough oxygen (between 85 and 90%) is an area where a pulse oximeter inaccuracy of ±5% can be of real concern.

A comparative study on oximeter bias in healthy subjects by Nickerson et al.[27] demonstrated that Spo_2 values from four different oximeters differed from CO-oximeter measured saturation by an average difference (bias) that ranged from −0.4 to −2.6% (Figure 22–5). This means that Spo_2 values from two different oximeters on the same patient could differ by nearly 3%, based on oximeter bias alone. As saturation levels decreased, oximeter bias often changed dramatically in one direction or another.

Oximeter bias can be clinically important because many hospitals use different brands of oximeters. Most hospitals have many (we have more than 10) makes and models of pulse oximeters, each of which has particular benefits and weaknesses and a bias that may be different from the next. The clinician is presented with a dilemma when trying to interpret oxygen saturation results from different makes or models of pulse oximeters. Furthermore, the intermittent use of different oximeters on the same patient increases the chances of making an error in judgment. One must also be cautioned against intermixing probes between oximeter brands, since this may lead to severe burns, as demonstrated by Murphy et al.[28] and pictured in Figure 22–6.

As recommended by Choe et al.,[29] the clinician's job of interpreting pulse oximeter results would be much easier if standardized oximeter calibration was the rule. Because standardized calibration is not widely used, we recommend the following steps:

1. Where practical, attempt to standardize pulse oximetry make and model throughout the hospital so that an Spo_2 in one area or patient can be compared more accurately to an Spo_2 in others.
2. If standardization throughout the hospital is not possible, use only one make or model of pulse oximeter on a given unit.
3. Do not alternate use of different oximeters (especially different makes) to follow trends in a given patient.
4. Test your oximeter bias in your clinical situation to develop a feeling for how Spo_2 relates to Sao_2 under various circumstances.

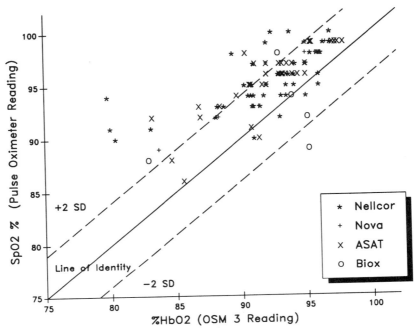

FIG 22–5.
Bias of four different pulse oximeters. (*From Nickerson et al. Chest 1988; 93:515–517. Used by permission.*)

If dyshemoglobins such as carboxyhemoglobin or methemoglobin are present, even in moderate amounts, pulse oximetry saturations misrepresent Sao_2 (Table 22–3). In clinical practice, dyshemoglobin levels of 2 to 3% are common. For example, 100 blood samples from nonsmokers in our institution produced mean carboxy plus methemoglobin levels of 2.3%. This kind of error will cause pulse oximeters to overestimate substantially the actual arterial oxyhemoglobin (Hbo_2) saturation. In some unusual cases dyshemoglobins can produce drastically erroneous results.[30, 31]

The inability of two-wavelength oximeters to segregate accurately oxyhemoglobin, carboxyhemoglobin, and methemoglobin limits the value of pulse oximetry in suspected smoke inhalation, heavy cigarette smoking, or when there is a risk of increased dysfunctional hemoglobin levels.[32, 33]

Poor perfusion states can be particularly troublesome when inconsistent Spo_2 values or pulse oximeter saturations are unavailable.[34, 35] Reflectance oximeter sensors have been touted to be preferable in low perfusion states, and we have found that reflectance oximetry on the forehead or cheek can sometimes produce accurate Spo_2 values when transmittance pulse oximetry fails. However, because reflectance oximetry is more labor-intensive (finding the appropriate site and securing the sensor can be difficult) and more awkward to apply than

TABLE 22–3.
Physiologic Factors Interfering with Pulse Oximeter Reliability

Factor	Source	Interfering Mechanism	Possible Solutions
Carboxyhemoglobin[30]	Tobacco smoke, smoke inhalation injury	Interference with light absorption at pulse oximeter wavelengths	Evaluate CO with exhaled CO monitor or CO oximeter
Methemoglobinemia[31,32]	Well water, dialysis baths, nitrate medications	Interference with light absorption at pulse oximeter wavelengths	Measure metHb with a blood oximeter
Poor perfusion	Low BP, vasoconstrictors, decreased temperature, thick digits, inflated BP cuff	Oximeter needs to sense pulsatile blood flow	Change sensor site, vasodilation (warm)
O_2 dissociation curve shifts	Variations in temperature, pH, P_{CO_2}, 2–3 DPG, Hb species	Pulse oximeter can only detect spectrophotometric O_2 saturation	Obtain ABG if question abnormality

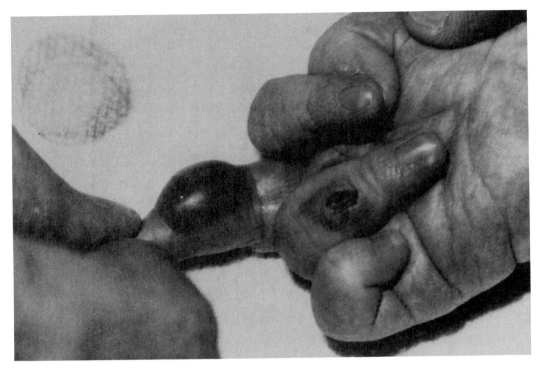

FIG 22–6.
Severe burn as a result of mixing oximeter probes between brands. (*From Murphy KG, Secunda JA, Rockoff MA:* Anesthesiol *1990; 73:350–352. Used by permission.*)

finger oximetry, it is likely to have more limited application. Physical and mechanical factors can also adversely affect the reliability of reflectance oximetry readings (Table 22–4).

Clinical Use of Pulse Oximetry

The clinical significance of the limitations of the pulse oximeter may go unrecognized unless viewed with a critical eye. Many clinicians remain less comfortable with the concept of arterial oxygen saturation[39] and pulse oximetry saturation than with Pao_2.

As already discussed, the limitations of pulse oximetry accuracy demonstrate why Spo_2 does not equal Sao_2, but pulse oximetry saturations are often assumed to be equivalent to Sao_2 and are widely accepted as an accurate indication of oxygenation. The flaw in this assumption is nicely demonstrated by Carlin et al.,[40] who showed that Medicare guidelines using Spo_2 for reimbursement of continuous oxygen therapy are inappropriate. Medicare guidelines state that an arterial Po_2 of 55 mm Hg or less, or either an arterial or spectrophotometric saturation of 85% or less (now 88%) indicates hypoxemia and justifies continuous oxygen therapy.[41] Carlin et al.[40] tested more than 50 patients with the Biox IIA pulse oximeter and compared their saturations with arterial Po_2 values. Overall, 80% of the patients with $Po_2 \leq 55$ mm Hg had pulse oximeter saturations greater than 85% (Fig 22–7). In these instances, if pulse oximetry

TABLE 22–4.
Physical Factors Interfering with Pulse Oximeter Reliability

Factor	Source	Interfering Mechanism	Possible Solutions
Vascular dyes[33]	Methylene blue, indocyanine green, indigo carmine	Interference with light absorption at pulse oximeter wavelengths	Do not rely on pulse oximeter during or near dye dosing
Skin pigmentation[36]	Darkly pigmented skin	Interference with light absorption at pulse oximeter wavelengths	Suspect inaccuracy, ABG prn
Nail colorings[37] or coverings[38]	Dark nail polish (black, blue, green, brown-red), synthetic nails	Interference with light absorption at pulse oximeter wavelengths	Remove nail color or coverings or choose alternative site
Ambient light	Sunlight, xenon, infrared or fluorescent light	Interference with light absorption at pulse oximeter wavelengths	Shield sensor from extraneous light
Motion	Sensor or patient movement	Interference with signal processing and pulse sensing with some "pulsating" light sources	Choose alternate site; calm patient; evaluate pulse signal, waveform, or synchronize with ECG

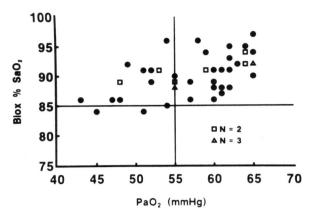

FIG 22–7.
The relationship between resting arterial oxygen tension Pao₂ and oxygen saturation measured by a Biox IIA pulse oximeter. *Solid lines:* Pao₂ of 55 mm Hg; and Spo₂ of 85% (now 88%) represent current Medicare criteria for long-term oxygen therapy prescription. (*From Carlin BW, Clausen JL, Ries AL:* Chest *1988; 94:239–241. Used by permission.*)

alone were used to justify oxygen therapy, these patients would have inappropriately been denied Medicare coverage.

King and Simon[3] used a pulse oximeter protocol for tapering oxygen therapy in pulmonary ward patients. Using an Spo₂ value of 90%, they demonstrated that patients could be weaned from oxygen faster and with fewer blood gases by pulse oximetry than a control group, but failure to correlate Spo₂ with arterial oxygen saturations in this study could lead to incorrect oxygen prescriptions.

A different approach for assessing oxygen therapy by pulse oximetry was taken by Smoker and Hess.[42] The amount of oxygen necessary to obtain an Spo₂ of 95% was established. Arterial blood gases were obtained if CO_2 retention was suspected. The value of this approach is that it allows the clinician to judge the significance of variations in Fio₂ and how they relate to changes in Spo₂. It also provides a margin of safety by establishing a liberal target value for Spo₂ of 95%. This avoids the risk that Spo₂ will underestimate true arterial oxygen saturation because of bias, dyshemoglobins, or oxygen dissociation curve shifts.

Recommendations for Pulse Oximetry Spot Checks
The following recommendations can be made when monitoring patients intermittently or by spot checks with pulse oximetry.

1. Before attempting to spot check oxygenation in a patient by pulse oximetry, evaluate the risks and benefits to the patient of a noninvasive versus invasive procedure.
2. Consider the likelihood of increased dyshemoglobin levels. For example, is the patient a smoker? Is smoke inhalation a possibility? Has the patient been exposed to carbon monoxide? Does the patient use medications such as nitroglycerin, nitroprusside,

amyl nitrate, dapsone, or benzocaine? If so, then an ABG *and* CO-oximetry should be used to evaluate oxygenation and dyshemoglobin levels.

3. Evaluate the patient's previous ABGs. This may help determine whether CO_2 retention or an abnormal pH is likely to shift the dissociation curve and affect oxygen uptake or unloading at the tissues. If no previous ABGs are available, the risk/benefit relationship of utilizing pulse oximetry must be evaluated.

4. Know the bias of the oximeter you are using in various saturation ranges and consistently use the same oximeter on a particular patient.

5. Evaluate the patient and pulse oximeter interface to rule out interference by movement, extraneous light, and interfering absorbers (nail polish, skin pigmentation). Assure a consistent strong signal before taking the pulse oximeter reading.

6. Keep the Spo_2 reading $\geq 95\%$ if no blood gas or CO-oximetry has been obtained for comparison.

Recommended Clinical Uses of Pulse Oximetry

Pulse oximetry is most valuable as a surveillance tool to monitor for a hypoxemic event that might be precipitated by a variety of patient conditions, as well as diagnostic or therapeutic procedures. Intermittent blood gases are of little value in this monitoring role.

Because pulse oximetry is simple and can continuously monitor and trend relative oxygenation status, it is proving to be very useful in the following clinical settings.

Tapering Supplemental Oxygen.—After initial ABG or CO-oximetry evaluation is performed in conjunction with pulse oximetry, the patient's oxygen requirement can be established by following continuous pulse oximetry trends as oxygen is tapered. Remember that many patients requiring supplemental oxygen may have significant ventilation-perfusion mismatching and thus their oxygenation equilibration time may be prolonged. The practice of changing O_2 and watching pulse oximeter readings for only a few minutes places the patient at risk of desaturating as time passes. A minimum of 10 to 15 minutes is normally sufficient after an O_2 therapy change to assure stabilization at the new Fio_2. However, if less than 10 minutes is allowed for stabilization, an additional pulse oximeter reading should be taken with the same oximeter after an hour has passed to assure that progressive desaturation has not occurred.

Pulmonary Rehabilitation.—Escourrou et al.[43] have recently demonstrated that although arterial blood saturations and pulse oximetry saturations were significantly different in 101 chronic pulmonary patients, both at rest and at maximal exercise, pulse oximetry reliably estimated the changes in arterial saturation and was clinically useful. Besides its usefulness in evaluating COPD patients at rest and exercise such as walking and stair climbing, pulse oximetry has been useful in determining the oxygen requirements of COPD patients (as well as sleep apnea patients) during sleep. The pulse oximeter has also been used effectively as a biofeedback tool in training chronic pulmonary disease patients to improve oxygenation through pursed lip breathing.[44]

Though pulse oximetry saturations should not be substituted for Po_2 in prescribing home oxygen therapy, they can be very useful in determining requirements for supplemental or additional oxygen during exercise (Fig 22–8). The continuous trending capabilities of pulse oximetry make it a useful tool in following changes in oxygenation status that occur as a result of a therapeutic intervention.

Diagnostic Procedures. — Various diagnostic procedures place the patient at risk of desaturation because of required positioning, as well as the procedure itself. As far back as 1976, the value of ear oximetry monitoring during bronchoscopy was reported.[45] Since the advent of simpler pulse oximetry, continuous monitoring of oxygenation status during certain diagnostic procedures has become routine. Because bronchial lavage and suctioning can cause significant

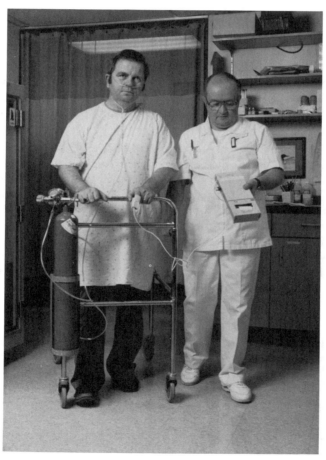

FIG 22–8.
Pulse oximetry may demonstrate oxygen desaturation during exercise.

desaturation, Spo_2 monitoring during therapeutic and diagnostic bronchoscopy should be universal (Fig 22–9).

Cardiac catheterization may lead to arterial hypoxemia. Dodson et al.[46] found that 38% of their cardiac catheterization patients often fell below 90% on the pulse oximeter during the catheterization procedure. They felt that continuous pulse oximetry monitoring should be considered during cardiac catheterization and they recommended continuous pulse oximetry or supplemental oxygen in patients with decreased left ventricular function, low baseline Spo_2 values, or patients expected to have a long procedure.

Pulse oximetry saturations have been monitored during bronchial challenge. A modest drop in Spo_2 of 3% was found by Stewart et al.[47] in patients who had a positive response. It is doubtful that the risk of desaturation during bronchial challenge and many other diagnostic procedures necessitates[48] the use of pulse oximetry, so pulse oximetry monitoring should be selective.

General Floor Sedation and Analgesia

Because the primary concern with the use of sedatives and narcotics on the general floors is suppression of respiratory drive and hypoventilation, continuous pulse oximetry has often been recommended and used to detect desaturation due to hypoventilation. If continuous pulse

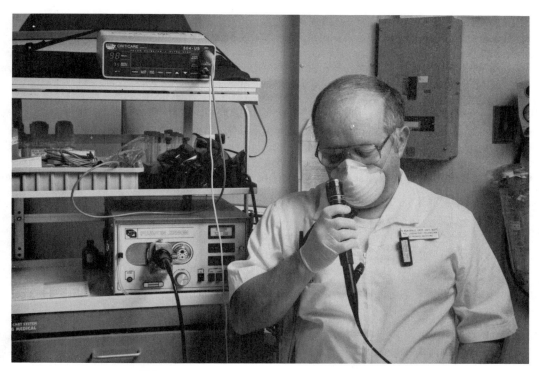

FIG 22–9.
Routine monitoring during fiber-optic bronchoscopy.

oximetry monitoring were to be used for all postoperative patients, or patients requiring sedation and/or pain relief, the cost of this increased monitoring would be considerable. Yet, it is evident that diminished pulmonary function and the risk of postoperative atelectasis, shunting, and hypoxemia is real. McKenzie[49] found that the clinical assessment of oxygenation and the need for oxygen therapy was inadequate in his New Zealand hospital. Within the first six postoperative days after abdominal surgery, 29 of 100 patients had a total of 51 episodes of Spo_2 less than or equal to 90% on daily pulse oximetry checks, and 13 patients displayed saturations less than or equal to 85% (Table 22–5).

McKenzie[49] recommended that pulse oximetry could be used on a surgical ward in the same way as thermometers, as a vital sign. Choi et al.[50] demonstrated that half of the women receiving either parenteral narcotics or epidural morphine in the postpartum ward after cesarean delivery experienced significant desaturation defined by an Spo_2 less than or equal to 85%. They found that significant desaturation occurred as late as 23 hours after epidural morphine, and they recommended continuous pulse oximetry monitoring as an alternative to expensive continuous supervision by a nurse.

Realizing the limitations in accuracy of pulse oximetry, especially at lower Spo_2 values, and the fact that no one has demonstrated a difference in outcome because of these intermittent saturations, it is impossible to know if these desaturations are significant.

Long-Term Ventilator-Dependent Patients. — Critical care units are reserved for acutely ill patients. Many patients are compromised with chronic respiratory failure due to injury, such as high cervical fractures, neuromuscular disease, or COPD. These patients are frequently managed on general wards and may require ventilatory support. How useful is pulse oximetry in their management?

Often, these long-term ventilator patients have good oxygenation but decreased respiratory muscle strength that limits ventilation. Though pulse oximetry cannot measure ventilation, it may nevertheless be useful when hypoventilation or lack of ventilation is the prime concern. For example, Marzocchi et al.[51] demonstrated that pulse oximetry detected 13 of 13 brief tracheostomy occlusions during sleep of six central apnea patients with diaphragm pacemakers. Conversely, none of the tracheostomy occlusions was detected by a transthoracic impedance/

TABLE 22–5.
Lowest Saturation Recorded in Patients During the Perioperative Period*

Oxygen Saturation	Number of Patients
≤94%	79
≤92%	51
≤90%	29
≤88%	20
≤85%	13
≤80%	5

* From McKenzie AJ: *Anesthesia Intens Care* 1989; 17:412–417. Used by permission.

heart rate (TI/HR) monitor, while paced diaphragmatic contractions continued to cause breaths to register and HR to increase on the TI/HR monitor. Despite this apparent usefulness of pulse oximetry in monitoring hypoventilation, Verhoeff and Sykes,[52] using a computer simulation, contend that oxygen saturation may reach dangerous levels when a paralyzed patient is disconnected from a breathing circuit before a pulse oximeter alarm is activated. Careful clinical monitoring and a low-pressure alarm remain necessities for the mechanically ventilated patient.

Emergency Department.—Emergency department patients are frequently acutely ill and require short-term intensive care and careful monitoring. The role of pulse oximetry in this setting has been studied and is increasing in popularity because of its ease of use and ability to evaluate oxygenation status quickly.[53, 54] It is certainly valuable to be able to noninvasively check an acutely ill patient's oxygenation status and get feedback within seconds. In patients with respiratory distress presenting in the emergency department, the ability of pulse oximetry to detect unsuspected changes in oxygenation, as well as hypoxemia during intubation, suctioning, and various other interventions, can greatly increase the efficiency of acute therapy (Fig 22–10).

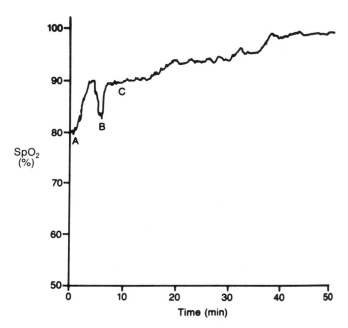

FIG 22–10.
Record of continuous oxygen monitoring in an ER patient with pulmonary edema showing changes in oxygenation associated with **A,** administration of oxygen, **B,** tracheal suctioning, **C,**diuresis with IV furosemide, and improvement in SpO2 as pulmonary edema was reduced. (*From Narang VPS:* Anesthesiol *1986; 65:239–240. Used by permission.*)

While the pulse oximeter is a useful surveillance tool in this acute care setting, the possibility of false-negative and false-positive values (based on the accuracy limitations of pulse oximetry, the possibility of undetected dyshemoglobinemias, shifts in the oxyhemoglobin curve, and artifacts), especially in this emergency setting, makes it risky to rely solely on pulse oximetry without selective ABG or CO-oximetry measurements.

Plethysmographic Uses of Pulse Oximetry. — The pulse monitoring capabilities of pulse oximeters have led to the investigation of a host of plethysmographic uses that could have clinical applications. It is often helpful to monitor heart rate as well as oxygen saturation in clinical situations, such as during diagnostic procedures and exercise, therapeutic interventions, and emergency care.

The amplitudes of pulse oximeter signals have been compared to Doppler determinations of arterial blood pressure[55, 56] and have been used to assess the adequacy of chest compressions in CPR.[57] Several studies have compared the use of a pulse oximeter for pulse detection versus the conventional Allen test to check the adequacy of collateral circulation in the hand,[58-62] although study results are mixed and inconclusive.

Pulse oximeter placement on the toe of a child was found to be useful in locating the femoral artery for cannulation.[63] Partridge described the use of pulse oximetry as a noninvasive indicator of volume status.[64] Menick[65] found the pulse oximeter useful to monitor perfusion of a muscle flap and skin graft site after surgery. He referred to the pulse oximeter as a "microvascular surgeon's sleep aid." Although pulse oximetry is useful in determining oxygenation status and appears sensitive in detecting pulsatile flow, there are limits to its usefulness as a monitor of tissue perfusion. Lawson et al.[66] reminds us that "the presence of a functioning pulse oximeter should not be construed as evidence of adequate tissue oxygenation or oxygen delivery to vital organs." Although more reports of plethysmographic uses of pulse oximetry are sure to come, currently, the uses are of unproven value and mostly anecdotal in nature.

Conclusions

The ability of pulse oximetry to monitor oxygenation status simply and continuously in the noncritically ill hospitalized patient lends itself to many clinical applications. The availability of real-time oxygenation data can help guide clinical interventions and decrease the incidence of patient hypoxia in many clinical settings (Table 22–6). However, the presence of monitoring equipment demands the attention of qualified personnel or the monitor is of no use. The value of monitoring in the general care areas can be limited by inattention to the oximetry results or inability to interpret saturation changes adequately.

Overall, many questions must be addressed and answered before pulse oximetry can be recommended as a "fifth vital sign" in general patient care settings (see Chapter 10 for details).

CO$_2$ MONITORING

For more than 100 years, attempts have been made to collect and analyze exhaled carbon dioxide (CO$_2$).[67] However, carbon dioxide monitoring has never gained widespread acceptance in adult general care despite significant technological improvements. One of the primary

TABLE 22–6.
Clinical Uses of Pulse Oximetry in General Care

Valuable Uses of Pulse Oximetry
- Monitoring therapeutic interventions
- Monitoring diagnostic procedures
- Pulmonary rehabilitation monitoring
- Tapering supplemental oxygen
- Emergency department monitoring

Possible Uses for Pulse Oximetry
- Monitoring conscious sedation/analgesia
- Monitoring long-term ventilator patients
- Pulse rate and amplitude detection

Pulse Oximetry Cautions
- Spot checks
- Dysfunctional hemoglobins
- Shifts in O_2 dissociation curve
- Poor perfusion
- Light absorption errors
- Motion

reasons it is not as popular as pulse oximetry is that increased carbon dioxide levels rarely cause death. Data from our outpatient pulmonary clinic indicate that patients remain functional with a broad range of CO_2 values (Fig 22–11). Knowledge of carbon dioxide tension alone has limited value. We need arterial blood gases to provide pH in order to determine if a value reflects an acute or chronic process.

End-tidal CO_2 monitoring is technically difficult and time-consuming compared to pulse oximetry, and the instruments require calibration. Much has been done to improve equipment operation, but end-tidal CO_2 monitoring requires a much greater understanding of physiology if it is to be used appropriately.

Transcutaneous CO_2 Monitoring

Transcutaneous Po_2 monitoring has never achieved widespread use in the adult general floor population. With its inherent problems of calibration, fear of burns, fragile sensors, and physiologic complexity, the monitor was unappealing and was quickly replaced by pulse oximetry.

The story is different with transcutaneous CO_2 monitoring. Here the competition between end-tidal CO_2 and transcutaneous CO_2 ($Ptcco_2$) is greater. Neither is easy to use, and both require a fairly sophisticated understanding of physiology. $Ptcco_2$ is reported to be as accurate as end-tidal CO_2 by Palmisano and Severinghaus[22] who conducted a large multi-center trial. The accuracy of transcutaneous CO_2 monitoring in their diverse patient population is displayed in Figure 22–12. Furthermore, there are cases where transcutaneous CO_2 monitoring is the only feasible CO_2 trending mechanism.

We monitored 21 patients being ventilated for nonanesthesia-related reasons[68] with a SensorMedics Transend monitor (SensorMedics Corp, Anaheim, CA) and a Novametrix 7000

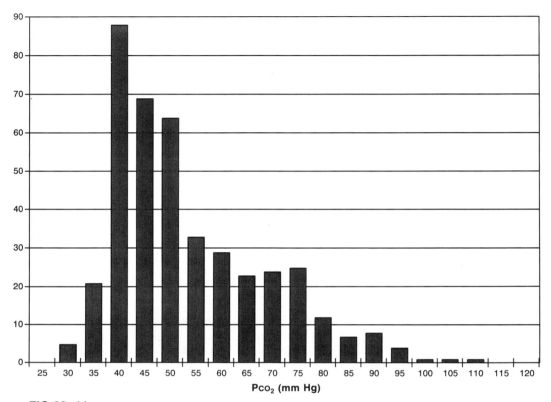

FIG 22–11.
Range of $Paco_2$ in 415 nonhospitalized COPD patients at Maine Medical Center, Portland, Maine.

combination mainstream $Petco_2$ monitor/pulse oximeter (Novametrix Medical Ssytems, Inc, Wallingford, CT). Combination transcutaneous Pco_2 and pulse oximetry monitors are currently available (Fig 22–13). Our findings in this setting were that in the majority of patients who had substantial respiratory distress, $Ptcco_2$ more accurately reflected $Paco_2$ and provided a better indication of ventilation status than $Petco_2$.

In the patient with chronic obstructive lung disease, transcutaneous monitoring is preferable to end-tidal CO_2 monitoring. These patients typically have high arterial CO_2, which is primarily a result of perfused areas that are underventialted. The $Paco_2 - Petco_2$ gradient is often wide because of increased dead-space, and emptying of the lungs is hampered by constricted airways and loss of elasticity. Transcutaneous monitoring more closely tracks arterial CO_2 in these patients.

$Ptcco_2$ would seem ideally suited for monitoring of patients receiving noninvasive ventilatory support. This equipment requires a mask that fits tightly over the nose and therefore eliminates the possibility of using end-tidal monitors. A report by Meduri et al.[69] presented a case of face

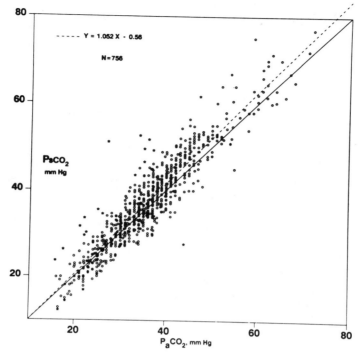

FIG 22–12.
The relationship of Ptcco$_2$ (Psco$_2$) to Paco$_2$, *n* = 756. The solid line is the identity. (*From Palmisano BW, Severinghaus JW: J Clin Monit 1990; 6:189–195. Used by permission.*)

mask ventilation that resulted in respiratory alkalosis with subsequent seizures and intubation (see Chapter 11 for details).

End-Tidal CO$_2$

In patients with normal ventilation-perfusion ratios, managing carbon dioxide levels is not difficult and CO$_2$ tensions are rarely the source of concern. In these patients alveolar carbon dioxide (P$_A$co$_2$) approximates Paco$_2$. On the other hand, when ventilation-perfusion mismatch occurs and ventilation exceeds perfusion, problems with end-tidal CO$_2$ monitoring occur. P$_A$co$_2$ does not equal Paco$_2$, and the end-tidal measurement reads lower than Paco$_2$. However, there are reports [70, 71] of cases and conditions in which the end-tidal CO$_2$ measurement is higher than the Paco$_2$. Patients whose perfusion exceeds ventilation may have a Pv̄co$_2$ greater than Paco$_2$ because there is more time for equilibration to take place between Pv̄co$_2$ and Paco$_2$. The unsophisticated user is often left confused and unable to explain these findings.

It is possible to monitor end-tidal CO$_2$ in nonintubated patients; reports of this application

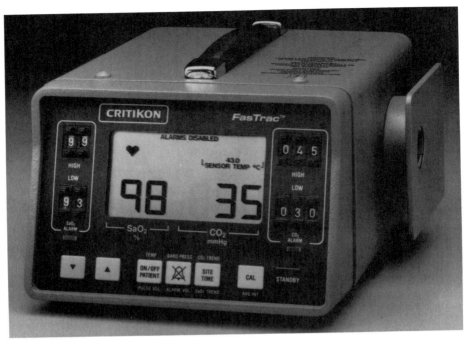

FIG 22–13.
Critikon combination transcutaneous CO_2 monitor–pulse oximeter. (*Courtesy of the Critikon Company.*)

have received mixed reviews. Patients who are in borderline ventilatory failure are poor candidates for end-tidal CO_2 monitoring because of the need to know the pH. Although end-tidal CO_2 monitoring has been described as an adjunct monitor during CPR in cardiac arrest and intubation, these applications apply to the ICU rather than general patient care areas.

End-tidal monitoring has been championed by some as the best disconnect alarm for patients who are mechanically ventilated on the general floors. Disconnects do happen and have been responsible for patient deaths. One common scenario is that the patient becomes disconnected and the patient ventilator circuit falls against the chest allowing pressure to be generated so that the low-pressure alarm does not sound. An oximeter might give an alarm depending on the FIO_2 requirements of the patient. A disconnect would be picked up immediately by an end-tidal CO_2 monitor. However, as an alarm it would be very expensive. The unit would have to be turned on and appropriately set and heard to be useful.

In circumstances when distinguishing a quantitative change in CO_2 is not necessary, other alternatives are available. Simple exhaled CO_2 monitors attached as nasal cannulas have been used as apnea monitors—usually in the neonatal population. A small plastic pH-sensitive device, which produces a color change in the presence of CO_2, is manufactured by Fenem, Inc. (Hollis, NY) and may be effective for detecting esophageal intubations.[72] This device may have application in cardiac arrest situations on the general floors (Fig 22–14). It is likely that the frequency of esophageal intubation is under-reported, making cost-benefit analyses difficult. The device can be stocked on a code cart and used during all intubations.

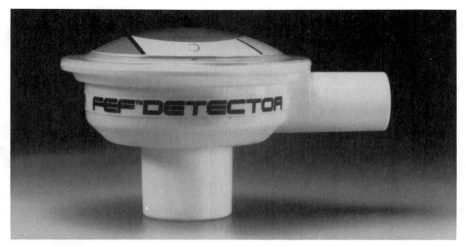

FIG 22–14.
Fenem Petco$_2$ detector (*Courtesy of Fenem Airway Management System, Hollis, NY.*)

The Ideal Place for CO$_2$ Monitoring

We believe that there is an appropriate place for CO$_2$ monitoring. The optimal setting would be an intermediate care unit for pulmonary patients. Krieger, Ershowsky, and Spivak[7] described a year's experience with a noninvasive monitoring unit. This unit accepted patients who still required close monitoring but who no longer needed intensive nursing care. Although they did not specifically address CO$_2$ monitoring, they used numerous types of monitoring with apparent success. This type of unit would seem appropriate for CO$_2$ monitoring. CO$_2$ monitoring will not take the place of blood gases, but in this setting it can reduce the number of blood gases drawn. Other uses for CO$_2$ monitoring are listed in Table 22–7.

It is appropriate to monitor exhaled CO$_2$ in the patient who requires emergency intubation as long as the complexity of the equipment does not compromise the rapidity of delivery of life-saving measures. An endotracheal tube in the esophagus requires immediate detection and

TABLE 22–7.
Uses of Carbon Dioxide Monitoring in General Care—by Technique

Transcutaneous CO$_2$ trending
Nasal CPAP/BiPAP
Nasal ventilation
Chronic hypoventilation
End-Tidal CO$_2$ trending
Weaning ventilated general care patients
End-Tidal CO$_2$ detector
Recognizing esophageal intubation

correction. A quick and simple color change indicator of CO_2 will halp guarantee appropriate endotracheal tube placement for the trained observer and help optimize care during these emergencies (see Chapters 12 and 23 for details).

MONITORING VENTILATORY MOVEMENT

Direct patient observation is the traditional and most practical method of monitoring and evaluating ventilatory movement. Ventilatory movement monitoring can be used to assess respiratory rate, tidal volume, ventilatory pattern, and the patient's work of breathing. Evaluation of these parameters may provide the clinician with valuable information concerning the changing respiratory status of the patient on the general floors. Patient observations are, by necessity, intermittent. Monitors are now available that can continuously monitor ventilatory excursions with varying degrees of reliability. Though many devices such as bellows pneumographs, linear differential transducers, mercury-in-silastic strain gauges, magnetometers, impedance pneumographs, and respiratory inductive plethysmographs are available, only the last two have been widely applied clinically.

The widespread use of impedance pneumography in infants at risk of sudden infant death syndrome came about prior to appropriate evaluation of the technique and understanding of its limitations.[73] The popularity of impedance pneumography has decreased because of its inability to adjust adequately to patient position changes. Alterations in chest lead position causes changes in electrical impedance. Cardiac impulse may mimic the impedance of a respiration and thus a respiratory rate may be indicated even in apnea.[74]

Respiratory inductance plethysmography (RIP) can continuously monitor and record respiratory rate and tidal volume without an artificial airway or mouthpiece in place (Fig 22–15). Shortcomings that dramatically affect the use of RIP in the general care areas include difficulty in assuring that trained personnel are available to calibrate the equipment and to monitor its performance. The cost of RIP units may range from over $5000 to near $100,000 for a four-bed self-calibrating unit. Krieger et al.[7] and Bone and Balk[6] described the use of centrally monitored RIP in a noninvasive respiratory monitoring unit as a cost-effective alternative to intensive care, especially in long-term ventilator patients. Although RIP monitoring in an intermediate intensive care setting is less expensive than intensive care, it is doubtful that this monitoring could be financially justified for chronic respiratory patients currently being monitored on the general floors of most hospitals. Respiratory inductive plethysmography may also prove to be of some use in monitoring postanesthesia recovery or respiratory depression in patients receiving sedation and analgesia.[74]

Besides these specific niches, we do not believe that monitoring by respiratory inductive plethysmography has a place on the general care floors at this time. It is presently more practical to monitor transcutaneous CO_2 tensions and perform bedside spirometry. There may be value in monitoring respiratory rate by impedance pneumography in adults at risk of respiratory arrest after they have made their way to the general floor areas. However, the possibility of maintaining the leads in the correct position and limiting false alarms seems remote in a nonintensive care setting.

In general, little case can be made for the continuous monitoring of ventilatory movement in the general care setting by use of impedance pneumography or respiratory inductive plethysmography. Observation by a clinician remains the most practical and appropriate (though not most accurate or continuous) method of monitoring ventilatory movement in the general care areas.

MONITORING PULMONARY FUNCTION AT THE BEDSIDE

Bedside measurements of flow rates and maximum respiratory pressures and volumes are important clinical tools for the diagnosis and monitoring of the patient with compromised respiratory status. Simple bedside spirometry consists of forced vital capacity (FVC) and forced expiratory volume (FEV_1) measurements. Peak flow rates, maximum inspiratory pressure (MIP), and maximum expiratory pressure (MEP) are also monitored at the bedside.

Spirometry

The intermittent use of bedside spirometry is a common method of objectively following the functional abilities of the patient at risk of respiratory compromise (Fig 22–16). Though bedside spirometry is often utilized as a diagnostic tool and compared to predictive nomograms, it is also valuable in objectively monitoring disease stability or progression, as well as monitoring response to therapeutic modalities. Making this easier are simple and relatively accurate hand-held spirometers.

According to Fallat,[75] spirometric monitoring in the nonintubated patient should probably be done more frequently than is currently practiced. He belives that as much can be learned about the chronic obstructive pulmonary disease patient by using the FEV_1/FVC ratio as an ABG measurement. FEV_1 can be a good indicator of decreased respiratory function and more sensitive to functional changes than ABG measurements. For example, increased P_{CO_2} values are infrequently seen in asthmatics until FEV_1 is less than 25% of predicted.[76] Changes in bedside spirometry normally precede other objective measures in identifying changes in pulmonary function and observable clinical symptoms.

The comparison of current spirometry with previous spirometry data allows for quantification of change in the patient's condition and can provide valuable guidance in titrating therapy. The FEV_1 indicates the degree of airway obstruction and verifies the benefit of therapy. A post-bronchodilator response greater than or equal to 15% (or 12% by the American Thoracic Society) is considered significant. Because the degree of respiratory impairment does not always correspond with the patient's subjective sensation of dyspnea, objective spirometric data can help adjust inhaled bronchodilators to optimal dosage and schedule.[77]

Peak Flows

The routine measurement and monitoring of peak expiratory flow rates (PEFR) is most often used to monitor response to bronchodilator treatment, particularly in asthmatic patients.[78]

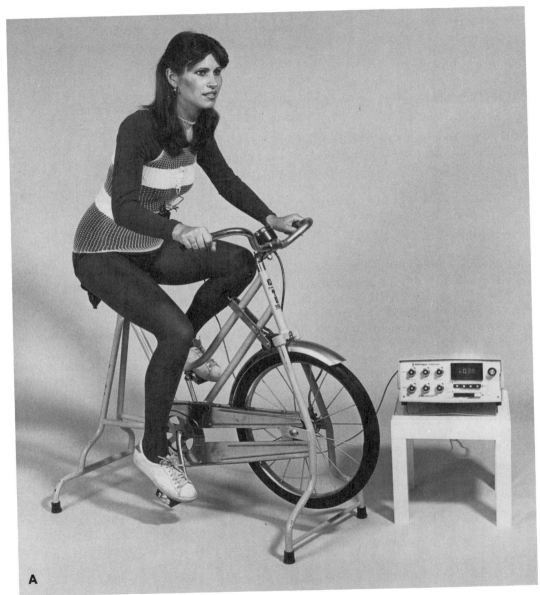

FIG 22–15.
Respiratory inductive plethysmography by the Respitrace monitor in **A**, active and **B**, inactive applications.
(*Courtesty of Ambulatory Monitoring, Inc, Ardsley, NY.*)

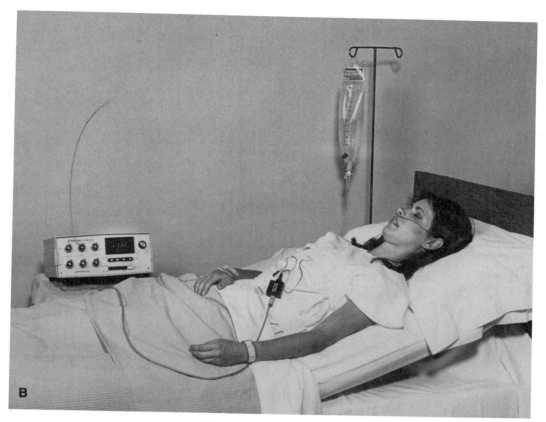

FIG 22–15. Continued

Peak flows are more variable than FEV_1 measurements because they are more effort-dependent. However, the simplicity and portability of relatively inexpensive peak flowmeters has made them a valuable objective measure of airway obstruction (Fig 22–17). In Europe, peak expiratory flow rates (PEFRs) are often monitored routinely as a fifth vital sign in airway obstruction. Asthmatic patients monitoring their PEFR were shown to use medication less often and to use fewer alternative non-drug therapies than a control group not monitoring PEFR.[79] European studies have suggested that patients can reliably keep their own peak flow records while hospitalized, thus saving nursing time and providing valuable clinical information.[80, 81]

It appears that despite its lack of precision when compared to more expensive and complicated FEV_1 measurement, PEFR could be effectively utilized as an objective measure of the course of obstructive disease and the response to bronchodilator therapy for many general floor patients.

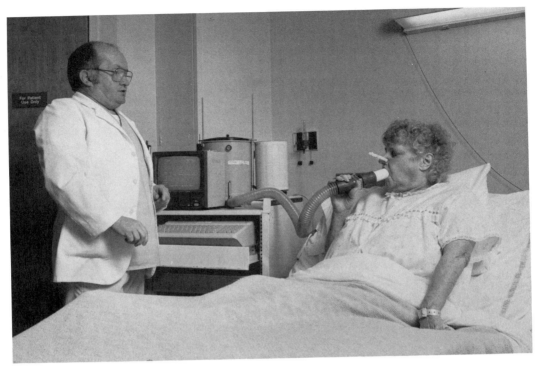

FIG 22–16.
Bedside spirometry—diagnostic and monitoring tool.

Uses of Bedside Pulmonary Function

Clinical evaluation may be unreliable in detecting airway obstruction.[82] For this reason, patients with obstructive lung disease should be monitored objectively for the presence and degree of airway obstruction in order to evaluate their need for and response to therapy. Too often patients are treated with varying dosages of systemic or inhaled anti-inflammatory or bronchodilator medications based on vague symptoms and no objective evidence of degree of obstruction or response to therapy. If airway obstruction were monitored by objective measurements such as spirometry or peak flows, a practical and effective regimen could be developed that would eliminate unnecessary treatment and optimize beneficial therapy.

Monitoring of bedside pulmonary function is often very useful in the neuromuscular disease patient as well as in the patient with obstructive lung disease. Monitoring of respiratory muscle weakness by use of bedside spirometry (primarily forced vital capacity and maximum voluntary ventilation) can provide valuable data for the assessment of the progression of neuromuscular weakness.[83] As discussed next in this section, maximal static respiratory pressures are the most appropriate measurements for monitoring respiratory muscle strength in the neuromuscular disease patient.

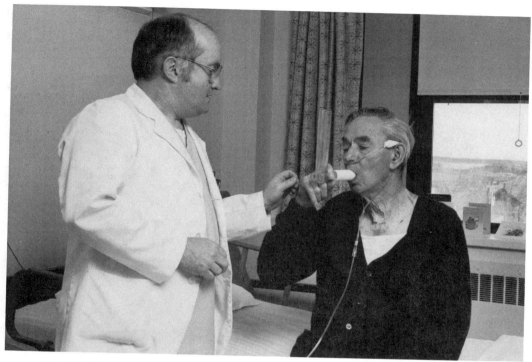

FIG 22–17.
Measurement of peak flow is simple though less precise and useful than spirometry.

Monitoring Respiratory Muscle Strength

Maximum inspiratory pressure (MIP, $P_{I_{max}}$) and maximum expiratory pressure (MEP, $P_{E_{max}}$) measurements are simple, direct indications of muscle strength, and they can be particularly useful in assessing respiratory reserve in general patient care areas (Fig 22–18). In practice, this monitoring is most often used on the general floors to measure the strength of respiratory muscles in patients with neuromuscular disease.[82]

Recent studies in critical care patients suggest the need for standardization of MIP and MEP measurement because of its technique sensitivity and effort dependency. For example, Branson et al.[84] and Kacmarek et al.[85] demonstrated that when an expiratory one-way valve and a 15- to 20-second airway occlusion was used, greater inspiratory pressures were generated in intubated patients and results were more repeatable than when other methods were used.

Standardization may be even more important in the nonintubated patient. It is more difficult to measure maximum inspiratory pressure and maximum expiratory pressure accurately in the general floor patient who does not have an artificial airway than in a patient with a cuffed tracheal tube. In a patient without an artificial airway, it is very important that a controlled

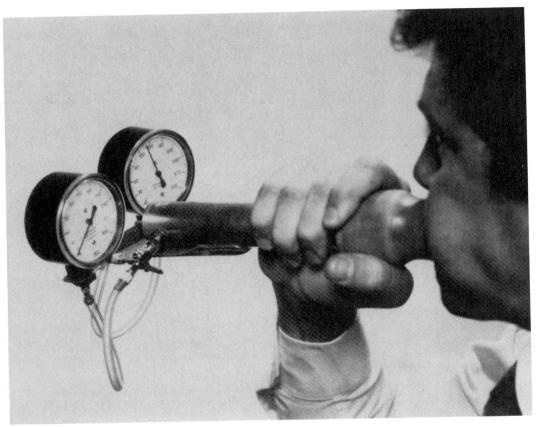

FIG 22–18.
A mouthpiece assembly and pressure gauges used to measure maximal inspiratory and expiratory respiratory pressures. (*From Enright PL, Hyatt RE:* Office Spirometry. *Philadelphia, Lea and Febiger, 1987, pp 13–22. Used by permission.*)

procedure be performed correctly and consistently in order to recognize trends and follow muscle strength.

Black and Hyatt,[82] who standardized MIP and MEP measurement, demonstrated its usefulness in a small group of neuromuscular disease patients with abnormal MIP an MEP values who had normal spirometry. Thus, it has been suggested that the measurement of maximum respiratory pressures are more accurate than vital capacity measurement in neuromuscular disease patients.[77] Besides being useful as a measure of inspiratory muscle strength in neuromuscular disease, MIP can be useful in quantitating the degree of respiratory muscle impairment in other conditions. MIP will be decreased by hyperinflation in emphysema. MIP may also be decreased in severe chest wall deformities, due to certain drugs and other conditions affecting diaphragm and inspiratory muscle function. MIP is also frequently utilized to monitor and assess the readiness to wean in the chronic ventilator patient.

A decreased MEP is seldom a cause for respiratory failure since expiration is generally passive. However, MEP can be helpful in evaluating a patient's ability to maintain a patent airway and clear secretions. A MEP greater than 40 cm H_2O is necessary to generate an effective cough.[86]

A normal value for MIP in adult men is greater than -100 cm H_2O. In adult women, the normal limit is -70 cm H_2O. MEP pressures of >200 cm H_2O in men and 140 cm H_2O in women are considered normal.[77] Some authors believe that these guidelines may exceed reasonable normal values,[86] and because of the extreme effort dependency, the lower limits of normal may be only one-third of the cited normals.[77]

The use of MIP and MEP measurements is recommended in evaluating patients with neuromuscular disease and potential respiratory muscle involvement.[82] In Guillain-Barre syndrome, myasthenia gravis, and other progressive neurological disorders, simple serial measurement of MIP and MEP can easily characterize the progression of the disease if a consistent procedure (Table 22–8) and a maximal effort is assured. Other circumstances in which the measurement of MIP and/or MEP is useful on the general floors include evaluating patients with unexplained dyspnea or respiratory failure, muscle dysfunction secondary to overinflation, and chest deformities.

MIP/MEP measurements are not normally used as a preoperative screening tool since they provide less information and demonstrate no clear advantage over routine spirometry.[87]

TABLE 22–8.
Procedure for MIP and MEP Measurement in Nonintubated Patients

---

1. Stress (and assure) maximal effort
   A. There is a considerable learning effect—subsequent numbers may be improved simply with practice
2. Position the patient sitting upright (or standing) for optimal efficiency
   A. Greater pressures can be obtained when there is no restriction from position
   B. Assure consistency in position on all subsequent efforts
3. Use a system with a small leak, an easily sealed rubber mouthpiece (or scuba-type mouthpiece), and a three-way valve to help assure maximal effort
4. For MIP Measurement:
   A. Use a nose clip
   B. Have the patient:
      1. Exhale to residual volume (three-way valve open to atmosphere)
      2. Place lips inside large rubber mouthpiece or tightly sealed around mouthpiece (turn three-way valve open to pressure gauge)
      3. Draw in as quickly and as hard as possible for 15 to 20 seconds
      4. Perform the manuever (and take measurements) three times
5. For MEP Measurement:
   A. Have the patient:
      1. Inhale to total lung capacity
      2. Place lips inside rubber mouthpiece
      3. Blast out air as quickly and as hard as possible
      4. Perform test three times if possible
   B. Test can be very uncomfortable—may not need (or be possible) to perform three times
6. Triplicate tests of MIP and MEP should be within 20% of each other

---

However, when neuromuscular disease or respiratory muscle weakness is of concern, MIP and MEP measurement is recommended.

INDIRECT CALORIMETRY ON GENERAL MEDICAL-SURGICAL FLOORS

For the most part, patients on the general wards are nourished orally, as formulated through consultation with dietary staff and the application of predictive caloric nomograms. However, a subgroup of individuals does exist whose clinical presentation and course renders the usual nutritional evaluation and prescription inaccurate and/or imprecise.

Patients identified as being at risk for complications from inappropriate nutritional support include patients with COPD, cancer, sepsis, burns, renal failure, malabsorption disorders, and those patients receiving long-term or parenteral feeding, as well as those recovering from major surgical procedures. For these patients, an approach that is somewhat more direct than that derived from regression models is indicated. Indirect calorimetry provides an accurate determination of caloric needs through the measurement of resting energy expenditure (REE). While there is no compelling need for continuously monitoring the caloric requirements of this patient group, the use of indirect calorimetry can be valuable and informative in the initial and post-treatment phases of nutritional support.[88] Available data suggest that measuring REE is more accurate than estimating REE. Foster et al.[89] studied 100 hospitalized patients and found that the nonprotein caloric requirements for total parenteral nutrition (TPN) based on measured caloric expenditure had minimal relationship to recommended caloric supply as calculated from published guidelines. According to their study, following the published guidelines on predicting energy expenditure would have resulted in the administration of 6947 excess liters of TPN per year.

In our institution, nonventilated patients located on general floors comprise approximately 5% of the population of patients undergoing measurement of REE by indirect calorimetry. These patients have been representative of the caseload as described above. Predominant diagnoses for this group have ranged from abdominal/GI sepsis and malabsorptive conditions, e.g., cystic fibrosis and inflammatory bowel syndromes, to metabolic disturbances associated with burn recovery and equivocal thyroid states. The current generation of open-circuit indirect calorimeters with mixing chambers and head hoods or canopies allows for the comfortable, well-tolerated, and precise measurement of REE in such patients and this has been our general experience. Our choice of equipment, Deltatrac Metabolic Monitor (SensorMedics Corp, Loma Linda, CA), operates on the dilution principle and requires that patients be free of supplemental oxygen and have the ability to tolerate placement under a canopy for exhaled gas collection for about 15 minutes (Fig 22–19). Canopy measurements with the Deltatrac on floor patients have yielded stable and precise clinical estimations of caloric requirements.

Major problems limiting the use of calorimetry on the general floors have been the initial cost of the instrument ($20,000 to $60,000), as well as the cost of training and maintaining a skilled operator to perform this technique-sensitive test. Surveys of institutions owning such metabolic carts have suggested that appropriate utilization of the service is maximized when

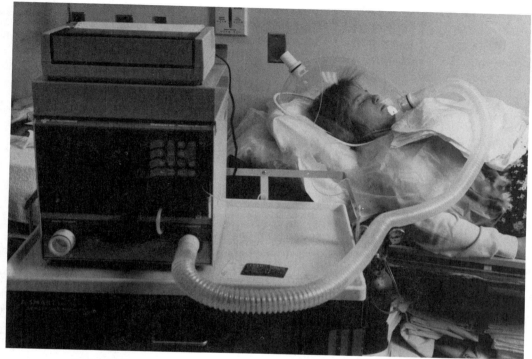

FIG 22–19.
Gas collecting canopy used for indirect calorimetry in nonintubated patients.

specialized personnel operate and maintain the instruments and when a team approach is employed in the interpretation and application of data. In addition, to assure that the technology is not overutilized just because it is available, or underutilized because it is uncommon, developing protocols for patient selection based on a predetermined criteria help to guide the clinical practice appropriately.[90]

It has been suggested that measurement of the oxygen cost of breathing (OCB) by indirect calorimetry may be used as a predictor of weaning success.[88] Calorimetry equipment may prove useful in evaluating OCB in long-term ventilator patients and may be useful in predicting caloric requirements and measuring CO_2 production. Additional research is required in order to evaluate the usefulness of indirect calorimetry for this application.

The use of indirect calorimetry has changed the nutritional management of a very small number of patients on our general floors. The equipment is expensive and requires specially trained individuals to assure consistency of this technique-sensitive technology. At this point in time, it is our opinion that this equipment can be best justified in centers engaged in research designed to identify the specific patient population that will most clearly benefit from the data generated. Larger centers with the financial and personnel resources available can do the medical community a service by identifying the group of patients whose nutritional status could be improved by monitoring indirect calorimetry-generated data. A tentative list of disease entities that could benefit from indirect calorimetry monitoring is given in Table 22–9.

In reality, most patients with severe gastrointestinal or metabolic disturbances who would benefit from monitoring with indirect calorimetry are cared for in critical care units. However, circumstances do arise in general care areas where the assessment of metabolic parameters by indirect calorimetry is beneficial (see Chapter 13 for details).

SUMMARY

Basic bedside evaluation by means of vital signs and physical exam remains the cornerstone of the monitoring structure in general patient care wards. Respiratory monitoring may frequently necessitate the use of arterial blood gases and other laboratory studies to aid in the identification of the causes or the extent of respiratory dysfunction. By necessity, monitoring on the general floors is usually intermittent; a clinician cannot be at the patient's side at all times. Noninvasive monitoring equipment such as pulse oximeters and transcutaneous and end-tidal CO_2 monitors can be more precise than clinical assessment and thus improve clinical decision-making, patient safety, and patient care. However, mechanical monitoring, even if noninvasive, cannot be recommended for the majority of general care respiratory patients. The amount of monitoring should be proportional to the patient's potential risk. This risk for general care patients, as opposed to intensive care patients, is minimal. Yet, risks will vary from patient to patient, from unit to unit and from situation to situation. The clinician's assessment of the need for monitoring ideally should be based on a demonstrated improvement in patient outcome when monitoring is utilized, but supportive "outcome" studies are sparse. The establishment of consistent policies and protocols for the appropriate use of monitoring on the general floors would help stem the arbitrary and unrestrained use of these modalities.

Indirect calorimetry, monitoring of ventilatory movement, and noninvasive CO_2 monitoring on the general floors seem indicated only in a specific small number of patients. The cost, as well as the complexity, of the equipment further relegates their more general use to intermediate or intensive care areas.

The effectiveness of bedside pulmonary function monitoring on the general floors as an

TABLE 22–9.
Potential Indications for Indirect Calorimetry Monitoring in General Care Areas

Abdominal/gastrointestinal disturbances
GI sepsis
Cystic fibrosis
Inflammatory bowel syndromes
Metabolic disturbances
Burn recovery
Thyroid abnormalities

objective measure of airway obstruction is well established. Pulmonary function monitoring allows the evaluation of functional respiratory impairment, as well as an assessment of response to bronchodilator therapies and other interventions.

The use of pulse oximetry has mushroomed in general care areas because of its ease of use, portability, and relatively low cost. The sanctity of adequate oxygenation fuels the belief that every unit needs a pulse oximeter. The value of trending and monitoring oxygen saturation in the anesthetized patient, critically ill patient, or patient undergoing diagnostic procedures is well established. However, the use of pulse oximeter saturations to replace arterial blood gases is wrought with problems and is discouraged, primarily based on pulse oximetry's inaccuracy.

One cannot pick up a newspaper today without reading about spiraling health care costs. It is important that we do our part and not allow for careless proliferation of technology. The goal of technology is to improve patient care. We need to be sure that the equipment we employ does, in fact, make a significant contribution to patient outcome before it becomes a standard of care.

Acknowledgments

We would like to thank Nancy Scarborough, John Dziodzio, and the pulmonary staff for their assistance in the preparation of this chapter, and the Maine Medical Center audio-visual department for their photographic work.

REFERENCES

1. Banta D: Technology assessment in health care in Jonus S (ed): *Health Care Delivery in the United States, ed 3. New York, Springer Publishing Co, 1986.*
2. Knox R: "'Free-choice' Rhetoric Isn't the Answer," *Boston Globe*, February 17, 1991, p 75.
3. King T, Simon RH: Pulse oximetry for tapering supplemental oxygen in hospitalized patients: evaluation of a protocol. *Chest* 1987; 92:713–716.
4. Joseph S, Kellerman AL, Cofer CA, Hackman BB: Impact of portable pulse oximetry on arterial blood gas analysis in an urban emergency department (abstract). *Ann Emerg Med* 1989; 18:458.
5. Finkler SA: The distinction between cost and charges. *Ann Intern Med* 1982; 96:102–109.
6. Bone RC, Balk RA: Noninvasive respiratory unit: A cost effective solution for the future. *Chest* 1988; 93:390–394.
7. Krieger BP, Ershowsky P, Spivack D, et al: Initial experience with a central respiratory monitoring unit as a cost saving alternative to the intensive care unit for Medicare patients who require long term ventilator support. *Chest* 1988; 93:395–397.
8. Kelleher JF; Pulse oximetry. *J Clin Monit* 1989; 5:37–62.
9. Hamilton WK: We monitor too much. *J Clin Monit* 1986; 2:264–267.
10. Block FE: We don't monitor enough. *J Clin Monit* 1986; 2:267–269.
11. MacIntyre NR: Respiratory monitoring without machinery. *Respir Care* 1990; 35:546–556.
12. Sapira JD: Vital signs in *The Art and Science of Bedside Diagnosis*. Baltimore, Urban and Schwarzenberg, 1990, pp 85–104.
13. McFadden JP, Price RC, Eastwood HD, et al: Raised respiratory rate in elderly patients. A valuable clinical sign. *Br Med J* 1982; 284;626–627.
14. Kory RC: The routine measurement of respiratory rate. An expensive tribute to tradition. *JAMA* 1957; 165:448–450.

15. Gravelyn TR, Weg JG: Respiratory rate as an indicator of acute respiratory dysfunction. *JAMA* 1980; 244:1123–1125.
16. Tandberg D, Sklar D: Effect of tachypnea on the estimation of body temperature by an oral thermometer. *N Engl J Med* 1983; 308:945–946.
17. Neff J, Ayoub J, Longman A, et al: Effect of respiratory rate, respiratory depth and open versus closed mouth on sublingual temperature. *Res Nurs Health* 1989; 12:195–202.
18. Wollam GI: *Hypertension Management: Clinical Practice and Therapeutic Dilemmas.* Chicago, Year Book Medical Publishers, 1988.
19. Bowton D, Scuderi P, Harris L, Haponik E. Pulse oximetry monitoring outside the intensive care unit: progress or problem. *Ann Intern Med* 1991; 115:450–454.
20. Severinghaus JW, Astrup PB: History of blood gas analysis. VI. Oximetry. *J Clin Monit* 1986; 2:270–288.
21. Tremper KK, Shomaker W: Transcutaneous oxygen monitoring of critically ill adults with and without low flow shock. *Crit Care Med* 1981; 9:709.
22. Palmisano BW, Severinghaus JW: Transcutaneous PCO_2 and PO_2. A multi-center study of accuracy. *J Clin Monit* 1990; 6:189–195.
23. Lukkari-Routiarinen E, Lepantalo M, Pietila J: Reproducibility of skin blood flow, perfusion pressure and oxygen tension measurements in advanced lower limb ischemia. *Eur J Vasc Surg* 1989; 3:345–350.
24. Cote CJ, Goldstein EA, Cote MA, et al: A single blind study of pulse oximetry in children. *Anesthesiol* 1988; 68:184–188.
25. *Operators Manual—Nellcor N-200 Pulse Oximeter*, Nellcor Inc, Hayward, CA, 1989.
26. Severinghaus JW, Naifeh KH: Accuracy of response of six pulse oximeters to profound hypoxia. *Anesthesiol* 1987; 67:551–558.
27. Nickerson BG, Sarkisian C, Tremper K: Bias and precision of pulse oximeters and arterial oximeters. *Chest* 1988; 93:515–517.
28. Murphy KG, Secunda JA, Rockoff MA: Severe burns from a pulse oximeter. *Anesthesiol* 1990; 73:350–352.
29. Choe H, Tashiro C, Fukumitsu K, et al: Comparison of recorded values from six pulse oximeters. *Crit Care Med* 1989; 17:678–681.
30. Barker SJ, Tremper KK: The effects of carbon monoxide inhalation on pulse oximetry and transcutaneous PO_2. *Anesthesiol* 1987; 66:677–679.
31. Barker SJ, Tremper KK, Hyatt J, et al: Effects of methemoglobinemia on pulse oximetry and mixed venous oximetry (abstract). *Anesthesiol* 1987; 67:A171.
32. Eisenkraft JB: Pulse oximeter desaturation due to methemoglobinemia. *Anesthetiol* 1988; 68:279–282.
33. Kessler MR, Eide T, Humayum B, et al: Spurious pulse oximeter desaturation with methylene blue injection. *Anesthesiol* 1986; 65:435–436.
34. Costarino AT, Davis DA, Keon TP: Falsely normal saturation reading with a pulse oximeter. *Anesthesiol* 1987; 67:830–831.
35. Evans ML, Geddes LA: An assessment of blood vessel vasoactivity using photoplethysmography. *Med Instrum* 1988; 22:29–32.
36. Ries AL, Prewitt LM, Johnson JJ: Skin color and ear oximetry. *Chest* 1989; 96:287–290.
37. Cote CJ, Goldstein EA, Fushman WH, et al: The effect of nail polish on pulse oximetry. *Anesth Analg* 1988; 67:683–686.
38. New W: Pulse oximetry. *J Clin Monit* 1985; 1:126–129.
39. Dear PRF: Monitoring oxygen in the newborn: saturation or partial pressure? *Archives Child Dis* 1987; 62:879–881.
40. Carlin BW, Clausen JL, Ries AL: The use of cutaneous oximetry in the prescription of long term oxygen therapy. *Chest* 1988; 94:239–241.

41. Criteria for Medicare coverage of oxygen services in the home. *Federal Register*, April 5, 1985, p 50.
42. Smoker JM, Hess DR, Frey-Zeiler VL, et al: A protocol to assess oxygen therapy. *Respir Care* 1986; 31:35–39.
43. Escourrou PJL, Delaperche MF, Visseaux A: Reliability of pulse oximetry during exercise in pulmonary patients. *Chest* 1990; 97:635–638.
44. Tiep BL, Burns M, Kas D, et al: Pursed lip breathing training using ear oximetry. *Chest* 1986; 90:218–221.
45. Berman L, Jones NL: Fiberoptic bronchoscopy: Monitoring oxygenation with ear oximetry (letter). *Am Rev Respir Dis* 1976; 114:651.
46. Dodson SR, Hensley FA, Martin DE, et al: Continuous oxygen saturation monitoring during cardiac catheterization in adults. *Chest* 1988; 94:28–31.
47. Stewart IC, Parker A, Catterall JR, et al: Effect of bronchial challenge on breathing patterns and arterial oxygenation in stable asthma. *Chest* 1989; 95:65–70.
48. Adams KS, Branson, RD, Hurst M: Monitoring of oxygenation by pulse oximetry during diagnostic procedures (abstract). *Respir Care* 1985; 30:859.
49. MacKenzie AJ: Perioperative hypoxemia detected by intermittent pulse oximetry. *Anesth Intens Care* 1989; 17:412–417.
50. Choi HJ, Little MS, Garber SZ, et al: Pulse oximetry for monitoring during ward analgesia: Epidural morphine versus parenteral narcotics. *J Clin Monit* 1989; 5:87–89.
51. Marzocchi M, Brouillette RT, Weese-Mayer DE, et al: Comparison of transthoracic impedance/ heart rate monitoring and pulse oximetry for patients using diaphragm pacemakers. *Pediatr Pulmonol* 1990; 8:29–32.
52. Verhoeff F, Sykes MK: Delayed detection of hypoxic events by pulse oximeter: computer simulations. *Anesthesia* 1990; 45:103–109.
53. McGuire TJ: Evaluation of a pulse oximeter in the pre-hospital setting. *Ann Emerg Med* 1988; 17:1058–1062.
54. Jones J, Heiselman D, Cannon L, et al: Continuous emergency department monitoring of arterial saturation in adult patients with respiratory distress. *Ann Emerg Med* 1988; 17:463–468.
55. Korbon GA, Wills MH, D'Lauro F, et al: Systolic blood pressure measurement: Doppler vs pulse oximeter. (abstract). Anesthesiol 1987; 67:A188.
56. Wallace CT, Baker JD, Alpert CC, et al: Comparison of blood pressure measurement by Doppler and by pulse oximetry techniques. *Anesth Analg* 1987; 66:1018–1019.
57. Narang VPS: Utility of the pulse oximeter during cardiopulmonary resuscitation. (letter). *Anesthesiol* 1986; 65:239–240.
58. Nowak GS, Moorthy SS, McNiece WL: Use of pulse oximetry for assessment of collateral arterial flow. (letter). *Anesthesiol* 1986; 64:527.
59. Hovagim AA, Katz RI, Poppers PJ: Pulse oximetry for evaluation of radial and ulnar blood flow. (abstract). *Anesth Analg* 1988; 67:594.
60. Matsuki A; A modified Allen's test using a pulse oximeter (letter). *Anesth Intens Care* 1988; 16:126–127
61. Laur KK, Cheng EY, Stommel KA, et al: Pulse oximetry evaluation of the palmar circulation. (abstract). *Anesth Analg* 1988; 67:S129.
62. Raja R. The pulse oximeter and the collateral circulation. (letter). *Anesthesia* 1986; 47:781–782.
63. Introna RPS, Silverstein PI: A new use for the pulse oximeter. (letter). *Anesthesiol* 1986; 65:342.
64. Partridge BL: Use of pulse oximetry as a noninvasive indicator of intravascular volume status. *J Clin Monit* 1987; 3:263–268.
65. Menick FJ: The pulse oximeter in free muscle flap surgery: "A microvascular surgeon's sleep aid." *J Reconstructive Microsurg* 1988; 4:331–334.
66. Lawson D, Norley I, Korbon G, et al: Blood flow limits and pulse oximeter signal detection. *Anesthesiol* 1987; 67:599–603.

67. Tyndall J: Action of an intermittent beam of radiant heat upon gaseous matter. *Nature (London)* 1881; 23:374–377.

68. Blanchette T, Harris K, Dziodzio J: Transcutaneous PCO_2 vs end tidal PCO_2 in ventilated adults. (abstract). *Respir Care* 1990; 35:1132.

69. Meduri G, Conoscenti C, Menashe P, et al: Noninvasive face mask ventilation in patients with acute respiratory failure. *Chest* 1989, 95:865–870.

70. Shankar KB, Mosely H, Kumar Y, et al: Arterial to end-tidal carbon dioxide difference during Caesarean section anaesthesia. *Anaesthesia* 1986; 41:698–702.

71. Fletcher R, Jonso B: Deadspace and the single breath test for carbon dioxide during anaesthesia and artificial ventilation. *Br J Anaesth* 1984; 56:109–119.

72. Hess D: Capnometry and capnography. *Respir Care* 1990; 35:557–576.

73. National Institutes of Health Consensus Development Conference Statement. Infantile apnea and home monitoring. US Department of Health and Human Services; National Institute of Health Publication No. 87-2905, 1987.

74. Tobin MJ: Noninvasive evaluation of respiratory movement, in Nochomovitz ML, Cherniak (eds): *Noninvasive Respiratory Monitoring.* New York, Churchill Livingstone; 1986, pp 29–57.

75. Fallat RJ: Bedside pulmonary function and ICU monitoring: Indications and interpretation, in Wilson AF (ed): *Pulmonary Function Testing.* Orlando, Grune and Stratton, 1985, p 296.

76. McFadden ER, Jr, Lyons HA: Arterial blood gas tensions in asthma. *N Engl J Med* 1968; 278:1027.

77. Enright PL, Hyatt RE: *Office Spirometry.* Philadelphia, Lea and Febiger, 1987, pp 13–22.

78. Klaustermeyer WB, Kurohara M, Guerra GA: Predictive value of monitoring expiratory peak flow rates in hospitalized adult asthma patients. *Ann Allergy* 1990; 64:281–284.

79. Plymat KR, Bunn CL: Monitoring asthma with a Mini-Wright peak flow meter. *Nurse Pract* 1985; 10:25–27.

80. Jansen-Bjerklie S, Shnell S: Effect of peak flow information on patterns of self care in adult asthma. *Heart-Lung* 1988; 17:543–549.

81. Hetzel MR, Williams IP, Shakespeare RM: Can patients keep their own peak-flow records reliably? *Lancet* 1979; 1(8116):597–599.

82. Black LF, Hyatt RE: Maximum static respiratory pressures in generalized neuromuscular disease. *Am Rev Respir Dis* 1971; 103:641–650.

83. Dawson A: Spirometry, in: Wilson AF (ed): *Pulmonary Function Testing.* Orlando, Grune and Stratton, 1985.

84. Branson RD, Hurst JM, Davis K, et al: Measurement of maximal inspiratory pressure: A comparison of three methods. *Respir Care* 1989; 34:789–794.

85. Kacmarek RM, Cycyk-Chapman MC, Young-Palazzo PJ, et al: Determination of maximal inspiratory pressure: A clinical study and literature review. *Respir Care* 1989; 34:868–878.

86. Collier CR: Elastic recoil and compliance, in Wilson AF (ed): *Pulmonary Function Testing.* Orlando, Grune & Stratton, 1985, p 132.

87. Gilbert R, Auchinocloss JH, Bleb S: Measurement of maximal inspiratory pressure during routine spirometry. *Lung* 1978; 155:23–32.

88. Branson RD: The measurement of energy expenditure: instrumentation, practical considerations and clinical applications. *Respir Care* 1990; 35:640–659.

89. Foster GD, Knox LS, Dempsey DT, et al: Calorie requirements in total parenteral nutrition. *J Am Coll Nutr* 1987; 6:231–253.

90. Ritz R: Resource management for noninvasive monitoring. *Respir Care* 1990; 35:729–739.

Chapter 23

Monitoring in Anesthesia

Takahisa Goto, M.D.

Jeffrey B. Cooper, Ph.D.

INTRODUCTION

Patient care in the operating room has different objectives from that in the intensive care unit (ICU). This places different demands on the monitoring as well. Surgery is a continuous trauma to the body. It requires anesthesia, a reversible pharmacologic intervention to keep the patient comfortable and stable during this period of trauma by inducing unconsciousness and/ or blocking the nerve impulses. Alterations of the patient's condition by anesthesia and surgery should be monitored in addition to the disease itself.

The objectives of monitoring in the operating room can be described in three categories:

1. Monitoring of the depth of anesthesia
2. Physiological monitoring
3. Safety monitoring.

The monitoring technologies used in the operating room are not so different from those used in other clinical settings. There are few technologies that are peculiar to anesthesia. In this chapter, we will focus on why the various forms of monitoring are used. Discussion of how monitors work has been presented in other chapters, although some special technologies peculiar to anesthesia are discussed below.

WHAT IS ANESTHESIA?

There are roughly three approaches to producing anesthesia, i.e., general, regional, and local. General anesthesia implies that the patient is rendered unconscious by the anesthetics. Regional anesthesia means that sensory (and frequently motor) nerve fibers are blocked by the epidural, spinal, or major nerve block technique so that the patient, although awake, does not feel pain or discomfort. Local anesthesia means infiltration of local anesthetics such as Xylocaine to numb the surgical field. In the following discussion, the term *anesthesia* refers to general anesthesia unless otherwise specified.

In current clinical practice, there are roughly two types of general anesthesia: inhalational and balanced (or narcotic) anesthesia.

In the inhalational anesthesia technique, one of the potent inhalational anesthetics such as halothane, enflurane, or isoflurane is given to render the patient unconscious, usually in combination with nitrous oxide. Nitrous oxide itself is also an inhalational anesthetic, but too weak to be used as a single anesthetic for all but the most minor procedure, e.g., dental extractions. But it is very useful because, in contrast to other potent inhalational agents, it has no significant cardiovascular depressive effect and also provides very rapid awakening. For the inhalational technique, 60 to 70% nitrous oxide in oxygen is typically administered with one of the potent inhalational agents.

Balanced anesthesia consists of nitrous oxide in oxygen, narcotics such as morphine, fentanyl, etc., and a muscle relaxant. The word "balanced" comes from the concept of the "components of general anesthesia," which include (1) analgesia, (2) amnesia, (3) muscle relaxation, and (4) blunted reflexes[1-3] (Table 23–1). In balanced anesthesia, nitrous oxide is used for amnesia and narcotics for analgesia.[4] Thus, each component of anesthesia is controlled by different drugs and the well-controlled combination of those medications provides satisfactory anesthesia.

Monitoring the Depth of Anesthesia

Unfortunately, there are no reliable monitors of amnesia (unconsciousness), the first component of anesthesia. The electroencephalogram (EEG) is not useful because different drugs produce different EEG patterns.[5] Changes in carbon dioxide, oxygen, body temperature, sensory stimulation, and blood pressure also influence the EEG.[6] It is therefore unrealistic to expect any simple relationship between the EEG pattern and clinical depth of anesthesia. The major use of EEG monitoring today is to ascertain adequacy of cerebral perfusion, such as during a carotid endarterectomy.

The only "monitor" of amnesia routinely used is the patient's postoperative statement that he or she had no recall of the intraoperative events or conversations.[7] A dose of drug is normally chosen that provides a lack of recall in all patients. Unfortunately, there are occasions on which an insufficient dose is used.

TABLE 23–1.
Goals of Anesthesia

Analgesia
Amnesia
Muscle relaxation
Blunted reflexes

Muscle relaxation, the second component of anesthesia, has been used to determine the potency of inhalational anesthetics, i.e., the *minimum alveolar concentration* (MAC).[8, 9] MAC is the concentration of an inhalational anesthetic in the alveoli, which suppresses the motor response to the initial surgical incision in 50% of the subjects. In general, patients who do not move under inhalational anesthesia have no recall of the surgical events. Therefore, the concentration of inhalational anesthetics needed to provide immobilization is normally high enough to guarantee amnesia. During balanced anesthesia, immbolization is usually provided by a muscle relaxant because even a massive dose of narcotic cannot guarantee immobilization. In this case, muscle relaxation does not mean amnesia because muscle relaxants do not affect consciousness.

Monitoring of reflexes or responses to noxious stimuli is also essential during anesthesia. The "responses" in this context refer to visceral and autonomic responses, i.e., respiratory (breath-holding, coughing), hemodynamic (hypertension, tachycardia), sweating, tearing, and hormonal (increased serum level of catecholamines and various other stress hormones). The respiratory pattern can be observed easily during inhalational general anesthesia when the patient is breathing spontaneously. This is one of the most important monitors of the depth of anesthesia. An adequately anesthetized patient breathes regularly with reduced tidal volume and at a relatively fast rate. As anesthesia becomes lighter and the patient enters the so-called "second" (or excitatory) stage, the respiration becomes irregular with intermittent sighs, and breath-holding, coughing, or laryngospasm may occur. Those signs not only suggest light anesthesia, but may impair gas exchange leading to precipitous oxygen desaturation. In a balanced technique, this useful monitor is lost because the respiratory muscles are paralyzed by the muscle relaxant.

Hemodynamic responses to the surgical stimuli are relied on heavily for assessing the depth of anesthesia. The inhalational anesthetic concentration required to suppress the hemodynamic responses to surgical incision in 50% of the patiens is about 45 to 60% higher than MAC.[10] Clearly, anesthetic depth sufficient to suppress hemodynamic responses to stimuli is also deep enough to prevent the patient from moving, which again should correlate with amnesia during inhalational anesthesia.

Sweating and tearing are also good indicators of light anesthesia and should be watched for carefully. Hormonal responses to stress are very difficult and unrealistic to monitor directly. They are monitored indirectly by blood pressure and heart rate.

In summary, under inhalational anesthesia, hemydynamic monitoring and, if spontaneous respiration is present, the observation of respiration are most important in monitoring depth of anesthesia, because a greater concentration of anesthetics is required to control these parameters than to provide muscle relaxation and amnesia. Under balanced anesthesia, again the indices of stress responses such as blood pressure, heart rate, sweating, and tearing are monitored. Immobilization is achieved by a muscle relaxant, which can be monitored by an electronic nerve stimulator. There is no means to monitor amnesia. In fact, balanced anesthesia is known to carry a significant risk of postoperative recall, and this problem remains to be solved.[11]

Thus, assessment of anesthetic depth has traditionally relied on monitoring of physical signs. While technological advances have modernized cardiovascular monitoring, they have not produced practical means of monitoring the depth of anesthesia.

PHYSIOLOGICAL MONITORING

Hemodynamic Monitoring

Hemodynamic monitoring has become more important in today's anesthesia because, with the advancement of monitoring, anesthetic drugs and management techniques, increasing numbers of seriously ill patients present for surgery.

Stethoscope

Monitoring heart and breath sounds via either a precordial or esophageal stethoscope is one of the basic and most useful monitors because it is continuous, noninvasive, easy-to-use, inexpensive, and covers both respiratory and cardiovascular systems simultaneously. Absent or diminished breath sounds, wheezing, or rhonchi from secretions may suggest inadequate ventilation or oxygenation. Heart sounds are also important. In the face of a flat ECG or unobtainable blood pressure, the presence of heart sounds should be checked immediately to rule out cardiac arrest. A precordial stethoscope and pulse oximeter may be sufficient monitors to start induction of anesthesia for a crying and scared child.

Blood Pressure

Blood pressure reflects not only the physiologic state (i.e., heart function, vascular tone, perfusion of vital organs, intravascular blood volume), but also the depth of anesthesia. A rapid fall in blood pressure may also reflect anesthetic overdose and so serves a safety function. Because anesthetics (especially inhalational) are potent cardiovascular depressants, some patients cannot tolerate the anesthetizing dose and experience severe hypotension. Indeed, by Keenan's report[13] of intraoperative cardiac arrests due to anesthesia, 6 of 27 occurred in patients with unstable hemodynamics from either sepsis or heart disease. Other studies of anesthetic mortality also point to "cardiovascular collapse"[13] or "failure of circulatory homeostasis"[14] occurring after administration of a conventional dose of anesthetic.

Blood pressure is usually checked with a blood pressure cuff at least every five minutes during anesthesia, although manual measurements are often replaced by an automatic noninvasive blood pressure monitor. An arterial catheter (A-line) is placed if beat-to-beat measurement is necessary. Operations for which an arterial catheter is usually placed are:

1. Cardiac and major vascular surgery (e.g., aortic aneurysm resection, carotid endarterectomy)
2. Neurosurgery, especially craniotomy (e.g., removal of brain tumor, hematoma or AVM, cerebral aneurysm clipping)
3. Lung resection (partly because frequent arterial blood gas analysis is required)
4. Operations in which massive blood loss or fluid shift is expected (e.g., hepatic resection, extensive abdominal or pelvic surgery)

5. Operations in which deliberate hypotension is planned to reduce blood loss or to facilitate surgery (e.g., total hip replacement, Harrington rod for scoliosis).

ECG

Intraoperative monitoring of the ECG is aimed at the detection of arrhythmias, myocardial ischemia, heart block, and pacemaker function. Standard limb lead II is always monitored during anesthesia for the detection and diagnosis of arrhythmias and heart block because P waves are most prominent in this lead. The presence or absence of P waves and the relationship of P and QRS waves are essential in diagnosing arrhythmias. The reported incidence[15] of arrhythmias during anesthesia is 60 to 84%, although life-threatening arrhythmias occur in less than 1%. When arrhythmias are diagnosed, both underlying abnormalities and hemodynamic instabilities should be treated. Junctional rhythms are common under anesthesia. Marked hypotension can occur with loss of P waves, especially in patients with heart disease who depend highly on atrial contractions for their cardiac output. (For example, atrial contraction accounts for up to 40% of cardiac output in patients with aortic stenosis, in contrast to 15 to 20% in normal subjects.) Tachycardia and premature ventricular contractions are also common and predisposed by hypoxia, hypercarbia, electrolyte abnormalities, or myocardial ischemia. Bradycardia is the most deleterious arrhythmia in infants, usually caused by hypoxia or vago-vagal reflex, resulting in a proportional decrease in cardiac output and blood pressure. The ECG is also useful in diagnosing myocardial ischemia.

Continuous monitoring of a 12-lead ECG in the operating room is impractical. Standard limb lead II used for detection of arrhythmias can also identify ischemia of the inferior wall. However, the more common anterior or lateral wall ischemia may be missed. Blackburn and Raymundo[16] showed that 89% of ischemic episodes during the exercise tolerance test were identified in lead V5, while the combination of II, aVF, V3 through V6 covered almost all ischemic events. London et al.[17] confirmed these findings by recording the 12-lead ECG intraoperatively. They showed that sensitivity was greatest in V5 (75%) and V4 (61%) while the combination of II, V4, and V5 was 96% sensitive. Therefore, the combination of II and V4 and V5 is usually selected if the patient is at high risk of myocardial ischemia.[18] Obviously, if the lead in which ischemic changes are most likely to occur is known preoperatively, that lead should be monitored during anesthesia.

The ECG has some limitations as a monitor of myocardial ischemia. Various conditions such as left bundle branch block, left ventricular hypertrophy, digitalis administration, or electrolyte imbalance distort the baseline ECG and make ST-T analysis more difficult and less sensitive. ECG changes are not the earliest signs of myocardial ischemia; they usually appear 30 to 60 seconds after acute ischemic injury. Myocardial wall motion abnormalities have been shown to occur much earlier,[19–21] which can be detected by transesophageal echocardiography.

Automatic ST-segment trend monitoring is useful for some procedures, e.g., cardiac or vascular surgery.[22] ST depression/elevation is monitored automatically and an alert is provided to subtle changes not easily recognized on conventional ECG monitors.

Central Venous Catheter and Pulmonary Artery Catheter

Central venous pressure (CVP) is monitored to assist in the evaluation of fluid status when the patient with normal cardiopulmonary function undergoes surgery with large blood loss or fluid shift, especially when urinary output is unreliable, e.g., radical cystectomy, radical prostatectomy, patients with renal dysfunction or on chronic diuretic therapy. The subclavian approach is usually avoided for catheter placement because of higher risk of pneumothorax. This is of particular concern during anesthesia because positive pressure ventilation may cause tension pneumothorax if the pleural space is accidentally punctured during catheter placement. The internal jugular, external jugular, or basilic vein (in antecubital fossa) are the commonly used insertion sites.

A central venous catheter is also used to treat air embolism. Especially during surgery in the posterior fossa (cerebellum) in the sitting position, subatmospheric pressure may develop in dural venous sinuses because the surgical site is well above the level of the heart, and air may be drawn into the venous circulation. Massive air embolization in the pulmonary vasculature causes hypotension by impairing blood return to the left heart. When air embolism is suspected, the central venous catheter can be aspirated to remove air from the right atrium.

A pulmonary artery (PA) catheter is usually indicated to reflect left-sided filling pressures and cardiac output of the patient with poor cardiopulmonary function when large fluid shifts or blood loss is expected during surgery. In the presence of chronic obstructive pulmonary disease, pulmonary hypertension, or left ventricular dysfunction, CVP correlates poorly with left-sided filling pressures.

A PA catheter may be used more frequently in the operating room than in the ICU setting because anesthesia and surgery affect the patient's baseline cardiovascular function. Anesthetics depress the heart and cause vasodilation, which may not be tolerated by the patient with marginal cardiac function and almost no reserve, e.g., the patient with congestive heart failure at rest or with minimal exercise, or severe valvular disease. When such patients develop hypotension during anesthesia, it is often difficult to know whether it is derived from hypovolemia, depressed contractility of the heart, or low vascular tone. Blood loss and fluid shift make the problem more complicated. The cardiac output and PCWP need to be measured with a PA catheter in such a situation.

A PA catheter is used routinely for cardiac surgery at many institutions. A unique feature of cardiac surgery is the use of cardiopulmonary bypass (CPB). During CPB, the heart is isolated from the systemic circulation, arrested or fibrillated, and emptied. The blood flow to the myocardium is stopped and body temperature may be lowered. Although every effort is made to protect the heart from ischemic injury during this period, heart function is depressed at the end of the CPB. On weaning from CPB, catecholamine and fluid therapy is guided under PA monitoring to optimize the contraction and filling of the heart as well as to counteract the vasodilation caused by rewarming.

Early reports implied that a PA catheter could detect myocardial ischemia earlier than the ECG by the elevation of PCWP or changes in the PCWP waveform,[23] but recent studies have shown that these signs are too insensitive and nonspecific[24, 25]

The limitation of PCWP to evaluate heart function is that PCWP is only an indirect measurement of left ventricular end-diastolic volume (which reflects left-sided preload) and does not necessarily correlate with it. Mitral valve dysfunction, positive pressure ventilation, positive end-expiratory pressure (PEEP), cardiac tamponade, changes in stiffness of the heart after heart surgery, acute myocardia ischemia or sepsis make interpretation of PCWP difficult.[26, 27] Echocardiography can monitor the size and contraction of the heart under direct vision and has been recently introduced for intraoperative use.

Transesophageal Echocardiography

Echocardiography offers advantages over the ECG and the PA catheter for the followings:

1. Earlier and more sensitive detection of myocardial ischemia than the ECG by detecting segmental wall motion abnormalities (SWMAs) of the heart[28]
2. Direct evaluation of the size and ejection of the heart
3. By combining with the Doppler technique, blood flow through valves can be clearly visualized; thus, stenosis and regurgitation can be quantitatively evaluated.

Surface echocardiography, which requires the probe to be placed on the anterior chest wall, is often impractical during surgery. With the introduction of a probe that can be positioned in the esophagus, intraoperative two-dimensional echocardiography has become a practical diagnostic tool for anesthesiologists.[29] Transesophageal echocardiography is performed via a gastroscope with a small probe mounted on its tip (Fig 23–1).

Transesophageal echocardiography, however, has not become a common monitor because of several limitations. Quantitative evaluation may require a computer-assisted video review system, which is too time-consuming for use in the operating room. Reproducibility of quantitative findings is critically dependent on highly skilled operators.[30] SWMAs are sensitive but not specific markers of myocardial ischemia. Their value in predicting outcome is controver-

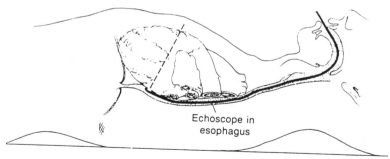

Echoscope in
esophagus

FIG 23–1.
Two-dimensional echocardiography monitoring in the operating room. Illustration of transesophageal probe placement. (*From deBruijn NP, Clements FM:* Transesophageal Echocardiography, *Boston, Martinus Nijhoff Publishing, 1987, p 6. Used by permission.*)

sial; new or worsened intraoperative SWMAs have been reported to correlate poorly with postoperative cardiac complications.[31]

RESPIRATORY MONITORING

Effects of Anesthesia on Respiratory Function

Why do we monitor respiratory function during anesthesia even in a patient with healthy lungs?

1. Safety monitoring; the majority of anesthesia incidents are associated with respiratory events. This will be discussed further in the section of safety monitoring.
2. Anesthesia and surgery impair gas exchange even in normal lungs by the mechanisms discussed in the following sections.

Decrease in Functional Residual Capacity

Functional residual capacity decreases by 0.5 to 1.0 L merely by changing from the upright to supine position because of a 4-cm cephalad displacement of the diaphragm by the abdominal viscera. Surgical positions such as Trendelenburg, kidney, or lithotomy also decrease FRC. The diaphragm of the awake patient keeps the abdominal contents out of the thorax by passive stretch and neurally medicated active tension. With anesthesia and paralysis, these two mechanisms are lost and the diaphragm shifts more cephalad, leading to further decreases in FRC. Thus, induction of general anesthesia is consistently accompanied by a 15 to 20% decrease in FRC, leading to a decrease in the oxygen reserve. Reduction in FRC also decreases lung compliance and increases airway resistance, which predisposes to hypoventilation, airway collapse, and atelectasis. Brismer et al.[32] showed via CT scan that atelectasis occurs in the dependent portion of the lungs within five minutes after the induction of general anesthesia even in healthy patients, which could be reversed by the application of 10 cm H_2O PEEP. The FRC reduction continues into the postoperative period and correlates well with an increase in the alveolar-arterial gradient in oxygen partial pressure, $P(A\text{-}a)o_2$.

Motion of the Diaphragm

The motion of the diaphragm of anesthetized and paralyzed subjects with mechanical ventilation differs from that of spontaneously breathing patients with or without anesthesia. With spontaneous breathing in the supine position, the greatest motion of the diaphragm is in dependent parts, where the radius or curvature is smaller so that the diaphragm excursion occurs more efficiently. With muscle paralysis and positive pressure ventilation, the diaphragm moves passively, and nondependent parts move more than dependent parts because abdominal contents push the diaphragm with greater force in the dependent parts by the hydrostatic pressure.[33] So the alveoli in the nondependent parts of the lungs receive more ventilation during mechanical ventilation than the dependent parts, while the pulmonary blood flow tends to go to the dependent parts of the lungs because of gravity. This descrepancy between ventilation and perfusion causes greater $P(A\text{-}a)o_2$ and predisposes to hypoxia.

Inhibition of Hypoxic Pulmonary Vasoconstruction

Decreased regional alveolar partial pressure of oxygen causes regional pulmonary vasoconstriction, which diverts blood flow away from hypoxic regions of the lungs to the better ventilated normoxic regions. This mechanism minimizes venous admixture from the under- or nonventilated lung regions. Inhalational anesthetics inhibit this protective reaction.

Decreased Removal of Secretions

If the patient is intubated, cool and dry gas bypasses the pharynx and reaches the lower airway without being warmed and humidified. This reduces the clearing of secretions by increasing viscosity and by reducing mucociliary flow. This is minimized by adding a humidifier to the breathing circuit. Endotracheal cuff inflation has been shown to suppress tracheal mucous velocity.[34] Halothane has also been shown to decrease mucociliary clearance, which is probably due to depression of ciliary activity.[35]

Physical Signs

Continuous monitoring of breath sounds via a stethoscope, frequent observation of chest wall excursion, and, if the patient is breathing spontaneously, palpation or observation of the reservoir breathing bag are essential. The first signs of hypoxia or hypercarbia during anesthesia may be those of increased sympathetic tone such as hypertension, tachycardia, or arrhythmias. If any of these signs appear, the adequacy of ventilation and oxygenation must be checked immediately. It is often appropriate to increase ventilation and FI_{O_2} as a first response because inadequate respiration can lead to disaster quickly.

It is also very important to observe the color of skin, mucous membrane, and blood in the surgical field, and at least part of the patient's skin should be kept undraped for observation. However, dangerous levels of hypoxia can occur without cyanosis.

Pulse Oximetry

Pulse oximetry was accepted quickly after its introduction as an essential monitoring device in the operating room and, more recently, in the postanesthesia recovery room because it provides a real-time, beat-to-beat, noninvasive, continuous, and virtually risk-free assessment of the arterial oxygen saturation. Another advantage is that pulse oximetry can monitor the adequacy of circulation. Heart rate can be measured with less interference by the electrocautery than ECG. Large respiratory variations in the intensity of pulsatile signals may suggest intravascular volume depletion. Pulse oximetry fails when pulsatile signals are inadequate due to hypotension, hypovolemia, or peripheral vasoconstriction. Severingaus and Spellman[36] have shown that pulse oximetry fails when systolic blood pressure falls to 42 mm Hg when the brachial artery is progressively occluded and at 58 mm Hg when arterial vasoconstriction by nor-epinephrine infusion is added to the brachial artery occlusion. Thus, pulse oximetry provides a rough estimate of peripheral perfusion. These advantages make pulse oximetry extremely useful during anesthesia and explain why it has been accepted with such enthusiasm.

A recent clinical study by Cote' et al.[37] has confirmed the necessity of Sp_{O_2} (oxygen saturation measured by pulse oximetry) during pediatric anesthesia. One hundred and fifty-two patients were continuously monitored with Spo$_2$ during anesthesia. In half of these patients, the Spo$_2$ data were "unavailable" to the anesthetic team. A major desaturation event was defined as Spo$_2$ < 85% for 30 seconds or longer. There were 24 major events in 76 cases when Spo$_2$ data were "unavailable," and only 11 when the Spo$_2$ data were "available." There was no relationship between visible cyanosis and desaturation documented by the oximeter. Vital signs were of little value in diagnosing desaturation. The incidence of major hypoxic events was not related to the experience of the anesthetist or to the duration of anesthesia, although sicker patients were more likely to experience major events.

Cooper et al.[38] studied recovery-room impact events (RRIEs), defined as an "unanticipated, undesirable, possibly anesthesia-related event that required intervention, was pertinent to recovery-room care, and did or could cause at least moderate morbidity." The incidence of RRIEs, especially the hypotensive and hypovolemic RRIEs, decreased significantly after the introduction of pulse oximetry.

The use of pulse oximetry during anesthesia has several limitations. Hypothermia, which occurs very frequently during anesthesia, causes peripheral vasoconstriction leading to inadequate pulsatile signals and pulse oximetry failure. Ambient light, infrared irradiation, motion, and surgical light (especially xenon arc lamps) are known to interfere with pulse oximetry.[39–41] Dyes commonly used in the operating room such as methylene blue or indocyanine green cause transient decrease in the Spo$_2$ reading.[42, 43] Hypoventilation may go undetected by pulse oximetry if a patient is breathing supplemental oxygen.

Too frequent false-positive alarms are distracting. A recent prospective study[44] in a pediatric hospital noted that alarms (principally of pulse oximetry) sounded an average of 10 times per case, every 4.5 minutes. Seventy-five percent of the alarms were false, while only 3% indicated possible patient risk. An instrument that alarms or drops to zero frequently due to motion or weak signals may fail to alert the physician when real desaturation has occurred.[45]

As an anesthesia monitor, pulse oximetry is particularly useful in the following situations:

1. Thoracotomy, especially when one-lung ventilation is employed. It is common during a thoracotomy to ventilate only the nonoperative lung and keep the operative side quiet to facilitate the surgery. Hypoxia occurs easily because the blood flowing through the operative (nonventilated) lung cannot be oxygenated and serves as a shunt. Pulse oximetry has been shown to be an accurate and useful monitor during one-lung ventilation.[46]

2. Patients with significant lung diseases.

3. Pediatric cases. Children are more susceptible to hypoxia than adults because of high oxygen consumption and low FRC (i.e., low oxygen reserve). Preterm infants younger than 44 weeks gestational age are at risk of retrolental fibroplasia (RLF) if given high Fio$_2$'s. RLF may lead to retinal detachment and blindness. The risk of developing RLF increases in direct proportion to the duration of exposure to oxygen, and the inspired oxygen concentration should be carefully controlled to avoid unnecessary hyperoxia. The safe level of arterial partial pressure of oxygen is now considered to be 50 to 70 mm Hg[47]. Fortunately, pulse oximetry is accurate in newborns who have a large amount of hemoglobin F (fetal hemoglobin). Anesthesiologists now usually control oxygen delivery to maintain Spo$_2$ around 90% in preterm babies. This is hazardous without a continuous monitor such as pulse oximetry because, due to the

sigmoid shape of the hemoglobin-oxygen dissociation curve, a small decrease in arterial partial pressure of oxygen causes a significant drop in oxygen saturation if it is below 90%.

4. Postanesthesia care unit (PACU). Reduction in FRC and atelectasis persist in the postoperative period; FRC decreases by as much as 70% after upper abdominal or thoracic surgery. Sedated patients are prone to airway obstruction. Residual anesthetics and muscle relaxant depress respiration. Only 0.1 MAC of isoflurane has been shown to impair significantly the ventilatory response to hypoxia. At 1.1 MAC, the response to hypercarbia is also suppressed.[48] Narcotics also depress respiratory drive via the opioid-receptor mediated mechanisms. A $Paco_2$ of 50 to 60 mm Hg is commonly seen in the spontaneously breathing patient receiving narcotics. Up to 55% of patients in the PACU have been found to have $Spo_2 < 90\%$ while up to 13% were noted to have $Spo_2 < 80\%$ when continuously monitored with a pulse oximeter.[49] Even during the transfer to the PACU while patients breathe room air after general anesthesia, 28.1% of the children were found to have $Spo_2 < 90\%$, with 45% of those desaturated demonstrating observable cyanosis.[50] In a similar study[51] of adult patients, 35% were found to have $Spo_2 < 90\%$, and 12% had $Spo_2 < 85\%$. Additional information is found in Chapter 10 and excellent reviews.[52, 53.]

Monitoring Carbon Dioxide Concentration

Monitoring the concentration of carbon dioxide in the airway is the best noninvasive means for quantitatively assessing the adequacy of ventilation. This is strongly encouraged in the standards for basic intraoperative monitoring adopted by the American Society of Anesthesiologists.[54] It is now required that placement of an endotracheal tube be confirmed by the presence of carbon dioxide in the exhaled gas, most easily done via capnometry (the measurement of CO_2 concentration) or capnography (the display of the concentration waveform). Capnography or capnometry serve as an anesthesia disaster early warning system. When the diagnostic utility of capnography was prospectively studied in 331 pediatric patients, 35 events, 20 of which were potentially life-threatening, were detected—while only two events were simultaneously diagnosed clinically.[55] For example, breathing circuit disconnection, accidental extubation, or complete airway obstruction are detected by capnography before hypoxia occurs. Rebreathing of CO_2 due to an exhausted CO_2 absorber or a malfunctioning exhalation valve in the anesthesia circuit can be diagnosed from the capnogram. Partial airway obstruction from kinking of tubing or a breathing circuit leak normally creates a sudden drop of the end-tidal CO_2 with a poor alveolar plateau in the capnographic waveform.[56] Detailed analysis of capnography waveforms is discussed in Chapter 12 and other excellent reviews.[57, 58] A few examples of curves of special interest in anesthesia are shown in Figure 23–2.

Esophageal intubation is still one of the major problems in anesthesia morbidity and mortality. Detection of exhaled CO_2 by capnometry or capnography in combination with direct visualization of the vocal cords is the most reliable method to determine proper tube placement.[59] Easily identifiable CO_2 curves are obtained with ventilation through the trachea when the tube is in the proper position. Carbon dioxide can be detected initially with esophageal intubation when expired CO_2 has been forced into the stomach during mask ventilation. However, the end-tidal CO_2 is low in such cases, the wave pattern irregular, and CO_2 levels

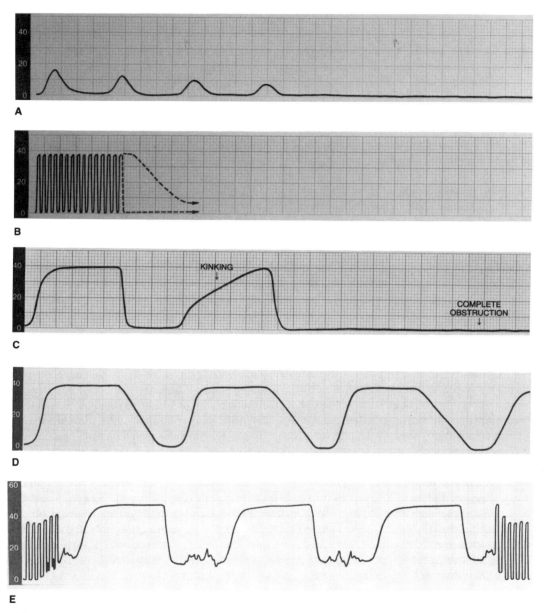

A

B

C

KINKING

COMPLETE
OBSTRUCTION

D

E

FIG 23–2.

Illustrations of capnographic waveforms idealized (i.e., not actual clinical samples): **A,** A likely capnographic pattern resulting from intubation of the esophagus. **B,** Disconnection of the patient from the breathing system at the connection to the tracheal tube can be rapidly recognized via the capnogram, although disconnection of the sampling line must be ruled out. **C,** A capnogram of kinking of the tracheal tube and eventual complete obstruction. **D,** A likely capnographic pattern in restrictive pulmonary disease. **E,** Possible pattern of capnogram within a defective exhalation valve in the anesthesia breathing system. (*From a Hewlett-Packard brochure. Andover, MA, Hewlett-Packard Company Medical Products Group, October, 1986. Used by permission.*)

rapidly diminish with repeated ventilation, making it easy to distinguish between intratracheal and intraesophageal tracings. Auscultation of bilateral breath sounds has been shown to be unreliable. Ventilation via the tube placed in the esophagus often creates bilaterally equal, but ambiguous breath sounds. A recent study of closed malpractice claims revealed that in 48% of esophageal intubations in which auscultation of breath sounds allegedly had been performed, this confirmatory maneuver led to the erroneous conclusion that the tracheal tube had been correctly placed in the trachea.[60]

Capnometry and capnography are particularly useful in certain clinical settings.

Neurosurgery

In neurosurgery, hyperventilation is frequently employed to induce cerebral vasoconstriction and thereby lower the intracranial pressure. $Paco_2$ is usually maintained at 25 to 30 mm Hg. Capnometry or capnography helps to estimate $Paco_2$ after hyperventilation is started, and the difference between $Paco_2$ by ABG analysis and end-tidal CO_2 is determined. The end-tidal CO_2 value is typically several mm Hg below $Paco_2$ and follows changes fairly well under most conditions.

Capnography is a very useful diagnostic tool of air embolisms because a sudden drop in end-tidal CO_2 is one of the earliest signs.

Laparoscopy

Laparoscopy is a very common procedure in gynecology. The peritoneal cavity is insufflated with carbon dioxide, which is absorbed to the systemic circulation and raises the $Paco_2$ unless offset by increased ventilation. Increased abdominal pressure by this CO_2 insufflation and occasional use of the extreme Trendelenburg position make the patient more prone to hypoventilation. The end-tidal CO_2 should be monitored to prevent hypercarbia.

Asthmatic Patients

Management of the asthmatic patient is always a challenge to anethesiologists. Life-threatening bronchospasm can be triggered by endotracheal intubation, light anesthesia, or surgical stimulation. Inhalational anesthetics are very potent bronchodilators and still the mainstay in anesthetizing the asthmatic. When bronchospasm occurs, the expiratory upstroke and alveolar plateau on the capnogram become slanted. This morphology of the capnogram and auscultation of the wheeze help to evaluate the severity of bronchospasm as well as the efficacy of the treatment such as deepening of anesthesia by inhalational anesthetics.

Malignant Hyperthermia

Malignant hyperthermia is a fulminating hypermetabolic crisis triggered by anesthetic agents (especially volatile anesthetics and succinylcholine), which carries a mortality rate of 70% if not recognized and treated promptly. Fever is actually a late sign and carries a poor prognosis if therapy has not yet been started. Monitoring of CO_2 is a very valuable diagnostic tool because respiratory acidosis due to increased carbon dioxide production is one of the earliest and most reliable signs of malignant hyperthermia.

Prolonged Apnea on Emergence from General Anesthesia

If spontaneous respiration does not return at the end of general anesthesia with controlled ventilation, the end-tidal CO_2 should be checked first by just manually inflating the lungs. If the end-tidal CO_2 is high, an anesthetic overdose (especially of narcotics) or incomplete reversal of muscle relaxant is likely. If it is low, it is appropriate to wait for the $Paco_2$ to rise. Desaturation may occur during this period especially in the patient with reduced FRC from obesity, lung disease, upper abdominal surgery, etc. Intermittent breaths may be needed under the guidance of pulse oximetry.

Regional Anesthesia and Monitored Anesthesia Care (MAC)

Under these circumstances, the awake, nonintubated, spontaneously breathing patient may become apneic due to the effects of intravenous sedatives or regional anesthetics. Midazolam and fentanyl, the two most common sedatives during regional anesthesia, have been reported to cause a high incidence of apnea and hypoxia if used in combination.[61] More than half of the cardiac arrests during spinal anesthesia may have been caused by unappreciated respiratory insufficiency due to heavy IV sedation.[62] By placing an IV catheter to the end of a sidestream gas sampling tubing of a capnometer or capnograph and attaching this IV catheter to the face mask or nasal prongs, the expired CO_2 can be detected, although the absolute values are misleading.

Several technologies can be used for measuring carbon dioxide concentration. These are described in detail in Chapter 12. In the anesthesia setting, interference from anesthetics is a concern and must be addressed in the design of the instrument.

Monitoring the Concentration of Inhalation Anesthetics

The exact concentration of inhalational anesthetics delivered to the patient is difficult to estimate because it depends on the uptake by the patient (which changes with time), fresh gas flow, and even the characteristics of the vaporizer. Monitoring the anesthetic concentration is very useful for safety monitoring to avoid absolute overdose, as a guide to more rapid awakening and as an estimate of anesthetic depth. The limitation of using anesthetic concentrations as indicators of anesthetic depth is the wide individual variability in dose-response curves. It yields good additional information, but never substitutes for the careful monitoring of the simple clinical data discussed earlier.

Like capnography, inhalation anesthetic concentration can be monitored via analyzers based on infrared sensing technologies or via a mass spectrometer. The latter has the advantage of differentiating between anesthetics, while most infrared techniques implemented to date require that the operator identify which anesthetic is being introduced into the anesthesia system.

Temperature Monitoring

Hypothermia is common perioperatively. Vaughan, Vaughan, and Cork[63] reported that tympanic membrane temperature averaged 35.6 ± 0.1°C (mean ± SEM) on admission to the recovery room and that 60% of the patients had temperatures of less than 36.0°C. Temperature is regulated by central structures (primarily the hypothalamus). Heat production is greatly impaired during anesthesia due to the inability to shiver and lower metabolic rate. Heat loss is even greater because the operating room is often cold for the comfort of surgeons, intravenous fluids are cold, and heat loss by evaporation from an exposed body cavity (for example, peritoneal cavity during abdominal surgery) is large. General anesthesia decreases the thermo-regulatory threshold (i.e., the temperature at which the body initiates thermoregulation) for hypothermia by 2.5°C; responses to maintain temperature are absent until body temperature decreases to 34.5°C. Thus, the anesthetized patient is very prone to hypothermia.[64] Anesthesi-ologists must monitor body temperature and take appropriate precautions to avoid wide deviations from normal temperature.

The hypothermic patient shivers vigorously on emergence from general anesthesia. Shiv-ering increases oxygen consumption by as much as 400 to 500%,[64] which may not be well tolerated when respiration is still depressed by the residual anesthetic effects. Peripheral vasoconstriction secondary to hypothermia becomes less marked as the temperature returns toward normal, and rewarming hypotension results. Vigorous fluid administration may be necessary.

Hyperthermia is not as common as hypothermia during anesthesia. Malignant hyperthermia is a rare but potentially lethal disorder triggered by anesthetics. High temperature may be a late manifestation, but temperature should be monitored as a guide to therapy.

Electronic thermometers are used commonly in the operating room.[64] The sites of intraoper-ative temperature monitoring are the tympanic membrane, pulmonary artery, nasopharynx, esophagus, rectum, bladder, and axilla; the nasopharynx or esophagus is most often used. Skin and peripheral temperatures are unreliable because they can be unpredictably lower than the temperature of the well-perfused organs (core temperature) such as brain, heart, liver, and kidneys. Tympanic membrane temperature is a good indicator of core temperature because it is close to what the hypothalamus senses and attempts to regulate. The bladder probe reflects the kidney temperature only if the urinary output is adequate. Esophageal and nasopharyngeal probes reflect the temperature of the blood in the aorta and carotid artery, respectively, and are very accurate monitors of core temperature.

Deliberate hypothermia down to 25°C or lower is routinely achieved during cardiopulmo-nary bypass to protect vital organs (especially the brain) by reducing metabolism. Temperature is controlled by cooling or warming the blood flowing through the cardiopulmonary byass pump. It is well known that rectal and nasopharyngeal temperatures differ significantly on cooling and rewarming; rectal temperature tends to change more slowly. Nasopharyngeal temperature reflects the temperature of the brain and other well-perfused organs, whereas the rectal temperature monitors the less well-perfused muscle-fat tissues that constitute most of the body's mass and thermal inertia. Both temperatures are monitored during deliberate hypothermia.

Monitoring the Neuromuscular Junction

Monitoring the neuromuscular junction with a nerve stimulator has proven to be useful during anesthesia involving the use of neuromuscular blocking drugs. These devices permit administration of muscle relaxants such that optimal surgical relaxation is achieved while permitting timely drug reversal either spontaneously or with antagonists. The muscle relaxant dosage can be titrated against the patient's response to nerve stimulation. This is particularly important because of the tremendous variability in patient response to muscle relaxants.

Two electrodes of a nerve stimulator are usually placed at the wrist over the ulnar nerve, and the evoked tension of the adductor pollicis muscle is estimated by feeling for thumb adduction or measured and recorded through a strain gauge attached to the thumb. The advantage of the ulnar-nerve/adductor-pollicis system is that the results are not complicated by direct muscle activation because no muscles involved in the movement of the thumb are directly stimulated by those electrodes on the ulnar side of the wrist.

The four commonly used patterns of stimulation for monitoring neuromuscular blockade are single twitch, train-of-four, sustained tetanus, and post-tetanic stimulation. Train-of-four is used most commonly (Fig 23–3). Four supramaximal stimuli at a frequency of 2 Hz are repeated at intervals no less than 10 seconds apart. In the presence of nondepolarizing neuromuscular blockade, the height of the fourth twitch should be less than the first twitch, allowing calculation of a train-of-four ratio. With deeper blockade, the fourth, the third, and then the second twitch begins to disappear. Thus, a wide range of neuromuscular blockade can be evaluated easily by counting the number of twitches to four successive stimuli or estimating the train-of-four ratio.

The advantages of train-of-four monitoring are: (1) it is more sensitive than single twitch, (2) it does not require a control twitch height recorded before the administration of muscle relaxant, (3) it correlates well with clinical signs of muscle relaxation, and (4) it is not as painful as tetanic stimulation.

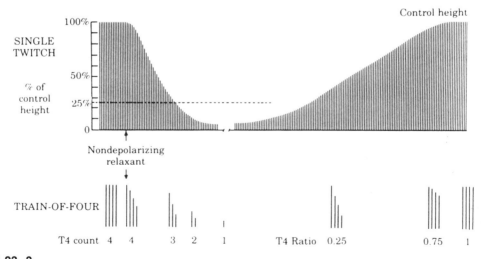

FIG 23–3.
Schematic illustration of recordings during monitoring of neuromuscular blockade via the train-of-four technique. (*From Firestone LL, Lebowitz PW, Cook CE (eds):* Clinical Procedures of the Massachusetts General Hospital, *ed 3. Boston, Little, Brown & Co, 1988, p 183. Used by permission.*)

Muscle relaxants also paralyze respiratory muscles. At the end of an anesthetic, the recovery of respiratory muscle function (especially the diaphragm) from neuromuscular blockade is of the greatest concern. Full recovery from neuromuscular blockade monitored by a nerve stimulator does not always guarantee adequate recovery of diaphragmatic function because the sensitivities of the diaphragm and other skeletal muscles to muscle relaxants are different. Therefore, clinical tests of adequate respiration as well as skeletal muscle function should always be undertaken before the patient is extubated. These tests include adequate a vital capacity more than 15 to 20 mL/kg body weight, maximum inspiratory pressure greater than 25 cm H_2O, good respiratory pattern without use of accessory muscles, the ability to open the eyes or mouth widely, tongue protrusion, grip strength, and sustained head lift for five seconds.

MONITORING THE ANESTHESIA MACHINE

A discussion of anesthesia monitoring would not be complete without mention of the many devices that monitor the anesthesia machine and its associated apparatus. Space does not permit a lengthy discussion of the design of anesthesia machines and the reader is referred to any one of several basic or more detailed descriptions.[65, 66] Briefly, the role of the anesthesia machine is to deliver controlled flows and concentrations of anesthetic gases and vapors. This is done through a system of plumbing not too dissimilar from the basic concept of a critical care ventilator with the addition of various apparatus for adding nitrous oxide and inhalational anesthetics.

The anesthesia breathing system is the interface between the drug delivery system and the patient and is very similar to that in ICU ventilators with the exception that provisions are made for recirculation of gases, primarily for economy. This requires a means for absorption of carbon dioxide, which is accomplished via a chamber containing an absorbant material, usually soda-lime. A series of unidirectional valves assures that gases will not be rebreathed and an exhaust valve is also provided to allow escape of excess gas. The anesthesia breathing system also includes a reservoir bag for holding gases between breaths and provides an independent means for assisting ventilation. This describes the basic circle system (Fig 23–4), which is the most common in the United States, although other types of breathing systems are used, particularly for infants.

The anesthesia machine can create many hazardous situations either due to its own failure or from errors in its use. Thus, many monitors are employed to monitor the anesthesia machine in the same way that monitors are used to monitor the patient, i.e., the monitors serve the dual purpose of setting the machine to deliver desired rates of drugs and to monitor the safety of the machine. An oxygen analyzer is required to assure delivery of an adequate concentration of oxygen. A mechanical pressure gauage monitors the breathing system pressure and, on all modern machines, electronic means are used to monitor machine and ventilator pressures and include alarms to warn of deviations from desired values. A spirometer is used in the same manner as in the critical care setting. The two most common anesthesia machines in the United States employ either a rotating turbine or impeller type of spirometer with either direct mechanical or electronic coupling. Capnography can be said to serve a dual role in monitoring

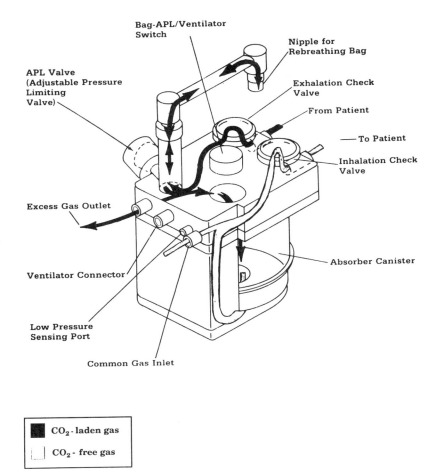

FIG 23–4.
Diagram of a typical circle breathing system. (*From Bowie E, Hauffman LM:* The Anesthesia Machine—Essential for Understanding. *Madison, WI, Ohmeda, 1985, p 132. Used by permission.*)

the patient's physiologic status as well as detecting many types of breathing system failures, e.g., disconnection, unidirectional valve failure, exhaustion of carbon dioxide absorbant (see Fig 23–2).

The Anesthesia System

What has been described so far is a collection of monitoring modalities that are typically used during anesthesia. The increasing proliferation of measurements has created several problems for the anesthesiologist by the presentation of so much information that it is difficult to assimilate it quickly to arrive at an accurate diagnosis. The arrangement of instruments and the nonstandardization of alarms are themselves problems. Until recently, it was most common for individual devices to be mounted on the frame of the anesthesia machine. This still occurs to some extent, but during the 1980s, integrated anesthesia systems were created by manufacturers. The intent is to better organize the presentation of information and the display of alarm messages. One example of a machine that represents an intermediate step in this evolutionary process is shown in Figure 23–5. In this case, the capnometer and ventilator are integrated into the body of the machine while other individual instruments, produced by different manufactures are mounted in various locations. More recent machine designs fully integrate almost all monitoring functions and provide a central display of alarm and warning information.

SAFETY MONITORING

Anesthetics are potentially dangerous drugs; they are potent depressants of the central nervous, cardiovascular, and respiratory systems. They make the patient insensible to surgical stimuli, but at the same time they deprive the patient of the ability to respond to and protect him/herself from lethal events before vital organ functions are damaged. For example, the anesthetized patient has such a blunted ability to respond to hypoxia that it may go undetected until sudden cardiac arrest and irreversible brain damage occur. In contrast, awake subjects never have cardiac arrest or brain damage due to hypoxia without responding to hypoxia itself first by complaining of shortness of breath and increasing ventilation.

What do statistics reveal about the safety of anesthesia? Death due to anesthesia is the most commonly used marker of anesthesia safety. Studies since World War II involving more than 100,000 anesthetics report incidences of anesthetic deaths of 0.7 to 3.7 per 10,000 anesthetics (Table 23–2). These data imply that an anesthesiologist who administers 1000 anesthetics annually can expect to experience personally one anesthesia-related death every 5 to 10 years. On a nationwide basis, 2000 or more may die of causes attributable to anesthesia among the approximately 20 million patients anesthetized annually in the United States. This is relatively high when compared with the mortality of commercial aviation (approximately 125 deaths/year among 200 million passenger boardings). In both cases, injured parties have no direct responsibility for or practical defense against injury. Thus, in both cases, extraordinary measures may be warranted to minimize the risk. Also a common view is that anesthesia risk should be zero because anesthesia itself is not therapeutic but a "necessary evil" to make the patient comfortable and to facilitate surgery. This rationale and the financial cost of an accident to an otherwise healthy individual demand perfection as the goal of anesthesia administration.

Etiology of Anesthesia Accidents and Near Misses

Many studies, including the mortality studies in Table 23–2, support the finding that ventilation/oxygenation problems are the single most frequent cause of anesthesia accidents, accounting for more than half of anesthetic disasters.[73, 74] In Keenan's report[13] of intraoperative cardiac arrest, 11 of the 20 "avoidable" cases were caused by failure to ventilate (Table 23–3).

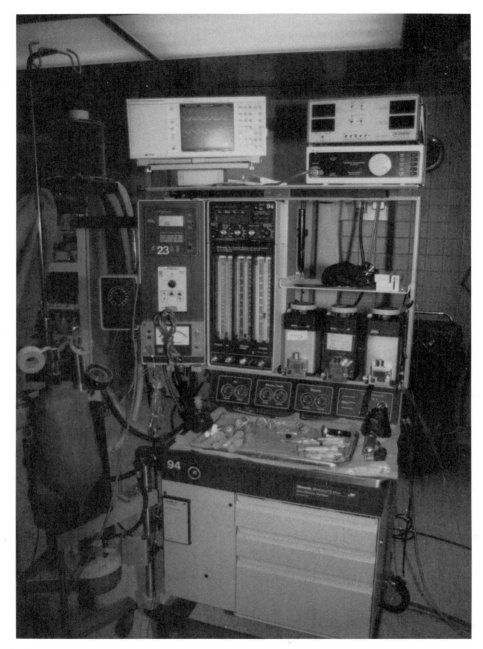

FIG 23–5.
Photograph of a common model anesthesia machine onto which other monitors have been mounted. Note the anesthesia ventilator control panel, anesthetic vaporizers, breathing system, neuromuscular monitor, cardiovascular monitor, continuous noninvasive blood pressure monitor, pulse oximeter, and capnograph.

TABLE 23–2.
Studies of Anesthetic Mortality in Hospitals

Year	Authors	Anesthetics	Deaths	Deaths/10,000
1954	Beecher, Todd[67]	599,584	224	3.7
1956	Hingson et al.[68]	136,043	23	1.7
1963	Clifton, Hotton[69]	205,640	34	1.6
1975	Bodlander[13]	211,130	15	0.7
1978	Harrison[14]	240,483	53	2.2
1980	Turnbull et al.[70]	195,232	29	2.0
1980	Hovi-Viander[71]	338,934	67	2.0
1985	Keenan, Boyan[12]	163,240	14	0.9
1986	Tiret et al.[72]	198,103	25	1.3

Eichhorn reported that seven of 11 major intraoperative accidents solely attributable to anesthesia were due to unrecognized hypoventilation and another was due to delivery of a hypoxic mixture.[73] He also felt that these 8 accidents would have been prevented by earlier warnings that would have been generated by adherence to the Harvard minimal monitoring standards (see Appendix following this chapter).

More recently, analysis of anesthesia-related closed malpractice claims showed that (1) respiratory events constituted the single largest group of claims of injury (522 of 1541 cases; 34%); (2) 85% of these events resulted in death or brain damage; (3) inadequate ventilation, esophageal intubation, and difficult intubation accounted for three-fourths of these events; (4) 72% of these respiratory accidents were considered preventable with better monitoring, e.g., pulse oximetry and capnography; and (5) the median cost of settlement or jury award was $200,000, which was significantly higher than that of nonrespiratory events ($35,000).[60]

TABLE 23–3.
Causes of Anesthetic Cardiac Arrest*

Avoidable   20
　Failure to ventilate 11
　　Unable to ventilate or intubate 4
　　Unrecognized esophageal intubation 4
　　Unrecognized ventilator disconnection 2
　　Displaced endotracheal tube 1
　Absolute overdose of inhalational anesthetics 9
　Questionable 6
　Relative overdose...6
　　Cardiac dysfunction 3
　　Sepsis 3

Unavoidable   1
　Failure to ventilate due to severe asthma 1

* From Keenan RL, Boyan CP: *JAMA* 1985; 253:2373–2377. Used by permission.

Another study of closed claims revealed that 31.5% of all the negative outcomes could have been prevented by application of additional monitors, and that pulse oximetry and capnometry were considered potentially preventive in 93% of the preventable mishaps.[75]

Analyses of near misses or "critical incidents" indicated that the single most common preventable incident was breathing circuit disconnection, and that 7 of the 10 most common incidents would have resulted in hypoxia.[76, 77] It was also found that 82% of the incidents involved human errors, while true equipment failure was rare.

In summary, hypoxia due to human errors such as hypoventilation, esophageal intubation, endotracheal tube displacement, or breathing circuit disconnection is the underlying cause of most anesthetic disasters, the majority of which are considered to be preventable.

The critical incident studies also looked into "associated factors," which conceivably could have contributed to the occurrence of an error or to a failure to detect an error promptly.[77] Multiple factors were found to be involved in most serious incidents. On average, each incident that caused a substantive negative outcome (SNO) such as death, cardiac arrest, procedure cancellation, extended hospital or ICU stay were found to involve 3.4 factors, while each non-SNO incident involved 2.5 factors. In a New South Wales study of deaths under anesthesia, an average of 4.3 "errors" per case was identified.[78] One problem or error generally does not lead to patient harm. Accidents are complex events and usually involve several errors, distraction, and/or system inadequacies that combine in a way to prevent prompt detection and correction.[79] Better monitoring is one of the important strategies of breaking the chain of accident evolution and recovering without negative outcomes. Capnography, oxygen concentration monitoring, and airway pressure monitoring are examples of tactics for detecting the start of accident evolution, while pulse oximetry detects the final common pathway, i.e., hypoxia.

Role of Monitoring as a Vigilance Aid in Anesthesia

Monitoring of the patient and equipment serves at least two functions—it provides information on which to base clinical decisions for controlling the depth of anesthesia and maintaining homeostasis and, if appropriate displays and alarms are operating, warns of deviations that may go unnoticed by clinical observation alone.[80] In other words, monitoring serves as an aid for decision-making and for vigilance.

Patient safety requires the detection of a deviation from the desired physiologic state. This requires prediction and vigilance—the ability to sustain attention. By understanding the patient's condition and the effects of surgery and anesthesia, and making thorough anesthetic plans beforehand, an anesthetist can predict many intraoperative changes, detect and treat them promptly, and avoid negative outcomes even though these changes tend to occur very rapidly during anesthesia. However, no matter how perfect the anesthetic plan, unexpected changes can still occur, and vigilance is critically important to detect them early enough to avert actual harm to the patient.

Most vigilance tasks are generally performed at the level of 90% accuracy.[81] Obviously, this leaves an unacceptable margin of error in anesthesia practice, because anesthetic accidents tend to be lethal and costly. Furthermore, vigilance can be adversely affected by many factors.[82]

Sleep deprivation, fatigue, and noise lower one's ability to sustain attention. Boredom not only reduces vigilance but also generates the false sense of security through the expectation of a low rate of adverse events. Alarms used in the operating room are susceptible to artifact. Frequent false-positive alarms may distract the observer from more clinically significant information. Excessive work load also diminishes vigilance. An anesthetist must carry out many diverse tasks that often require both visual attention and manual dexterity. Using a secondary (subsidiary) task paradigm, Gaba and Lee[83] found that spare capacity to attend to the additional tasks requiring inspection or attention and manual response was compromised in 40% of the time during an anesthetic procedure.

Thus, vigilance needs to be supplemented with appropriate monitoring[84]. In recent years, in particular, this role has become widely recognized, in part because of the impact of increasing malpractice rates resulting from anesthetic-related injuries. Pulse oximetry and capnometry play key roles as vigilance aids as do several types of anesthesia machine monitors, e.g., breathing system pressure monitors, oxygen analyzers, etc.

Monitoring is a supplement to or extension of the anesthetist's senses. The responsibility of the anesthetist is to play the role of the patient's brain and nervous systems because, by anesthetizing them, the anesthetist deprives the patient of his/her own ability to monitor and maintain homeostasis. The anesthetist must monitor what the patient's nervous system senses and regulates and has to make every effort to do this as smartly as the patient would do him/herself. Even the most careful observation of the patient using the anesthetist's senses alone may not be enough, and monitors are added to improve the quality of this observation, provide better patient care, and enhance the safety of anesthesia.

Is it always better to have more monitors for the safety of anesthesia? For example, does an arterial catheter, in addition to a blood pressure cuff, always enhance patient care and safety? The benefits of additional monitoring should always be weighed against the added risks. A blood pressure cuff has great advantages over the anesthetist's finger on the pulse with minimal disadvantages. It provides very accurate measurement with almost no harm to the patient, and its malfunction is rare. However, the comparison of an A-line and blood pressure cuff is not so simple. An A-line provides beat-to-beat measurement of blood pressure, which is obviously unnecessary for a healthy patient undergoing minor surgery. The A-line is invasive, and causes discomfort on insertion. Several complications are associated with the A-line including thrombosis, infection, and even loss of extremity. Finally, the A-line can provide artifacts and inaccurate data, possible causes of which are numerous. Kinking of a catheter or conducting tubing, a loose connection, clotting, air in tubing, malfunction of a transducer, cable, or display, improper transducer position, calibration, or zeroing must be considered. False data may lead to confusion or misjudgment and actual harm to the patient. Merely getting the monitor to function properly may require the anesthetist's attention when it is badly needed elsewhere. Not rarely, a vasopressor is administered to treat hypotension shown in the A-line display when the true blood pressure is reasonable, or the treatment of true hypotension is delayed by checking the A-line itself.

A study of performance of anesthesia residents in a comprehensive anesthesia simulator showed that 16 of 132 unplanned incidents during 19 simulations were fixation errors with monitor displays, with the subjects persistently misinterpreting artifact for patient data or vice versa.[85] Unfortunately, very few studies about the risk-benefit of monitors have been done from this aspect. Reliance on technology is a double-edged sword. Achieving the optimum use of technology means understanding the operation of devices, including their flaws and limitations.[80]

The decision to employ advanced monitors should be based on the benefit-risk evaluation in each individual patient. However, from the previous discussion of anesthetic accidents, it is the belief of most anesthesia professionals that a certain minimal level of monitoring is required for every anesthetic.

Standards for Basic Intraoperative Monitoring

In 1985, the first minimal monitoring standards were published by the Department of Anaesthesia of the Harvard Medical School.[86–88] The motivation for the standards arose from the concern over mounting malpractice liability costs related to anesthesia problems. Although relatively rare, anesthetic losses tended to be very expensive per event. A committee of the Harvard Anaesthesia Department was formed and anesthetic accidents were thoroughly reviewed. Adequate monitoring of the patient and the anesthesia delivery system was felt to be the most prominent issue amenable to remediation. It was decided to first address the area of monitoring by establishing a set of basic standards.

The first standard requires that anesthesia personnel be present in the operating room. This standard emphasizes that the anesthetist is the key to all monitoring.

Measurement of blood pressure and heart rate at least every five minutes, continuous display of ECG, use of breathing system disconnect monitoring with audible alarm during mechanical ventilation, use of an oxygen analyzer, and availability of a means to measure temperature were included in the standards.

The essence of monitoring standards is the requirement for continuous monitoring of ventilation and circulation. The standards are written to stress unequivocally that intermittent observations alone are insufficient. Since the underlying cause of most anesthetic accidents is hypoxia due to airway problems, even diligent monitoring of vital signs and recording of blood pressure and heart rate every five minutes may not detect various untoward developments until relatively late in the evolution of the incident. The need for the earliest possible warning of adverse events led to mandating capnography continuous monitoring.

Fifteen months later, the American Society of Anesthesiologists (ASA) adopted slightly more demanding monitoring standards that were based on the original Harvard standards. There is a clear preference for quantitative rather than qualitative methods. The standards have been revised several times and currently require pulse oximetry in all cases and capnography for verifying correct placement of an endotracheal tube (see the Appendix at the end of this chapter)[54]. These standards are reasonable minimal requirements for anesthesia practice, although there is no clearcut evidence showing that they have improved anesthesia safety. Anesthetists should avoid a false sense of security from the use of monitors. Monitoring strategies are based on the assumption that correct interpretation and response will follow the early warning provided. The anesthetist is still the key to the safe conduct of anesthesia. No machines can substitute for a well-trained, dedicated, and vigilant anesthetist who is capable of utilizing all information appropriately and responding promptly.

MONITORING IN THE POSTANESTHESIA CARE UNIT

The postanesthesia care unit (PACU), which was previously referred to as the recovery room, is a specialized area where monitoring and nursing care are applied to all patients emerging from general or regional anesthesia. A PACU service is considered a necessity to any hospital undertaking modern surgical therapy. Although recovery from anesthesia is a smooth, uneventful process for most patients, a small but significant number of patients suffer complications that are or can be life-threatening. This problem was first addressed by the 1947 report of the Anesthesia Study Commission of the Philadelphia County Medical Society.[89] This 11-year study reported on 307 patients who died within 24 hours of surgery. Nearly half of these deaths were classified as preventable and, in 63% of this group, death was considered to be primarily a result of unrecognized airway obstruction. All occurred in the immediate postanesthesia period. Recent studies[38, 90–92] have indicated that events requiring intervention occur relatively frequently in the PACU and that the overall complication rate may range from 3.7 to 30%. Hypotension, airway obstruction, nausea/vomiting, and mental status alteration were the leading complications seen in the PACU, while more serious problems such as myocardial infarction, aspiration, or cardiac arrest were relatively rare.

There are two special concerns in the PACU; emergence from anesthesia and the acute phase of recovery from the surgery. In other words, the PACU care should be given to the patient until the effects of the residual anesthetics become minimal, pain is under reasonable control, and the medical condition is stabilized so that no acute problems are carried over to the ward.

Common complications by the residual anesthetics are mainly respiratory. The airway of the unconscious patient often obstructs partially or completely. Nausea and/or vomiting is another common complication after anesthesia and aspiration may occur if the patient vomits while not fully awake. Hypoxia as a PACU problem has already been discussed in the section on pulse oximetry. Clinical signs of hypoxia are variable and difficult to detect because circulatory and respiratory responses to hypoxia are modified by residual anesthesia. Severe hypoxia ($Pao_2 = 30$ mm Hg) during light halothane anesthesia rapidly induced cardiac or respiratory arrest in dogs.[93] On the other hand, a study using pulse oximetry in children showed that wakefulness did not correlate with hypoxia, indicating the multifactorial character of postoperative hypoxia and usefulness of pulse oximetry in the PACU.[94] Hypoventilation and resultant hypercarbia is most often seen after anesthesia using narcotics, but can also be a significant problem after inhalational anesthesia or incomplete reversal of the muscle relaxant. Narcotic anesthesia can produce a biphasic respiratory depression.[95] Intraoperative respiratory depression caused by the administration of narcotics dissipates on arrival in the PACU only to be followed by a second period of respiratory depression. This phenomenon may be explained by the varying intensity of stimulation during the recovery period. When entering the PACU, the patient may be stimulated by the initial evaluation by the nurses and the rapid elimination of nitrous oxide. This is usually followed by a relatively quiet period, and then the patient who was apparently awake and breathing well may fall back to sleep and stop breathing.

Establishing adequate pain control is another important component of the PACU care. IV narcotics are most commonly used, which again cause respiratory depression and sedation.

What should be monitored in the PACU? Blood pressure, heart rate and rhythm, fluid balance (urinary output, output from the drains, dryness of the dressing, etc.), respiratory rate and pattern, breath sounds, consciousness, and temperature are usually observed. If the patient has additional monitoring from the operating room such as a CVP line, it should continue in the PACU if required by the patient's condition. After regional anesthesia, the recovery of sensory and motor function is also evaluated. The major difference from patient care in the operating room is that a nurse in the PACU usually observes two to three patients simultaneously, whereas an anesthetist in the operating room cares for only one patient throughout the case. Therefore, uninterrupted observation of the patient in the PACU is both impractical and impossible, and continuous monitoring devices with alarms are very useful. Invasive monitors such as an A-line or CVP line should be continuously displayed on the screen with high- and low-pressure alarms activated. Pulse oximetry is also useful from this aspect. Monitoring ventilation is a more complicated problem. End-tidal CO_2 measurement by capnometry or capnography is difficult in awake, extubated patient and is rarely performed in the PACU. Apnea monitors have too high a rate of false-positive alarms to be used routinely in this setting. The patient tends to have frequent physical movements from shivering, pain, or agitation, which causes artifacts in the apnea monitor and reduces its reliability.

A scoring system to evaluate the postanesthesia recovery is widely used. The scoring system of the PACU of Massachusetts General Hospital is presented in Table 23–4. Seven basic parameters (airway, respiration, skin perfusion, consciousness, blood pressure, cardiac

TABLE 23–4.
Postanesthetic Recovery Scoring System

Airway	Clear airway	−2
	Needs airway	−1
	Guarded airway or trached	−1
	Needs ET tubes	−0
Respiration	Clear bilateral breath sounds with adequate tidal volume	−2
	Dyspnea or inadequate TV	−1
	No spontaneous respirations	−0
Skin perfusion	Pink and dry	−2
	Pale, dusky, mottled, diaphoretic	−1
	Cyanotic	−0
Consciousness	Alert and oriented × 3	−2
	Arousable	−1
	Disoriented	−1
	Unresponsive	−0
Blood pressure	Syst BP ± −20 mm Hg preanesthetic level	−2
	Syst BP ± −20 to 40 mm Hg preanesthetic level	−1
	Syst BP >40 mm Hg preanesthetic level	−0
Cardiac rhythm	Same as preanesthetic	−2
	Newly abnormal—no therapy required	−1
	Newly abnormal—requiring therapy	−0
Activity	Moves all four extremities	−2
	Moves all unblocked extremities	−1
	Moves no extremities	−0

rhythm, and activity) are assessed and scored as either point 0, 1, or 2. The patient is considered ready for discharge when the total score is 13 or above. This scoring system helps prevent the medical staff from overlooking problems likely to be seen in the PACU and also facilitates follow-up of the delayed component of the recovery process.

APPENDIX: STANDARDS FOR BASIC INTRAOPERATIVE MONITORING

(Approved by ASA House of Delegates on October 21, 1986, and last amended on October 23, 1990)[54]

These standards apply to all anesthesia care although, in emergency circumstances, appropriate life-support measures take precedence. These standards may be exceeded at any time based on the judgment of the responsible anesthesiologist. They are intended to encourage high quality patient care, but observing them cannot guarantee any specific patient outcome. They are subject to revision from time to time, as warranted by the evolution of technology and practice. This set of standards addresses only the issue of basic intraoperative monitoring, which is one component of anesthesia care. In certain rare or unusual circumstances, (1) some of these methods of monitoring may be clinically impractical and (2) appropriate use of the described monitoring methods may fail to detect untoward clinical developments. Brief interruptions of continual monitoring may be unavoidable. Under extenuating circumstances, the responsible anesthesiologist may waive the requirements marked with an asterisk (*); it is recommended that when this is done, it should be so stated (including the reasons) in a note in the patient's medical record. These standards are not intended for application to the care of the obstetric patient in labor or in the conduct of pain management.

(Note that *continual* is defined as "repeated regularly and frequently in steady, rapid succession" whereas *continuous* means "prolonged without any interruption at any time.")

Standard I

Qualified anesthesia personnel shall be present in the room throughout the conduct of all general anesthetics, regional anesthetics, and monitored anesthesia care.

Objective

Because of the rapid changes in patient status during anesthesia, qualified anesthesia personnel shall be continuously present to monitor the patient and provide anesthesia care. In the event there is a direct known hazard (e.g., radiation) to the anesthesia personnel, which might require intermittent remote observation of the patient, some provision for monitoring the patient must be made. In the event that an emergency requires the temporary absence of the person primarily responsible for the anesthetic, the best judgment of the anesthesiologist will be exercised in comparing the emergency with the anesthetized patient's condition and in the selection of the person left responsible for the anesthetic during the temporary absence.

Standards II

During all anesthetic, the patient's oxygenation, ventilation, circulation, and temperature shall be continually evaluated.

Oxygenation

Objective

To ensure adequate oxygen concentration in the inspired gas and the blood during all anesthetics.

Methods

1. Inspired gas: During every administration of general anesthesia using an anesthesia machine, the concentration of oxygen in the patient breathing system shall be measured by an oxygen analyzer with a low oxygen concentration limit alarm in use.*
2. Blood oxygenation: During all anesthetics, a quantitative method of assessing oxygenation such as pulse oximetry shall be employed.* Adequate illumination and exposure of the patient is necessary to assess color.*

Ventilation

Objective

To ensure adequate ventilation of the patient during all anesthetics.

Methods

1. Every patient receiving general anesthesia shall have the adequacy of ventilation continually evaluated. While qualitative clinical signs such as chest excursion, observation of the reservoir breathing bag, and auscultation of breath sounds may be adequate, quantitative monitoring of the CO_2 content and/or volume of expired gas is encouraged.
2. When an endotracheal tube is inserted, its correct positioning in the trachea must be verified by clinical assessment and by identification of carbon dioxide in the expired gas.* End-tidal CO_2 analysis, in use from the time of endotracheal tube placement, is encouraged.
3. When ventilation is controlled by a mechanical ventilator, there shall be in continuous use a device that is capable of detecting disconnection of components of the breathing system. The device must give an audible signal when its alarm threshold is exceeded.

4. During regional anesthesia and monitored anesthesia care, the adequacy of ventilation shall be evaluated, at least, by continual observation of qualitative clinical signs.

Circulation

Objective

To ensure the adequacy of the patient's circulatory function during all anesthetics.

Methods

1. Every patient receiving anesthesia shall have the electrocardiogram continuously displayed from the beginning of anesthesia until preparing to leave the anesthetizing location.*
2. Every patient receiving anesthesia shall have arterial blood pressure and heart rate determined and evaluated at least every 5 minutes.*
3. Every patient receiving general anesthesia shall have, in addition to the above, circulatory function continually evaluated by at least one of the following: palpation of a pulse, auscultation of heart sounds, monitoring of a tracing of intra-arterial pressure, ultrasound peripheral pulse monitoring, or pulse plethysmography or oximetry.

Body temperature

Objective

To aid in the maintenance of appropriate body temperature during all anesthetics.

Methods

There shall be readily available a means to continuously measure the patient's temperature. When changes in body temperature are intended, anticipated, or suspected, the temperature shall be measured.

REFERENCES

1. Woodbridge PD: Changing concepts concerning depth of anesthesia. *Anesthesiol* 1957; 18:536–550.
2. Pinsker MC: Anesthesia: A pragmatic construct. *Anesth Analg* 1986; 65:819–820.
3. Prys-Roberts C: Anesthesia: A practical or impractical construct? (editorial) *Br J Anaesth* 1987; 59:1341–1345.
4. Dodson BA, Miller KW: Evidence for dual mechanism in the anesthetic action of an opioid peptide. *Anesthesiol* 1985; 62:615–620.
5. Clark DL, Rosner BS: Neurophysiologic effects of general anesthetics: I. The electroencephalogram and sensory evoked responses in man (review). *Anesthesiol* 1973; 38:564–582.
6. Donegan JH, Rampil IJ: The electroencephalogram, in Blitt CD (ed): *Monitoring in Anesthesia and Critical Care Medicine*, ed 2. New York, Churchill Livingstone, 1990, pp 431–459.

7. Aldrete VA: Concerning the acceptability of awareness during surgery. *Anesthesiol* 1985; 63:460–461.

8. Eger EI, Saidman LJ, Brandstater B: Minimum alveolar anesthetic concentrations: A standard of anesthetic potency. *Anesthesiol* L965; 26:756–770.

9. Merkel G, Eger EI: A comparative study of halothane and halopropane anesthesia. Including method for determining potency. *Anesthesiol* 1963; 24:346–357.

10. Roizen MF, Horrigan RW, Frazer BM: Anesthetic doses blocking adrenergic (stress) and cardiovascular responses to incision—MAC BAR. *Anesthesiol* 1981; 54:390–398.

11. Russell IF: Balanced anesthesia: Does it anesthetize? *Anesth Analg* 1985; 64:941–944.

12. Keenan RL, Boyan CP: Cardiac arrest due to anesthesia. A study of incidence and causes. *JAMA* 1985; 253:2373–2377.

13. Bodlander FMS: Deaths associated with anaesthesia. *Br J Anaesth* 1975; 47:36–40.

14. Harrison GG: Death attributable to anaesthesia. *Br J Anaesth* 1978; 50:1041–1046.

15. Bertrand CA, Steiner NV, Jameson AG, et al: Disturbances of cardiac rhythm during anesthesia and surgery. *JAMA* 1971; 216–1615–1617.

16. Blackburn H, Raymundo K: What electrocardiographic leads to take after exercise? *Am Heart J* 1964; 67:184–185.

17. London MJ, Hollenberg M, Mangano DT, et al: Intraoperative myocardial ischemia: Localization by continuous 12-lead electrocardiography. *Anesthesiol* 1988; 69:232–241.

18. Kaplan JA, King SB: The precordial electrocardiographic lead (V5) in patients who have coronary-artery disease. *Anesthesiol* 1976; 45:570–574.

19. Upton MT, Rerych SK, Jones RH, et al: Detecting abnormalities in left ventricular function during exercise before angina and ST-segment depression. *Circulation* 1980; 62:341–349.

20. Horowitz RS, Morganroth J, Pauletto FJ, et al: Immediate diagnosis of acute myocardial infarction by two-dimensional echocardiography. *Circulation* 1982; 65:323–329.

21. Clements FM, de Bruijn NP: Perioperative evaluation of regional wall motion by transesophageal two-dimensional echocardiography (review). *Anesth Analg* 1987; 66:249–261.

22. Kotrly KJ, Kotter GS, Mortara D, et al: Intraoperative detection of myocardial ischemia with an ST-segment trend monitoring system. *Anesth Analg* 1984; 63:343–345.

23. Kaplan JA, Wells PH: Early diagnosis of mycardial ischemia using the pulmonary arterial catheter. *Anesth Analg* 1981; 60:789–793.

24. Haeggmark S, Hohner P, Lowenstein E, et al: Comparison of hemodynamic, electrocardiographic, mechanical, and metabolic indicators of intraoperative myocardial ischemia in vascular surgical patients with coronary artery disease. *Anesthesiol* 1989; 70:19–25.

25. Van Daele MERM, Sutherland GR, Roelandt JRTC, et al: Do changes in pulmonary capillary wedge pressure adequately reflect myocardial ischemia during anesthesia? A correlative preoperative hemodynamic, electrocardiographic, and transesophageal echocardiographic study. *Circulation* 1990; 81:865–871.

26. Hansen RM, Viquerat CE, Chatterjee K, et al: Poor correlation between pulmonary arterial wedge pressure and left ventricular end-diastolic volume after coronary artery bypass graft surgery. *Anesthesiol* 1986; 64:764–770.

27. Calvin JE, Driedger AA, Sibbald WJ: Does the pulmonary capillary wedge pressure predict left ventricular preload in critically ill patients? *Crit Care Med* 1981; 9:437–443.

28. Smith JS, Cahalan MK, Shiller NB, et al: Intraoperative detection of myocardial ischemia in high-risk patients: Electrocardiography versus two-dimensional transesophageal echocardiography. *Circulation* 1985; 72:1015–1021.

29. Schueter M, Langenstein BA, Hanrath P, et al: Transesophageal cross-sectional echocardiography with a phased array transducer system. Technique and initial clinical results. *Br Heart J* 1982; 48:67–72.

30. Cahalan MK, Litt L, Botvinick EH, et al: Advances in noninvasive cardiovascular imaging: Implications for the anesthesiologist (review). *Anesthesiol* 1987; 66:356–372.

31. London MJ, Tubau JF, Mangano DT: The "natural history" of segmental wall motion abnormalities in patients undergoing noncardiac surgery. *Anesthesiol* 1990; 73:644–655.

32. Brismer B, Hedenstierna G, Lundquist H, et al: Pulmonary densities during anesthesia with muscular relaxation—a proposal of atelectasis. *Anesthesiol* 1985; 62:422–428.

33. Froese AB, Bryan AC: Effects of anesthesia and paralysis on diaphragmatic mechanics in man. *Anesthesiol* 1974; 41:242–255.

34. Sackner MA, Hirsch J, Epstein S: Effect of cuffed endotracheal tubes on tracheal mucous velocity. *Chest* 1975; 68:774–777.

35. Forbes AR: Halothane depresses mucociliary flow in the trachea. *Anesthesiol* 1976; 45:59–63.

36. Severinghaus JW, Spellman MJ: Pulse oximeter failure threshold in hypotension and vasoconstriction. *Anesthesiol* 1990; 73:532–537.

37. Cote' CJ, Goldstein EA, Ryan JF, et al: A single-blind study of pulse oximetry in children. *Anesthesiol* 1988; 68:184–188.

38. Cooper JB, Cullen DJ, Veneble C, et al: Effects of information feedback and pulse oximetry on the incidence of anesthesia complications. *Anesthesiol* 1987; 67:686–694.

39. Brooks TD, Paulus DA, Winkle WE: Infrared heat lamps interfere with pulse oximeters. *Anesthesiol* 1984; 61:630.

40. Costarino AT, Davis DA, Keon TP: Falsely normal saturation reading with the pulse oximeter. *Anesthesiol* 1987; 67:830–831.

41. Hanowell L, Eisele JH, Downs D: Ambient light affects pulse oximeters. *Anesthesiol* 1987; 67:864–865.

42. Kessler MR, Eide T, Humayun B, et al: Spurious pulse oximeter desaturation with methylene blue injection. *Anesthesiol* 1986; 65:435–436.

43. Schller MS, Unger RJ, Kelner MJ: Effects of intravenously administered dyes on pulse oximetry readings. *Anesthesiol* 1986; 65:550–552.

44. Kestin IG, Miller BR, Lockhart CH: Auditory alarms during anesthesia monitoring. *Anesthesiol* 1988; 69–106–109.

45. Severinghaus JW: Personal communication, 1990.

46. Brodsky JB, Shulman MS, Swan M, et al: Pulse oximetry during one-lung ventilation. *Anesthesiol* 1985; 63:212–214.

47. Steward DJ (ed): Retrolental fibroplasia, in *Manual of Pediatric Anesthesia*, ed 2. New York, Churchill Livingstone, 1985, p 9.

48. Knill RL, Kieraszewicz HT, Dodgson BG, et al: Chemical regulation of ventilation during isoflurane sedation and anaesthesia in humans. *Can Anaesth Soc J* 1983; 30:607–614.

49. Moller JT, Wittrup M, Johansen SH: Hypoxemia in the postanesthesia care unit; an observer study. *Anesthesiol* 1990; 73:890–895.

50. Pulleritis J, Burrows FA, Roy WL: Arterial desaturation in healthy children during transfer to the recovery room. *Can Anaesth Soc J* 1987; 34:470–473.

51. Tyler IL, Tantisira B, Winter PM, et al: Continuous monitoring of arterial oxygen saturation with pulse oximetry during transfer to the recovery room. *Anesth Analg* 1985; 64;1108–1112.

52. Alexander CM, Teller LE, Gross JB: Principles of pulse oximetry: Theoretical and practical considerations. *Anesth Analg* 1989; 68:368–376.

53. Tremper KK, Barker SJ: Pulse oximetry. *Anesthesiol* 1989; 70:98–108.

54. American Socitey of Anesthesiologists, Park Ridge, IL, 1990.

55. Cote' CJ, Liu LMP, Szyfelbein SK, et al: Intraoperative events diagnosed by expired carbon dioxide monitoring in children. *Can Anaesth Soc J* 1986; 33:315–320.

56. Riley RH, Marcy JH: Unsuspected endobronchial intubation—detection by continuous mass spectrometry. *Anesthesiol* 1985; 63:203–204.
57. Swedlow DB: Capnometry and capnography: The anesthesia disaster early warning system. *Seminars in Anesthesia* 1986; 5:194–205.
58. Fairley HB: Respiratory monitoring, in Blitt CD (ed): *Monitoring in Anesthesia and Critical Care Medicine*, ed 2. New York, Churchill Livingstone, pp 339–372.
59. Birmingham PK, Cheney FW, Ward RJ: Esophageal intubation: A review of detection techniques. *Anesth Analg* 1986; 65:886–891.
60. Caplan RA, Posner KL, Ward RJ, et al: Adverse respiratory events in anesthesia: A closed claims analysis. *Anesthesiol* 1990; 72:828–833.
61. Bailey PL, Pace NL, Stanley TH, et al: Frequent hypoxemia and apnea after sedation with midazolam and fentanyl. *Anesthesiol* 1990; 73:826–830.
62. Caplan RA, Ward RJ, Posner KL, et al: Unexpected cardiac arrest during spinal anesthesia: A closed claims analysis of predisposing factors. *Anesthesiol* 1988; 68:5–11.
63. Vaughan MS, Vaughan RW, Cork RC: Postoperative hypothermia in adults: Relationship of age, anesthesia, and shivering to rewarming. *Anesth Analg* 1981; 60:746–751.
64. Cork RC: Temperature monitoring, in Blitt CD (ed): *Monitoring in Anesthesia and Critical Care Medicine*, ed 2. New York, Churchill Livingstone, 1990, pp 557–573.
65. Dorsch JA, Dorsch SE: *Understanding Anesthesia Equipment*, ed 2. Baltimore, Williams and Wilkins, 1984.
66. Petty C: *The Anesthesia Machine*. New York, Churchill Livingstone, 1987.
67. Beecher HK, Todd DP: A study of the deaths associated with anesthesia and surgery based on a study of 599,548 anesthesias in ten institutions 1948–1952, inclusive. *Ann Surg* 1954; 140:2–35.
68. Hingson RA, Holden WD, Barnes AC: Mechanisms involved in anesthetic deaths. A survey of operating room and obstetric delivery room related mortality in the University Hospitals of Cleveland, 1945–1955. *NY State J Med* 1956; 56:230–236.
69. Clifton BS, Hotten WJT: Deaths associated with anesthesia. *Br J Anaesth* 1963; 35:250–259.
70. Turnbull KW, Fancourt-Smith PF, Banting GC: Death within 48 hours of anaesthesia at the Vancouver General Hospital. *Can Anaesth Soc J* 1980; 27:159–163.
71. Hovi-Viander M: Death associated with anaesthesia in Finland. *Br J Anaesth* 1980; 52:483–489.
72. Tiret L, Desmonts JM, Hatton F, et al: Complications associated with anaesthesia—a prospective survey in France. *Can Anaesth Soc J* 1986; 33:336–344.
73. Eichhorn JH: Prevention of intraoperative anesthesia accidents and related severe injury through safety monitoring. *Anesthesiol* 1989; 70:572–577.
74. Taylor G, Larson CP, Prestwich R: Unexpected cardiac arrest during anesthesia and surgery. An environmental study. *JAMA* 1976; 236:2758–2760.
75. Tinker JH, Dull D, Caplan RA, et al: Role of monitoring devices in prevention of anesthetic mishaps: A closed claims analysis. *Anesthesiol* 1989; 71:541–546.
76. Cooper JB, Newbower RS, Long CD, et al: Preventable anesthesia mishaps: A study of human factors. *Anesthesiol* 1978; 49:399–406.
77. Cooper JB, Newbower RS, Kitz RJ: An analysis of major errors and equipment failures in anesthesia management: Considerations for prevention and detection. *Anesthesiol* 1984; 60:34–42.
78. Holland R: Special committee investigating deaths under anaesthesia: Report on 745 classified cases, 1960–1968. *Med J Aust* 1970; 1:573–594.
79. Gaba DM: Human error in anesthetic mishaps. *Int Anesthesiol Clin* 1989; 27:137–147.
80. Cooper JB, Gaba DM: A strategy for preventing anesthesia accidents. *Int Anesthesiol Clin* 1989; 27:148–152.

81. Paget NS, Lambert TF, Sridhar K: Factors affecting an anaesthetist's work: Some findings on vigilance and performance. *Anaesth Intens Care* 1981; 9:359–365.
82. Weinger MB, Englund CE: Ergonomic and human factor affecting anesthetic vigilance and monitoring performance in the operating environment. *Anesthesiol* 1990; 73:995–1021.
83. Gaba DM, Lee T: Measuring the workload of the anesthesiologist. *Anesth Analg* 1990; 71:354–361.
84. Gaba DM, Maxwell M, DeAnda A: Anesthetic mishaps: Breaking the chain of accident evolution. *Anesthesiol* 1987; 66:670–676.
85. DeAnda A, Gaba DM: Unplanned incidents during comprehensive anestehsia simulation. *Anesth Analg* 1990; 71:77–82.
86. Eichhorn JH, Cooper JB, Cullen DJ, et al: Standards for patient monitoring during anesthesia at Harvard Medical School. *JAMA* 1986; 256:1017–1020.
87. Hornbein TF: The setting of standards of care (editorial). *JAMA* 1986; 256:1040–1041.
88. Eichhorn JH, Cooper JB, Cullen DJ, et al: Anesthesia practice standards at Harvard: A review. *J Clin Anesth* 1988; 1:55–65.
89. Ruth HS, Haugen FP, Grove DD: Anesthesia study commission: Findings of eleven years' activity. *JAMA* 1947; 135:881–884.
90. Cohen MM, Duncan PG, Pope WDB, et al: A survey of 112,000 anaesthetics at one teaching hospital (1975–1983). *Can Anaesth Soc J* 1986; 33:22–31.
91. Gewolb J, Hines R, Barash PG: A survey of 324 consecutive admissions to the post-anesthesia recovery room at a university teaching hospital (abstract). *Anesthesiol* 1987; 67:A471.
92. Zelcer J, Wells DG: Anaesthetic-related recovery room complications. *Anaesth Intens Care* 1987; 15:168–174.
93. Cullen DJ, Eger EI II: The effects of halothane on respiratory and cardiovascular responses to hypoxia in dogs: A dose response study. *Anesthesiol* 1974; 41:350–360.
94. Soliman IE, Patel RI, Ehrenpreis MB, et al: Recovery scores do not correlate with postoperative hypoxemia in children. *Anesth Analg* 1988; 67:53–56.
95. Becker LD, Paulson BA, Eger EI II, et al: Biphasic respiratory depression after fentanyl-droperidol or fentanyl alone used to supplement nitrous oxide anesthesia. *Anesthesiol* 1976; 44:292–296.

Chapter 24

Monitoring in the Home and the Outpatient Setting

Mary E. Gilmartin, B.S.N., R.R.T.

INTRODUCTION

Home care for patients with respiratory disease and the use of highly sophisticated life support equipment in the home has evolved over the past decade.[1-12] Many mechanically ventilated patients are sent home with specific alarm systems to monitor equipment function and other devices such as oxygen analyzers or respirometers to monitor their response to ventilatory support. Many patients with chronic obstructive pulmonary disease or interstitial lung disease on continuous oxygen in the home now have the availability of liquid oxygen systems and more compact portable units, as well as transtracheal oxygen. These systems have allowed patients to travel away from the home and to function more effectively at work or in the community. Some of these patients have used pulse oximeters to monitor their response to oxygen therapy. In the pediatric population, apnea impedance monitors have been used extensively on infants at home to detect changes in respiratory rate and pattern and alert caregivers to episodes of apparent life-threatening events.

Extensive technology is now available to monitor patients and equipment function in the home. However, what level of monitoring is really needed in the home and the outpatient setting, and what use is made of the results of the functions that are monitored? In addition, is it possible that overmonitoring can be more deleterious? This chapter focuses on these questions related to monitoring of respiratory care in the home and outpatient settings.

OXYGEN THERAPY IN THE HOME

Oxygen therapy alone, or in conjunction with other respiratory care modalities, constitutes the largest element of respiratory care provided in the home. The data from the Nocturnal Oxygen Therapy Trial[13] and the British Medical Research Council Trial[14] have been used by medical insurance programs as the basis for establishment of guidelines for the reimbursement of the costs of oxygen therapy in the home.[15] Originally, an oxygen saturation via pulse oximeter (SpO_2) of <85% or an arterial oxygen partial pressure (PaO_2) of <55 mm Hg while breathing room air, were necessary for reimbursement. However, Carlin, Clausen and Ries[16] demonstrated that using SpO_2 data alone would essentially deny oxygen to a majority of patients. They found that 80% of the 55 patients studied would qualify for oxygen if an arterial blood gas were done since they had a resting PaO_2 of <55 mm Hg but would not qualify if pulse oximetry were used since their SpO_2 was >85%. (Fig 24–1). Medicare has since changed their reimbursement guidelines. Now an arterial oxygen saturation (SaO_2) or SpO_2 of <88% qualifies a patient for reimbursement.[17]

Studies,[18, 19] of oximetries have established the 95% confidence interval for agreement with CO oximetry at ±4.0 to 5.0% at saturations of >70%. These studies have shown that pulse oximetry should not be used to establish the need for oxygen therapy unless data from a given pulse oximeter are correlated to arterial blood gas (ABG) results.[18–21]

Table 24–1 lists patient and equipment monitoring requirements when oxygen is used in the home. Spot checks with pulse oximetry can be helpful in assessing a patient's overall status, as well as changes during exercise, or sleep disturbances. If desaturations are noted, it must

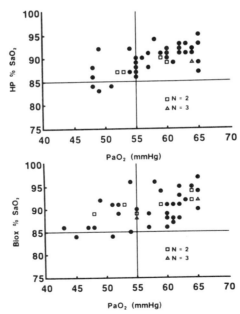

FIG 24–1.
The relationship between resting arterial oxygen tension (PaO_2) and arterial oxygen saturation (SaO_2) measured by a Hewlett-Packard HP 47201A (*top*) or a Biox IIA (*bottom*) ear oximeter. The solid lines (PaO_2 55 mm Hg; SaO_2 85%) represent original Medicare criteria for long-term oxygen therapy. (*From Carlin BW, Clausen JL, Ries AL:* Chest 1988; 94:239–244. Used by permission.)

TABLE 24–1.
Oxygen Therapy in the Home

Patient Monitoring
Spo_2—intermittent: during rest, exercise, and
  sleep
ABG—intermittent
Clinical status
  Lung sounds
  Vital signs
  Sputum production
  Breathing patterns
  Presence of dyspnea
Equipment Monitoring
Stationary and portable oxygen flow rate
  accuracy
Fio_2—concentrators
Pulse oximeter—accuracy
Inlet filters—cleanliness and need for
  replacement
Humidifiers—cleanliness and function

---

be determined if they are a result of a change in the patient's clinical status or a result of the inaccuracy of oxygen delivery equipment, the inaccuracy of the oximeter, or if the change is simply a result of a different oximeter being used for the assessment.[21] If the patient is symptomatic, a visit to the hospital or doctor's office may be warranted. An ABG and other diagnostic testing may be done to assess the reasons for the change in the oxygen prescription or the need for other therapeutic interventions. If the patient is not acutely sick and the home care company is equipped to do an ABG or other diagnostic testing in the home, this may be more cost-effective than a visit to the hospital. As the patient's clinical status stabilizes, a reassessment of oxygen therapy is needed. When a patient (who comes into the clinic or in follow-up by the home care practitioner) is noted to have symptomatology of nighttime desaturation, continuous nighttime recording of Spo_2 may be warranted but only after a daytime ABG is checked.

After hospitalization for an acute exacerbation, patients should have Spo_2 spot checks to determine the continued need for the discharge oxygen prescription.[21] All spot checks of Spo_2 in the home or outpatient setting should be correlated with the patient's overall clinical status.

At this time, there seems to be no rational need for the use of continuous pulse oximetry in the home, either for adults or children, if they are stable. Encouraging a patient to buy a pulse oximeter is counterproductive to safe, effective care since many patients may have momentary changes in Spo_2 secondary to stress, coughing, or a routine need for bronchodilator therapy, which are of no clinical significance. The presence of continuous pulse oximetry may actually cause patients to change their oxygen therapy prescription based on momentary changes or to perceived changes in Spo_2 that are frequently a result of inappropriate probe placement, decreased circulation or temperature changes in the hand. They may not only be causing themselves harm by increasing their O_2 liter flow, but also increasing their anxiety level. Pulse oximetry is a sophisticated tool available to the health care professional, but it can be misused if not correlated with data obtained from a good history, physical examination, and ABG results (see Chapter 10 for details).

Monitoring the accuracy of the patient's stationary and portable oxygen delivery device may be far more beneficial and cost-effective since many times flowmeter calibration is lacking and, as a result, the patient may not be receiving the ordered oxygen dose. This inaccuracy may be the sole culprit in the patient's change in oxygen saturation.

When using an oxygen concentrator in the home, proper function and understanding of the particular unit are very important. There are two basic types of oxygen concentrators. One employs a set of polymer membranes through which air is filtered. Since oxygen and water vapor are more permeable than nitrogen, the resulting gas delivered to the patient is higher in oxygen. This type of concentrator only delivers 40% oxygen and, as a result, it is infrequently used. With these devices patients need a high concentrator gas flow rate to achieve adequate Spo_2 levels.

Other concentrators use a molecular sieve to remove nitrogen from air. The sieve beds are periodically purged to release the nitrogen as exhaust. This type of concentrator can deliver 90 to 95% oxygen at low flow rates (1 to 2 L/min) but falls to 80 to 90% at higher flow rates.[22, 23] Because of these limitations in operation the Fio_2 should be monitored at frequent intervals along with the Spo_2. This is especially important when patients require higher liter flows since the Fio_2 may decrease more at higher delivered flows. In patients where oxygen requirements have increased, an alternate oxygen source may be warranted. However, when the patient or an insurance company has bought the oxygen concentrator, adequate monitoring of the machine may not be performed and if the patient needs a different delivery system, the insurance carrier may resist providing reimbursement for the newer system. The physician and home care provider will need good documentation of need to justify reimbursement for any change in delivery system.

CONTINUOUS POSITIVE AIRWAY PRESSURE

As our understanding of obstructive sleep apnea (OSA) increases and technology changes, we will see more and more patients at home using continuous positive airway pressure (CPAP). More recently, patients with severe tracheobronchomalacia have had CPAP prescribed during sleep, chest physical therapy, and/or with exercise to prevent airway collapse. Patients with severe COPD may also have CPAP prescribed for use during exercise to prevent or counteract intrinsic PEEP.[24] CPAP, in the home environment, is normally provided by a nasal mask and blower. When nasal CPAP was first used, the masks were not very comfortable and the devices unwieldy; now, with the development of more comfortable masks and head gear and smaller, simpler, and quieter blowers, patients tend to be more compliant. Figure 24–2 shows some of the current CPAP devices. The level of CPAP is usually set by the sleep lab or the home care provider and, depending on the CPAP model, may not be easily readjusted by the patient. A humidifier can be incorporated into the setup if needed.

With the increase in the use of nasal CPAP, it has become more important that we be able

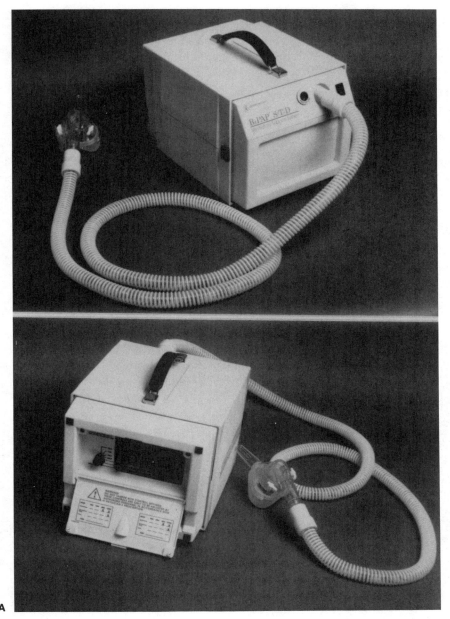

A

FIG 24–2.
CPAP Devices for use in the home: **A,** BiPAP S/TD model, Respironics, Inc, Monroeville, PA. **B,** Remstar Choice, Respironics, Inc, Monroeville, PA. **C,** Healthdyne Tranquility Plus, Healthdyne, Marietta, GA. **D,** Puritan Bennett Companion 318, Puritan Bennett, Lenexa, KS. (*Used by permission.*)

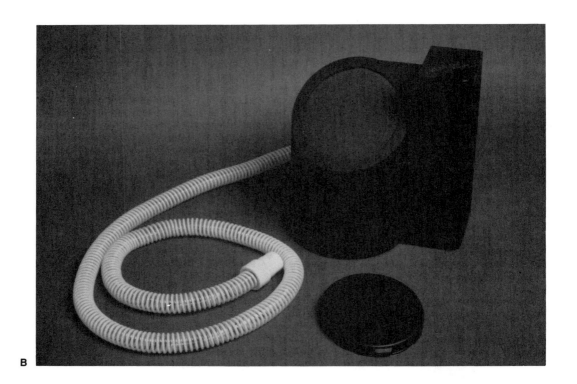

B

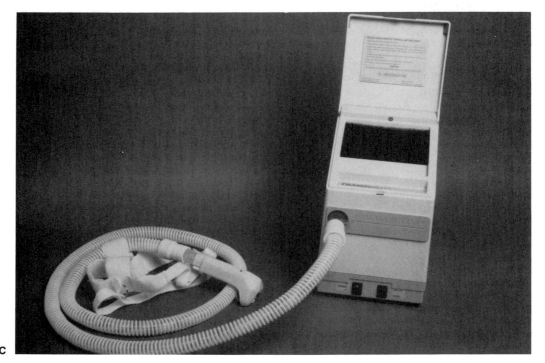

C

FIG 24–2. Continued

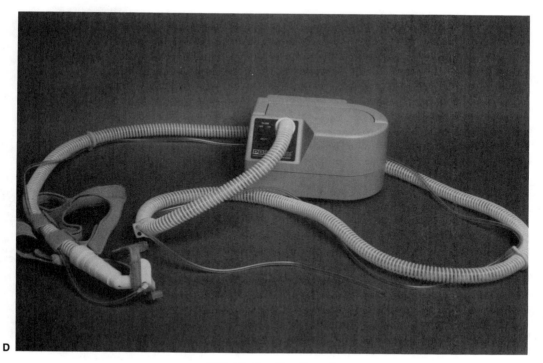

D

FIG 24–2. Continued

to monitor the patient's response to therapy and the accuracy of the CPAP device. Table 24–2 summarizes patient and equipment monitoring necessary with nasal CPAP. The patient's clinical status is assessed for their daytime functioning, presence of hypersomnulence, cor pulmonale, polycythemia, arrhythmias, and/or spouse's report of disturbed sleep patterns. If the patient is symptomatic, it is important to determine if the patient is using the CPAP every night and for how many hours. These patients should have periodic assessment of sleep quality and adequacy of oxygenation by continuous nighttime Spo_2, and/or modified sleep studies in the home. The portable sleep apnea screening devices (Fig 24–3) now available allow for up to eight channels of physiologic data collection[25]; including heart rate, respiratory rate, Spo_2, chest impedance, nasal and oral flow, and electro-ocular, electromyographic, and electroencephalographic activity. As noted in Table 24–3, sleep studies in the home may be indicated in conditions other than sleep apnea. These monitors may be appropriate to use as a screening tool prior to a formal sleep study, as follow-up after therapy has been initiated and when sleep disturbances secondary to hypoxemia are suspected.[26, 27] Sleep monitoring in the home for primary diagnosis of sleep apnea is indicated in geographic locations where formal sleep labs are scarce and there are long waiting lists. However, these studies must be under the direction of a physician and performed by a home care practitioner with expertise in setting up the equipment in the home.

TABLE 24–2.
CPAP in the Home

Patient Monitoring
SpO$_2$—nighttime recording
Modified sleep study
Clinical status
   Presence of hypersomnulence
   Cor pulmonale
   Daytime functioning
   Disturbed sleep patterns
   Morning headaches
   Vital signs
   Arrythmias
Equipment Monitoring
Preset and delivered CPAP pressure
Record hours of use
Change filters
Incorporate low-pressure alarm

Of equal importance is monitoring the accuracy of the CPAP device.[28] The devices currently on the market do not have intrinsic alarms to alert the user of changes in pressure, circuit disconnections, or failures of the device. If needed, pressure monitoring alarms are available for placement in the circuit. These monitors should be set with a pressure and time threshold so that momentary changes in pressure do not activate the alarm. Figure 24–4 is an example of one such pressure monitor. The home care company should periodically monitor the level of CPAP delivered to patients with an in-line manometer. In addition, filters need to be changed frequently or blowers may either overheat or adequate pressure may not be delivered to the patient circuit.

APNEA IMPEDANCE MONITORS IN INFANTS

Monitoring of infants with diagnosed or suspected pathologic apnea has been available for about 15 years via apnea impedance monitors; however, whether infant mortality has decreased as a result is controversial.[29, 30] Apnea impedance monitors (Fig 24–5) function by measuring chest wall movement and, therefore, can be influenced by the chest wall movement caused by cardiac impulses.[31] These monitors are not sensitive to periods of obstructive apnea since chest wall movement continues in the absence of airflow.[32] Many infants experience mixed apneic episodes—a combination of central and obstructive events. A premature infant may be prone to central apnea because of incomplete maturation of the respiratory center and blunted responses to hypoxemia and hypercarbia.[33, 34]

    Upper airway obstruction can occur because of the immaturity of the upper airway reflexes and decreased muscle tone of the tongue and pharynx, and a compliant chest wall affects the

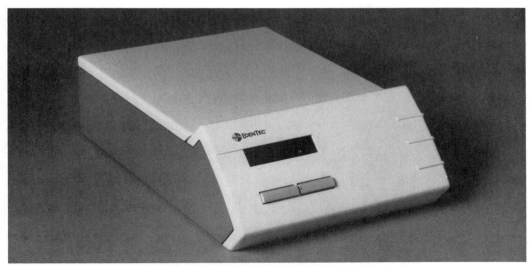

A

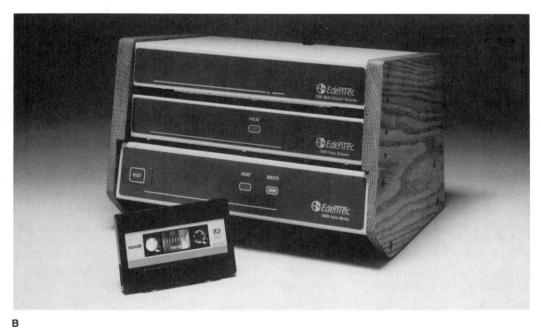

B

FIG 24–3.
Portable sleep apnea screening device: **A,** EdenTrace II. **B,** EdenTec Multichannel Recorder, Pulse Oximeter, Apnea Monitor, EdenTec, Eden Prairie, MN. (*Used by permission.*)

TABLE 24–3.
Sleep Monitoring in the Home

Diagnosis and Follow-up
  OSA
  Central sleep apnea
  COPD
  Tracheobronchomalacia
  Central hypoventilation
  Apnea of infancy
  ALTE
  Muscular skeletal disease (i.e., kyphoscoliosis,
    diaphragmatic paralysis)
  Hypoxemia
Epidemiologic Studies of OSA
Unavailability of Formal Sleep Labs
Monitoring Response to Therapy
  Noninvasive ventilation
    negative pressure
    positive pressure [nasal, mouth]
  CPAP
  Pharmocologic interventions
  Oxygen prescription

infant's ability to maintain airway tone.[35] Because infants have a large head and short neck, airway obstruction can occur secondary to flexion of the neck.[34] Since these devices are used mainly by parents or caretakers in the home, the user must thoroughly understand the function of the monitor and how to troubleshoot its operation.[30] Frequent assessment of the accuracy of the device is mandatory.

Apnea impedance monitors can only alert caregivers to changes in the infant's status, but are not a guarantee of infant survival. The family needs to be well educated in specialized procedures such as cardiopulmonary resucitation.[30] They must be able to recognize the differences between periodic breathing (three or more respiratory pauses that persist for more than 3 seconds, with intervals of respiration between pauses that are no longer than 20 seconds), which may be normal in young infants, and pathologic apnea (a cessation of breathing 20 seconds or longer accompanied by bradycardia, cyanosis, and/or limpness).[30] Table 24–4 lists patient and equipment functions that need timely monitoring in this setting. More extensive monitoring such as a four-channel pneumocardiogram, which evaluates nasal airflow, thoracic impedance, heart rate, and oxygen saturation, or a polysomnography (sleep study) may be warranted if problems are suspected. With any monitoring device used in the home, if the alarms are sounding frequently for no apparent reason they easily become ignored or turned down or off with resultant disastrous consequences.

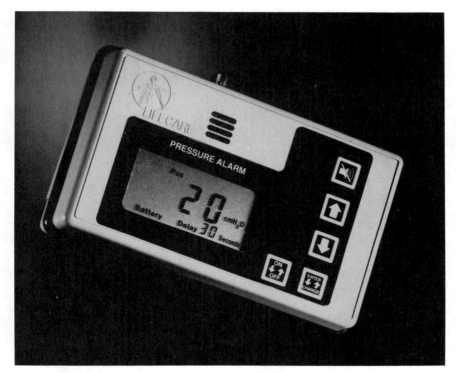

FIG 24–4.
Pressure Monitor, Life Care, Lafayette, CO. (*Used by permission.*)

MECHANICAL VENTILATION

Continuous Mechanical Ventilation in Adults

Most patients who require continuous ventilatory support have a tracheostomy, though there is a small population of patients maintained on continuous positive pressure ventilation with the use of noninvasive techniques.[36] Most of these patients required ventilation after an acute event and failure to wean. Some require continuous support (24 hours/day) as their disease progressed. Many of these patients have no spontaneous respiratory efforts, nor do they have the ability to reconnect themselves to the ventilator if inadvertently disconnected. As a result, disconnect without appropriate alarm function has disastrous consequences. Therefore, these patients need secondary and remote alarms incorporated into the ventilator system. Table 24–5 lists patient status and equipment functions that require monitoring.

The ventilator's intrinsic and secondary alarms should be assessed daily by the patient and/or caregivers. Each time the patient is disconnected for suctioning, the low-pressure alarm

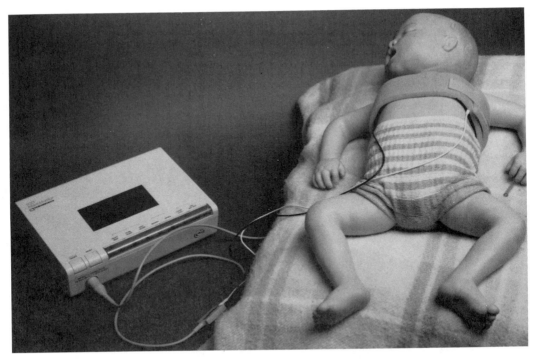

FIG 24–5.
Corometrics 500 Infant Monitor, Corometrics, Wallingford, CT. (*Used by permission.*)

TABLE 24–4.
Apnea Impedance Monitoring in the Home

Infant Monitoring
Spo₂—intermittent nighttime recording
Clinical status
  Vital signs
  Breathing patterns
  Growth and development
Pneumocardiogram (four channel)
Polysomnography

Equipment Monitoring
Alarm settings
Alarm function
Electrode placement

TABLE 24–5.
Continuous Mechanical Ventilation of Adults
in the Home

Patient Monitoring
SpO_2—intermittent
ABG—intermittent
Clinical status
   Vital signs
   Lung sounds
   Sputum production
Compliance
Airway resistance—pre- and post-
   bronchodilator
Presence of intrinsic PEEP
$PetCO_2$—intermittent, by therapist
Spontaneous ventilatory parameters [selected
   patients]
   V_T
   VC
   MIP
Tracheostomy site
Tracheostomy cuff
   Pressure
   Volume
Equipment Monitoring
Ventilator function—at routine therapist visit
Alarm settings—daily
Alarm function—daily
Peak inspiratory pressure—daily and at routine
   therapist visit
Pressure manometer calibration—at routine
   therapist visit
Ventilator settings—daily
   V_T—machine delivered
   Rate
   Sensitivity
   FIO_2—monthly, at routine therapist visit
   Flow rate and/or inspiratory time
Leaks in the systems
Integrity of the circuit
Hours of use—at routine therapist visit
Inlet filters—per manufacturer's
   recommendations
Bacteria filters—monthly
Accessory equipment function

function can be checked for the time interval before alarming. The calibration of the pressure manometer needle must be checked routinely by the home care provider; if this is out of calibration the alarms settings may not be accurate. The average peak inspiratory pressure (PIP) should be checked, the low- and high-pressure alarm settings may need periodic readjustment based on PIP.

Alarms that are activated frequently are commonly readjusted inappropriately by the patient and/or caregiver. This may result in lack of appropriate ventilation due to leaks in the system, loose connections, or holes in the circuits. The caretakers or patient should be taught to check the ventilator system on a daily basis. The caretakers can be shown how to adjust temporarily the high-pressure alarm and pressure release to 100 cm H_2O followed by occlusion of the circuit at the tracheostomy swivel to assess the presence of small system leaks. The patient and caregiver can also learn to assess leaks in the system by listening to the ventilator function. Small leaks can cause a whistling or hissing sound and bubbling of water at the leak site. Leaks in the humidifier jar can cause a high- or low-pitched sound with each ventilator breath.

Currently, the continuous use of monitors to assess gas exchange in the home environment is not recommended,[1, 2] even though we have the technology to monitor all aspects of physiological response. Patients discharged to the home should be medically stable and not in need of continuous monitoring. If their condition changes, then clinical signs of deterioration should be detected and appropriate measures taken. Simple monitoring, such as pulse oximetry and Holter monitoring, as well as end-tidal carbon dioxide ($Petco_2$), sleep studies, portable xray, ultrasounds, and ABG, can be periodically performed in the home. Periodic spot checks of Spo_2 and $Petco_2$ may be done based on the patient's clinical status or during routine therapist visits, provided baseline arterial blood gases are available for comparison and the provider understands the problems with reliability and accuracy of the instruments.[20, 37] The accuracy of $Petco_2$ is dependent on the patient's underlying lung disease.[38] In our experience[8] with more than 70 patients maintained at home with mechanical ventilation, $Petco_2$ was never indicated and only rarely was Spo_2 monitoring needed. If patients have problems, they are seen in the outpatient setting where an ABG and detailed physical assessment can be performed. The use of $Petco_2$ does not contribute to the care of ventilator-dependent patients, but does increase the anxiety of the patient and caretaker as well as cost.

The periodic assessments by the home care provider should consist of monitoring the function of the equipment, as well as monitoring the patient's response to therapy. Exhaled tidal volume and inspired oxygen concentration should be checked at routine visits to the home. Patient assessment may include lung and chest wall static compliance, airway resistance, and spontaneous breathing effort. The provider should observe these measurements before and after a bronchodilator treatment and suctioning to determine the response to therapy. The patient's general condition, including vital signs, chest assessment, and sputum production, should be monitored. In selected patients, spontaneous ventilatory parameters (vital capacity, maximum inspiratory pressure, and tidal volume) may be assessed.

Continuous Use of Mechanical Ventilation in Infants and Children

The reasons for monitoring infants and children on mechanical ventilators in the home differ greatly from adults. This is, in part, due to changes in ventilatory and oxygen needs as they grow, the use of uncuffed tracheostomy tubes, their weaning capabilities, and the type of ventilatory assistance used in the home.[25] Whether these situations justify continuous monitoring is controversial. In a review of the literature, many authors list various monitors in their equipment list for home care but do not specify which infants need them.[12, 39, 40] Other authors indicate the need for apnea monitors,[5] gas exchange monitors,[1] or tidal volume measurement devices.[1] One gets the sense that all are avoiding making a specific statement regarding monitoring of ventilation and oxygenation function in the home. Continuous monitoring of gas exchange greatly increases the cost of home care for infants and children, transforms the home into an intensive care unit,[12] and adds to the stress of the family and caregivers. Guidelines are needed to ensure safety but to also allow for individualization. Two factors—age and the disease process—may be the determinants for how much monitoring is needed and the type of monitoring devices used. Other factors, such as patient stability, coexisting disease, type of ventilatory assistance, artificial airway, and alterations in growth and development, also play a role in establishing guidelines.

Table 24–6 separates ventilatory support under two major disease categories: respiratory distress syndrome/bronchopulmonary dysplasia (RDS/BPD), and congenital anomalies/neuromuscular dysfunction. Children under one year of age with primary pulmonary disease, an uncuffed tracheostomy tube, and pressure-limited ventilation may need more continuous or frequent monitoring, especially for oxygenation. However, I have rarely seen an indication for continuous pulse oximetry. Children with congenital anomalies or neuromuscular disease who are under one year of age may need continuous $Petco_2$ monitoring, but the feasibility of this is questionable since there are many issues related to using this device in the home (see Chapter 12).

In general, a sidestream sampling capnometer cannot be used in pediatrics since, in order to achieve frequency response, sidestream flows between 125 and 500 mL/min are required. The mainstream sampling units are more accurate, but the sampling port clogs with mucous and water.[37, 38] With these units, the transducer increases the weight on the airway. In addition, the effectiveness of measuring $Petco_2$ is dependent on the degree of ventilation/perfusion abnormality.[39] The practitioner setting up the device and monitoring the data needs to under-

TABLE 24–6.
Continuous Mechanical Ventilation of Infants and Children

Infants with Respiratory Distress Syndrome or bronchopulmonary dysplasia

Age <1 year	>1 year
Monitor	
Spo_2—continuous?	Spo_2—intermittent
Fio_2—continuous?	Fio_2—intermittent
$Petco_2$—intermittent	$Petco_2$—intermittent
Apnea impedance	Apnea impedance
VT_{exh}—continuous versus hourly	VT_{exh}—daily
Pressure (ventilator)	Pressure (ventilator)

Infants or children with congenital anomaly or neuromuscular disease

Monitor	
Spo_2—intermittent	Spo_2—intermittent
$Petco_2$—intermittent	$Petco_2$—intermittent
Fio_2—intermittent	Fio_2—intermittent
Apnea impedance	Apnea impedance

stand the device completely and be able to interpret the data. Any changes noted must be related to other clinical data and equipment malfunction must be ruled out.[38] Since infants have uncuffed tracheostomy tubes, the leak around the tube may cause lower Petco$_2$ readings; this needs to be addressed if capnometry is being used. When using these monitors, the data must be correlated with arterial blood gases. As a result of the many problems related to using these monitors, I would not recommend the use of Petco$_2$ monitors on a continuous basis. If the infant or child is so unstable as to require continuous monitoring of Petco$_2$, he or she should be hospitalized.

Monitoring exhaled tidal volume (V$_{T_{exh}}$) when using pressure-controlled ventilation should be done routinely since many changes can take place during ventilation that alter the tidal volume (i.e., secretions, airway resistance, changes in compliance, or atelectasis). Whether these measurements are done continuously or intermittently depends on the patient and the equipment available. Although remember that anything placed in-line on the ventilator circuit adds to the complexity of the device, may become disconnected, increases dead-space, and increases the weight on the artificial airway. Guidelines must be established for each patient specifying within what range changes are considered safe and when the physician should be called. These parameters must be very specific when the caretakers are nonprofessionals.

As with adults, all children require additional monitoring by a skilled respiratory care practitioner. The ventilator and accessory equipment must be closely monitored to detect problems as discussed with adult patients. As the infant or child grows, reassessment of ventilatory parameters need to be performed, either in the hospital or in the home. Modifications in ventilator settings and equipment and the tracheostomy tube need to be periodically performed. Nutritional status in relation to growth and development of the child also requires periodic evaluation.[40]

Intermittent use of Mechanical Ventilation in the Home

Generally, most patients on nighttime ventilation, with or without intermittent daytime use, are maintained on noninvasive ventilatory support. This may include nasal or mouth positive-pressure ventilation, negative-pressure ventilation, diaphragmatic pacing, or the use of a pneumobelt or rocking bed. Table 24–7 lists the periodic monitoring needs of these patients. The type and degree of monitoring necessary for these patients depends on the underlying disease process and the device they are using. Patients on nighttime ventilatory assistance for central alveolar hypoventilation, kyphoscoliosis, post-polio syndrome, or muscular dystrophy, may need periodic assessment of the adequacy of ventilation by obtaining morning and evening ABG to determine their ability to maintain the desired Paco$_2$ level during the day. If the patient is on a device without an inherent alarm for low pressure or disconnect, then an alarm should be incorporated into the system to alert the patient and/or caretaker of problems. A patient with diaphragmatic pacing may need an apnea impedance monitor to alert the caregiver to inadequate respiratory excursions.

If the patient on nighttime ventilation is complaining of symptoms indicative of alteration in sleep such as morning headaches, daytime somnulence, frequent wakefulness, and an increase in dyspnea, then additional monitoring may be necessary. If the patient has edema or other signs of right heart failure, periodic nighttime Spo$_2$ monitoring may be warranted.

TABLE 24–7.
Intermittent Mechanical Ventilation in the Home

Patient Monitoring
Spo_2—spot checks or nighttime recording
ABG—early morning and evening (periodic)
Clinical status
   Vital signs
   Lung sounds
   Sputum production
   Signs of cor pulmonale
   Morning headaches
Modified sleep study
$Petco_2$—spot checks
Spontaneous ventilatory parameters
Compliance
Airway resistance
Skin integrity of face and nose—nasal mask
   ventilation
Lips and oral mucosa—mouth ventilation
Skin integrity of chest and abdomen—negative
   pressure ventilation
Tracheostomy site
Equipment Monitoring
Ventilator function—monthly
Alarm settings—daily
Alarm function—daily
Peak inspiratory pressure—daily and monthly
Pressure manometer calibration—monthly
Ventilator settings:
   V_T
   Rate
   Sensitivity
   Flow rate and/or inspiratory time
   Fio_2 [monthly]
Leaks in system—daily
Hours of use—monthly
Inlet filters—per manufacturer recommendation
Bacteria filters—monthly
Accessory equipment function

This could be done with a modified sleep study performed in the home, and if abnormalities are detected then the patient may be admitted for further evaluation, readjustment of ventilator settings, and/or an increase in ventilatory assistance. If the patient is on nasal ventilation, he or she may need a chin strap to prevent excess mouth leak. Other patients may need a change in the type of ventilatory support; patients with a pneumobelt, rocking bed, or a negative-pressure ventilator may need to be switched to a positive-pressure device and other patients may need to be tracheostomized as their disease progresses. These assessments are very important in patients who have a progressive neuromuscular disease or in the aging patient with a decrease in lung and chest wall compliance.

Patients on intermittent ventilatory support also need periodic assessment of spontaneous ventilatory mechanics, including tidal volume, minute ventilation, vital capacity, and maximal inspiratory and expiratory pressures. These can be performed in the home and reported to the prescribing physician. Routine therapist visits should include recording the total hours that the ventilator has been used. If the patient is having increased problems, it may be related to inadequate time receiving ventilatory support. Routinely checking the time meter is also important for determining when preventive maintenance is due.

When patients are receiving nasal ventilation, they must be routinely assessed for nasal passage or sinus pathology. If they develop sinusitis, are they routinely cleaning the ventilator circuits and humidifier or changing the artificial nose? If on mouth positive pressure, their lips and mouth must be checked for lesions or pressure sores secondary to the mouthpiece. When patients are using a negative-pressure device, the chest and abdomen must be checked for pressure sores.

PATIENT AND CAREGIVER REACTION TO HOME RESPIRATORY CARE

When a patient is sent home with any type of respiratory support device, from something as simple as oxygen therapy to a mechanical ventilator, there is always a certain degree of anxiety related to having the equipment in the house. When we add to the complexity of the equipment, we add to the degree of anxiety. If monitors are used, then strict guidelines must be given for each individual situation possible. We cannot expect the patient or caregiver to act and think like a trained clinician. In my experience, when patients are given extra alarms for back up, they are never used because they were a nuisance to the family. When oximeters, oxygen analyzers, and respirometers are sent home with the patient, we are asking nonclinicians to make medical judgments based on the data they collect and these data may be skewed because of calibration and application problems. If we try to monitor at home as we would in the hospital, the patient and family get the impression that the patient should not be in the home. As a result, family members may refuse to take on the responsibility for caring for the individual and, ultimately, an excellent home care candidate may never get home.

When we use "high-tech" monitoring equipment in the home, we must be willing to teach unskilled caregivers how to react to changes noted on the monitor and make adjustments to the ventilator according to these changes. We must be prepared to accept all the phone calls from caregivers when monitor alarms are activated or measurements change slightly from prior values. Most likely, we will be placing an unnecessary burden on the caretaker by incorporating continuous monitoring in the home and increasing the level of anxiety with resultant fatigue of the caretaker, which may result in lack of appropriate response when the patient's condition actually is critical. Also, not that cost should be the driving force, but when excessive equipment and monitors are placed in the home, the cost-effectiveness of home respiratory care is greatly decreased.

Individualized patient care is important, though guidelines are necessary to provide direction for the overall patient population. If the patient is to be at home, we must not treat him as if he is still in the intensive care unit (ICU). If ICU-level care is needed, the patient should not

TABLE 24–8.
Monitoring Equipment Potentially Used in
the Home

Stethoscope
Blood pressure cuff
Respirometer
Oxygen analyzer
Pulse oximeter
Pressure manometer
Apnea impedance monitor
Capnograph, capnometer
Recorders
Polysomnography
Holter monitor
Transcutaneous oxygen and carbon dioxide
    monitor
Portable x ray
Ultrasound

be at home. Table 24–8 lists some of the monitoring equipment that potentially could be ordered for home care use. This list is endless and intimidating to the patient and family, and it does not include the nonrespiratory care equipment needed for patient care such as feeding pumps or special beds and mattresses.

For many patients, the home care respiratory company and the nursing agency will be responsible for monitoring the patient. The referring physician needs to be very specific when writing discharge orders regarding monitoring. As technology increases and we have more and more equipment available for patient care, we will need to be more vigilant with our home care patients and use this technology appropriately.

The future direction for monitoring of respiratory care in the home must be outcome based and quality of life issues must be addressed. Establishing guidelines for monitoring in the home should be the goal of all home care practitioners. A consensus homecare conference on monitoring to assist in establishing these guidelines is gravely needed.

REFERENCES

1. O'Donohue WJ, Giovannoni RM, Goldberg AL, et al: ACCP ad hoc committee report. Long-term mechanical ventilation guidelines for management in the home and at alternate community sites. *Chest* 1986; 90(suppl):1s–37s.
2. Gilmartin ME, Make BJ, (eds): Mechanical ventilation in the home: Issues for health care providers. *Probs Respir Care* 1988; 1:155–290.
3. Bach JR, Alba AS, Bohatiuk G, et al: Mouth intermittent positive pressure ventilation in the management of post-polio respiratory insufficiency. *Chest* 1987; 91:859–864.
4. Burr BH, Guyer B, Todres ID, et al: Home care for children on respirators. *N Engl J Med* 1983; 309:1319–1323.

5. Schreiner MS, Donar ME, Kettrick RG: Pediatric home mechanical ventilation in children. *Pediatr Clin North Am* 1987; 34:47–60.
6. Gilmartin ME: Long term mechanical ventilation. Patient selection and discharge planning. *Respir Care* 1991; 36:205–216.
7. Sivak ED, Cordasco EM, Gibson WT, et al: Home care ventilation: The Cleveland Clinic experience from 1977–1985. *Respir Care* 1986; 31:294–302.
8. Make BJ, Gilmartin ME: Mechanical ventilation in the home. *Crit Care Clin* 1990; 6:785–796.
9. Make BJ: Long-term management of ventilator assisted individuals: The Boston University experience. *Respir Care* 1986; 31:303–310.
10. Kerby GR, Mayer LS, Pingleton SK: Nocturnal positive pressure ventilation via nasal mask. *Am Rev Respir Dis* 1987; 137:738–740.
11. Posch CM, Edwards PA: The ventilator-dependent child: Challenge and opportunity. *Rehab Nurs* 1988; 13:15–18.
12. Donar ME: Community care: Pediatric home mechanical ventilation. *Holistic Nurs Pract* 1988; 2:68–80.
13. Nocturnal Oxygen Therapy Trial Group. Continuous or nocturnal oxygen therapy in hypoxemic chronic obstructive lung disease: A clinical trial. *Ann Intern Med* 1980; 93:391–398.
14. British Medical Research Council Working Party. Long term domiciliary oxygen therapy in chronic hypoxic cor pulmonale complicating chronic bronchitis and emphysema. *Lancet* 1981; 1:681–686.
15. Criteria for Medicare coverage of oxygen services in the home. *Federal Register* April 5, 1985; p 50.
16. Carlin BW, Clausen JL, Ries AL: The use of cutaneous oximetry in the prescription of long-term oxygen therapy. *Chest* 1988; 94:239–244.
17. Transmittal to the Medicare coverage issue. Manual No. 32: Section 60-4, Home use of O_2 therapy. June 1989.
18. Tweedale PM, Douglas NJ: Evaluation of Biox IIA ear oximeter. *Thorax* 1985; 40:825–827.
19. Kagle DM, Alexander CM, Berko RS, et al: Evaluation of the Ohmeda 3700 pulse oximeter: Steady-state and transient response characteristics. *Anesthesiol* 1987;66:376–380.
20. Severinghaus KW, Naifch KH, Kohl SO: Errors in 14 pulse oximeters during profound hypoxemia. *J Clin Monit* 1989; 5:72–81.
21. Welch JP, DeCasare R, Hess D: Pulse oximetry: Instrumentation and clinical applications. *Respir Care* 1990; 35:584–601.
22. McPherson SP: Respiratory home care equipment. Dubuque, IA, Kendall/Hunt, 1988.
23. Ward JJ: Equipment for mixed gas and oxygen therapy, in Barnes TA (ed) *Respiratory Care Practice*. Chicago, Mosby Year Book, 1988.
24. O'Donnell DE, Sanii R, Younes M: Improvement in exercise endurance in patients with chronic airflow limitations using continuous positive airway pressure. *Am Rev Respir Dis* 1988; 138F:1510–1514.
25. Kacmarek RM: Noninvasive monitoring of respiratory function outside of the hospital. *Respir Care* 1990; 35:719–727.
26. Hoelscher TJ, Erwin CW, Marsh GR, et al: Ambulatory sleep monitoring with the Oxford-Medilog 9000: Technical acceptability, patient acceptance and clinical indications. *Sleep* 1987; 10:606–607.
27. Wilkinson RT, Mullaney D: Electroencephalogram recording of sleep in the home. *Postgrad Med J* 1976; 52(suppl):92–96.
28. Millman RP, Kipp GJ, Deadles SC, et al: A home monitoring system for nasal CPAP. *Chest* 1988; 93:730–733.
29. Yount JE: Reduction in SIDS after selective use of home monitoring among infants who weigh less than 2 kg at birth. *Pediatr Res* 1981; 15:734–739.
30. Consensus statement: National Institutes of Health Consensus Development Conference on infantile apnea and home monitoring. Sept. 29–Oct. 1, 1986. *Pediatr* 1986; 79:292–299.

31. Lewis R, Thompson S, Coldberg A: Respiratory care for the infant and child, in Burton G, Hodgkin J Ward J (eds): *Respiratory Care. A Guide to Clinical Practice*, ed 3. Philadelphia, JB Lippincott Co, 1991.
32. Brouillette RT, Morrow AS, Weese-Maye DE, et al: Comparison of respiratory inductive plethysmography and thoracic impedence for apnea monitoring. *J Pediatr* 1987; 111–377–383.
33. Grisemer AN. Apnea of prematurity: Current management and mursing implications. *Pediatr Nurs* 1990; 16:606–611.
34. Martin RJ, Miller MJ, Carlo WA: Pathogenesis of apnea in preterm infants. *J Pediatr* 1986; 109:733–741.
35. Spitzer AR, Fox WW: Infant apnea. *Pediatr Clin NA* 1986; 33:561–581.
36. Bach JR, Alba AS: Management of chronic alveolar hypoventilation by nasal ventilation. *Chest* 1990; 97:52–57.
37. Hess D: Capnometry and capnography: Technical and physiologic aspects and clinical applications. *Respir Care* 1990; 35:557–576.
38. Clark JS, Votteri B, Ariagno RL, et al: Non-invasive assessment of blood gases. *Am Rev Respir Dis* 1992; 145:220–232.
39. Kacmarek RM, Thompson JE: Respiratory care of the ventilator-assisted infant in the home. *Respir Care* 1986; 31:605–614.
40. Kettrick RG, Donar ME: Ventilator-assisted infants and children. *Probs Respir Care* 1988; 1:269–278.

Chapter 25

Unattended Monitoring for Respiratory Events

Kingman P. Strohl, M.D.

Michael J. Decker, C.R.T.T.

Susan Redline, M.D., M.P.H.

INTRODUCTION

This chapter will review the potential role of unattended monitoring for respiratory events for diagnosis and management of pulmonary disease. The term *unattended monitoring* is meant to define technology that does not require continuous human surveillance for the collection of physiologic data. Historically this type of clinical monitoring is best exemplified by the use of Holter monitoring for cardiac rate, rhythm, and electrogram morphology. The ability of a continuously monitored heart rate was demonstrated in the 1950s, and the usefulness of ambulatory EKG monitoring for the recognition of lethal arrhythmias in the usual environment of the patient was quickly recognized by the medical community. This allowed diagnosis of events related to sudden changes in cardiac rhythm and eventually led to better management of patients with pharmaceutical agents or exercise prescription[1-3] and more recently to prospective identification and treatment of individuals at high risk.[4-6] In the past 10 years, particularly with the recognition of sleep disorders, much activity has occurred in the technological development of unattended monitoring for continuous evaluation of patients with hypertension, insomnia, hypersomnia, gastroesophageal reflux, and behavior disorders.[7-13] This technology now includes the assessment of blood pressure,[14, 15] temperature,[16, 17] electroencephalogram,[12, 16, 18] esophageal pH,[19] body position and movement,[16, 20] penile tumescence,[21] and certain stress-related autonomic events.[22] This list is, moreover, not exhaustive; new applications are proposed or demonstrated every few months.

The purpose of this chapter is to review the principles and implications of unattended monitoring in regard to respiratory events. In general, it should be evident that clinical decision-making, defined as ascertainment of therapeutic need and its relationship to beneficial patient outcome, ideally should be made in the normal environment for the patient. Technology to measure respiratory rate, rhythm, and certain variables related to gas exchange, such as Pao_2, $Paco_2$, pH, and oxygen saturation, are now sufficiently advanced to allow for such assessment outside a specialized laboratory and without constant attendance. Certainly, measurements that are made in a hospital or laboratory setting provide information that is derived contextually from an environment that is much different from that of the patient's own daily life. Therefore, unattended monitoring will have less potential to affect patient lifestyle than inpatient monitoring. Since the former allows for monitoring patients outside of the hospital-based laboratory, a better definition of the diurnal variation or chronobiology of the disease process can be obtained. Finally, it may be possible to reduce costs for diagnosis of disease by reducing personnel or space requirements or by limiting the number of variables needed to define a disease or to define a beneficial outcome for any therapeutic intervention.

Unattended monitoring includes two separate but related types of technology. The first would be defined as *ambulatory monitoring*, the technology that allows the patient free movement throughout the day. Such examples of this would be Holter monitoring, in which devices are light and portable to allow patients of all ages to move freely, to be able to go home, and to go about their daily activities, returning the equipment either the next day or the next week. Another form of unattended monitoring would be that of *portable monitoring*. This technology would be taken to the bedside of the patient. In general, portable monitors are more bulky and heavier than ambulatory monitors and limit to some degree the ability of the patient to move around freely in the environment. Usually portable monitoring is performed at a specific location, such as the bedside at home, a general hospital ward, or a nursing home.

ADVANTAGES AND DISADVANTAGES OF UNATTENDED MONITORING

Unattended monitoring will be utilized according to both the needs of the system and the cultural sensitivities of the patient-physician environment. In Europe unattended monitoring has gained wider acceptance than in the United States; and, in general, there is much more clinical research activity in both ambulatory and portable monitoring for respiratory events in Europe and Australia than in the United States. One force for developing unattended monitors is the relative lack of specialized laboratories within hospitals and the rationing of such expensive resources in medical systems by central agencies. However, economic rationing probably does not completely explain the differences in attitude between physicians in the United States and Europe. Home assessment of patients, lifestyle assessments and their changes with disease, and patient sensitivities have been more routinely assessed in European medicine than in American medicine. This bias, therefore, tends to shed a favorable light on unattended monitoring by Europeans, while in America the literature emphasizes the problems associated with unattended monitoring. These problems include a greater incidence of technically uninterpretable data, technologic and patient difficulties in data acquisition, and the limitations of this approach to patient care as opposed to using a "gold standard," such as clinical polysomnography.

More specific advantages and disadvantages for ambulatory and portable monitoring are listed in Table 25–1. Both ambulatory and portable monitoring allow the assessment of the patient in their home environment or in their usual clinical environment. In addition, they can allow monitoring in unusual conditions such as during space flight[14] or cross-country hiking.[17] Such monitoring has shown patterns of respiratory rate and rhythm in disease states. One example of this is in the transient hyperpnea and tachycardia at rest in patients with anxiety syndromes including occupational stress. In addition, both ambulatory and portable monitoring have been shown to have a minimal effect on sleep-wake cycles in contrast to a specialized in-hospital laboratory where the first night in the laboratory can have a significant effect on some of these variables.[7, 23, 24] Studies of patient acceptance have shown that unattended monitoring is preferable to specialized laboratory monitoring in terms of reduced anxiety and of greater patient willingness to undergo repeated studies. There are relative advantages of ambulatory monitoring in terms of the free mobility of the patient and of the ability to record continuously events over a day and, therefore, to define diurnal events in the course of disease. Portable monitoring, which does not allow such free range motion of the subject throughout their daily activities, does not allow this assessment. Portable monitoring can be useful in monitoring bedridden patients in nursing homes or in those that have limited mobility because of existing disease. Certainly unattended monitoring has less space cost than hospital-based specialized laboratories. However, at the present time, the personnel costs involved in continuous monitoring of patients for 8 to 10 hours may not be eliminated by unattended technologies since the time to analyze unattended monitoring records can be considerable and, at present, poorly summarized by automatic analysis.

At the present time, a general problem of unattended monitoring for respiratory events is the lack of standards and guidelines for clinical use by the professional societies. In general,

TABLE 25–1.

ADVANTAGES

Free mobility of patient (A)
Record diurnal events (A)
Minimal first night effect (A,P)
Patient acceptance (A,P)
Monitoring in clinical/unusual environments
  (A,P)
Less personnel cost than hospital or inpatient
  laboratories (A,P)

DISADVANTAGES

Lack of standards or guidelines for clinical use
  (A,P)
Lack of technical requirements (software and
  hardware) (A,P)
Durability and equipment reliability (A,P)
Patient comfort (A,P)
Physician acceptance (A,P)

A = Ambulatory; P = Portable.

the medical community has yet to agree on the minimum number of variables to monitor and, equally important, on the criteria for scoring sleep-related physiologic variables. Hence, there is no consensus on how to utilize unattended recordings. In all fairness, this problem also applies to polysomnography laboratory studies. This lack of general consensus could be because patients who present to their primary physician with signs or symptoms of sleep-related breathing disorders can be referred to either a neurologist, pulmonologist, or psychiatrist. Since each of these specialized fields of medicine has its own diagnostic dilemmas, as well as its own criteria to determine thresholds of disease, differences exist between disciplines as to what variables should be monitored, scored, and interpreted.

Because of the interdisciplinary differences in recording and scoring of sleep-related physiologic variables, manufacturers have pursued a number of different pathways in the development of unattended monitoring systems. Some monitoring devices offer an array of interchangeable sensors and recording parameters. Unfortunately, while the recording devices can be altered to be acceptable to most clinicians, primary problems remain with standardized criteria to distinguish a physiologic event from pathological states or artifactual signals. Without accepted criteria, there can be no development of the time-saving, automated analysis of collected data.

A certain amount of potential subjective bias will exist in the scoring of recorded events and the determination of clinical relevance. For instance, inter-rater reliability on polysomnograms is 60 to 80%, even when the different observers are trained to score similarly. Once common scoring criteria do exist, the next step is to determine their diagnostic sensitivity. Since analysis of respiratory-related signals can be complex, empirical studies are needed to equate changes in breathing patterns with clinical severity.

While the technology for portable and ambulatory recording has been feasible for several years, there is a lack of stated requirements for both the hardware and software aspects of this equipment. This lack of standardization is another reason for skepticism by physicians since, in general, the understanding of this technology is not a part of the general education of the clinician. This technology is new and in many instances the operating procedures are not few nor the manuals easy to follow. Some of the equipment for reading or reviewing the collected data can be expensive, and neither the handling of the equipment by the patient or by the technician is currently user-friendly. For instance, the playback of data may require considerable personnel time and input. This is the case not only for respiratory monitoring but also for Holter monitoring for arrhythmias or cardiac ischemia. Finally, in both ambulatory and portable monitoring, durability and equipment longevity have rarely been assessed. For all these reasons, physician acceptance of unattended monitoring has been a problem in spite of the intellectual attractiveness for patient care.

THE CRITERIA FOR TECHNOLOGY ASSESSMENT

There are at lease five clinically available systems for either portable or ambulatory monitoring of airflow, respiratory effort, and/or gas exchange (Table 25–2). Some of these packages are fairly well developed and offer an array of variables, often including measurements of body position and movement that may also be useful in assessment of sleep-related respiratory events. Other systems are not so packaged but can be constructed from available technology

TABLE 25–2.

Commercial Monitor	Respiratory Airflow	Effort	Oxygen Saturation	Options
CNS	P	P	X	X
Eden Tec	P	X	X	X	EKG, HR
Oxford Medilog*	A	X	X	X	EEG, BP, POS, AC, Lite, EKG, O_2
Sleep Trace	P	X	X	X	
Vitalog	A	X	X	X	POS, AC

A = Ambulatory; P = Portable; EKG = electrocardiography; BP = blood pressure; HR = heart rate only; POS = body position; O_2 = transcutaneous O_2; AC = activity; CO_2 = carbon dioxide levels; Lite = light intensity for day-night.
* Four or eight channels of data acquisition. EEG = electroencephalography

to allow similar measurements. All of these systems require sensors, a recording device, and a playback device. Each of these components will need to be assessed technologically as well as for its cost-effectiveness in clinical decision-making.

There are differences in evaluating diagnostic tests as opposed to therapy.[25, 26] First, the process of diagnosis can be complex. The monitoring of a patient suspected of sleep apnea can have, as an example, a certain cost and perhaps even some risk in terms of the equipment or of the patient-equipment interaction. There will be benefit if the monitoring results in a pattern of abnormality that is diagnostic of sleep apnea, an event most likely in those people who have major abnormalities in respiratory events. However, not all individuals will have specific patterns or even have sleep apnea. At the present time we do not have the information to predict which of the many candidate patients are more or less likely to receive an advantage. Also, diagnostic tests do not stand on their own merits as do therapeutic technologies sometimes. Therapy is assessed by the patient as either giving relief with some degree of acceptable nuisance and by the doctor as having an effect on morbidity and mortality. A single diagnostic measurement may not be as sufficient or as quantifiable. Moreover, an accurate test for an untreatable condition has limited merit, while an inaccurate test for a treatable disease adds costs to the system.

Sox[27] has placed the information needed to assess technology into four categories: biologic plausibility, technical feasibility, diagnostic accuracy, and clinical impact.

For respiratory events the biologic reasons for measuring such variables as airflow, respiratory effort, and oxygen saturation certainly are well established (refer to previous chapters). There are certain clinical syndromes, such as sleep apnea, in which a constellation of these measurements provides a definition of the number, type, and severity of breathing abnormalities. There are other syndromes, however, such as chronic lung disease, in which the severity of breathing abnormalities may not be as clearly defined. However, in general, these signals are useful for both specialized in-hospital laboratories as well as for unattended monitoring. Monitoring of these variables has disclosed correlations with clinical syndromes (sleep apnea, hypoventilation, "blue-bloater," etc.) and has provided the basis for clinical decisions for interventions, such as nasal CPAP, tracheostomy, or supplemental oxygen therapy. In addition, some of these measurements are now part of our definitions or standards of care in the community. Therefore, a strong biological plausibility exists for measuring oxygen saturation, airflow, and respiratory effort in individuals over time with known or suspected pulmonary disease.

With regard to technical feasibility, the measurement of respiratory events—airflow, effort, and gas exchange—has different degress of application for unattended monitoring. The signals are relatively easy to monitor and to record with sensors that can be easily applied; however, they cannot be quantitated easily. More importantly, measurements of airflow and respiratory effort are affected by the body and by sensor position; therefore, their output can vary independently from changes that might occur because of pathophysiological events. On the other hand, pulse oximetric measurements of oxygen saturation as one index of oxygenation have an inherent ability to provide calibrated, quantitative data. The signal for oxygen saturation is expressed in a voltage proportional to the saturation. Changes in that voltage output as well as changes in the pulse waveform from which values are calculated can be stored and assessed at the time of playback. With pulse oximetry it is more possible to distinguish artifact from physiologically relevant changes in the sensed signal.[28, 29] Unfortunately, pulse oximetry monitors are currently quite bulky and more often incorporated into portable monitors than ambulatory monitors.

Besides the technical feasibility of measurement of respiratory events, one must also consider the technical feasibility of the data storage and data retrieval portions of these monitoring devices. At the present time we, as a laboratory, have chosen to examine data collected on tape rather than on a memory chip. Originally, this was due to a current limitation of the amount of real-time data that could be stored in digital memory. Tape recording allows us to collect multiple channels of data continuously and then sort and test for relevant correlations after full data retrieval. However, the analog tape player is subject to mechanical breakdown, to the need for greater battery requirements, and to more mechanical upkeep; therefore, ultimately the cost of recording for these variables may prohibit its application to a larger number of patients.

With the advent of multiple-channel, continuous digital recording, there will be a greater need for standards in signal processing and definition of optimal storage and retrieval systems for these signals. Respiratory events are, in general, low frequency in nature and, therefore, should require little preprocessing of data, allowing for real-time collection. However, the simultaneous measurement of such variables, such as EMG or EEG, which require greater amounts of memory for real-time collection or greater amounts of signal processing, may put a limit on memory available for the respiratory variables. We believe that the respiratory variables should be monitored at least at 10 Hz to be able to provide definition of the measured variables. At the present time, we believe real-time collection and so-called "full disclosure" is still needed for diagnostic decision-making.

Another area is that of data retrieval. While the cost of the monitor may be relatively inexpensive, data retrieval systems at the present time are costly and, as with the data collection devices, the standards and requirements for the technology have not been explicitly formulated. This is an area that should receive more attention. A related area is that of the summary of collected data. Certainly display or real-time data provides an overall assessment and quality assurance of the data collection. However, other sorts of analyses, such as display of values, distribution of values, and the quantification of the number of events, for instance, apneas and hypopneas, are needed for better definition of patients and categorization of levels of physiologic abnormality. As a laboratory, we are paying more attention to this aspect of ambulatory monitoring for two reasons. First of all, data summary would allow for an objective description of physiological tracts among many different patients and for a more targeted approach to signal collection and data processing. Secondly, we believe that physician decision-making skills can be better assessed by interpretation of a summary of data than on real-time collection and that correlations in larger numbers of subjects may allow for more insight into how clinical decisions can be made better.

The final criterion for technological feasibility is patient use. With the advent of both portable and ambulatory monitoring, the ease of instrumentation has received attention only recently. As the need for an application of this technology increases, there will be a greater need for patient involvement in the design of sensors and in their use, particularly in the area of patient instruction and technical ease of application.

The diagnostic accuracy of unattended monitoring has received some attention, but it is an area needing substantial work in order to establish the validity and cost-effectiveness of such instrumentation to both traditional physicians and medical agencies. Emsellem and associates[21] studied 67 patients referred to a sleep laboratory with polysomnography and simultaneous monitoring with a portable recorder (Eden-Trace, Eden Prairie, MN) of airflow, chest wall impedance, ECG, and oximetry. The portable tracing was inadequate for evaluation in three instances (4% of studies). Among the remainder of studies, the polysomnogram and portable sleep study similarly characterized the presence or absence of sleep apnea (as defined by greater than or equal to five respiratory disturbances/hour estimated sleep). We also have found an excellent level of agreement between the number of respiratory disturbances identified with this portable monitor (used in home as well as hospital settings) and in-hospital polysomnography ($r = 0.96$) in a population that included healthy or minimally impaired subjects as well as subjects referred for evaluation of a sleep disorder.[30] Portable technology also has been used to characterize breathing disturbances in the geriatric population, a group with a high prevalence of increased numbers of sleep-disordered breathing disturbances as well a periodic leg movements. In this population, Ancoli-Israel and associates[31] have demonstrated that a system that recorded respiratory and abdominal inductance plethysmography, bilateral tibialis EMG, and wrist movement (a modified Oxford Medilog system) correctly classified respiratory disturbances in the majority of subjects studied with portable and hospital-based technologies. These studies, however, have not specifically addressed the ability of portable technology to distinguish central from obstructive events, to assess the degree of positional or sleep stage dependance of the respiratory disturbance, or to characterize sleep architecture. Unfortunately, little consensus exists yet regarding the degree to which this additional information would impact on clinical decision-making. Further understanding of what physiological data are minimally necessary to screen, diagnose, and treat sleep-disordered breathing is needed.

The utility of a physiological tool not only relates to the ability of the tool to provide accurate and unbiased results, but also relates to the reliability of the tool; i.e., the reproducibility and interobserver agreement associated with the technology. As previously discussed, the night-to-night reproducibility of sleep monitoring may be poor because of prominent "first-night" effects or because of inherent variability in physiological behaviors that may be influenced by such conditions as body posture, medication/sedative/stimulant use, nasal stuffiness, etc. However, although prominent first-night effects have been described with the use of hospital-based studies,[23] first-night effects do not appear to be prominent in studies performed in settings familiar to the subject. In this regard, Ancoli-Israel et al.,[31] Redline et al.,[30] and Gyulay et al.,[32] have found no differences in the number of respiratory disturbances identified with first *versus* subsequent night studies. These investigators report that sleep-associated breathing disturbances are reclassified on the basis of subsequent studies in between 3 to 15% of subjects undergoing repeat testing. However, differences in the "number" of events reported to occur night to night may measure only one aspect of the sleep-related respiratory disturbance. The issue of night-to-night variability in interpretation of a "number" may be addressed with development of guidelines for interpreting multiple physiologic parameters (i.e., degree of desaturation associated with respiratory events, number of arousals, length of apneas, etc.) and incorporation of these data with information regarding a patient's symptoms, physical findings, age, etc., in a clinical decision-making paradigm.

Interobserver agreement, for both in-hospital and home studies, appears to be much better for summary measures of respiration (i.e., the respiratory disturbance index) that it is for more specific parameters such as hypopneas and apnea, central and obstructive events, or duration of events.[33, 34] If such specification is determined to be clinically important (see below), then better standardization of measurement techniques and scoring procedures would be needed both for laboratory and portable technologies.

A final area of technology assessment is *whether* and, if so, *how* the test has an effect on the clinical management of respiratory disease.[35] Does the technology improve patient outcome? Do patients live longer, are they happier, and is medical management more cost-effective or efficient in regard to these technologies? In terms of sleep apnea, unattended monitoring may have immediate use in follow-up assessment of patients treated for sleep-disordered breathing, particularly where events such as changes in oxygen saturation or airflow and respiratory efforts can be monitored after initiation of therapy such as nasal CPAP. In this instance a follow-up study within a specialized laboratory of a hospital and the use of increased personnel and technology resources can be obviated. Also, if the treatment results are correlated with clinical symptoms, the analysis of the record may not have to be as rigorous in contrast to the undifferentiated patient where the diagnosis is not made. Another area where unattended monitoring has a particular advantage is in the assessment of those patients who are not good candidates for specialized laboratory assessment, either because of multiple clinical problems or their particular individual sensitivities. For example, patients with quadriplegia,[36] who are prone to sleep-disordered breathing, often require intensive nursing management, which would make it impractical to bring them to the sleep laboratory. Alternatively, in elderly patients or those who are in nursing homes, an assessment in a specialized laboratory can sufficiently disrupt their routine or disrupt the sleep laboratory to make it unwise to study those patients in any environment other than their routine one.

Although several methodologies can satisfy one or two of these areas, at the present time there has been no systematic evaluation of any one modality in all four categories. Although it is possible to have a useful test that may not satisfy all four criteria, failure to assess technology in all four areas should serve as a warning that there may be problems with this diagnostic technology. At the present time, the role of unattended monitoring for respiratory events in patient management is unsettled. However, it took more than two decades for Holter monitoring to become an accepted diagnostic technique; therefore, we should look forward to the definition of this technology in pulmonary medicine in the forthcoming years.

EXAMPLES OF CLINICAL APPLICATION

In this section we will present four examples of the use of unattended monitoring for identification of patterns of disease and insight into diurnal variations in respiratory events.

Sleep Apnea with Daytime Attacks

We have utilized ambulatory monitoring to assess diurnal variations in oxygen saturation in patients with sleep apnea. The disease of obstructive sleep apnea syndrome (OSAS) is characterized by multiple, repetitive apneas during sleep. The mechanism for these apneas is pharyngeal closure, which occurs only when the patient is asleep. Apneas during sleep are terminated by arousals; and, with the repetitive events, the resulting sleep fragmentation leads to the excessive daytime sleepiness seen in these patients. In turn, the patient experiences daytime sleep attacks, which result in sleepiness, sleep apnea, and hypoxemia occurring throughout the 24-hour period. An example in Figure 25–1 shows a 24-hour tracing of oxygen saturation over time in a 52-year-old man who presented with rather minor complaints of

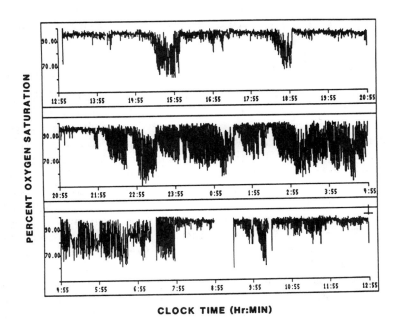

CLOCK TIME (Hr:MIN)

FIG 25–1.
This figure displays oxygen saturation data collected by ambulatory monitoring of a patient presenting with symptoms suggestive of sleep apnea syndrome. The horizontal axis is military time; the vertical axis is percent oxygen saturation. An activity diary kept by the patient indicated self-reported sleep between the hours of 21:55 and 08:00. Marked changes in oxygen saturation coincide with sleep onset and terminate upon awakening. Two episodes of abrupt changes in oxygenation occurring at 15:55 and 18:55 correspond with naps reported in the patient diary.

daytime sleepiness and heavy snoring. The tracings show periods at night in which changes in oxygen saturation occur on a repetitive basis. This pattern is characteristic of apneas seen during polysomnography. Also seen are two bursts of desaturation during self-reported wakefulness. Upon further questioning of this patient, it appears that these really were unintended naps. These unintended naps during the daytime are accompanied by hypoxemia as severe as that seen during sleep.

Figure 25–2 shows this patient's distribution of the oxygen saturation values from the record displayed in Figure 25–1. In this patient, during the entire 24-hour recording period, 30% of the recording time (approximately 8 hours) was spent at an oxygen saturation equal to or below 85%. Figure 25–2, B, is a second oxygen saturation profile from the same patient after the use of nocturnal nasal CPAP, which prevented apneas and, as a consequence, hypoxemic events.

We believe that this example illustrates three points. First, ambulatory monitoring is feasible in patients that have unexpected sleep attacks and can be performed successfully in conditions such as obstructive sleep apnea. Second, such monitoring discloses unexpected bouts of hypoxemia during the daytime that correlate with sleep attacks. This example illustrates that the hypoxemia during naps can be similar to that seen at nighttime. Third, hypoxemia and the total burden of sleep apnea are not necessarily assessed by nocturnal polysomnography alone. Events occur outside the normal sleep time and such events could relate to the development of hypoxic complications. It would be interesting to determine if the appearance of hypoxemia throughout a 24-hour period could be one objective criterion of disease severity.

COPD and Oxygen Therapy

Unattended monitoring has also been used in the evaluation of the patient with obstructive lung disease. Ambulatory assessment of oxygen saturation over time affords the opportunity to catch patients in their normal environment and may disclose changes in oxygen saturation that could occur with changes in activity or unattended therapeutic failure such as cessation of supplemental oxygen therapy. For example, a 66-year-old woman presented with dyspnea and was found to have severe chronic obstructive lung disease (FEV_1-FVC ratio of 42% and an FEV_1 of 0.78 L) and an arterial blood gas of pH 7.43, PCO_2 of 43, and PO_2 of 61. Furthermore, daytime resting oximetry did not disclose values less than 88%. Therefore, this patient does not meet the strict criteria for low-flow oxygen therapy. The 24-hour oxygen profile shown in Figure 25–3, A, illustrates that the patient spends a significant amount of time below 88% saturation, which is ameliorated by 2 L/min in nasal cannula (Fig 25–3, B). Also note the normative data shows that less than 2% of the time, oxygen saturation is less than 88% for normal subjects. This sort of quantitative assessment of oxygen saturation over time can be a tool for understanding how hypoxemic complications develop. If such data were available, then we would be better able to choose when and how to treat patients.

Quadriplegia

Another application of unattended monitoring is for diagnostic assessment of patients unable to come to the polysomnography laboratory. A patient with quadriplegia is vulnerable to hypoxemia because of low lung volumes and inactivity of respiratory muscles of the chest wall.

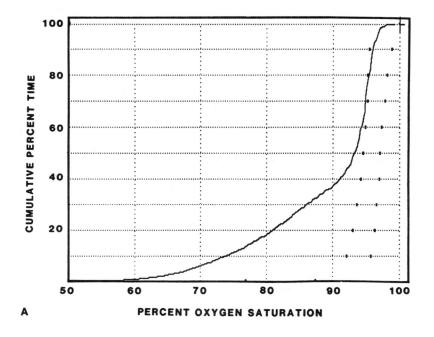

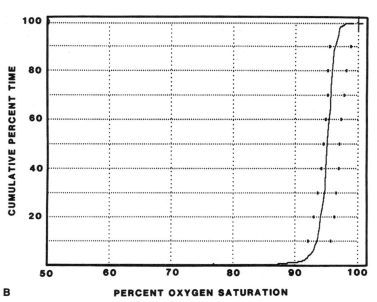

FIG 25–2.
A, Oxygen saturation values from Figure 25–1 are presented as percent oxygen saturation (horizontal axis) versus cumulative percent recording time (vertical axis). Normative values of oxygen saturation are defined as falling within the small darkened squares between 90 and 100% range on the horizontal axis. This quantitative presentation of the data indicates that 30% of the total recording time was spent at or below an oxygen saturation of 85%. **B,** Distribution of oxygen saturation values over time in the same patient following initiation of nasal CPAP therapy. The rightward shift of the data to within the normative limits reflects improved oxygen saturation values with the use of nasal CPAP.

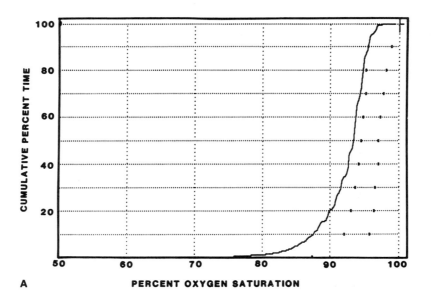

A

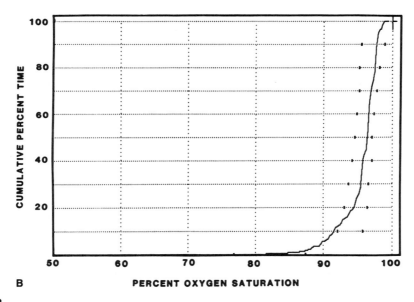

B

FIG 25–3.
Values of oxygen saturation measured in a patient with chronic obstructive pulmonary disease are presented in the same format as in Figure 25–2. The data in **A** were collected with an ambulatory monitor while the patient maintained her daily routine; no supplemental oxygen was used. **B,** The oxygen saturation profile of the same patient, once again collected by ambulatory monitoring; however, during this recording session, oxygen at 2 L/min was continually administered. The therapeutic effect of improved oxygen saturation values related to supplemental oxygen administration is documented by the rightward shift of values to within the normative range.

In many instances, a sleep disorder can be suspected in these patients based on daytime sleepiness, fatigue, or other neuropsychiatric complaints; however, the ability to distinguish between sleep apnea and other consequences of the chronic illness independent of respiratory events is often difficult by clinical history. Indeed, many quadriplegic patients complain of snoring and restless sleep. Monitoring these patients in a specialized sleep laboratory is often difficult because of their intense nursing needs. We have used unattended monitoring to show that episodes of repetitive desaturations can be monitored at the bedside and, therefore, be an adjunct to the assessment of these patients (Fig 25–4).

Other examples in which unattended monitoring is used for special populations include nursing home studies, which have shown that an increased number of apneic events during sleep is associated with premature death. We can conceive that other patient populations, such as those with cerebral palsy or Down's syndrome, may be better monitored in their home environment than in a specialized laboratory.

Epidemiologic Research

Another example of the usefulness of unattended monitoring is in the description of physiologic and pathophysiologic events in general clinical and nonclinical populations.[37] Such research requires that the tools for assessment be easily performed and be applied to large numbers of subjects and, preferably, to the general population. Studies of subjects in a population referred to a clinic or hospital or confined to those willing to be studied in a specialized laboratory may have inherent selection bias. In our hands there is a concordance between unattended monitor-

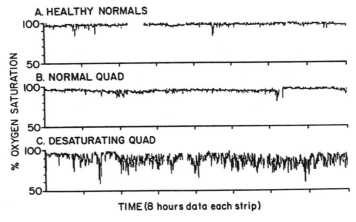

FIG 25–4.
Patterns of oxygen saturation observed during sleep obtained by ambulatory monitoring in **A,** one healthy subject and **B** and **C** bedside monitoring in two quadriplegic patients are presented. In both the healthy subject and the "normal" quad patient, tracings are rather monotonic. However, repetitive cyclic desaturations similar to those observed in sleep apneic patients were also observed within this patient population, **C.** (*Used by permission.*)

ing and polysomnographic studies of 0.88, indicating fairly good agreement between the two methods. We are using unattended monitoring in defining familial patterns of sleep-disordered breathing in family members. When such patterns are identified, more complex assessment can be used to disclose patterns of familial or nonfamilial transmission of physiologic traits. Figure 25–5 shows a family tree of a group of subjects studied using both unattended monitoring as well as polysomnographic studies.

AREAS OF FUTURE DEVELOPMENT

We anticipate that there are three roles for unattended monitoring in the field of respiratory medicine. One is the use of this technology for clinical decision-making in patients with diseases, such as sleep apnea or COPD, in which improvement in oxygenation is a goal of therapy. We think that ambulatory monitoring will allow for more cost-effective follow-up of patients treated for diseases such as sleep apnea as well as make a more rational assessment of the needs for oxygen therapy in areas such as chronic lung disease, both obstructive and restrictive. Second, such monitoring is currently the only cost-effective way to identify preclinical traits and diseases in the community. Epidemiologic research will provide clues to the understanding of clinical expression of the complications of apnea or of breathing abnormalities

FAMILIAL AGGREGATION
OF RESPIRATORY DISTURBANCES
DURING SLEEP

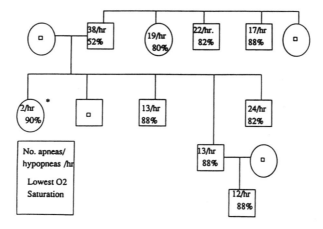

FIG 25–5.
In this figure, the number of apneas/hypopneas per hour of sleep as well as the lowest recorded oxygen saturation value are displayed for each subject. Circles represent female subjects; squares, male subjects. The open symbols with no values displayed represent family members who were not studied.

during sleep/wakefulness. We assume that there are individuals in the community who have significant physiological abnormalities without overt clinical symptoms. The identification of such patients may give insight into why a disease develops and is brought to the attention of the doctor. Finally, while there is hope that such ambulatory monitoring will be cost-effective and allow better patient management, clearly an understanding of the requisite physiological data for clinical decision-making is limited at the present time. Further technological development will probably be influenced by issues of feasibility and cost. For example, if sleep apnea is found to be a risk factor for cardiovascular disease, in particular hypertension, the need to diagnose or recognize such individuals would rapidly overwhelm specialized laboratories such as sleep centers. Likewise the assessment of disease in the elderly would be facilitated by more low-cost and at-home assessment of respiratory events rather than by more specialized laboratories.

REFERENCES

1. Barr Taylor C, Kraemer HC, Bragg DH, et al: A new system for long term recording and processing of heart rate and physical activity in outpatients. *Comp Biomed Res* 1982; 15:7–17.
2. Mueller KJ, Gossard D, Adams FR, et al: Assessment of prescribed increases in physical activity: Application of a new method for microprocessor analysis of heart rate. *Am J Cardiol* 1986; 57:441–445.
3. Rogers F, Juneau M, Taylor CB, et al: Assessment by a microprocessor of adherence to home-based moderate-intensity exercise training in healthy, sedentary middle-aged men and women. *Am J Cardiol* 1987; 60:71–75.
4. Barry J, Campbell S, Nabel EG, et al: Ambulatory monitoring of the digitized electrocardiogram for detection and early warning of transient myocardial ischemia in angina pectoris. *Am J Cardiol* 1987; 60:483–488.
5. Deanfield JE, Shea M, Ribeiro P, et al: Transient ST-segment depression as a marker of myocardial ischemia during daily life. *Am J Cardiol* 1984; 54:1195–1200.
6. Rozanski A, Berman DS. Silent myocardial ischemia. I. Pathophysiology, frequency of occurrence, and approaches toward detection. *Am Heart J* 1987; 11:615–626.
7. Agnew HW, Webb WB, Williams RL. The first night effect: An EEG study of sleep. *Psychophysiol* 1966; 2:263–266.
8. Burnett KF, Taylor CB, Agras WS. Ambulatory computer-assisted therapy for obesity: A new frontier for behavior therapy. *J Consult Clin Psychol* 1985; 53: 698–703.
9. Miles LE, Rule RB: in Stott FD *et al* (eds): *Long Term Monitoring of Multiple Physiological Parameters Using a Programmable Portable Microcomputer*. London, Academic Press, 1982; pp 249–257.
10. Miyamoto, Shimokawa SH, Sumioki H, et al: Circadian rhythm of plasma atrial natriuretic peptide, aldosterone, and blood pressure during the third trimester in normal and preeclamptic pregnancies. *Am J Ob Gyn* 1988; 158:393–399.
11. Pickering TG: Strategies for the evaluation and treatment of hypertension and some implications of blood pressure variability. *Circulation* 1987; 76:177–182.
12. Sewitch DE, Kupfer DJ. A comparison of the telediagnostic and medilog systems for recording normal sleep in the home environment. *Psychophysiol* 1985; 22:718–726.
13. Wildschiødtz G, Clausen J, Langemark M. The Somnolog system: Home monitoring of sleep-EEG, other physiologic data, and sound, in Miles LE, Broughton RJ (eds): *Medical Monitoring in the Home and Work Environment*. New York, Raven Press, 1990; pp 285–294.
14. Connell LJ, Graeber RC. Ambulatory monitoring in the aviation environment, in Miles LE, Broughton RJ (eds): *Medical Monitoring in the Home and Work Environment*. New York, Raven Press, 1990; pp 175–185.

15. Halberg F, Cornelissen G, Halberg J, et al: The sphygmochron for blood pressure and heart rate assessment: A chronobiologic approach, in Miles LE, Broughton RJ (eds): *Medical Monitoring in the Home and Work Environment*. New York, Raven Press, 1990; pp 85–98.

16. Broughton RJ, Stampi C, Dunham W, et al: Ambulant monitoring of sleepwake state, core body temperature and body movement, in Miles LE, Broughton RJ (eds): *Medical Monitoring in the Home and Work Environment*. New York, Raven Press, 1990; pp 139–150.

17. Mermin JH, Czeisler CA: Continuous body temperature monitoring at varying levels of physical exertion in cross-country bicyclists, in Miles LE, Broughton RJ (eds): *Medical Monitoring in the Home and Work Environment*. New York, Raven Press, 1990; pp 165–174.

18. Smith JR. Transferring EEG polysomnography to the home environment, in Miles LE, Broughton RJ (eds): *Medical Monitoring in the Home and Work Environment*. New York, Raven Press, 1990; pp 219–229.

19. Orr WC: Ambulatory monitoring from the gastrointestinal tract, in Miles LE, Broughton RJ (eds): *Medical Monitoring in the Home and Work Environment*. New York, Raven Press, 1990; pp 301–307.

20. Burnett KF, Taylor CB, Thoresen CE, et al: Toward computerized scoring of sleep using ambulatory recordings of heart rate and physical activity. *Behav Assess* 1985; 7:261–271.

21. Emsellem HA, Corson WA, Rappaport BA, et al: Verification of sleep apnea using a portable sleep apnea screening device. *South M J* 1990; 83:748–752.

22. Gander PH, Connell LJ, and Graeber RC. Masking of the circadian rhythms of heart rate and core temperature by the rest-activity cycle in man. *J Biol Rhythms* 1986; 1:119–135.

23. Bliwise DL, Carey E, and Dement WC. Nightly variation in sleep-related respiratory disturbances in older adults. *Exper Aging Res* 1983; 9:77–80.

24. Mendels J, Hawkins DR: Sleep laboratory adaptation in normal subjects and depressed patients ("first-night effect"). *Electroencephogr Clin Neurophys* 1967, 22:556–558.

25. Institute of Medicine: *Assessing Medical Technologies*. Washington, DC, Academy Press, 1985.

26. Sox HC, Blatt MA, Higgins MC, et al: *Medical Decision Making*. Boston, Butterworths, 1988.

27. Sox HC (ed): *Common Diagnostic Tests: Use and Interpretation*. Philadelphia, American College of Physicians, 1987.

28. Decker MJ, Hoekje PL, Strohl KP: Ambulatory monitoring of arterial oxygen saturation. *Chest* 1989; 95:717–722.

29. Flick MR, and Block AJ. Continuous *in vivo* monitoring of arterial oxygenation in chronic obstructive lung disease. *Ann Intern Med* 1977; 86:725–730.

30. Redline S, Boucher MA, and Millman RP. Validity and reproducibility of using an ambulatory sleep monitor. *Am Rev Respir Dis* 1990; 141:A855.

31. Ancoli-Israel S, Kripke DF, Mason W, et al: Comparison of home sleep recordings and polysomnograms in older adults with sleep disorders. *Sleep* 1981; 4:283–291.

32. Gyulay S, Gould D, Sawyer B, et al: Evaluation of a microprocessor-based portable home monitoring system to measure breathing during sleep. *Sleep* 1987; 10:130–142.

33. Bliwise D, Bliwise NG, Kruemer HC, et al: Measurement error in visually scored electrophysiological data: respiration during sleep. *J Neurosci Methods* 1985; 12:49–56.

34. Nino-Murcia G, Bliwise DL, Kennan S, et al: The assessment of a new technology for evaluating respiratory abnormalities in sleep. *Int. J. Technol Assess Health Care* 1987; 3:427–445.

35. Schwartz JS, Ball JR, and Moser RH. Safety, efficacy and effectiveness of clinical practices: A new initiative. *Ann Intern Med* 1982; 96: 246–247.

36. Cahan C, Gothe B, Decker MJ, et al: Arterial oxygen saturation over time and sleep studies in quadriplegic patients (abstract). *Am Rev Respir Dis* 1989; 139:A81.

37. Ancoli-Israel S. Epidemiology of sleep disorders. *Clin Ger Med* 1989; 5:347–362.

Chapter 26

Monitoring in High-Altitude Environments

Nausherwan K. Burki, M.D., Ph.D., F.R.C.P.

INTRODUCTION

Exposure to the high-altitude environment poses particular hazards. Certain physiologic changes are invariable, and monitoring of bodily function should be considered mandatory at altitudes above 10,000 ft (3048 m) because of the expected adverse effects of the environment. Many of the physiologic responses to high-altitude exposure are not understood very clearly and some of these may be life-threatening. This chapter will first review the known effects of high-altitude exposure on man and then discuss monitoring techniques in this situation.

PHYSIOLOGIC RESPONSES TO HIGH-ALTITUDE EXPOSURE

The primary environmental change that occurs at high altitude is hypobaric hypoxia; the decrease in barometric pressure that occurs with increasing altitude results in a decrease in ambient P_{O_2}. Table 26–1 indicates the relationship between altitude, atmospheric pressure, and expected arterial P_{O_2}, assuming either no change in ventilation (arterial P_{CO_2} = 40 mm Hg) in a normal human subject or increases in ventilation (decrease in arterial P_{CO_2}). Note that in the absence of any change in alveolar ventilation, severe hypoxemia would result at altitudes above 13,000 ft (3963 m). However, the normal response to high-altitude exposure is an increase in ventilation, which results in a lower arterial P_{CO_2} and a higher alveolar and arterial P_{O_2}, allowing man to survive without supplemental O_2, even on the summit of Mt. Everest.[1]

The effects of high-altitude exposure can be considered systematically in terms of the respiratory, cardiovascular, endocrine and renal systems, cerebral function, hematologic changes, and general effects.

TABLE 26–1.

Calculated Changes in Alveolar and Arterial Po_2 with Altitude, with and without Changes in Alveolar Ventilation

Altitude, feet (meters)	P_B* mm Hg	PAo_2 mm Hg ($Paco_2$ = 40 mm Hg)	Pao_2 mm Hg ($Paco_2$ = 40 mm Hg)	PAo_2 mm Hg	Pao_2 mm Hg
Sea Level	760	101.7	91.7		
5000	650	78.6	68.6	84.6	74.6
(1524)				($Paco_2$ = 35 mm Hg)	
10,000	540	55.5	45.5	67.5	57.5
(3048)				($Paco_2$ = 30 mm Hg)	
15,000	430	32.4	22.4	50.4	40.4
(4572)				($Paco_2$ = 25 mm Hg)	
20,000	360	17.7	7.7	41.7	31.7
(6096)				($Paco_2$ = 20 mm Hg)	
25,000	280	0.9	-0-	36.9	26.9
(7620)				($Paco_2$ = 10 mm Hg)	

P_B = Barometric pressure; PAo_2 = alveolar Po_2, calculated from the alveolar air equation; Pao_2 = arterial Po_2, assuming $PAo_2 - Pao_2$ = 10 mm Hg.
* P_B is approximated relative to altitude since it will vary with climatic conditions.

Respiratory System

The primary effect of high-altitude exposure on the respiratory system is on ventilatory control. Minute ventilation ($\dot{V}E$) and, hence, alveolar ventilation are consistently increased (Table 26–2) and changes in ventilatory pattern occur (Table 26–3). The increase in minute ventilation is entirely attributable to an increase in respiratory frequency.[2]

The mechanism of the increase in ventilation is not clearly understood. It is likely that it is due to a combination of peripheral chemoreceptor (carotid body) stimulation from the hypobaric hypoxia and a resetting of the central nervous system respiratory controller.[2-4] Interestingly, the acute induction of hyperoxia at high altitude (HA) has no immediate effect on $\dot{V}E$ (Table 26–4; Ref. 1); on return to sea level (SL) the increased $\dot{V}E$ may persist for several days. In the majority of subjects, lung structure or mechanics do not alter at HA unless, of course, pulmonary edema occurs.

Cardiovascular System

Hypoxia is a potent stimulus to pulmonary vasoconstriction, and exposure to high altitude is known to result in pulmonary vasoconstriction (Fig 26–1) and an increase in the pulmonary arterial pressure.[5-7] At rest, there is no change in the cardiac output on exposure to high altitude.[7] Prolonged exposure to high altitude results in right ventricular hypertrophy, due to the pulmonary hypertension and, while the pulmonary vasoconstriction appears to be reversible in the initial stages, after a prolonged sojourn at high altitude it may become permanent.

TABLE 26–2.
Effects of High-Altitude (3940-m) Exposure on Pulmonary Gas Exchange Parameters*

Variable	Low Altitude	High Altitude					
		Day 1		Day 2		Day 3	
Patm, mm Hg	743.7	474		452		453	
PA_{O_2}, mm Hg	100.0			47.5	$P < 0.05$	49.1	$P < 0.05$
	±3.2			±4.4		±2.4	
Pa_{CO_2}, mm Hg	38.2			31.0	$P < 0.05$	29.9	$P < 0.05$
	±2.7			±3.6		±2.0	
$\dot{V}_{O_2}$, L/min	0.273	0.290 NS		0.283	NS	0.302	NS
	±0.106	±0.073		±0.074		±0.049	
$\dot{V}_{CO_2}$, L/min	0.191			0.235	NS	0.234	NS
	±0.006			±0.072		±0.041	
R	0.70			0.83	NS	0.77	NS
	±0.09			±0.08		±0.04	

* From Burki NK: *J Appl Physiol* 1984; 56:1027–1031. Used by permission.
Values are means ±SD. Patm, atmospheric pressure; PA_{O_2} = alveolar P_{O_2}; Pa_{CO_2} = arterial P_{CO_2}; $\dot{V}_{O_2}$ = O_2 uptake, STPD; $\dot{V}_{CO_2}$ = CO_2 production, STPD; R = respiratory exchange ratio; NS = Not significant. *P* values based on Newman-Keuls analysis of variance; NS = $P >0.05$.

The heart rate is consistently increased following acute exposure to high altitude, but after a prolonged sojourn, the heart rate tends to drop toward sea level values. Structural changes in the pulmonary vasculature have been noted: After a prolonged HA sojourn some, but not all, subjects develop increased thickness and hypertrophy of the media of the pulmonary veins.[8] Other studies indicate no significant changes in the alveolocapillary membrane.[9]

Cerebral Vascular Changes

The exact changes in human cerebral blood flow in response to high-altitude hypoxia have, for obvious reasons, not been measured. However, it is believed that there is an initial increase in cerebral blood flow in response to the hypoxia, which is probably damped by the opposite effects of hypocapnia (which causes cerebral vasoconstriction) and that, with time (four to five days), the cerebral blood flow returns to sea level baseline values.[10–12]

The mental effects of high-altitude exposure are dependent on the rate at which exposure develops: the more rapid the change in altitude, the more likely it is that the subject will become confused and disoriented. Subtle changes in cognitive function are common but not easily detectable. Sudden exposure to extreme altitudes may result in unconsciousness.[13]

Endocrine and Renal Effects

It has been suggested that the normal response to high-altitude exposure is the development of a diuresis.[14] However, our own data[15] indicate that this is unlikely to be true and renal

TABLE 26–3.
Effects of Acute High-Altitude (3940-m) Exposure on Ventilatory Parameters*

Variable	Low Altitude	High Altitude					
		Day 1		Day 2		Day 3	
V_E, L/min	9.94 ±1.78	12.44 ±2.09	$P < 0.05$	14.29 ±3.31	$P < 0.05$	14.25 2.67	$P < 0.05$
V_T, L	0.60 ±0.21	0.53 ±0.17	NS	0.55 ±0.21	NS	0.61 ±0.12	NS
f, breaths/min	15.6 ±3.5	24.5 ±5.0	$P < 0.05$	27.6 ±5.8	$P < 0.05$	23.8 ±6.2	$P < 0.05$
T_I, s	1.03 ±0.25	0.84 ±0.22	$P < 0.05$	0.80 ±0.21	NS	0.93 0.12	NS
V_T/T_I, L/s	0.58 ±0.09	0.63 ±0.04	NS	0.68 ±0.16	NS	0.66 ±0.07	NS
T_E, s	2.58 ±0.53	1.68 ±0.27	$P < 0.05$	1.45 ±0.26	$P < 0.05$	1.73 ±0.52	$P < 0.05$
T_I/T_E	0.40 ±0.08	0.49 ±0.09	$P < 0.05$	0.55 ±0.09	$P < 0.05$	0.57 ±0.14	$P < 0.05$
$P_{0.1}$, cm H_2O	1.05 ±0.27	1.30 ±0.35	NS	1.41 ±0.44	NS	1.43 ±0.51	NS
$V_E/P_{0.1}$, L · min^{-1} · cm H_2O^{-1}	9.56 ±1.41	9.62 ±2.32	NS	9.72 ±2.07	NS	9.97 ±2.47	NS

* From Burki NK: *J Appl Physiol* 1984; 56:1027–1031. Used by permission.
Values are means ±SD; $n = 6$. V_E = expired minute ventilation, BTPS; V_T = tidal volume; f = Respiratory frequency; T_I and T_E = inspiratory and expiratory time per breath, respectively; V_I/T_I = Mean inspiratory airflow; $P_{0.1}$ = inspiratory pressure developed at the mouth 0.1 s after onset of inspiratory effort against a total occlusion at function residual capacity; $V_E/P_{0.1}$ = ratio of V_E to $P_{0.1}$; NS = not significant. P values based on Newman-Keuls analysis of variance; NS = $P > 0.05$.

TABLE 26–4.
Effects of Acute Induction of Hyperoxia at High Altitude (3940 m) on Ventilatory Parameters*

	Control	100% O_2	P
V_E, L/min	13.87	13.86	NS
	±2.93	±3.51	
V_T, L	0.56	0.62	NS
	±0.21	±0.28	
f, breaths/min	26.8	25.1	NS
	±7.3	±7.6	
T_I, s	0.87	0.96	NS
	±0.23	±0.35	
T_E, s	1.53	1.60	NS
	±0.48	±0.39	
V_T/T_I, L/s	0.63	0.62	NS
	±0.10	±0.10	

* From Burki NK: *J Appl Physiol* 1984; 56:1027–1031.
Values are means ±SD; *n* = 6. V_E = minute expired ventilation; V_T = tidal volume; *f* = Respiratory frequency; T_I = Inspiratory time; T_E = Expiratory time; V_T/T_I = Mean inspiratory airflow.

function, as with other bodily functions, is very dependent on the rate at which high-altitude exposure develops. Many studies have been performed on the endocrine aspects of high-altitude exposure; however, no definite statements regarding the hormonal response to high altitude exposure can be made.[16, 17] Our own data (Fig 26–2) indicate that there are changes in various hormones, but that the only significant change consistently noted by most workers is a significant decrease in plasma renin activity. The implications of these hormonal changes on salt and water balance are unclear.

Hematologic Effects

It has been well established that hypoxia is a stimulus to erythropoiesis, and exposure to high altitude results in the rapid development of polycythemia. A reticulocytosis in the peripheral blood is evident within two to three days of HA exposure and the blood hematocrit increases within the first week at high altitude.[18, 19] Some workers have suggested that changes in the blood coagulation system occur, but these have not been definitely documented.[20]

General Effects

Immediately following arrival at high altitude, somnolence and anorexia develop. The somnolence is presumably related to altered cerebral blood flow/metabolism.

Subjects exposed to high altitude generally tend to lose weight in spite of an adequate caloric intake.[21] The cause of this weight loss is unknown.

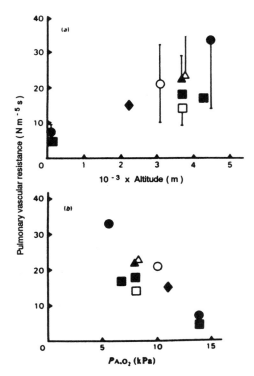

FIG 26–1.
Measured increase in pulmonary vascular resistance with altitude (*upper graph*) and decrease in alveolar
Po$_2$ (*lower graph*) from six different studies. (*From Lockhart A, Saiag B:* Clin Sci *1981; 60:599–605. Used
by permission.*)

Retinal hemorrhages and retinal edema develop in many subjects during HA exposure.[22]
These are related to the hypoxia but the exact mechanism is unclear and the long-term effects
are also not known. An increase in capillary fragility as a mechanism for the retinal hemorrhages
has been suggested.[23]

Sleep disturbances are a usual feature of HA exposures.[24–26] These consist primarily of insomnia
and the development of Cheyne-Stokes respiration, which may be quite marked, with repeated
awakenings at the nadir of ventilation.[27] Again, the precise mechanism is unclear.

Exercise capacity is surprisingly well maintained, despite hypoxia at HA. Since

$$\dot{V}O_2 = Hb(SaO_2 - S\bar{v}O_2) \times 1.34 \times CO$$

(where Hb = hemoglobin concentration; SaO$_2$ and SvO$_2$ = arterial and mixed venous O$_2$
saturation; respectively, 1.34 is the O$_2$ in milliliters carried by 1 G of fully saturated Hb, and
CO = cardiac output), it is clear that maximal $\dot{V}O_2$ and, hence, maximal exercise capacity will
be limited at HA because of the decrease in SaO$_2$. Nevertheless at HA, tissue extraction of O$_2$

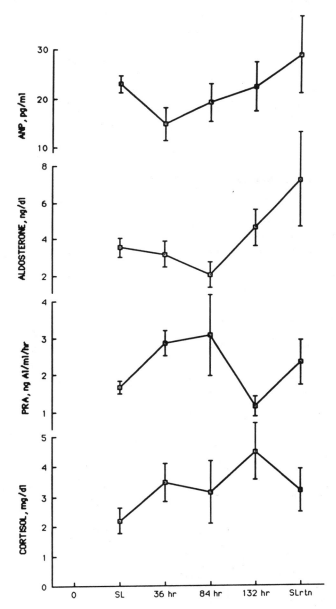

FIG 26–2.
Changes in plasma hormones following high-altitude (4450 m) exposure. ANP = Atrial natriuretic peptide; PRA = Plasma renin activity; SL = sea level. Only PRA changed significantly ($p < 0.05$) after 36 hours at HA. (*From McConnell JW, et al:* Am Rev Respir Dis *1988; 137:177. Used by permission.*)

appears to be better than at sea level, resulting in lower $S\bar{v}o_2$, and muscle energy stores are well maintained.[28, 29] The physiology of high-altitude exposure in subjects born and living at high altitude (highlanders) is different to that of lowlanders acutely exposed to high altitude. In highlanders, the pulmonary arterial pressure is higher than that of lowlanders, although, following exposure to high altitude, the pulmonary arterial pressure in lowlanders approximates that of the highlanders.[7] Right ventricular hypertrophy is present in highlanders and the pulmonary vasculature shows evidence of muscularization.[7, 8] At rest, highlanders have a lower heart rate than lowlanders acutely exposed to high altitude.[7] However, the ventilatory responses, i.e., level of alveolar ventilation and arterial oxygenation are similar to lowlanders acutely exposed to high altitude.

THE PATHOLOGY OF HIGH-ALTITUDE EXPOSURE

High-altitude exposure may result in a benign, though debilitating syndrome of acute mountain sickness, or in more life-threatening syndromes, such as acute pulmonary edema and/or acute cerebral edema. In addition, chronic mountain sickness may develop in subjects sojourning at high altitude for long periods of time.

Acute Mountain Sickness

Acute mountain sickness (AMS) occurs about 6 to 12 hours after arrival at high altitude and is characterized by severe headache, anorexia, nausea, and vomiting.[30] This benign but unpleasant and debilitating condition is self-limited, usually resolving in 48 to 72 hours. The precise cause(s) of AMS is unclear, although many workers have implicated alterations in fluid balance as a major factor.[14] However, our own studies do not support this.[31]

The development and severity of AMS in a given subject cannot be predicted; it does not appear to be related to physical conditioning or to other known factors. Our own experience indicates that some degree of AMS is invariably present in all subjects who are acutely exposed to high altitude.[31]

Pulmonary and Cerebral Edema

In a small proportion of subjects exposed to high altitude (ranging from 1.2 to 4.3%), a malignant syndrome of pulmonary and/or cerebral edema may occur and is frequently fatal.[32–34]

Pulmonary edema is heralded by increasing tachypnea and shortness of breath, usually occurring any time from 48 hours after arrival at HA up to two weeks later. Physical examination may reveal the presence of inspiratory crackles over the lung bases. The condition, if untreated, progresses rapidly with cough, and frothy, blood-tinged sputum production, increasing cyanosis, hypoxemia, and death.[35]

Cerebral edema also develops over the same time period as pulmonary edema and is heralded by increasing mental confusion and somnolence, passing into coma, which is usually irreversible.[34]

Studies in patients who die of cerebral and/or pulmonary edema indicate widespread thromboses in the pulmonary vessels, as well as infarctions of the brain.[35] Pulmonary edema is considered to be an increased permeability edema with high protein content in the edema fluid.[33] The exact mechanism of these two malignant syndromes is unknown.

MONITORING OF SUBJECTS EXPOSED TO HIGH ALTITUDE

The brief discussion above of the physiologic and pathologic effects of high-altitude exposure should indicate the importance of at least a minimal degree of monitoring of subjects exposed to high altitude.

Monitoring of subjects at high altitude can be performed with various levels of sophistication. In the majority of cases, clinical observation with some simple tests should suffice. In a few instances, it may be necessary to monitor in more detail, while in other instances specific forms of monitoring may be required.

PREEXPOSURE EVALUATION

In subjects likely to be subjected to HA exposure, preliminary screening of general health is prudent. As broad guidelines, in subjects over 40 years of age and in younger subjects with any history of cardiopulmonary disease, a minimum assessment should consist of medical history and physical examination, and a noninvasive assessment of arterial O_2 saturation, using a pulse oximeter.[36] Depending on the findings of this initial assessment, an electrocardiogram and more detailed pulmonary function assessment may be indicated.

Prudence would dictate that subjects with a history of cardiac disease should be cautioned against exposure to altitudes above 3000 m; there is a paucity of data in this regard and recommendations must necessarily be made on the basis of good medical practice. In the stable subject with a prior history of myocardial infarction/ischemia and no evidence of heart failure or arrhythmia, there are no data to indicate any increased risk of cardiac malfunction at altitudes up to 3000 m. It is the author's experience that high-altitude exposure tends to exacerbate preexisting arrhythmias.

In patients with purely pulmonary deficits, a review of Table 26–1 and the application of the alveolar-air equation will indicate the maximum altitude to which such a subject can be exposed without supplemental O_2. Patients with ventilatory defects who may be unable to increase ventilation would be at particular risk of severe hypoxemia.

MONITORING AT HIGH ALTITUDE

In all subjects exposed to high altitude, a certain basic level of monitoring should be considered mandatory, especially at altitudes above 10,000 ft (3050 m). Clinical monitoring is especially crucial during the first few days of arrival at high altitude. After the first week, assuming there are no complications, it would probably be adequate to monitor at weekly and, later, monthly intervals.

Monitoring Equipment at High Altitude

The high-altitude environment poses special hazards for equipment: apart from the general hazards of field work, temperature and barometric pressure particularly need to be considered.

As a rule, the author has attempted to use battery-powered equipment. However, while this may be adequate for low-current-drain devices, equipment requiring long-term use or high-current requirements usually cannot be sustained on battery power alone. For these items, a power generator is necessary. Requirements will clearly vary depending on the sophistication and detail of monitoring required for an individual project. An appropriate minimum output for a power generator would be 500 W; it is important to ensure that the voltage output matches the requirements of the equipment to be used.

For projects requiring prolonged (greater than one or two days) sojourn at HA (>10,000 ft, 3000 m), it would be appropriate to have the following minimum equipment available:

1. Stethoscope, ophthalmoscope, sphygmomanometer
2. Weighing machine, barometer
3. Pulse oximeter with heart rate monitor
4. CO_2 gas analysis meter
5. CO_2 calibrating gas

Additional equipment, depending on requirements:

1. Electrocardiograph
2. O_2 gas analysis meter
3. Gas volume meter
4. Spirometer with calibration syringe
5. Physiologic recorder
6. Douglas bags, mouthpieces, accessories
7. Power generator

Simple Observation

Mentation

Subjects should be tested for level of consciousness, orientation to time, place, and person, and a simple test of attention, such as a digit span. Somnolence usually occurs after arrival at high altitude and should be considered a normal finding; however, excessive somnolence may be a cause for concern since this may be the first indication of cerebral edema.[34] If the subject shows any indication of depressed consciousness and confusion, a more detailed neurologic examination should be undertaken, including in particular examination of the retinal fundi for papilledema. Any unusually depressed level of consciousness, confusion, or any hint of papilledema should be an indication for immediate removal of the subject to lower altitudes since it may be indicative of cerebral edema, which, if not rapidly treated, would result in progression to coma and death.

Dyspnea

Some level of dyspnea is normal and to be expected after arrival at high altitude, but an excessive degree of dyspnea, especially at rest, might be the herald of pulmonary edema. The assessment of dyspnea in a given subject, and whether it is unusual or not, can only be made in comparison to other subjects and from the observer's own previous experience at that altitude. However, this may be the most sensitive indicator of early pulmonary edema.

Cyanosis

Depending on the altitude to which the subject is exposed, cyanosis may be a normal finding. However, the subject should be checked against his peers at altitude for excessive cyanosis, which would be an indicator of untoward hypoxemia at that altitude.

Clinical Examination

Cardiovascular Examination

Tachycardia is a usual finding at high altitude; however, in our experience, at altitudes up to 15,000 ft (5000 m), the resting pulse rate rarely exceeds 110/min. Higher pulse rates might indicate cardiac decompensation and should prompt a more detailed cardiovascular evaluation. The jugular venous pressure should be examined; if it is elevated it would indicate right heart failure. Blood pressure is usually not affected by exposure to high altitude and any abnormalities should be evaluated. Similarly, the heart sounds should remain normal and the development of any new murmurs or other abnormalities in the heart sounds should be evaluated further. A point to note is that some subjects develop an irregular pulse due to ventricular ectopic beats at high altitude; the significance of these is unknown.

Respiratory Examination

Apart from examination for assessment of dyspnea and cyanosis as noted earlier, careful percussion and auscultation of the lungs should be carried out. The presence of any inspiratory crackles or crepitations would be suggestive of pulmonary edema and should prompt immediate measures to remove the subject to a lower altitude.

The daily urine output should be monitored. While it has been claimed that subjects with reduced urine output may be more prone to developing acute mountain sickness, our own experience suggests that the oliguria may be related to dehydration.[31]

Measurements

A second level of sophistication in terms of monitoring would involve instrumentation and measurement.

Weight

Daily measurement of weight might provide some information on pending abnormalities. For example, previous workers and ourselves have found that a fall in weight after arrival at high altitude is usual.[31] An excessive fall in weight might indicate the need for better hydration and food intake. Second, an increase in weight might herald the onset of pulmonary edema, although this has not been documented.

Electrocardiogram

In subjects with excessive tachycardia or irregular pulse, an electrocardiogram should be measured to assess for ventricular ectopics or other abnormalities of the cardiac rhythm. While high-altitude exposure has not been blamed for the development of ischemic heart disease, preexisting coronary artery disease might, in the presence of high-altitude hypoxia, result in the development of cardiac ischemia, with resultant changes on the electrocardiogram. The finding of such changes should obviously prompt an immediate return to lower altitude.

Respiratory Monitoring

Apart from monitoring of respiratory rate as above, measurements of arterial oxygen saturation and arterial Pco_2 can be made noninvasively.[2, 37]

Arterial oxygen saturation can be monitored with a pulse oximeter[36]; most of the available pulse oximeters also measure the pulse rate. Noninvasive oximetry has been compared to directly measured arterial O_2 saturation (Sao_2) at sea level[36] in patients and at high altitude[38] and has been found to be accurate to levels of Sao_2 as low as 65%. Problems specific to oximeters at high altitude are related to vasoconstriction and the ambient temperature. The usual response to hypoxia and to the colder temperatures at high altitude is peripheral vasoconstriction. If this is marked, the pulse oximeter may not be able to monitor the arterial oxygen saturation. However, this problem can usually be overcome by vigorously rubbing the area to be monitored (ear, nose, lip, etc.) with resulting hyperemia and an adequate oximeter signal.

A more common finding at high altitude is that the oximeter will not provide a stable reading, with the digital readout swinging wildly above and below the true arterial oxygen saturation. The reason for this is that most of the available pulse oximeters are rated for correct function within a relatively narrow range of ambient temperatures. At very low temperatures such as at high altitude, or at high temperatures (as may occur within a tent when the sun is out), the oximeter will not read properly. The observer should be aware of this problem, which can be corrected by bringing the oximeter to an appropriate ambient temperature by placing the machine in a shady, well-ventilated area, or in a warmer environment, as necessary. The arterial oxygen saturation at any given altitude varies widely between subjects. However, at any given altitude, the lower the arterial oxygen saturation, the more likely it appears that the subject will develop symptoms of mountain sickness.[31] Furthermore, the development of pulmonary edema would be heralded by a further fall in the arterial oxygen saturation and provide an early indication for prompt action.

The arterial Pco_2 can be monitored either by the end-tidal Pco_2 in subjects with normal lungs,[37] or by measurement of the mixed venous Pco_2 from which the arterial Pco_2 can be derived.[37, 39] A number of CO_2 analysis meters are available; it is useful to select one that is lightweight yet accurate and has a pump mechanism for drawing gas in to the machine (many of the CO_2 analysis machines on the market are meant for in-line placement with patients on ventilators and are inappropriate for HA purposes). A calibrated CO_2 gas cylinder should be available to calibrate the CO_2 analysis meter, as well as a barometer to convert gas concentration to pressure.

The arterial P_{CO_2} should be appropriately decreased at high altitude due to alveolar hyperventilation. Again, there is a wide variance between subjects (Table 26–2), but an unusually high arterial P_{CO_2} at any given altitude should be cause for concern, indicating the development of relative hypoventilation.

More sophisticated monitoring can be performed at high altitude, depending on special requirements. These would include monitoring during exercise and noninvasive measurements of cerebral blood flow.[11, 12] In addition, direct measurements of arterial blood gases and measurements of serum electrolytes and hormones can be made, although these are usually for experimental purposes.

Monitoring during sleep is usually not necessary. However, in subjects suspected to be developing high-altitude pulmonary or cerebral edema, sleep monitoring may be necessary while awaiting removal to a lower altitude. In its simplest form, continuous monitoring of arterial O_2 saturation by pulse oximetry and of respiratory rate and rhythm by observation should suffice. End-tidal CO_2 concentration at the mouth provides a monitor not only of alveolar ventilation, but also of air flow at the mouth and, therefore, respiratory rate.

ADVERSE EFFECTS OF HIGH-ALTITUDE EXPOSURE

Prevention

It has long been recognized by mountaineers and high-altitude inhabitants that gradual ascent prevents or ameliorates the symptoms of AMS. For example, ascent to 5000 ft (1500 m) from SL usually presents no problems, but further ascent should, if possible, be gradual; ascent to 10,000 ft should take another two to three days. Similarly, further ascent should not be at a rate greater than 1000 ft per day. An old axiom is "climb high, sleep low" implying that it is useful to descend a few thousand feet every night to sleep, going up again during the day.

With acute HA exposure the chances of developing AMS are greatly increased. Our experience[31] is that a change in altitude form 4000 ft to 15,000 ft over an 8-hour period results invariably in the development of AMS.

Treatment

Drug treatment of AMS is only partially successful. The most established drug in this regard is acetazolamide (250 mg bid or 500 mg daily). Acetazolamide is a carbonic anhydrase inhibitor that causes an acidosis; in man it results in an increase in ventilation at HA with a higher S_{aO_2} and lower P_{aCO_2}.[31, 40] The increase in S_{aO_2} has been cited as the mechanism for its beneficial effects in AMS.[40] The drug should be started 24 hours before ascent and continued for the first few days at HA. Experience shows that it ameliorates, but does not fully prevent the development of AMS.[31, 40, 41]

Other drugs claimed to be effective are dexamethasone[42] and phenytoin.[43] These are not yet generally accepted as treatments of choice for AMS.

The development of pulmonary edema at HA is a medical emergency and the most effective treatment is to remove the subject immediately to altitudes below 3000 ft (<1000 m). Failing this, supplemental O_2 must be given. The role of steroids and diuretics is unclear, but they are probably not effective. Recent studies suggest that nifedipine, a calcium channel blocking agent that acts as a pulmonary vasodilator, might be useful in the treatment of HA pulmonary edema.[44] The development of high-altitude cerebral edema (HACE) also constitutes a medical emergency and should prompt immediate evacuation to lower altitudes below 3000 ft (<1000 m). There is no known specific therapeutic modality for HACE.[34]

REFERENCES

1. West JB: Climbing Mt. Everest without oxygen: An analysis of maximal exercise during extreme hypoxia. *Respir Physiol* 1983; 52:265–279.
2. Burki NK: Effects of acute exposure to high altitude on ventilatory drive and respiratory pattern. *J Appl Physiol: Respirat Environ Exercise Physiol* 1984; 56:1027–1031.
3. Forster HV, Dempsey, JA, Vidruk E, et al: Evidence of altered regulation of ventilation during exposure to hypoxia. *Respir Physiol* 1974; 20:379–392.
4. Busch MA, Bisgard GE, Forster HV: Ventilatory acclimatization to hypoxia is not dependent on arterial hypoxemia. *J Appl Physiol* 1985; 58:1874–1880.
5. Rotta A, Canepa A, Hurtado F, et al: Pulmonary circulation at sea level and at high altitudes. *J Appl Physiol* 1956; 9:328–330.
6. Kronenberg RS, et al: Pulmonary artery pressure and alveolar gas exchange in man during acclimatization to 12,470 ft. *J Clin Invest* 1971; 50:827–837.
7. Lockhart A, Saiag B: Altitude and the human pulmonary circulation. *Clin Sci* 1981; 60:599–605.
8. Wagenvoort CA, Wagenvoort N: Pulmonary veins in high-altitude residents: A morphometric study. *Thorax* 1982; 37:931–935.
9. Hogan J, Smith P, Heath D, et al: The thickness of the alveolar capillary wall in the human lung at high and low altitude. *Br J Dis Chest* 1987; 80:13–18.
10. Severinghaus JW, et al: Cerebral blood flow in man at high altitude. *Circ Res* 1966; 19:274–282.
11. Huang SY, et al: Internal carotid and vertebral arterial flow velocity in men at high altitude. *J Appl Physiol* 1987; 63:395–400.
12. Huang SY, et al: Internal carotid flow velocity with exercise before and after acclimatization to 4,300 m. *J Appl Physiol* 1991; 71:1469–1476.
13. Milledge JS: Physiological effects of hypoxia, in Clarke C, Ward M, Williams E (eds): *Mountain Medicine and Physiology*. London, Alpine Club, 1975, p 73.
14. Hackett PH, et al: Fluid retention and relative hypoventilation in acute mountain sickness. *Respir* 1982; 43:321–329.
15. McConnell JW, Hollister AS, Liles R, et al: Plasma atrial natriuretic peptide levels during acute high altitude exposure. *Am Rev Respir Dis* 1988; 137:177.
16. Colice GL, Ramirez G: Aldosterone response to angiotensin II during hypoxemia. *J Appl Physiol* 1986; 61:150–154.
17. Milledge JS, et al: Effect of prolonged exercise at altitude on the renin-aldosterone system. *J Appl Physiol* 1983; 55:413–418.

18. Eckardt K-U, et al: Rate of erythropoietin formation in humans in response to acute hypobaric hypoxia. *J Appl Physiol* 1989; 66:1785–1788.
19. Winslow RM, et al: Different hematologic responses to hypoxia in Sherpas and Quechua Indians. *J Appl Physiol* 1989; 66:1561–1569.
20. Andrew M, O'Brodovich H, Sutton J: Operation Everest II: Coagulation system during prolonged decompression to 282 Torr. *J Appl Physiol* 1987; 63:1262–1267.
21. Boyer SJ, Blume FD: Weight loss and changes in body composition at high altitude. *J Appl Physiol* 1984; 57:1580–1585.
22. Frayser R, Houston CS, Bryan AC, et al: Retinal hemorrhage at high altitude. *N Engl J Med* 1970; 282:1183–1184.
23. Hunter DJ, Smart JR, Whitton L: Increased capillary fragility at high altitude. *Br Med J* 1986; 292:98.
24. Ravenhill TH: Some experience of mountain sickness in the Andes. *J Trop Med Hygiene* 1913; 16:313–320.
25. Reite M, Jackson D, Cahoon RL, et al: Sleep physiology at high altitude. *Electroenceph Clin Neurophysiol* 1975; 38:463–471.
26. Nicholson AN, et al: Altitude insomnia: Studies during an expedition to the Himalayas. *Sleep* 1988; 11:354–361.
27. Berssenbrugge A, et al: Mechanisms of hypoxia induced periodic breathing during sleep in humans. *J Physiol* 1983; 343:507–524.
28. Reeves JT, Groves BM, Sutton JR, et al: Operation Everest II: Preservation of cardiac function at extreme altitude. *J Appl Physiol* 1987; 63:531–539.
29. Sutton JR, Reeves Jt, Wagner PD, et al: Operation Everest II: Oxygen transport during exercises at extreme simulated altitude. *J Appl Physiol* 1988; 64:1309–1321.
30. Hackett PH, Rennie D, Levine HD: The incidence, importance, and prophylaxis of acute mountain sickness. *Lancet* 1976; ii:1149–1154.
31. Burki NK, Khan SA, Hameed MA: The effects of acetazolamide on the ventilatory response to high altitude hypoxia. *Chest* 1992; 101:736–741.
32. Houston CS: Acute pulmonary edema of high altitude. *N Engl J Med* 1960; 263:478–480.
33. Schoene RB: Pulmonary edema at high altitude. Review of pathophysiology, and update. *Clin Chest Med* 1985; 6:491–507.
34. Hamilton AJ, Cymmerman A, Black PMcL: High altitude cerebral edema. *Neurosurgery* 1986; 19:841–849.
35. Dickinson J, Heath D, Gosney J, et al: Altitude-related deaths in seven trekkers in the Himalayas. *Thorax* 1983; 38:646–656.
36. Chaudhary BA, NK Burki: Ear oximetry in clinical practice. *Am Rev Respir Dis* 1978; 117:173–175.
37. Burki NK, Albert RK: Noninvasive monitoring of arterial blood gases: A report of the ACCP Section on Respiratory Pathophysiology. *Chest* 1983; 83:666–670.
38. McEvoy JDS, Jones NL, Campbell EJM: Mixed venous and arterial PCO_2. *Br Med J* 1974; 4:687–690.
39. Forte VA, et al: Operation Everest II: Comparison of four instruments for measuring blood O2 saturation. *J Appl Physiol* 1989; 67:2135–2140.
40. Lort DJ, et al: Acetazolamide in control of acute mountain sickness. *Lancet* 1981; ii:180.
41. Evans WO, Robinson SM, Horstman DH, et al: Amelioration of the symptoms of acute mountain sickness by staging and acetazolamide. *Aviat Space Environ Med* 1976; 47:512–516.
42. Levine BD, et al: Dexamethasone in the treatment of acute mountain sickness. *N Engl J Med* 1989; 321:1707–1719.
43. Wohns RNW, et al: Phenytoin and acute mountain sickness on Mount Everest. *Am J Med* 1986; 80:32–36.
44. Oelry O, et al: Nifedipine for high altitude pulmonary oedema. *Lancet* 1989; ii:1241–1244.

Index

DATE DUE

DEMCO 38-297